Sleisenger and Fordtran's

GASTROINTESTINAL AND LIVER DISEASE

REVIEW AND ASSESSMENT

Sleisenger and Fordtran's
Ninth Edition

GASTROINTESTINAL AND LIVER DISEASE

REVIEW AND ASSESSMENT

Edited by

Anthony J. DiMarino, Jr., MD
William Rorer Professor of Medicine
Chief, Division of Gastroenterology and Hepatology
Thomas Jefferson University and Hospital
Philadelphia, Pennsylvania

Robert M. Coben, MD
Associate Professor of Medicine
Academic Coordinator, GI Fellowship Program
Division of Gastroenterology and Hepatology
Thomas Jefferson University and Hospital
Philadelphia, Pennsylvania

Anthony Infantolino, MD
Associate Professor of Medicine
Director, Endoscopic Ultrasound
Division of Gastroenterology and Hepatology
Thomas Jefferson University and Hospital
Philadelphia, Pennsylvania

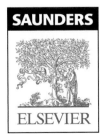

SAUNDERS

ELSEVIER

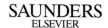

SAUNDERS
ELSEVIER

1600 John F. Kennedy Blvd.
Ste 1800
Philadelphia, PA 19103-2899

Sleisenger and Fordtran's GASTROINTESTINAL AND
LIVER DISEASE: REVIEW AND ASSESSMENT

ISBN: 978-1-437-70730-4

Notice

Knowledge and best practice in this field are constantly changing. As new research and experience broaden our understanding, changes in research methods, professional practices, or medical treatment may become necessary.

Practitioners and researchers must always rely on their own experience and knowledge in evaluating and using any information, methods, compounds, or experiments described herein. In using such information or methods they should be mindful of their own safety and the safety of others, including parties for whom they have a professional responsibility.

With respect to any drug or pharmaceutical products identified, readers are advised to check the most current information provided (i) on procedures featured or (ii) by the manufacturer of each product to be administered, to verify the recommended dose or formula, the method and duration of administration, and contraindications. It is the responsibility of practitioners, relying on their own experience and knowledge of their patients, to make diagnoses, to determine dosages and the best treatment for each individual patient, and to take all appropriate safety precautions.

To the fullest extent of the law, neither the Publisher nor the authors, contributors, or editors, assume any liability for any injury and/or damage to persons or property as a matter of products liability, negligence or otherwise, or from any use or operation of any methods, products, instructions, or ideas contained in the material herein.

The Publisher

Previous editions copyrighted 2007, 1999, 1996

Library of Congress Cataloging-in-Publication Data
Sleisenger and Fordtran's gastrointestinal and liver disease review and assessment / [edited by] Anthony J. DiMarino Jr., Robert Coben, Anthony Infantolino—9th ed.
     p. ; cm.
   Other title: Gastrointestinal and liver disease
   Rev. ed. of: Sleisenger & Fordtran's gastrointestinal and liver disease / edited by Mark Feldman, Lawrence S. Friedman, Lawrence J. Brandt. 8th ed. c2006.
   Includes bibliographical references and index.
   ISBN 978-1-4377-0730-4
   1. Gastrointestinal system—Diseases—Examinations, questions, etc. I. DiMarino, Anthony J. II. Coben, Robert. III. Infantolino, Anthony. IV. Sleisenger, Marvin H. V. Sleisenger & Fordtran's gastrointestinal and liver disease. VI. Title: Gastrointestinal and liver disease.
   [DNLM: 1. Gastrointestinal Disease. 2. Liver Diseases. WI 140 S6321 2010]
   RC801.G384 2010 Suppl.
   616.3′3—dc22

                                                                      2010005185

Acquisitions Editor: Druanne Martin
Developmental Editor: Virginia Wilson
Senior Project Manager: David Saltzberg
Design Direction: Steve Stave

Printed in the United States of America.

Last digit is the print number: 9 8 7 6 5 4 3 2 1

Dedicated to medical students, residents, fellows, and faculty who have a continuing quest for new knowledge in the field of gastroenterology and hepatology. Special appreciation to co-editors Robert Coben and Anthony Infantolino and to the section leaders—Cuckoo Choudhary, Sidney Cohen, Steven Herrine, David Kastenberg, Howard Kroop, David Loren, and Satish Rattan—and to our gastroenterology fellows, who participated in this project and raised many important questions and topics. Recognition is given to Donna Collins and Patricia Shaughnessy for their invaluable help in making this book a success.

Anthony J. DiMarino, Jr., MD

Contributors

Jeffrey A. Abrams, MD
Clinical Assistant Professor of Medicine, Division of Gastroenterology and Hepatology, Department of Medicine, Thomas Jefferson University, Philadelphia, Pennsylvania

Kristin Braun, MD
Fellow, Division of Gastroenterology and Hepatology, Department of Medicine, Thomas Jefferson University, Philadelphia, Pennsylvania

Cuckoo Choudhary, MD
Assistant Professor of Medicine, Division of Gastroenterology and Hepatology, Department of Medicine, Thomas Jefferson University, Philadelphia, Pennsylvania

Robert M. Coben, MD
Associate Professor of Medicine; Academic Coordinator, GI Fellowship Program, Division of Gastroenterology and Hepatology, Department of Medicine, Thomas Jefferson University, Philadelphia, Pennsylvania

Sidney Cohen, MD
Professor of Medicine; Director of Research Program, Division of Gastroenterology and Hepatology, Department of Medicine, Thomas Jefferson University, Philadelphia, Pennsylvania

Mitchell Conn, MD, MBA
Associate Professor of Medicine; Medical Director, GI/Transplant Service Line, Division of Gastroenterology and Hepatology, Department of Medicine, Thomas Jefferson University, Philadelphia, Pennsylvania

Anthony J. DiMarino, Jr. MD
William Rorer Professor of Medicine; Chief, Division of Gastroenterology and Hepatology, Division of Gastroenterology and Hepatology, Department of Medicine, Thomas Jefferson University, Philadelphia, Pennsylvania

Michael C. DiMarino, MD, MMS
Clinical Assistant Professor of Medicine, Division of Gastroenterology and Hepatology, Department of Medicine, Thomas Jefferson University, Philadelphia, Pennsylvania

Bob Etemad, MD
Medical Director of Endoscopy, Main Line Gastroenterology Associates PC, Main Line Health System, Wynnewood, Pennsylvania

Jonathan M. Fenkel, MD
Fellow, Division of Gastroenterology and Hepatology, Department of Medicine, Thomas Jefferson University, Philadelphia, Pennsylvania

Mara Goldstein-Posner, MD
Fellow, Division of Gastroenterology and Hepatology, Department of Medicine, Thomas Jefferson University, Philadelphia, Pennsylvania

Steven M. Greenfield, MD
Assistant Professor of Medicine, Division of Gastroenterology and Hepatology, Department of Medicine, Thomas Jefferson University, Philadelphia, Pennsylvania

Hie-Won L. Hann, MD
Professor of Medicine; Director, Liver Disease Prevention Center, Division of Gastroenterology and Hepatology, Department of Medicine, Thomas Jefferson University, Philadelphia, Pennsylvania

Nikroo Hashemi, MD
Fellow, Advanced Hepatology, Division of Gastroenterology and Hepatology, Department of Medicine, Thomas Jefferson University, Philadelphia, Pennsylvania

Christine M. Herdman, MD
Fellow, Division of Gastroenterology and Hepatology, Department of Medicine, Thomas Jefferson University, Philadelphia, Pennsylvania

Steven K. Herrine, MD
Professor of Medicine; Associate Director, Fellowship Program; Associate Medical Director, Liver Transplant Program, Division of Gastroenterology and Hepatology, Department of Medicine, Thomas Jefferson University; Assistant Dean, Academic Affairs, Jefferson Medical College, Philadelphia, Pennsylvania

Anthony Infantolino, MD, AGAF, FACG, FACP
Associate Professor of Medicine; Director, Endoscopic Ultrasound, Division of Gastroenterology and Hepatology, Department of Medicine, Thomas Jefferson University, Philadelphia, Pennsylvania

David Kastenberg, MD, FACP, AGAF
Associate Professor of Medicine, Division of Gastroenterology and Hepatology, Department of Medicine, Thomas Jefferson University, Philadelphia, Pennsylvania

Leo C. Katz, MD
Assistant Professor of Medicine, Division of Gastroenterology and Hepatology, Department of Medicine, Thomas Jefferson University, Philadelphia, Pennsylvania

Bryan Kavanaugh, MD
Fellow, Division of Gastroenterology and Hepatology, Department of Medicine, Thomas Jefferson University, Philadelphia, Pennsylvania

Thomas Kowalski, MD
Associate Professor of Medicine; Director, Gastrointestinal Endoscopy, Division of Gastroenterology and Hepatology, Department of Medicine, Thomas Jefferson University, Philadelphia, Pennsylvania

Patricia Kozuch, MD
Assistant Professor of Medicine, Division of Gastroenterology and Hepatology, Department of Medicine, Thomas Jefferson University, Philadelphia, Pennsylvania

Howard S. Kroop, MD
Clinical Associate Professor of Medicine, Division of Gastroenterology and Hepatology, Department of Medicine, Thomas Jefferson University, Philadelphia, Pennsylvania; Chief, Division of Gastroenterology, Department of Medicine, Underwood Memorial Hospital, Woodbury, New Jersey

David Loren, MD
Assistant Professor of Medicine; Director of Endoscopic Research, Division of Gastroenterology and Hepatology, Department of Medicine, Thomas Jefferson University, Philadelphia, Pennsylvania

Aarati Malliah, MD
Fellow, Division of Gastroenterology and Hepatology, Department of Medicine, Thomas Jefferson University, Philadelphia, Pennsylvania

Victor J. Navarro, MD
Professor of Medicine, Pharmacology and Experimental Therapeutics; Medical Director, Liver Transplantation, Division of Gastroenterology and Hepatology, Department of Medicine, Thomas Jefferson University, Philadelphia, Pennsylvania

Nicholas T. Orfanidis, MD
Fellow, Division of Gastroenterology and Hepatology, Department of Medicine, Thomas Jefferson University, Philadelphia, Pennsylvania

Jorge A. Prieto, MD
Clinical Assistant Professor of Medicine, Division of Gastroenterology and Hepatology, Department of Medicine, Thomas Jefferson University, Philadelphia, Pennsylvania

Satish Rattan, DVM
Professor of Medicine; Director of Basic Research, Division of Gastroenterology and Hepatology, Department of Medicine, Thomas Jefferson University, Philadelphia, Pennsylvania

Marianne Ritchie, MD
Assistant Professor of Medicine, Division of Gastroenterology and Hepatology, Department of Medicine, Thomas Jefferson University, Philadelphia, Pennsylvania

Susie Rivera, MD
GI Motility Coordinator, Division of Gastroenterology and Hepatology, Department of Medicine, Thomas Jefferson University, Philadelphia, Pennsylvania

Jason N. Rogart, MD
Fellow, Advanced Endoscopy, Division of Gastroenterology and Hepatology, Department of Medicine, Thomas Jefferson University, Philadelphia, Pennsylvania

Simona Rossi, MD
Assistant Professor of Medicine, Division of Gastroenterology and Hepatology, Department of Medicine, Thomas Jefferson University, Philadelphia, Pennsylvania

Emily Rubin, RD, BS
Clinical Dietician, Division of Gastroenterology and Hepatology, Department of Medicine, Thomas Jefferson University, Philadelphia, Pennsylvania

Ivan Rudolph, MD
Clinical Assistant Professor of Medicine; Director, Gastroenterology Clinic, Division of Gastroenterology and Hepatology, Department of Medicine, Thomas Jefferson University, Philadelphia, Pennsylvania

Bridget Jennings Seymour, MD
Fellow, Division of Gastroenterology and Hepatology, Department of Medicine, Thomas Jefferson University, Philadelphia, Pennsylvania; Gastroenterologist/Hepatologist, Department of Medicine, Merrimack Valley Hospital, Haverhill, Massachusetts; Gastroenterologist/Hepatologist, Department of Medicine, Anna Jaques Hospital, Newburyport, Massachusetts

Maya Spodik, MD
Fellow, Division of Gastroenterology and Hepatology, Department of Medicine, Thomas Jefferson University, Philadelphia, Pennsylvania

Preface

The Division of Gastroenterology and Hepatology at Jefferson Medical College and Thomas Jefferson University Hospital is honored to once again be given the opportunity to prepare this self-assessment text that accompanies the ninth edition of *Sleisenger and Fordtran's Gastrointestinal and Liver Disease*. We are pleased to have worked with Mark Feldman, MD; Lawrence S. Friedman, MD; Lawrence J. Brandt, MD; and the publisher, Elsevier Inc., to update the self-assessment companion text.

We hope that the readers will find the questions stimulating. We are happy to receive questions, comments, or critiques related to the content and hope that this text contributes to the lifelong commitment of obtaining new knowledge that improves the care of patients with gastrointestinal and liver disease.

Contents

Video Contents

Videos available at www.expertconsult.com

Ascaris lumbricoides in the colon

Clonorchis sinensis exiting the ampulla during endoscopic retrograde cholangiopancreatography

Enterobius vermicularis in the colon

Taenia saginata seen on video capsule endoscopy

Taenia solium seen on colonoscopy

All videos correspond to chapter 110—"Intestinal Worms"—from Sleisenger and Fordtran's Gastrointestinal and Liver Disease, *9e.*

CHAPTER

1

Biology of the Gastrointestinal Tract and Liver Disease

QUESTIONS

1 Several pathways play a role in gastrointestinal (GI) tumors. Recently this pathway has been recognized as a key regulator in prostaglandin synthesis that is induced in inflammation and neoplasia. No mutations have been identified, but inhibition with aspirin and nonsteroidal anti-inflammatory drugs is associated with reduced risk of colorectal adenoma and cancer. What is the pathway?
A. Cyclooxygenase-2 (COX-2)
B. Nuclear factor-κB
C. P13K/Akt
D. RAF

2 What is the major function of glucagon and glucagon-like peptide?
A. As a neurotransmitter
B. Mediator of satiety and food intake
C. To produce pancreatic fluid and pancreatic secretion
D. To regulate glucose homeostasis

3 Which of the following is the most populous cell of the lamina propria mononuclear cells?
A. Macrophages
B. Dendritic cells
C. Immunoglobulin A–positive (IgA⁺) plasma cells
D. Tumor necrosis factor (TNF)–secreting T cells

4 During a meal, nutrients interact with cells in the mouth and GI tract to regulate hunger and satiety. Which of the following does not play a major role in this complex interaction?
A. Cholecystokinin (CCK)
B. Glucagon-like peptide 1
C. Ghrelin
D. Leptin
E. Lipase

5 The Wnt pathway is important in which of the following processes?
A. Programmed cell death (apoptosis)
B. Senescence
C. Intestinal epithelial cell (IEC) proliferation
D. Pancreatic acinar cell proliferation

6 Adrenergic neurons originate in ganglia of the autonomic nervous system and synapse with enteric neurons. Adrenergic neurons only contain which of the following?
A. Norepinephrine
B. Acetylcholine
C. Neuropeptide Y and somatostatin
D. A and C

7 Which of the following neuromodulators has the following characteristics: a potent vasodilator that increases blood flow in the GI tract and causes smooth muscle relaxation and epithelial cell secretion; is expressed primarily in neurons of the peripheral/enteric and central nervous systems; has effects on many organ systems, although in the GI tract stimulates fluid and electrolyte secretion from intestinal epithelium and bile duct cholangiocytes; causes relaxation of gastric smooth muscle and therefore is an important modulator of sphincters in the GI tract?
A. Acetylcholine
B. Somatostatin
C. CCK
D. Gastrin
E. Vasoactive intestinal polypeptide

8 T cell differentiation is influenced by the microenvironment of the gut. This will influence development of cells and promotion of cytokines, thereby promoting or suppressing inflammation. Which of the following cytokines play a role in IgA secretion?
A. Interleukin (IL)-12
B. IL-4

C. IL-5
D. IL-6
E. A and B
F. C and D

9 CCK and somatostatin are both hormones that are released in the GI tract. They may work as which of the following?
A. Endocrine agent
B. Paracrine agent
C. Neurocrine agent
D. All of the above

10 The analog of which one of the following is used to treat conditions of hormone excess produced by endocrine tumors (including acromegaly, carcinoid tumors, islet tumors, and gastrinomas)?
A. Somatostatin
B. Gastrin
C. CCK
D. Secretin

11 Which of the following genes is deleted or mutated in pancreatic adenocarcinoma?
A. TP53
B. SMAD4
C. APC
D. MLH1

12 What is the phenomenon known as epithelial mesenchymal transition?
A. Polarized epithelial cells no longer recognize boundaries of adjacent epithelial cells and adopt features of migratory mesenchymal cells.
B. Degradation of the basement membrane followed by migration into perivascular stroma and creating capillary sprout
C. Clonal expansion after formation of a metastatic focus
D. Genetic pathway used to modulate Wnt pathway

13 Obesity has become an epidemic in the United States. Much research has been targeted to identify the mediators of satiety. Which one of the following may be the major mediator of satiety and food intake?
A. Somatostatin
B. Acetylcholine
C. Gastrin
D. CCK

14 The nature and form of the antigen play a large role in oral tolerance. Which of the following represents an antigen that is most effective at inducing tolerance?
A. Large amount of soluble carbohydrate
B. Large amount of aggregate lipids
C. Moderate amount of soluble protein
D. Moderate amount of aggregate protein

15 Which of the following statements describes the major contributing mechanism behind the controlled inflammation in the gut?
A. Lamina propria lymphocytes respond poorly when activated via their T cell receptor, failing to proliferate and providing a state of activation without expansion.
B. Antigen-specific nonresponse to antigens administered orally

C. Large potentially antigenic macromolecules are degraded so that potentially immunogenic substances are rendered nonimmunogenic.
D. Th3 cells that are activated in Peyer patches

16 Patients who have celiac disease may have a disruption in their oral tolerance. Which of the following does not affect the induction of oral tolerance?
A. Genetic factors
B. Nature of the antigen
C. Ethnicity
D. Age
E. Tolerogen dose

17 Point mutations in this gene have been identified in esophageal squamous carcinoma and adenocarcinoma, gastric carcinoma, pancreatic adenocarcinoma, hepatocellular carcinoma, and sporadic colon cancers. Interestingly, mutations are rarely identified in colonic adenomas. What is the gene?
A. SMAD4
B. TP53
C. APC
D. MLH1

18 The gut is the largest lymphoid organ in the body. It contains billions of organisms. Significant inflammation is not present in the intestine. What is this phenomenon known as?
A. Oral tolerance
B. The intestinal barrier
C. Relative chemotaxis
D. Controlled/physiologic inflammation

19 This gene is found on chromosome 5q and is associated with Gardner's syndrome. Both somatic and germline mutations appear in this gene and contribute to the development of polyps.
A. TP53
B. Multiple endocrine neoplasia (MEN1)
C. E-cadherin1 (CDH1)
D. Adenomatous polyposis coli (APC)

20 All GI peptides are synthesized via gene transcription of DNA into messenger RNA and subsequent translation of messenger RNA into precursor proteins known as preprohormones. The peptides that are destined to be secreted begin as proteins that are cleaved and the prepropeptide is then prepared for structural modifications. Modifications of the peptide hormone for the full biological activity occur in which organelle of the cell?
A. Mitochondria
B. Golgi apparatus
C. Endoplasmic reticulum
D. Cytoplasm

21 Which antibody is most abundant in mucosal secretions?
A. IgA
B. IgM
C. IgG
D. IgE

22 This test can be performed on archived colon tumor tissue and can be helpful in identifying those individuals with colon cancer in the setting of hereditary nonpolyposis colorectal cancer.

A. Stool DNA for *TP53*
B. Germline DNA analysis for *PTEN*
C. Microsatellite instability testing
D. Direct DNA sequencing

23 Which of the following seems to be overexpressed in patients with inflammatory bowel disease and may contribute to activate T lymphocytes?
A. Major histocompatibility complex class II molecules
B. Toll-like receptors
C. Peroxisome proliferator activated receptor-γ
D. All of the above

24 All of the following are tumor suppressor genes *except*:
A. *APC*
B. *TP53*
C. *SMAD4*
D. *C-Myc*

25 IECs are derived from the basal crypts and have many roles. Which of the following is not a role of the IECs?
A. Antigen trafficking
B. Secretion of cytokines and chemokines to control the spread of infection once a pathogen has been recognized
C. Binding of antigens and then transporting to Peyer patches
D. Expression of Toll-like receptors
E. IECs play a role in all of the above.

26 Which of the following characteristics is not associated with inherited GI cancer syndromes?
A. Individuals are at risk of tumors outside the GI tract.
B. Tumors carry a higher mortality.
C. Multiple primary tumors develop within the target tissue.
D. Tumors in affected individuals typically appear at a younger age.
E. Tumor often develops in the absence of predisposing environmental factors.

27 The PP/PYY/NPY (pancreatic polypeptide/peptide tyrosine tyrosine/neuropeptide Y) family of peptides function as which type of transmitter?
A. Endocrine
B. Paracrine
C. Neurocrine
D. All of the above
E. None of the above

28 Environmental factors play a role in tumorigenesis. Dietary and viral agents play a role in tumor. Which of the following viruses has been linked to gastric lymphoepithelial malignancies?
A. Human papillomavirus
B. Hepatitis B virus
C. Cytomegalovirus
D. Epstein-Barr virus

29 The lamina propria mononuclear cells and lamina propria lymphocytes (LPLs) are involved in several pathways. Which pathway may be defective in Crohn's disease?
A. Resistance of the LPLs to undergo apoptosis when activated inappropriately

B. Activation of nuclear factor-κB by IL-18
C. Ability of intraepithelial lymphocytes to secrete cytokines such as IL-7
D. All of the above

30 *Ras* genes are the most commonly detected oncogenes in the GI tract cancers. The highest frequency of mutation (90%) is found in which of the following tumors?
A. Colon cancer
B. Exocrine pancreas
C. Gastric cancer
D. Colon adenoma

31 Chemokines are secreted by IECs and they aid in the regulation of inflammation. Chemokines attract which of the following cells to sites of interest?
A. Lymphocytes
B. Macrophages
C. Dendritic cells
D. A and B
E. All of the above

32 What modulator is released from the extrinsic and intrinsic nerves and from the mucosal enterochromophin cells of the gut? It is important in epithelial secretion, bowel motility, nausea, and emesis. Identification of this hormone-specific receptor subtype has led to the development of selective agonists and antagonists for the treatment of irritable bowel syndrome and chronic constipation and diarrhea.
A. Norepinephrine
B. Acetylcholine
C. Serotonin
D. Histamine

33 Two pathways trigger cell apoptosis. One is mediated by activation of *TP53* and the other is mediated through death receptors. Which of the following is not a death receptor?
A. TNF receptor
B. DR5
C. Fas
D. Caspase receptor

34 In animal models, deletion of which of the following leads to colitis?
A. TNF
B. IL-6
C. IL-10
D. Transforming growth factor-β
E. A and B
F. C and D

35 Polio vaccine is one of the few orally administered vaccines that induces active immunity in the gut. Which of the following may contribute to why this oral vaccine provides immunity?
A. The virus binds to IECs.
B. The virus binds to microfold cells (M cells).
C. Disrupts tight junctions allowing antigen to pass into paracellular space
D. Activation of regulatory T cells

36 True or false: Somatic mutations lead to the expression of a gene in all cells within a tissue.

A. True
B. False

37 All of the following are gene mutations that can lead to colon cancer and can be tested for by immunohistochemistry *except*:
A. *MSH2*
B. *MLH1*
C. *MYH*
D. *LKB1*

38 Pain pathways within the GI tract are complex. Which of the following participate in pain pathways and modulate inflammation?
A. Substance P
B. Calcitonin gene–related peptide
C. Acetylcholine
D. None of the above
E. All of the above (A, B, C)

39 The primary origin of TNF is in the following cell types:
A. Macrophages, Th1, dendritic, endothelial
B. Macrophages only
C. Th2
D. Epithelial

40 Nuclear oligomerization domain 2 (NOD2)/CARD15 polymorphisms are associated with which of the following?

A. Ulcerative colitis
B. Crohn's disease
C. Celiac disease
D. Carcinoid

41 Which of the following is the principal regulator of cell cycle progression or movement from G_2 to M phase and G_1 to S phase in the cell cycle?
A. Cyclin
B. Retinoblastoma protein
C. P21
D. Cyclin dependent kinase
E. All of the above
F. A and D

42 A genetically unstable environment contributes to the development of cancer. Microsatellite instability involves which of the following?
A. Frequent alterations in smaller tracts of microsatellite DNA
B. Aneuploidy
C. Chromosomal deletions
D. Chromosomal duplication

43 All of the following are oncogenes *except*:
A. K-*ras*
B. C-*Src*
C. β-*Catenin*
D. *P53*

ANSWERS

1 **A** (S&F, ch3)
The COX-2 pathway plays an important role in GI tumors. The enzyme COX-2 is a key regulator of prostaglandin synthesis that is induced in inflammation and neoplasia. Although no mutations of COX-2 have been described, overexpression of COX-2 in colon adenomas and cancers is associated with tumor progression and angiogenesis, primarily through the induction of synthesis of prostaglandin E_2. Inhibition of COX-2 with a variety of agents (aspirin, nonsteroidal anti-inflammatory drugs, and COX-2 selective inhibitors) is associated with a reduced risk of colorectal adenomas and cancer.

2 **D** (S&F, ch1)
Glucagon and glucagon-like peptides are synthesized and released from the cells of the pancreas, ileum, and colon and are not neurotransmitters.

3 **C** (S&F, ch2)
Lamina propria mononuclear cells are a heterogeneous group of cells. The most populous cell type is the IgA+ plasma cell, but there are more than 50% T and B cells, macrophages, and dendritic cells.

4 **E** (S&F, ch1)
CCK is one of the most studied satiety hormones. CCK reduces food intake in animals. Glucagon-like peptide 1 is produced by the ileum and the colon. Glucagon-like peptide 1 receptors are found in parts of the brain that are important in the regulation of hunger. Leptin is considered a long-term regulator of energy balance. Ghrelin is the only GI

hormone to have arexigenic effects. Lipase is an enzyme released from the pancreas and does not seem to regulate hunger and satiety.

5 **C** (S&F, ch3)
The Wnt pathway is one important example of a signaling pathway that regulates the cell cycle machinery to control the proliferation of IECs (see figure).

6 **D** (S&F, ch1)
A single type of neuron contains and releases different chemical substances (e.g., adrenergic neurons of the enteric nervous system contain not only norepinephrine but also neuropeptide Y and somatostatin to modulate the smooth muscle intestinal contraction or secretion).

7 **E** (S&F, ch1)
Vasoactive intestinal peptide has broad significance in the GI tract, which is represented by the listed characteristics.

8 **F** (S&F, ch2)
IL-5 induces B cells expressing surface IgA to differentiate into IgA-producing plasma cells. IL-6 causes an increase in IgA secretion with little effect on either IgM or IgG synthesis.

9 **D** (S&F, ch1)
CCK and somatostatin are typical examples of chemical substances that can be released as hormones by the endocrine cells and transported to the target cells. In addition, these substances may also be released by the nearby cells and quickly act on

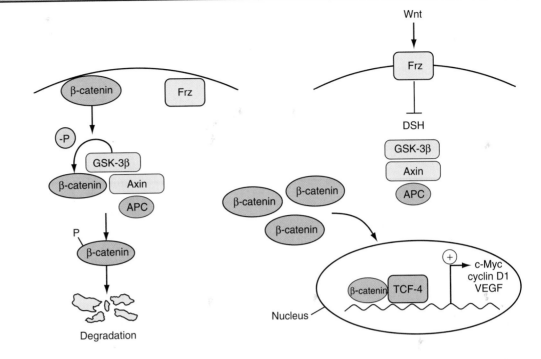

Figure for answer **5**

the neighboring cells and also be released as neu-rotransmitters. Somatostatin is a classic paracrine hormone, but, depending on where in the GI tract it is released, it can exert endocrine and neural effects.

10 A (S&F, ch1)
Because of its varied physiologic effects, somatostatin has several clinically important pharmacologic uses. Many endocrine cells possess somatostatin receptors and are sensitive to inhibitory regulation. Therefore, somatostatin and its analogs are used to treat conditions of hormone excess produced by endocrine tumors, including acromegaly, carcinoid tumors, and islet cell tumors. Its ability to reduce splanchnic blood flow and portal venous pressure led to somatostatin analogs being useful in treating esophageal variceal bleeding. The inhibitory effects on secretion have been exploited by using somatostatin analogs to treat some forms of diarrhea and reduce fluid output from pancreatic fistulas. Many endocrine tumors express abundant somatostatin receptors, making it possible to use radiolabeled somatostatin analogs, such as octreotide, to localize even small tumors throughout the body.

11 B (S&F, ch3)
SMAD4, also designated the deleted in pancreas cancer 4 gene, is a tumor suppressor gene located on chromosome 18q and is deleted or mutated in most pancreatic adenocarcinomas and a subset of colon cancers.

12 A (S&F, ch3)
Epithelial mesenchymal transition may be what promotes tumor progression. Clonal expansion after metastasis is a "survival of the fittest" model in which the metastatic focus proliferates. The Wnt pathway is an example of a signaling pathway that regulates the cell cycle machinery to control the proliferation of IECs.

13 D (S&F, ch1)
CCK has a major role in gallbladder contraction. It stimulates pancreatic secretion and has been shown to delay gastric emptying. Low levels of CCK have been noted in individuals with celiac disease and bulimia nervosa.

14 C (S&F, ch2)
Protein antigens are the most tolerogenic, whereas carbohydrates and lipids are less effective at inducing tolerance. The way in which the antigen is delivered is also critical. For example, a protein delivered in soluble form is quite tolerogenic, whereas aggregation of this protein reduces its potential to induce tolerance. The dose of antigen administered is critical to the form of oral tolerance generated; too little or too much is often not the correct dose to induce tolerance.

15 A (S&F, ch2)
The failure to produce GI pathology despite the activation state of intestinal lymphocytes is probably the consequence of regulatory mechanisms. The failure of LPLs to generate "normal" antigen receptor-mediated responses is an important factor in controlled inflammation. LPLs respond poorly when activated via their T cell receptor, failing to proliferate, although they still can produce cytokines. This is key to the maintenance of controlled inflammation. Answers **B** and **C** describe the concept behind oral tolerance, in which Th3 cells are thought to play a role.

16 C (S&F, ch2)
Factors affecting the induction of oral tolerance are the age of the host, genetic factors, the nature of antigen, and the tolerogen's form and dose. The state of the intestinal barrier affects oral tolerance, and when barrier function is reduced, oral tolerance decreases as well. Oral tolerance is difficult to achieve in the neonate, but early on, the intestinal

flora and the limited diet likely play a beneficial role in preventing a vigorous response to food antigen.

17 **B** (S&F, ch3)
TP53 is the gene responsible for the p53 protein. The p53 protein was detected in tumors as the product of a mutated gene that was mapped to chromosome 17p. Point mutations in *TP53* have been identified in 50% to 70% of sporadic colon cancers but only a small subset of colon adenomas. Mutations in *TP53* have also been found in esophageal squamous carcinoma and adenocarcinoma, gastric carcinoma, pancreatic adenocarcinoma, and hepatocellular carcinoma.

18 **D** (S&F, ch2)

19 **D** (S&F, ch3)
Genetic linkage analysis revealed markers on chromosome 5q21 that were tightly linked to polyp development in affected members of kindreds with familial adenomatous polyposis and Gardner's syndrome. The gene responsible for familial adenomatous polyposis is the adenomatous polyposis coli (*APC*) gene.

20 **B** (S&F, ch1)
For most of the peptides, including CCK, the final modification of the molecule (e.g., sulfation) occurs in the Golgi apparatus. The endoplasmic reticulum plays a critical role in the formation of the peptide; however, further modification occurs in the Golgi apparatus.

21 **A** (S&F, ch2)
Secretory IgA is the hallmark of mucosa-associated lymphoid tissue/gut-associated lymphoid tissue immune responses. Although IgG is the most abundant isotype in the systemic immune system, IgA is the most abundant antibody in mucosal secretions. In fact, given the numbers of IgA$^+$ plasma cells and the size of the mucosa-associated lymphoid tissue, IgA turns out to be the most abundant antibody in the body.

22 **C** (S&F, ch3)
The microsatellite instability test can be performed on archived colon tumor samples and serves as a useful screening test to identify individuals whose colon cancers may have developed as a manifestation of Lynch syndrome. Loss of hMSH (human Mut S homolog) 2, hMLH1, or hMSH6 protein by immunohistochemical staining may provide similar information. Emerging data suggest that the microsatellite instability status of a colon tumor may be predictive of the response to 5-fluorouracil–based chemotherapy.

23 **A** (S&F, ch2)
Increased expression of major histocompatibility complex class II molecules by IECs has been reported in patients with irritable bowel disease. Such overexpression would be expected to increase their potential to activate T lymphocytes. Drugs used to treat patients with irritable bowel disease such as 5-aminosalicylic acid preparations may reduce major histocompatibility complex class II expression on IECs.

24 **D** (S&F, ch3)
The c-Myc protein product is involved in critical cellular functions such as proliferation, differentiation, apoptosis, transformation, and transcriptional activation of key genes. Frequently, c-Myc is overexpressed in many GI cancers.

25 **C** (S&F, ch2)
Microfold cells bind antigens and transport them to Peyer patches. In addition to their function as a physical barrier in the gut-associated lymphoid tissue, IECs contribute to both innate and adaptive immunity in the gut and may play a key role in maintaining intestinal homeostasis. Classic antigen-presenting cells in the systemic immune system possess the innate capacity to recognize components of bacteria and viruses called pathogen-associated molecular patterns. Receptors for these pathogen-associated molecular patterns are expressed both on the cell surface (e.g., Toll-like receptors) and inside the cell. After invasion and engagement of Toll-like receptor 5, the IECs are induced to secrete cytokines and chemokines that attract inflammatory cells to the local environment to control spread of infection.

26 **B** (S&F, ch3)
Despite the variation in the type of tumor found in different inherited cancer syndromes, a number of features are common to all inherited GI cancer syndromes. Most importantly, the marked increase in risk of a particular tumor is found in the absence of other predisposing environmental factors. Multiple primary tumors often develop within the target tissue, and tumors in these affected members typically arise at a younger age. Finally, affected individuals are sometimes at risk of some types of tumors outside the GI tract.

27 **D** (S&F, ch1)
PP is the founding member of the PP family. The PP family of peptides includes NPY and PYY. PP is stored and secreted from specialized pancreatic endocrine cells (PP cells), whereas NPY is a principal neurotransmitter found in the central and peripheral nervous systems. PYY has been localized to enteroendocrine cells throughout the GI tract but is found in greatest concentrations in the ileum and colon. The PP/PYY/NPY family of peptides functions as endocrine, paracrine, and neurocrine transmitters in the regulation of a number of actions. PP inhibits pancreatic exocrine secretion, gallbladder contraction, and gut motility. PYY inhibits vagally stimulated gastric acid secretion. NPY is one of the most abundant peptides in the central nervous system and, in contrast to PYY, is a potent stimulant of food intake. Peripherally, NPY affects vascular and GI smooth muscle function.

28 **D** (S&F, ch3)
Viral agents can lead to disruption of normal genes by entry into the host genome, which may disrupt the normal gene sequence. HPV has been linked to squamous cell cancers of the esophagus and anus. Hepatitis B virus has been linked to hepatocellular carcinoma.

29 **A** (S&F, ch2)

LPLs are more prone to undergo apoptosis compared with their peripheral counterparts. This may be a regulatory mechanism limiting the potentially inflammatory effects of activated lymphocytes. A major defect reported in Crohn's disease is the resistance of LPLs to undergo apoptosis when activated inappropriately. The mechanism underlying this apoptotic phenomenon possibly relates to engagement of the death receptor Fas and its ligand on activated LPLs and by the imbalance between the intracellular anti-apoptotic and proapoptotic factors Bcl2 and Bax. Defects in this proapoptotic balance have been reported in patients with Crohn's disease.

30 **B** (S&F, ch3)

Virtually all *ras* mutations in GI malignancies that have been identified occur in the K-*ras* oncogene. The highest frequency is found in tumors of the exocrine pancreas; more than 90% of these tumors possess mutations in the K-*ras* gene. *Ras* genes have been identified in approximately 50% of colonic cancers as well as large benign colon polyps. Less than 10% of colon adenomas smaller than 1 cm have K-*ras* mutations.

31 **E** (S&F, ch2)

Many of the chemokines secreted in the gut-associated lymphoid tissue are produced by IECs. This is especially true in inflammatory bowel diseases in which the secretion of IEC-derived chemokines and cytokines is increased, contributing to the augmentation of mucosal inflammation. The chemokines have the capacity to attract inflammatory cells, such as lymphocytes, macrophages, and dendritic cells.

32 **C** (S&F, ch1)

The GI tract contains more than 95% of the total body serotonin, and serotonin is important in a variety of processes, including epithelial secretion, bowel motility, nausea, and emesis. Serotonin is synthesized from tryptophan and is converted to its active form in nerve terminals. Most plasma serotonin is derived from the gut, where it is found in mucosal enterochromaffin cells and the enteric nervous system. Serotonin mediates its effects by binding to a specific receptor. There are seven different serotonin receptor subtypes ($5-HT_1$ to $5-HT_7$) found on enteric neurons, enterochromaffin cells, and GI smooth muscle. Serotonin can cause smooth muscle contraction through stimulation of cholinergic nerves or relaxation by stimulating inhibitory nitric oxide–containing neurons. Serotonin released from mucosal cells stimulates sensory neurons, initiating a peristaltic reflex, secretion (via $5-HT_4$ receptors), and the serotonin released modulates sensation through activation of $5-HT_3$ receptors.

33 **D** (S&F, ch3)

One pathway is mediated through membrane-bound death receptors, which include TNF receptors, Fas, and DR5, whereas the other pathway involves activation of *TP53* expression by environmental insults such as ionizing radiation, hypoxia, and growth factor withdrawal with the subsequent

increase in the bax-to-bcl-2 ratio. Both pathways converge to disrupt mitochondrial integrity and release of cytochrome c.

34 **F** (S&F, ch2)

TNF and IL-6 are considered to be proinflammatory, while IL-10 and transforming growth factor-β are anti-inflammatory.

35 **B** (S&F, ch2)

Oral tolerance may also be associated with the cells serving as the antigen-presenting cells as well as the site of antigen uptake. Poliovirus binds to M cells, which may account for its ability to stimulate active immunity in the gut. The evidence of this comes from studies in mice. Orally administered reovirus type 3 is taken up in mice by M cells expressing reovirus type 3–specific receptors. This epithelial uptake by M cells induces an active IgA response to the virus. Reovirus type 1 infects IECs adjacent to M cells, and this uptake induces tolerance to the virus. Thus, the route of entry (M cell vs. IEC) of a specific antigen may dictate the type of immune response generated (IgA vs. tolerance).

36 **B** (S&F, ch3)

Whereas germline mutations may lead to altered expression of a gene in all cells within a tissue, subsequent additional somatic mutations generally occur only in a small, largely random subpopulation of cells.

37 **D** (S&F, ch3)

Immunohistochemistry can determine the presence or absence of a gene product in a tissue sample. Gene LKB1 is detected in Peutz-Jeghers syndrome. Loss of MSH2, MYH, and MLH1 protein can be detected by immunohistochemical staining.

38 **E** (S&F, ch1)

Bipolar neurons that project to the mucosa and myenteric plexus act as sensory neurons and contain the hormones listed.

39 **A** (S&F, ch2)

TNF is a cytokine that has its primary origin in macrophages, T cells, dendritic cells, and mesenchymal cells. It functions to increase apoptosis and nuclear factor.

40 **B** (S&F, ch2)

The significance of the ability of IECs to recognize pathogen-associated molecular patterns via surface Toll-like receptors or via intracellular nuclear oligomerization domains 1 and 2 (NOD1, NOD2) has been increasingly recognized over the past decade. The latter ability has been shown to contribute to intestinal inflammation because approximately 25% of patients with Crohn's disease have mutations in the NOD2/CARD15 gene, interfering with their ability to mount an appropriate immune response to bacterial stimuli.

41 **F** (S&F, ch3)

Regulation of cell cycle progression seems to be achieved principally by cyclins and cyclin-dependent kinase activity at the G_1/S and G_2/M phase transitions. Dysregulation can promote neoplasia.

42 **A** (S&F, ch3)
Chromosomal instability results in tumor cells that display frequent aneuploidy, large chromosomal deletions, and chromosomal duplications. Tumors that display microsatellite instability are often diploid or near-diploid on a chromosomal level but harbor frequent alterations in smaller tracts of microsatellite DNA.

43 **D** (S&F, ch3)
More than 80 oncogenes have been isolated. Most of these genes are widely expressed in many different types of tumor cells. Multiple oncogenes are commonly found within a single tumor.

Nutrition in Gastroenterology

QUESTIONS

44 Which of the following is considered protective against childhood obesity?
A. Maternal gestational diabetes
B. Maternal smoking during pregnancy
C. Breast-feeding
D. Reduced nighttime sleep for young children

45 Human proteins are comprised of amino acids. There are 20 different amino acids, some of which are considered essential because their carbon skeletons cannot be synthesized by the body. Which of the following amino acids are considered to be essential?
A. Histidine
B. Glycine
C. Serine
D. Alanine

46 A 3-year-old boy presents with crampy abdominal pain and diarrhea occurring within an hour of eating. He has a poor appetite and is in the 15th percentile for height and weight. Both a food-specific immunoglobulin E (IgE) antibody skin prick test and serum food-specific IgE antibody test are performed, and the results are positive. He is diagnosed as having a gastrointestinal allergy due to IgE-mediated hypersensitivity. Eliminating which of the following group of foods would most likely reduce this child's symptoms?
A. Milk, egg, peanuts
B. Barley, beef, lamb
C. Soy, wheat, potato
D. Shellfish, potato, wheat

47 A 50-year-old woman lost 60 pounds during the first four months after gastric bypass surgery for obesity. She now presents with new epigastric pain that begins about 30 minutes after a meal and is not relieved with antacids. What is the most likely explanation for this patient's symptoms?

A. Marginal ulcer
B. Internal hernia
C. Intestinal obstruction
D. Dumping syndrome
E. Cholelithiasis/biliary colic

48 A 30-year-old female executive has frequent lunch meetings during which she typically chooses salads and other low-calorie options. However, once a month, she returns home late at night and consumes several pints of ice cream, boxes of cookies, and several cans of soda. Immediately afterward, she becomes very anxious, takes several laxatives, and forces herself to vomit. This pattern has been repeating itself for the past 5 years. She is 5 feet 5 inches tall and weighs 130 pounds. Her diagnosis is most likely
A. Bulimia nervosa
B. Night-eating syndrome
C. Anorexia nervosa
D. Binge-eating disorder

49 Protein requirements are affected by the adequacy of essential amino acids in the protein source. What proportion of total protein requirements should be provided in the form of essential amino acids?
A. 5% to 10%
B. 15% to 20%
C. 30% to 40%
D. More than 50%

50 A 32-year-old woman is considering bariatric surgery. Which of the following would usually be recommended as part of her preoperative evaluation?
A. CT scan of the abdomen and pelvis
B. Abdominal ultrasonography
C. Esophagogastroduodenoscopy/upper endoscopy
D. Colonoscopy
E. Esophageal manometry

51 Which of the following statements regarding calcium absorption is most accurate?
A. Calcium absorption occurs primarily in the distal small intestine.
B. Calcium absorption occurs primarily in the proximal small intestine.
C. Calcium absorption occurs throughout the length of the small intestine.
D. Calcium absorption occurs primarily in the colon.

52 Diarrhea in a chronically malnourished population is often caused by a combination of factors, including increased GI secretions, decreased intestinal transit time, and osmotic stimulation of water secretion by unabsorbed contents of the food stream. The somatostatin analog octreotide acetate (Sandostatin) may be used in the management of diarrhea in malnourished patients. Which of the following statements regarding this medication is most accurate?
A. It decreases stool volume, sodium, and chloride output.
B. It decreases small intestinal transit time in patients with short gut syndrome.
C. It improves absorption of macronutrients and micronutrients.
D. It is typically administered by continuous infusion.

53 An 18-year-old girl with bulimia nervosa has a body mass index (BMI) of 15. She reports early satiety and postprandial abdominal pain and vomits twice daily. Over the past two months, she has been hospitalized twice for these symptoms and has lost 5 pounds. Endoscopy reveals scant food debris in the stomach. Treatment with a proton pump inhibitor results in minimal clinical improvement. Which diagnostic test would be most helpful at this time?
A. Breath test for bacterial overgrowth
B. Computed tomography scan of the abdomen
C. Gastric emptying scan
D. Esophageal manometry

54 A 50-year-old alcoholic man has been homeless for several months. He is evaluated in an emergency department and found to be confused and ataxic and to have abnormal eye movements. A computed tomography scan of the head reveals no acute abnormalities, and the results of a drug and alcohol screen are negative. Which of the following vitamin deficiencies best explains these symptoms?
A. Vitamin C deficiency
B. Riboflavin deficiency
C. Niacin deficiency
D. Pantothenic acid deficiency
E. Thiamine deficiency

55 A 2-month-old male infant presents with protracted vomiting and diarrhea. The infant was initially begun on a cow-milk formula and was then switched to a soy-based formula, which he tolerated for two days before his symptoms recurred. A small intestine biopsy specimen shows edema and an increased number of lymphocytes, eosinophils, and mast cells. What is this infant's most likely diagnosis?
A. Dietary protein-induced enterocolitis syndrome
B. Celiac disease

C. Dietary protein-induced enteropathy
D. Whipple's disease

56 Orlistat (Xenical), an orally administered weight reduction agent, prevents the absorption of fats from the diet, thereby reducing caloric intake. Which of the following statements regarding orlistat is true?
A. The mechanism of action is inhibition of pancreatic lipase.
B. It is available in the United States by prescription only.
C. Side effects are mostly related to excellent absorption of the drug via the GI tract.
D. It is effective whether taken before, during, or after a meal.

57 A 50-year-old woman presents to a primary care physician for a routine physical examination. Her medical history is significant for hypertension and diet-controlled diabetes. Her BMI is 42. What is her weight classification?
A. Ideal weight
B. Overweight
C. Obese
D. Morbidly obese

58 A 17-year-old girl with a history of binging and purging is diagnosed with bulimia nervosa. She reports to her dentist symptoms of heartburn, teeth discoloration, and sensitivity to extreme temperatures. The dentist observes rounded teeth and some dents. Which of the following best describes this complication of bulimia nervosa?
A. Dentinogenesis imperfecta
B. Gingivitis
C. Bruxism
D. Perimolysis

59 A 40-year-old man with a history of rhino-conjunctivitis, asthma, and atopic dermatitis presents with heartburn and dysphagia. Twice daily treatment with a proton pump inhibitor for six weeks does not improve his symptoms. Endoscopy reveals mucosal rings, ulcerations, and strictures throughout the esophagus. What is his most likely diagnosis?
A. Reflux esophagitis
B. Allergic eosinophilic esophagitis
C. Bile reflux
D. Candidal esophagitis

60 Undernutrition in children differs from that in adults because it affects growth and development. Which of the following is the most distinguishing feature appreciated during physical examination of a child with kwashiorkor compared with a child with marasmus?
A. Short stature
B. Small head circumference
C. Low weight
D. Peripheral edema

61 Aggressive nutritional support will not benefit every acutely ill patient. For which clinical scenario in a hospitalized patient would aggressive nutritional support be most beneficial?
A. Acute cholecystitis in an obese but otherwise healthy 45-year-old woman

B. Acute alcoholic hepatitis in a 45-year-old man without any other known medical problems

C. Acute coronary syndrome in a 60-year-old man with a history of hypertension

62 A 26-year-old woman with a recent diagnosis of diabetes mellitus and a BMI of 43 is referred by her gynecologist for treatment of obesity. An evaluation for infertility has led to a diagnosis of polycystic ovarian syndrome. Which of the following agents would be most optimal for treating this patient?
A. Orlistat
B. Metformin
C. Prozac
D. Wellbutrin

63 Which of the following agents is approved by the U.S. Food and Drug Administration (FDA) for long-term use in the pharmacologic treatment of obesity?
A. Amphetamine
B. Orlistat
C. Fenfluramine
D. Phentermine

64 A 30-year-old woman with a history of irritable bowel syndrome is seen in a dermatology clinic for evaluation of a papulovesicular rash on her elbows. A biopsy is performed and dermatitis herpetiformis is diagnosed. Her rash is likely to improve by excluding which of the following foods from her diet?
A. Wheat, soy, and dairy
B. Wheat, soy, and peanuts
C. Wheat, rye, and barley
D. Wheat, corn, and peanuts

65 A continuous supply of energy is required for normal organ function, maintenance of metabolic homeostasis, heat production, and performance of mechanical work. What is the largest contributor to the total (daily) energy expenditure (TEE)?
A. Resting energy expenditure
B. Energy expenditure of physical activity
C. Thermic effect of feeding

66 A 48-year-old woman with esophageal cancer has been undergoing chemotherapy and receives nutrition via a percutaneously placed gastrostomy tube. She was recently hospitalized for 5 days for treatment of pneumonia and subsequently developed severe diarrhea. Which one of the following is the best treatment for this patient's diarrhea?
A. Change the enteral feeding formula
B. Change the gastrostomy tube to a jejunostomy tube
C. Metronidazole
D. Ciprofloxacin

67 A 42-year-old man with a history of antrectomy and vagotomy for recalcitrant peptic ulcer disease presents with recurrent episodes of nausea, cramping, diaphoresis, and palpitations after meals. Upper endoscopy reveals normal postoperative findings without obstruction or peptic ulcer disease. Which intervention is most likely to improve this patient's symptoms?
A. Ingest frequent small meals.
B. Ingest simple sugars with meals.

C. Ingest large volumes of fluids with meals.
D. Start a prokinetic agent.

68 A 65-year-old woman with a history of diabetes and hypertension is admitted to the hospital with severe nausea, vomiting, and abdominal pain. Acute cholecystitis is diagnosed based on physical examination, imaging, and laboratory studies. Her weight is 150 pounds and her height is 5 feet 6 inches. Following cholecystectomy, the patient suggests that had her weight been lower she would not have developed gallbladder disease. Based on her BMI of 24.2, how would you best describe her nutritional status?
A. Moderately malnourished
B. Normal
C. Overweight
D. Obese

69 A 45-year-old woman presents for a "health maintenance" visit to your office. Based on her height and weight obtained by your medical assistant, you calculate her BMI to be 37. The patient informs you that she is extremely interested in losing weight with your help. Which of the following statements regarding weight reduction agents is correct?
A. Fluoxetine is approved by the FDA for weight reduction.
B. Fluoxetine is a good option for a long-term weight loss.
C. Wellbutrin has data to support off-label use for short-term weight loss.
D. Topiramate is ineffective for weight reduction.

70 A 19-year-old ballet dancer with a 10-year history of anorexia nervosa presents to the emergency department with confusion, headache, and diffuse weakness one day after a performance. The patient severely restricts her daily intake, keeping to a low-calorie diet for one week before each performance. Immediately after each performance, she quickly liberalizes her diet and starts eating a lot more calories in the form of carbohydrates. Her height is 5 feet 6 inches, and she weighs 100 pounds. The emergency department staff suspects refeeding syndrome. Which laboratory result is most commonly seen with refeeding syndrome?
A. Hyperphosphatemia
B. Hypophosphatemia
C. Hypercalcemia
D. Hypocalcemia

71 A 66-year-old man underwent a bariatric surgical procedure 8 years ago and now presents with fatigue, anemia, and diarrhea in addition to a greater than expected weight loss. Which of the following bariatric surgical procedures is most likely to lead to serious complications due to excessive malabsorption?
A. Biliopancreatic diversion/duodenal switch
B. Roux-en-Y gastric bypass
C. Laparoscopic adjustable gastric banding
D. Partial and sleeve gastrectomy

72 Sibutramine (Meridia), an orally administered agent for the treatment of obesity, suppresses appetite. Which of the following statements regarding sibutramine is true?

A. It has no side effects.

B. It acts directly on serotonin receptors in the brain.

C. It is a selective inhibitor of serotonin uptake.

D. It is not considered effective for maintenance of weight loss.

73 Protein energy malnutrition affects nearly every organ system. Which of the following abnormalities is found in the GI tract of a malnourished patient?

A. Proliferation of intestinal villi

B. Increased volume of gastric secretions

C. Increased number of facultative and anaerobic bacteria in the small bowel

D. Increased volume of bile

74 A 76-year-old man with a history of biliary obstruction due to cholangiocarcinoma presents to his primary care physician with fatigue and shortness of breath. He has a long-term indwelling external biliary drain that is functioning well. There is no scleral icterus. The serum bilirubin level is normal, but the patient is noted to have a severe hypochromic microcytic anemia. Which micronutrient deficiency best explains this patient's anemia?

A. Selenium deficiency

B. Zinc deficiency

C. Copper deficiency

D. Iodine deficiency

75 An 18-year-old female college freshman is evaluated at the student health center because she has never had a menstrual cycle. An aspiring gymnast, she has been preoccupied with maintaining a low weight for much of her life. The patient periodically diets by consuming only vegetables and fruit for several days. Her current weight is 100 pounds, and her height is 5 feet 8 inches. What is her most likely diagnosis?

A. Bulimia nervosa

B. Purging disorder

C. Anorexia nervosa

D. Binge-eating disorder

76 The central nervous system plays an important role in regulating food intake by receiving and processing information from the environment and internal milieu. A number of neurotransmitter systems, including monoamines, amino acids, and neuropeptides, are involved in modulating food intake.

Which of the following statements is the most accurate?

A. The stimulation of α_1-adrenergic receptors increases food intake.

B. The stimulation of serotonin receptors in the brain reduces fat intake, with little or no effect on the intake of protein or carbohydrates.

C. The stimulation of β_2 receptors in the brain increases food intake.

D. The stimulation of the H_1 receptor in the central nervous system increases food intake.

77 A cachectic 56-year-old schizophrenic man has been living on the streets for several months and is admitted to the hospital with pneumonia. He is treated with intravenous antibiotics, and total parenteral nutrition is started. He initially demonstrates clinical improvement but then becomes short of breath despite an improved chest radiograph. Which of the following deficiencies best explains his dyspnea?

A. Phosphorous

B. Calcium

C. Copper

D. Selenium

E. Zinc

78 Hormonal disturbances may occur with eating disorders. In patients with anorexia nervosa and bulimia nervosa, elevation of which specific hormone is most closely associated with secretion of growth hormone, stimulation of appetite and intake, induction of adiposity, and signaling to the hypothalamic nuclei involved in energy homeostasis?

A. Leptin

B. Serotonin

C. Cholecystokinin

D. Ghrelin

79 A 60-year-old woman living in an assisted care facility is admitted to the hospital with a hip fracture. During this hospitalization, the patient is observed to have hyperglycemia. Which micronutrient deficiency best explains this problem?

A. Chromium deficiency

B. Manganese deficiency

C. Copper deficiency

D. Iron deficiency

E. Selenium deficiency

ANSWERS

44 **C** (S&F, ch6)

Several factors are linked to postnatal weight and lifetime weight gain. Among the risks for obesity are maternal smoking and gestational diabetes. Infants who are breast-fed for more than three months may have a reduced risk of future obesity. Children who get more sleep tend to weigh less when they enter school than do those who sleep less.

45 **A** (S&F, ch4)

Histidine, isoleucine, leucine, lysine, methionine, phenylalanine, threonine, tryptophan, valine, and possibly arginine are considered to be essential amino acids because their carbon skeletons cannot be synthesized by the human body. The remaining amino acids (glycine, alanine, serine, cysteine, cystine, tyrosine, glutamine, glutamic acid, asparagine, and aspartic acid) are nonessential in most circumstances because they can be made from endogenous precursors or essential amino acids.

46   **A** (S&F, ch9)
Milk, eggs, and peanuts are the most common foods associated with food allergy due to IgE-mediated hypersensitivity. Symptoms may develop within minutes to two hours of consuming an implicated food and consist of nausea, abdominal pain, vomiting, and diarrhea. The other food choices are associated with non–IgE-mediated food hypersensitivities.

47   **E** (S&F, ch7)
Cholelithiasis is very commonly associated with rapid weight loss and occurs in as many as one third of patients after weight loss surgery. Although marginal ulcers may occur and cause postoperative pain in this patient population, cholelithiasis is much more common and does not respond to antacid therapy. Most experts recommend prophylactic treatment with ursodiol for the first six months postoperatively to prevent this complication.

48   **A** (S&F, ch8)
Bulimia nervosa is a recurrent binge-eating disorder accompanied by inappropriate behaviors to control weight or purge calories. These behaviors may include using laxatives or diuretics, vomiting, and excessive exercise. Binge-eating disorder is characterized by excessive intake of calories within a discrete period of time, without associated inappropriate compensatory behaviors to prevent weight gain. Anorexia nervosa is characterized by an unwillingness to maintain normal weight. Commonly, this is described as a failure to exceed 85% of the expected body weight in association with a fear of weight gain. Night-eating syndrome is defined as recurrent bouts of overeating during nighttime awakening, without necessarily binging. The syndrome is not associated with inappropriate compensatory behaviors to prevent weight gain.

49   **B** (S&F, ch4)
Proteins containing low amounts of essential amino acids are considered to be of low biologic quality. The total protein requirement is higher when the protein source is of low biologic quality. In normal adults, approximately 15% to 20% of the total protein requirement should be in the form of essential amino acids.

50   **C** (S&F, ch7)
Upper endoscopy is generally recommended for all patients who will be undergoing bariatric surgery. A high percentage of patients considering bariatric surgery will have clinically significant findings on endoscopy. The other listed options are only indicated for the evaluation of specific symptoms. A colonoscopy is a reasonable screening test for colon and rectal cancer but is not part of the routine preoperative evaluation for a young patient.

51   **C** (S&F, ch5)
Calcium absorption occurs throughout the length of the entire small intestine and is vitamin D dependent. During periods of restricted calcium intake, the colon may become more involved in calcium homeostasis by increasing its absorption.

52   **A** (S&F, ch4)
The somatostatin analog octreotide acetate (Sandostatin) can decrease small intestine secretions. Therapy with octreotide has been shown to decrease ostomy or stool volume, decrease sodium and chloride output, and prolong small intestine transit time in patients with short bowel syndrome. Octreotide therapy, however, usually does not improve absorption of macronutrients and other minerals; in fact, it may exacerbate the degree of fat malabsorption, presumably by inhibiting pancreatic secretions. In addition, octreotide is expensive, diminishes protein synthesis in the intestinal epithelium and exocrine pancreas, and may decrease appetite and increase the risk of gallstones. It is usually administered subcutaneously, often several times per day.

53   **C** (S&F, ch8)
Gastroparesis is associated with bulimia nervosa and anorexia nervosa, and presents with early satiety and postprandial abdominal pain. Upper endoscopy excluded structural abnormalities, but the finding of food in the stomach did suggest gastroparesis. Therefore, the gastric emptying scan would be the most helpful test at this point (see table at end of chapter).

54   **E** (S&F, ch5)
Thiamine is important for energy transformation as well as membrane and nerve conduction. Thiamine deficiency may cause Wernicke's encephalopathy, which is characterized by altered mental status, ataxia, and abnormal eye movements. Although common in alcoholic patients, this condition may occur in any severely malnourished patient. Treatment consists of immediate administration of thiamine.

55   **A** (S&F, ch9)
Dietary protein-induced enterocolitis syndrome occurs in infants between one and three months of age, presents with protracted vomiting and diarrhea (mild to moderate steatorrhea in ~80%), and may result in dehydration and poor weight gain. Cow's milk sensitivity is the most frequent cause of this syndrome, but it also has been associated with sensitivities to soy, eggs, wheat, rice, chicken, and fish. Loss of protein sensitivity, with resultant reduction in clinical reactivity, occurs frequently. In this case, a rice-based formula would be recommended. During breast-feeding, infants virtually never develop this syndrome. Celiac disease is due to an immunologic reaction to gliadin, which is found in wheat, rye, and barley. The biopsy typically has an infiltrate limited to lymphocytes and may demonstrate villous atrophy. Whipple's disease is a rare infectious disease resulting in weight loss, incomplete breakdown of carbohydrates and fats, and immune system dysfunction. Whipple's disease is treated with antibiotics.

56   **A** (S&F, ch6)
Orlistat is taken three times daily and specifically before meals. In the United States, orlistat is available in two strengths: a prescription dose of 120 mg (Xenical) and an over-the-counter dose of 60 mg

(Alli). Orlistat is poorly absorbed and acts by inhibiting the enzymatic action of pancreatic lipase. Subsequently, its side effects are those associated with maldigestion of fats including fecal incontinence, anal leakage, bloating, and borborygmi.

57 **A** (S&F, ch6)

Over the past 50 years, there has been a steady rise in the incidence of obesity. A useful tool for studying this trend is the BMI, defined as the weight (W) in kilograms divided by the height (H) in meters squared (W/H²). A BMI greater than 30 provides a useful operating definition of obesity.

BMI <18	Underweight
BMI 18-26.5	Ideal weight
BMI 26.6-29	Overweight
BMI 30-40	Obese
BMI >40	Morbidly obese

58 **D** (S&F, ch8)

Chronic vomiting, a feature of bulimia nervosa, may cause dental erosions or perimolysis. Neither gingivitis (irritation of the gums) nor bruxism (teeth grinding) is associated with bulimia nervosa or typically presents with dental erosions. Dentinogenesis imperfecta is a genetic disorder of tooth development that causes the teeth to be discolored (most often a blue-gray or yellow-brown color) and translucent and is not a feature of bulimia nervosa.

59 **B** (S&F, ch9)

The most likely diagnosis is allergic eosinophilic esophagitis. A biopsy specimen demonstrating a high number of eosinophils would be helpful in establishing a diagnosis. The symptoms may be confused with those of reflux. Endoscopic findings include mucosal rings, ulcerations, and strictures. The absence of clinical improvement despite proton pump inhibitor therapy makes reflux esophagitis less likely. The clinical presentation and endoscopic findings are not suggestive of bile reflux or candidal esophagitis.

60 **D** (S&F, ch4)

The presence of peripheral edema distinguishes children with kwashiorkor from those with marasmus and nutritional dwarfism.

61 **B** (S&F, ch4)

The prevalence of moderate to severe protein energy malnutrition is so high among patients admitted for acute alcoholic hepatitis and other forms of decompensated alcoholic liver disease that it is best to assume that all such patients are malnourished. Furthermore, patients with acute alcoholic hepatitis usually fall far short of their nutritional needs when allowed to eat ad libitum. Clinical trials demonstrate that the rates of morbidity and mortality and the speed of recovery are improved with prompt institution of enteral or parenteral nutrition in these patients.

62 **B** (S&F, ch6)

Metformin is a biguanide that is approved for the treatment of diabetes mellitus and often used in management of polycystic ovarian syndrome. It reduces hepatic glucose production, decreases glucose absorption from the GI tract, and enhances insulin sensitivity. As compared to sulfonylureas, clinical trials have demonstrated weight loss with metformin.

63 **B** (S&F, ch6)

Two agents are approved by the FDA for long-term treatment of obesity—sibutramine and orlistat. As monotherapy, both agents can produce weight loss of 8% to 10%. Orlistat promotes weight reduction by inhibiting the enzymatic action of pancreatic lipase. Sibutramine promotes satiety and possibly increases energy expenditure by blocking the reduction in metabolic rate that accompanies weight loss. Fenfluramine increases serotonin levels, resulting in a sense of fullness and loss of appetite. Phentermine acts on the hypothalamus to release norepinephrine and reduces hunger. Outside the brain, phentermine causes release of epinephrine, which acts to break down fat in adipose tissue, and reduces hunger. Fenfluramine, and a combination agent consisting of fenfluramine and phentermine ("fen-phen"), were withdrawn from the market after being shown to cause pulmonary hypertension and heart valve abnormalities.

64 **C** (S&F, ch9)

Dermatitis herpetiformis is a chronic blistering skin disorder associated with a gluten-sensitive enteropathy (celiac disease). It is characterized by a chronic, intensely pruritic, papulovesicular rash symmetrically distributed over the extensor surfaces and buttocks. Although many patients have minimal or no GI symptoms, biopsy of the small bowel generally confirms intestinal involvement. Elimination of gliadin, the alcohol-soluble portion of gluten found in wheat, rye, and barley, from the diet generally leads to resolution of skin symptoms and normalization of intestinal findings over several months. An increased incidence of celiac disease in individuals previously diagnosed with irritable bowel syndrome has been shown.

65 **A** (S&F, ch4)

Total (daily) energy expenditure (TEE) is composed of three components: the resting energy expenditure (~70% of TEE), the energy expenditure of physical activity (~20% of TEE), and the thermic effect of enteral or parenteral nutrition (~10% of TEE).

66 **C** (S&F, ch5)

The most common cause of diarrhea in patients receiving enteral feeds is *Clostridium difficile (C. difficile)*–induced colitis due to concurrent antibiotics. Metronidazole is usually an effective treatment for this infection. Changing the route of feeding to the jejunum would likely worsen this patient's diarrhea. Another acceptable option that was not included as an answer choice is oral vancomycin. Some patients have diarrhea after antibiotic therapy without *C. difficile* infection. This subset of patients may improve with probiotic supplementation after withdrawal of the original antibiotic.

67 | **A** (S&F, ch5)
This patient has symptoms of dumping syndrome, which is common in patients who have had a gastrectomy and vagotomy. These symptoms are caused by hypertonic gastric contents emptying rapidly into the small intestine. This causes a significant amount of the plasma volume to be shifted to the small intestine with resultant symptoms due mostly to hypovolemia. Nutritional therapy of this condition aims to deliver a lower osmolarity to the small intestine by frequent ingestion of small meals with *limited* simple sugars. Fluid intake should be restricted while eating solid food to avoid rapid gastric transit.

68 | **B** (S&F, ch4)
This patient's BMI based on her height and weight is 24.2. According to the table, she is considered normal (see table at end of chapter).

69 | **C** (S&F, ch6)
Fluoxetine is a selective serotonin reuptake inhibitor that blocks serotonin transporters, thus prolonging the action of serotonin. Fluoxetine is approved by the FDA for the treatment of depression. Approximately 50% of initial weight loss associated with fluoxitine is regained during the second six months of treatment, making this drug inappropriate for long-term treatment of obesity. Bupropion is approved for the treatment of depression and as an adjunctive agent for smoking cessation. Two multicenter clinical trials, one in obese subjects with depressive symptoms and one in uncomplicated overweight patients, evaluated the effectiveness of buproprion for weight loss. Nondepressed subjects may respond with more weight loss than those with depressive symptoms. Topiramate, an antiepileptic drug, was associated with weight loss in clinical trials for epilepsy.

70 | **B** (S&F, ch8)
Patients with anorexia nervosa are at risk of refeeding syndrome, a potentially life-threatening condition characterized by fluid and electrolyte disorders including hypophosphatemia, hypomagnesemia, and hypokalemia. This syndrome typically occurs within four days of introducing a healthy diet to a patient with anorexia nervosa. As a shift from fat to carbohydrate metabolism occurs, insulin levels increase, leading to increased cellular uptake of phosphate. Associated with intracellular movement of electrolytes is a decrease in the serum electrolytes, particularly phosphate, potassium, magnesium, glucose, and thiamine. Alteration in serum calcium levels is not commonly associated with refeeding syndrome (see table from answer **53**).

71 | **A** (S&F, ch7)
Biliopancreatic diversion/duodenal switch may result in serious complications due to excessive malabsorption resulting in malnutrition and a variety of vitamin deficiencies. This may present as excessive weight loss, anemia, and even diarrhea. This procedure has thus fallen out of favor because there are several other options that are highly effective with fewer long-term nutritional complications. All of the other choices, commonly performed in bariatric centers, are reasonable alternatives that are associated with fewer postoperative problems.

72 | **C** (S&F, ch6)
Sibutramine (Meridia) selectively inhibits reuptake of serotonin and norepinephrine into neurons but does not act on any known receptors. Sibutramine promotes satiety but may also increase energy expenditure by blocking the reduction in metabolic rate that normally accompanies weight loss.

73 | **C** (S&F, ch4)
Malnutrition is associated with structural and functional changes within the GI tract. Marked blunting of the intestinal villi, usually associated with loss of some or all of the brush border hydrolases, is often seen. There is a reduction in gastric and pancreatic secretions in association with lower concentrations of acid and digestive enzymes, respectively. In addition, the volume of bile, and the concentration of conjugated bile acids within the bile, is reduced. Increased numbers of facultative and anaerobic bacteria are found in the proximal small intestine, and this probably explains the increased proportion of free bile acids within the intestinal lumen.

74 | **C** (S&F, ch5)
Copper is necessary for iron utilization, hemoglobin formation and production, and survival of erythrocytes. Copper is excreted in the bile, and therefore patients with external biliary drainage are at high risk of copper deficiency. The daily copper requirement is 1.5 to 3 µg/day.

75 | **C** (S&F, ch8)
Anorexia nervosa is characterized by an unwillingness to maintain normal weight. Commonly, this is described as failure to exceed 85% of expected body weight in association with fear of gaining weight and amenorrhea. Bulimia nervosa is defined as recurrent binge eating accompanied by a variety of inappropriate purging behaviors, including laxatives, excessive exercise, diuretics, or vomiting to control weight gained during a binge. These behaviors must occur twice weekly for at least 3 months to meet diagnostic criteria. Binge-eating disorder is characterized by excessive intake of calories within a discrete period of time but is not associated with recurrent inappropriate compensatory behaviors to prevent weight gain. Purging disorder is defined by recurrent purging or elimination using laxatives, exercise, diuretics, or vomiting in the absence of clinically significant binge-pattern eating.

76 | **B** (S&F, ch6)
Stimulation of α_1-adrenergic receptors reduces all food intake, whereas stimulation of serotonin receptors in the brain selectively reduces fat intake, with little or no effect on the intake of protein or carbohydrate. Stimulation of β_2 receptors in the brain decreases food intake, and stimulation of the H_1 receptor in the central nervous system reduces feeding.

77 **A** (S&F, ch5)

Phosphorous deficiency may occur in malnourished patients who abruptly begin adequate nutrition. In these patients, the delivery of a glucose load after a period of starvation causes an increased serum insulin level. Insulin drives phosphorous, magnesium, and potassium into cells, with resultant very low serum levels of these electrolytes. This disorder is called refeeding syndrome, and may be life-threatening. Severe hypophosphatemia causes skeletal muscle dysfunction, and this effect may be most evident in the chest leading to hypoventilation and eventual tissue hypoxia. Severely malnourished patients should initially receive a reduced glucose load at a slow rate with close monitoring of all serum electrolytes.

78 **D** (S&F, ch8)

Ghrelin affects all of these regulatory functions and is elevated in anorexia nervosa and bulimia nervosa. The other hormones listed do not affect secretion of growth hormone. Leptin is associated with longer-term regulation of body fat stores and affects satiety through its binding to the ventromedial nucleus of the hypothalamus, an area known as the "satiety center." Altered serotonin function contributes to dysregulation of appetite as well as mood and impulse control in eating disorders. This abnormality persists after recovery from anorexia nervosa and bulimia nervosa, suggesting possible premorbid vulnerability. In bulimia nervosa, a blunted postprandial cholecystokinin (CCK) response impairs satiety. The findings regarding a relationship between pre- and postprandial CCK levels and anorexia nervosa are inconsistent.

79 **A** (S&F, ch5)

Chromium is necessary for the synthesis of glucose tolerance factor, a cofactor for insulin action. A deficiency in chromium can thus lead to glucose intolerance and elevated glucose levels.

Tables

Table for answer 53 **Selected Clinical Features and Complications of Behaviors in Patients with Eating Disorders**

	CLINICAL FEATURE OR COMPLICATION	
SYSTEM AFFECTED	ASSOCIATED WITH WEIGHT LOSS AND FOOD RESTRICTION OR BINGE-EATING IN ANOREXIA NERVOSA	ASSOCIATED WITH PURGING OR REFEEDING BEHAVIORS IN ANOREXIA NERVOSA, BULIMIA NERVOSA, OR EDNOS
Cardiovascular	Arrhythmia Bradycardia Congestive heart failure (in refeeding syndrome) Decreased cardiac size Diminished exercise capacity Dyspnea Hypotension Mitral valve prolapse Orthostasis Prolonged QT interval QT dispersion Syncope	Ventricular arrhythmia Cardiomyopathy (with ipecac use) Prolonged QT interval Orthostasis Syncope
Dermatologic	Brittle hair Dry skin Hair loss Hypercarotenemia Lanugo	Russell's sign (knuckle lesions from repeated scraping against the incisors)
Oral, pharyngeal	Cheilosis	Dental erosion and caries Sialadenosis Pharyngeal and soft palatal trauma Angular cheilitis Perimolysis Vocal fold pathology
Gastrointestinal*	Anorectal dysfunction Delayed gastric emptying Elevated liver enzyme levels Elevated serum amylase levels Gastroesophageal reflux Hepatic injury Pancreatitis Prolonged whole-gut transit time Rectal prolapse Slow colonic transit Superior mesenteric artery syndrome *During refeeding:* Acute gastric dilatation, necrosis, and perforation Elevated liver enzyme levels Hepatomegaly Pancreatitis	Abdominal pain Acute gastric dilatation Barrett's esophagus Bloating Constipation Delayed gastric emptying Diarrhea Dysphagia Elevated liver enzyme levels Elevated serum amylase levels Esophageal bleeding Esophageal ulcers, erosions, stricture Gastroesophageal reflux Mallory-Weiss tear Gastroesophageal reflux Gastric necrosis and perforation Hematemesis Pancreatitis Prolonged intestinal transit time Rectal bleeding Rectal prolapse

Continued

Table for answer 53 **Selected Clinical Features and Complications of Behaviors in Patients with Eating Disorders—Cont'd**

	CLINICAL FEATURE OR COMPLICATION	
SYSTEM AFFECTED	**ASSOCIATED WITH WEIGHT LOSS AND FOOD RESTRICTION OR BINGE-EATING IN ANOREXIA NERVOSA**	**ASSOCIATED WITH PURGING OR REFEEDING BEHAVIORS IN ANOREXIA NERVOSA, BULIMIA NERVOSA, OR EDNOS**
Endocrine and metabolic	Amenorrhea	Hypercholesterolemia
	Euthyroid sick syndrome	Hyperphosphatemia
	Hypercholesterolemia	Hypochloremia
	Hypocalcemia	Hypoglycemia
	Hypoglycemia	Hypokalemia
	Hyponatremia	Hypomagnesemia
	Hypothermia	Hyponatremia
	Low serum estradiol, low serum testosterone levels	Hypophosphatemia
		Metabolic acidosis
	Osteopenia, osteoporosis	Metabolic alkalosis
	Pubertal delay, arrested growth	Secondary hyperaldosteronism
	As part of the refeeding syndrome:	
	Hypomagnesemia	
	Hypophosphatemia	
	Acute kidney injury	Abnormal menses
Genitourinary and reproductive	Amenorrhea	Azotemia
	Atrophic vaginitis	Pregnancy complications (including low birth weight infant)
	Breast atrophy	
	Infertility	
	Pregnancy complications (including low birth weight, premature birth, and perinatal death)	
Neurologic	Cognitive changes	Stroke (associated with ephedra use)
	Cortical atrophy	Neuropathy (with ipecac use)
	Delirium (in refeeding syndrome)	Reduced or absent gag reflex
	Peripheral neuropathy	
	Ventricular enlargement	
Hematologic	Anemia	
	Leukopenia	
	Neutropenia	
	Thrombocytopenia	

EDNOS, eating disorder, not otherwise specified.

*Gastrointestinal complications associated with binge pattern eating in any of the eating disorders, are not all listed, and include weight gain, acute gastric dilatation, gastric rupture, gastroesophageal reflux, increased gastric capacity, and increased stool volume.

Table for answer 68 **Classification of Nutritional Status by Body Mass Index in Adults**

BODY MASS INDEX (KG/M^2)	**NUTRITIONAL STATUS**
<16.0	Severely malnourished
16.0-16.9	Moderately malnourished
17.0-18.4	Mildly malnourished
18.5-24.9	Normal
25.0-29.9	Overweight
30.0-34.9	Obese (class I)
35.0-39.9	Obese (class II)
≥40	Obese (class III)

CHAPTER

3

Topics Involving Multiple Organs

QUESTIONS

80 A 32-year-old nurse presents with symptoms of dizziness, jittery behavior, and headaches before meals. Which of the following supports the diagnosis of factitious hypoglycemia?
A. Elevated sulfonylurea levels
B. Normal proinsulin levels
C. Normal C-peptide levels
D. Plasma insulin-to-glucose ratio <0.3
E. All of the above

81 Foreign bodies and/or food boluses can lodge in the esophagus in any of the following four areas of narrowing *except*:
A. Hiatal hernia
B. Upper esophageal sphincter
C. Level of the aortic arch
D. Level of the mainstem bronchus
E. Gastroesophageal junction

82 Hypoproteinemia and edema are the principal clinical manifestations of protein-losing gastroenteropathy. Hypoproteinemia, the most common clinical sequela, manifests as a decrease in serum levels of albumin, fibrinogen, lipoproteins, α_1-antitrypsin, transferrin, and ceruloplasmin, and the following gamma globulins *except*:
A. Immunoglobulin A (IgA)
B. IgM
C. IgE
D. IgG

83 Which of the following is the most common complication after colonoscopy with polypectomy?
A. Perforation of the hollow viscus
B. Infection
C. Immediate postoperative bleeding
D. Cardiorespiratory complications
E. Delayed postoperative bleeding

84 A 20-year-old white woman who had hematochezia when she was five days old is seeking a second opinion. She has multiple cutaneous vascular lesions that have been present since five days of age. She has received blood transfusions on three occasions after hematochezia episodes. An emergent exploratory laparotomy showed a large pelvic vascular malformation, which was not treated. On physical examination, she is asthenic and appears pale but in no distress. She has multiple, bluish, nodular, soft, compressible, nontender lesions on her face, soft palate, arms, legs, hands, and trunk. No abdominal or rectal abnormalities are found on examination, and she is not orthostatic. All of the following statements about this young woman's diagnosis are true *except*:
A. Gastrointestinal (GI) bleeding is a rare feature of this condition.
B. Intussusception may be a presenting feature.
C. It can be transmitted in an autosomal dominant fashion.
D. The cutaneous nodules are venous malformations, for which no treatment is needed.

85 All of the following statements about eosinophilic gastroenteritis are true *except*:
A. It commonly presents between 20 and 60 years of age.
B. Peripheral eosinophilia is present in a majority of patients.
C. It most commonly affects the stomach and small bowel, but also can extend to the esophagus, colon, and rectum.
D. It affects primarily mucosa and pyloric obstruction and usually indicates alterative disease.

86 Which of the following statements regarding hepatitis B infection in pregnancy is true?

A. Most women of childbearing age with chronic hepatitis B have a high risk of the development of complications of their disease during gestation.
B. Maternal-fetal transmission is responsible for most cases of hepatitis B worldwide.
C. Mothers who test negative for the hepatitis B e-antigen cannot transmit the virus to their fetuses.
D. Women with hepatitis B can be treated with interferon during pregnancy.
E. Women with hepatitis B should not be treated with lamivudine during pregnancy.

87 Typhlitis can be the presenting manifestation of or be associated with
A. *Yersinia* infection
B. Acute leukemia
C. Crohn's disease
D. Cecal superinfection with cytomegalovirus (CMV)
E. **B** and **D**

88 All of the following statements about esophageal dilation during upper endoscopy are true *except*:
A. Patients with eosinophilic esophagitis (EE) should not undergo dilation because they are at very high risk of perforation.
B. The esophageal stricture should always be dilated to the size of an uninvolved lumen for symptom relief.
C. The greatest risk of esophageal dilation is perforation.
D. The type of dilator used during the procedure is a very important determinant of the risk of perforation.
E. Proximal esophageal strictures are more likely to perforate than mid or distal strictures.

89 Early mucosa-associated lymphoid tissue (MALT) lymphomas of the stomach can be difficult to distinguish from marked *Helicobacter pylori* gastritis. Histologic features of the mucosa to assist the differentiation include which of the following?
A. Follicular colonization and invasion of germinal centers of lymphoid follicles
B. Destruction of gastric folds by lymphoid infiltrate (lymphoepithelial lesion)
C. Presence of plasma cells with Dutcher bodies (periodic acid–Schiff–positive intranuclear inclusions)
D. All of the above

90 In a patient with a history of food bolus impaction, symptoms of retrosternal chest pain can localize the level of impaction to the middle of the esophagus.
A. True
B. False

91 A 54-year-old white man presents for a screening colonoscopy. He has not noticed any change in his bowel habits or any blood in the stool. He does not have any GI symptoms. His family history is significant for his father having colon cancer at 75 years of age. His laboratory test results show no abnormality in his complete blood count, metabolic panel, thyroid-stimulating hormone level, or prothrombin time/partial thromboplastin time. He reports taking 81 mg of aspirin daily for cardioprotective reasons and enalapril (Vasotec) for control of mild hypertension. Colonoscopy is performed to the cecal tip without difficulty and shows scattered diverticula in the left and transverse colon and a lesion in the cecum (see figure). Which of the following is a true statement about this lesion?
A. It should be treated with a heater probe to prevent occurrence of lower GI bleeding.
B. It indicates that the patient should undergo angiography after the colonoscopy to confirm that he does not have other similar lesions.
C. It indicates that the patient should be offered hormonal therapy.
D. It should be treated with argon plasma coagulation because this kind of lesion is a common cause of recurrent lower GI bleeding.
E. It does not require any treatment because the risk of bleeding from this lesion is very small.

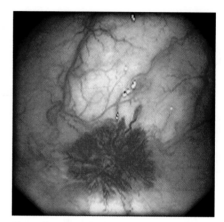

Figure for question **91**

92 A 54-year-old man who has undergone bilateral lung transplantation presents with midepigastric pain and nausea. He takes high-dose glucocorticoids and cyclosporine for acute rejection as well as a proton pump inhibitor (PPI). Which one of the following studies should be performed next?
A. Upper GI series
B. Upper endoscopy
C. Computed axial tomography (CAT) scan of the abdomen
D. Gastric-emptying scan

93 In polymyositis and dermatomyositis
A. Involvement is limited to skeletal muscle fibers.
B. Perforation of the esophagus and duodenal diverticulosis are frequent complications.
C. Dermatomyositis is associated with an increased prevalence of malignancy.
D. Malabsorption and pseudo-obstruction occur commonly.
E. The pathology is a result of antibodies against smooth muscle fibers.

94 A 21-year-old man presents to the hospital emergency department with food impaction while eating a steak dinner. As upper endoscopy is performed, the bolus spontaneously passes. Esophagogastro-duodenoscopy (EGD) shows no stenosis but longitudinal furrows in the distal esophagus with punctate white patches scattered over the mucosal surface. There is no history of preceding heartburn, but he has had multiple allergies in the past. All of the following statements about his diagnosis are true *except*:

A. Dilation of the distal esophagus can be readily performed to prevent further impaction.
B. Biopsy specimens of the distal and midesophagus are expected to show >15 eosinophils per high-power field.
C. Treatment with swallowed fluticasone should be effective.
D. There is a personal history of atopy in 50% of these patients.

95 A 32-year-old woman of Ashkenazi Jewish descent who is 15 weeks pregnant was just admitted by the high-risk obstetrics group because of multiple skin lesions and odynophagia. She denies abdominal pain, but has had nausea for two weeks. She has some constipation but has not noticed any blood in the stool. She states that she "was doing fine till three weeks ago when the skin lesions started." Her medical history is significant for appendectomy. She is otherwise healthy and takes prenatal vitamins. On physical examination, she is afebrile. There are multiple erosions and pustules over the skin on the arms, chest, abdomen, and thighs. Similar lesions are seen in the oral cavity and gingiva. All of the following statements about this illness are true *except*:

A. A definitive diagnosis of this condition is made by biopsy and demonstration of antibody and complement in the basement membrane zone by immunofluorescence.
B. Intravenous IgG has been used in the treatment of this disorder.
C. Patients with serum IgG and IgA antibodies are less likely to respond to medications.
D. Oral ulcerations are present in 100% of patients with this condition.
E. Glucocorticoid medications, both topical and systemic, have been used to treat this condition.

96 A 38-year-old woman who has been on oral contraceptive pills for 18 years presents with abdominal pain. A computed tomography (CT) scan shows peritoneal nodules, and laparoscopy reveals multiple small, rubbery nodules along the peritoneum. What is the most appropriate treatment?

A. Hormone withdrawal
B. Chemotherapy
C. Surgical debulking
D. Radiation

97 Which of the following is/are true regarding esophageal strictures resulting from caustic ingestion?

A. They commonly develop two months after injury.
B. Primary treatment is frequent dilation.
C. As many as 50% eventually need operative intervention.
D. **A** and **B**
E. All of the above

98 All of the following statements regarding hyperemesis gravidarum are true *except*:

A. It occurs in >15% of all pregnancies.
B. It is defined by the presence of ketonuria and a 5% decrease in prepregnancy weight.
C. As many as 20% of affected patients will have symptoms until delivery.
D. Symptoms may be exacerbated by higher levels of human chorionic gonadotropin (HCG) such as with multiple gestations, trophoblastic disease, and trisomy 21.
E. Symptomatic treatment and hydration are the mainstays of therapy.

99 Which of the following treatments is the least appropriate treatment of gastroesophageal reflux disease (GERD) in a pregnant patient?

A. Pantoprazole
B. Omeprazole
C. Ranitidine
D. Sucralfate
E. Lifestyle modifications

100 When considering GI bacterial infections in patients with acquired immunodeficiency syndrome (AIDS), all of the following are true *except*:

A. Small bowel bacterial overgrowth is common in AIDS patients.
B. *Salmonella*, *Shigella*, and *Campylobacter* have higher rates of bacteremia and antibiotic resistance.
C. They are more frequent and more virulent in human immunodeficiency virus (HIV)–infected patients.
D. The most common bacterial infection is *Clostridium difficile*.
E. Mycobacterial infection most commonly involves the duodenum and may be suspected at endoscopy by the presence of yellow mucosal nodules, seen in the clinical setting of malabsorption, bacteremia, and systemic infection.

101 All of the following are useful in the staging of MALT lymphoma *except*:

A. Endoscopic ultrasonography
B. CT scan of the chest and abdomen
C. Upper airway examination
D. Bone marrow biopsy
E. Positron emission tomography

102 All of the following statements about the relationship between somatostatin and carcinoid tumors are true *except*:

A. Somatostatin and its analogs inhibit synthesis and release of peptides produced by carcinoid tumors.
B. They do not block the effects of amines and peptides on target tissue.
C. Their role in carcinoid heart disease is unclear.
D. They have several side effects and are not very well tolerated by patients.
E. They are not effective in the treatment of abdominal pain due to carcinoid tumor.

103 A 46-year-old woman with type 2 diabetes, hypertension, and gastroparesis was recently started on nifedipine by her physician. She now presents with a vague feeling of epigastric distress and worsening early satiety. Her physical examination findings are unremarkable. An endoscopy performed two months earlier for dyspepsia showed no abnormalities, but an upper GI series with barium contrast shows a gastric-filling defect. What is the most likely diagnosis?

A. Gastric ulcer
B. Gastric cancer
C. Lymphoma
D. Pharmacobezoar
E. None of the above

104 A 60-year-old man is four months post–orthotopic liver transplantation (OLT). He presents with fever, malaise, myalgia, and an occasional cough. He is found to have elevated liver enzymes. His only medication is mycophenolate mofetil (MMF). Which treatment should be started for his condition?

A. Valgancyclovir
B. Ganciclovir
C. Acyclovir
D. Voriconazole

105 A 16-year-old college student presents with symptoms of abdominal pain, vomiting, and sporadic diarrhea. He has a serum albumin level of 2.3 g/dL and a creatinine level of 0.9 mg/dL. His blood smear shows microcytosis and peripheral eosinophilia. The stool specimen will most likely show which of the following?

A. *C. difficile* toxin
B. Charcot-Leyden crystals
C. *Giardia*
D. Ova and parasites

106 A consult is requested on a hospitalized 24-year-old white man with anemia and stools positive for occult blood. He had been admitted to the hospital because of a nonhealing ulcer over the left medial malleolus that had not improved after surgery for varicose veins on the left leg three years ago. His medical history is significant for recurrent ulcer over the left medial malleolus, and the patient's parents report that he walks with a limp. On physical examination, there are multiple varicose veins over the left lower limb. There is predominant left lower limb hypertrophy, with the left limb being longer and larger. An x-ray shows distinct soft tissue and osteohypertrophy of the left lower limb. A duplex scan of the left lower limb shows massive superficial venous varicosities and multiple anastomoses between the superficial and deep venous systems. An angiogram shows multiple arteriovenous fistulas. What is the most likely diagnosis?

A. Klippel-Trénaunay syndrome
B. Blue rubber bleb nevus syndrome
C. Parkes Weber syndrome
D. Diffuse intestinal hemangiomatosis
E. None of the above

107 A 29-year-old white woman who is 24 weeks pregnant presents with dysphagia and odynophagia that started about a week ago and have progressed in severity. She has pruritus and severe oral pain, for which she has started taking pain medication. She has no significant medical history, and before this, her only routine medication was a prenatal vitamin. On physical examination, she is alert and oriented but appears uncomfortable and has a temperature of 99.6°F. She has multiple lace-like lesions in her oral cavity with overlying ulcerations and small to medium, flat-topped pruritic and violaceous papules all over her skin. All of the following statements about her condition are true *except*:

A. Upper GI endoscopy will likely show erythema, ulcers, and webs in the proximal esophagus.
B. The condition should be treated with topical and systemic glucocorticoids.
C. The condition is associated with an increased prevalence of chronic liver disease.
D. Treatment of this condition will decrease the risk of the development of esophageal cancer.

108 A fragile, underweight 70-year-old woman is brought to the emergency department with right lower abdominal pain. An obstructive series suggests small bowel obstruction. An astute resident notes that her pain is felt into the medial aspect of the thigh with associated paresthesias. Hip flexion improves the pain, whereas extension of the hip and medial rotation increase the pain. What is her most likely diagnosis?

A. Unrecognized hip fracture
B. Femoral hernia
C. Obturator hernia
D. Sciatic foramen hernia

109 What is the most common gastric lesion causing severe protein loss?

A. Ménétrier's disease
B. *H. pylori* gastritis
C. Allergic gastroenteropathy
D. Systemic lupus erythematosus gastroenteropathy

110 Which one of the following diseases causes constipation?

A. Addison's disease
B. Hyperparathyroidism
C. Hyperthyroidism
D. Medullary carcinoma of the thyroid

111 True statements regarding the relationship between carcinoid tumor of the gut and urine levels of 5-hydroxyindoleacetic acid (5-HIAA) include all of the following *except*:

A. Urine excretion rates of 5-HIAA of >25 mg/24 hr are diagnostic.
B. The excretion rate of 5-HIAA in the urine corresponds well with a carcinoid tumor mass.
C. Midgut carcinoid tumors are associated with an increased excretion rate of 5-HIAA in urine.
D. Foregut carcinoids may be associated with normal urinary levels of 5-HIAA.
E. All of these statements are true.

112 Which of the following statements regarding management of carcinoid syndrome is most accurate?

A. Serotonin antagonists such as methysergide, ondansetron, and cyproheptadine provide excellent control of flushing episodes.

B. Hypertension is best treated with angiotensin-converting enzyme inhibitors.
C. Bronchospasm is best treated with β-adrenergic receptor agonists.
D. Ondansetron is very effective in controlling diarrhea due to carcinoid syndrome.
E. Glucocorticoids should not be given to a patient with carcinoid syndrome in whom hypotension develops.

113 Which of the following lists the correct sequence of damage to intestinal epithelium after ingestion of a caustic substance?
A. Necrosis, ulceration, fibrosis, stricture, carcinoma
B. Ulceration, necrosis, fibrosis, stricture, carcinoma
C. Necrosis, fibrosis, ulceration, stricture, carcinoma
D. Ulceration, fibrosis, necrosis, stricture, carcinoma
E. None of the above

114 A 29-year-old man with AIDS whose last CD4 count was 58 presents to the emergency department with a history of diarrhea for several days. He has not been taking his highly active antiretroviral therapy (HAART) medications. The diarrhea is large volume, nonbloody, and associated with nausea, but not with abdominal pain. What is the most likely cause of the patient's diarrhea?
A. *Campylobacter* species
B. *Microsporidium*
C. *Escherichia coli*
D. *Salmonella*
E. *Shigella*

115 Subacute periumbilical abdominal pain develops in a 30-year-old woman taking glucocorticoids for systemic lupus erythematosus. The pain is most likely due to which of the following?
A. Peritonitis
B. Budd-Chiari syndrome
C. Mesenteric ischemia
D. Pancreatitis
E. Any of the above

116 All of the following statements about post-traumatic diaphragmatic hernias are correct *except*:
A. They occur immediately after the trauma and should present within one week afterward when symptoms are not masked by other injury.
B. Eighty percent are due to blunt trauma, typically motor vehicle accidents.
C. The other 20% are due to penetrating trauma such as knife wounds to the chest below T4 to the umbilicus.
D. Spinal CT is useful in making the diagnosis.

117 A 40-year-old white man comes to the emergency department because of melena of two days' duration and dizziness. He has been taking over-the-counter nonsteroidal anti-inflammatory drugs (NSAIDs) for three days for a sports-related injury. He has multiple cherry-red spots on his lips and tongue. All of the following statements about this patient's condition are true *except*:

A. It is inherited.
B. It is characterized by telangiectasias that occur more commonly in the stomach and small intestines than in the colon.
C. The diagnosis is usually made by endoscopy.
D. Vascular involvement of the liver can present as a giant hemangioma.

118 The presence of *H. pylori* by histology in cases of gastric MALT lymphoma is
A. 90%
B. 75%
C. 60%
D. 50%

119 Ascites in multiple myeloma
A. Usually results from portal hypertension caused by tumor infiltration
B. Can result from tuberculous peritonitis
C. Can be secondary to dissemination of myeloma cells into the peritoneal cavity
D. Can be secondary to congestive heart failure
E. All of the above

120 A 49-year-old woman with a somatostatinoma that is being treated with octreotide presents with severe right upper quadrant and midepigastric pain along with fever and chills. Which treatment is most likely to benefit her?
A. Discontinuation of medications
B. Emergent laparotomy
C. Cholecystectomy
D. Insulin infusion
E. None of the above

121 A 69-year-old white man is transferred from another hospital with severe diarrhea, abdominal pain, weight loss, electrolyte disorder, and malnutrition. On physical examination, he appears well developed and well nourished and his vital signs are stable, but his mucous membranes are dry. He states that he was fine before the onset of symptoms six weeks ago and has never noticed gross blood in the stool. The most notable findings on physical examination include alopecia, onycholysis, and shedding of some of the nails. His wife has noticed increased pigmentation on the patient's upper arms and thighs. The patient's brother had colon cancer at the age of 70 years. Medical records from the outside hospital indicate that he had upper and lower endoscopies that showed multiple gastric and colon polyps; analysis of the multiple biopsy specimens that were taken indicated that these were hyperplastic in nature. The most likely diagnosis is which of the following?
A. Cowden's syndrome
B. Gardner's syndrome
C. Muir-Torre syndrome
D. Peutz-Jeghers syndrome
E. Cronkhite-Canada syndrome
F. Symptoms that can be associated with portal hypertension and variceal bleeding

122 A 40-year-old woman is admitted with a two-day history of nausea, vomiting, and abdominal distention. An obstruction series shows dilated loops of small bowel. On examination, the abdomen is soft with no local tenderness. A 2- to 3-cm indurated, tender nodule is felt in the right groin. The most likely diagnosis is which of the following?

A. Obstructing small bowel neoplasm with lymph node metastasis

B. Lymphoma presenting with inguinal adenopathy and perhaps small bowel involvement

C. Incarcerated femoral hernia

D. Small bowel obstruction with incidental inguinal adenopathy

123 GI stromal tumors (GISTs) can present in all of the following ways *except*:

A. Asymptomatic abdominal mass

B. Enlarged left supraclavicular (Virchow's) node

C. Gastric outlet obstruction

D. GI bleeding (intraluminal)

E. Intraperitoneal bleeding

124 All of the following statements regarding nonfunctioning pancreatic endocrine tumors (PETs) are true *except*:

A. An elevated plasma pancreatic polypeptide level establishes the diagnosis.

B. Treatment is directed at the tumor itself and includes surgical resection.

C. The prognosis depends on the size of the tumor and presence of metastasis.

D. The median survival is 75% at 4.5 years.

E. The majority are located in the pancreatic head.

125 A 45-year-old man who recently completed neoadjuvant chemotherapy and radiation treatment for gastric cancer presents with symptoms of increased abdominal girth, fatigue, and right upper quadrant abdominal pain. His examination reveals tender hepatomegaly, shifting dullness, and anicteric sclera. Laboratory findings are significant for an alkaline phosphatase level of 680 U/L, an aspartate aminotransferase (AST) level of 120 U/L, an alanine aminotransferase (ALT) level of 180 U/L, and a total bilirubin level of 1.2 mg/dL. The remainder of the laboratory test results are normal. A CT scan of the abdomen demonstrates no mass lesions or biliary obstruction. What is the most likely diagnosis in this patient?

A. Metastatic gastric cancer

B. Acalculous cholecystitis

C. Radiation-induced liver disease

D. Hepatic abscess

E. Primary biliary cirrhosis

126 Cholelithiasis, diarrhea, steatorrhea, diabetes, and hypochlorhydria are associated with which of these syndromes?

A. VIPoma

B. Somatostatinoma

C. Glucagonoma

D. Insulinoma

E. None of the above

127 All of the following statements about the pathology of diffuse, large B cell lymphoma of the stomach are true *except*:

A. *TP53* and *P16* mutations are found.

B. Initially these tumors can be confined to the mucosa.

C. Some areas of low-grade MALT lymphoma can be recognized intermixed with a predominantly large B cell population.

D. Large cell lymphoma discovered early may respond to antibiotic therapy occasionally.

128 Bouts of jaundice and upper abdominal pain with elevated liver enzymes in patients with sickle cell disease can be attributable to all of the following *except*:

A. Ischemic liver injury

B. Hepatitis B infection

C. Hepatitis C infection

D. Zinc deficiency

E. Cholecystitis

129 PETs are associated with all of the following inherited disorders *except*:

A. Multiple endocrine neoplasia type I (MEN-I)

B. Osler-Weber-Rendu disease

C. von Hippel-Lindau disease

D. Tuberous sclerosis

E. Neurofibromatosis 1 (NF1)

130 A 32-year-old man with acute myelogenous leukemia underwent hematopoietic cell transplantation (HCT) 20 days ago. He is now reporting severe pain near the anal canal, and this pain is worse with defecation. External examination of the perineum shows no abnormalities. Laboratory test results are significant for neutropenia. What should be done next?

A. Start acyclovir

B. Start ganciclovir

C. Obtain a CAT of the abdomen/pelvis

D. Perform a flexible sigmoidoscopy

131 Which of the following statements about anorectal disease in homosexual AIDS patients is true?

A. There is a higher frequency of anorectal squamous cell cancer in homosexual men than in others with AIDS.

B. The risk of squamous cell cancer increases as the HIV infection progresses.

C. Neoplasms result from human papillomavirus infections via sexual contact.

D. All of the above are true.

E. **A** and **B**

132 Eosinophils in the GI tract can be caused secondarily by other conditions, which must be excluded before a diagnosis of primary eosinophilic GI disease can be made. These possibilities include all the following *except*:

A. Parasite infection

B. Inflammatory bowel disease

C. Lymphoma of small bowel

D. Medications

E. Post-transplantation

133 Match each of the following skin disorders with its associated GI pathology.

Skin Disorder	GI Pathology
1. Dermatitis herpetiformis (DH)	**A.** Pancreatic tumor
2. Porphyria cutanea tarda	**B.** Crohn's disease
3. Necrolytic migratory erythema	**C.** Celiac disease
4. Erythema nodosum	**D.** Hepatitis C infection
5. Sister Mary Joseph nodule	**E.** Gastric cancer

134 The treatment of Mediterranean lymphoma (alpha heavy-chain disease) consists of which of the following methods?
A. Surgery + radiation
B. Radiation + chemotherapy
C. Antibiotics + chemotherapy
D. Surgery + chemotherapy

135 A 60-year-old man presents to the emergency department with a one-day history of epigastric and right chest pain of abrupt onset. It was accompanied by retching, with only a small amount of mucoid blood produced. He is unable to swallow food or fluids. There is no history of exertional chest pain. A chest x-ray and abdominal films show a retrocardiac air-filled structure. A nasogastric tube could not be passed. The epigastrium is mildly tender, but no abdominal guarding is observed. What is the best management at this time?
A. Direct admission to the cardiac care unit
B. Surgical consult and close observation for what may evolve into a surgical emergency
C. Intravenous PPI and a liquid diet
D. Intravenous fluids and close observation on the medical ward
E. Laparoscopic cholecystectomy

136 All of the following lymphomas are considered to be non–immunoproliferative small intestinal diseases *except*:
A. Alpha heavy-chain disease (Mediterranean lymphoma)
B. Diffuse large B cell lymphoma
C. Mantle cell lymphoma
D. Burkitt's lymphoma
E. Follicular lymphoma

137 What should patients with MEN-I/Zollinger-Ellison syndrome (ZES) be advised regarding surgery for their disease?
A. All patients should undergo an exploratory surgery for resection.
B. All metastatic lesions to the liver are considered nonoperable.
C. Patients should undergo a gastrectomy.
D. A vagotomy is indicated.
E. Surgical exploration is recommended if lesions greater than 2 cm are identified.

138 A 48-year-old woman who underwent OLT presents with three weeks of watery diarrhea. She is maintained on MMF for immunosuppression. The patient has no abdominal pain and is afebrile, and her stool study results are negative. What is the next step?
A. Colonoscopy
B. Stop MMF
C. Give loperamide (Imodium)
D. Reduce the dose of MMF

139 Which of the following statements about alpha heavy-chain disease (Mediterranean lymphoma) is incorrect?
A. It is most prevalent in North Africa, Israel, the Middle East, and other Mediterranean countries.
B. It is associated with a lack of sanitation and poor socioeconomic status.
C. It has been reported to be associated with *Campylobacter jejuni* infection.

D. The tumor secretes a polyclonal immunoglobulin.

140 Which of the following is the most common clinical manifestation of protein-losing gastroenteropathy besides hypoproteinemia?
A. Dependent edema
B. Anasarca
C. Increased susceptibility to infections
D. Coagulopathy

141 Bacterial overgrowth can manifest in which of the following?
A. Scleroderma
B. Marfan syndrome
C. Chronic renal failure
D. Fabry disease
E. All of the above

142 Which of the following is considered a useful tool in the diagnosis of insulinoma?
A. Detailed history
B. Hypoglycemia associated with fasting
C. Fasting glucose, insulin, and C peptide
D. Plasma proinsulin
E. All of the above

143 A 65-year-old man presents to his primary care physician reporting nocturnal regurgitation of food for several months. Symptoms have recently become worse, waking him up at night. He denies any dysphagia or odynophagia. His wife also noticed that his voice has been changing and has told him often that he has severe halitosis. He states that he has no other medical problems, but his current symptoms have affected his quality of life. Which of the following is the most useful diagnostic study?
A. Endoscopy
B. Barium swallow
C. pH monitoring for 24 hours
D. Esophageal manometry
E. CT scan of the chest

144 A 40-year-old alcoholic man is hospitalized with typical physical and radiographic findings of right lower lobe pneumonia. He has been started on an antibiotic medication. Gram-positive cocci are seen. On the second hospital day, he appears slightly jaundiced, and jaundice is worse the following day. Liver function test results are as follows: alkaline phosphatase, twice normal; AST, 55 U/L; ALT, 70 U/L; bilirubin, 5 mg% (direct, 3.5 mg%); gamma glutamyl transferase, twice normal. An ultrasound scan of the liver is unremarkable. What is the best next step in managing this patient's condition?
A. Test for hepatitis A and B, CMV, Epstein-Barr virus, and herpes simplex virus.
B. Perform urgent endoscopic retrograde cholangiopancreatography (ERCP).
C. Observe and reevaluate liver function daily.
D. Perform magnetic resonance imaging (MRI) and MRI with cholangiopancreatography.
E. Immediately change to another antibiotic medication.

145 An 84-year-old man has had a prolonged hospital course in the intensive care unit after penetrating abdominal trauma sustained during a motor-vehicle accident that caused a splenic laceration. He was initially treated with broad-spectrum antibiotics with improvement. However, 10 days into his hospital stay, recurrent fevers develop. A repeat CT scan shows the development of a 3.5- × 4.6-cm intra-abdominal abscess. Which of the following are the bacteria most likely associated with this infection?

A. Resistant gram-negative organisms, *Enterococcus* species, and yeast
B. *E. coli* and *Bacteroides*
C. *Candida*
D. Gram-positive staining and *Enterococcus* species

146 True statements about perforation during upper endoscopy include which of the following?

A. Patients with large cervical osteophytes are at an increased risk of perforation.
B. The incidence of perforation in upper endoscopy is 2 to 3 per 10,000 procedures.
C. Most perforations in the neck can be managed conservatively.
D. Perforation is more likely to occur if the stricture is in the proximal esophagus.
E. All of the above

147 A 25-year-old G1P0 at 30 weeks' gestation is brought to the emergency department by her husband after he noted jaundice and mild confusion. Her prenatal course had been uneventful thus far. Laboratory test results reveal a normal blood count with the exception of a hemoglobin level of 10.9. Chemistries are normal; however, her prothrombin time is 18.6, AST 900 U/L, and ALT 860. She undergoes a liver biopsy, which reveals intracytoplasmic inclusion bodies and areas of focal hemorrhage. What would likely be the most effective treatment for this patient?

A. Immediate delivery of the baby
B. Supportive care
C. Steroids
D. Acyclovir
E. Lamivudine

148 A 37-year-old woman with AIDS who is receiving antiretroviral therapy presents with increasing abdominal girth and fullness. She has a temperature of 100.8°F and ascites. Diagnostic paracentesis is performed, and straw-colored fluid is withdrawn. The patient's serum-to-ascites albumin gradient is 0.9; she has a low glucose level of 18 g/dL; and her white blood cell (WBC) count is 540,000 with 68% lymphocytes. Which of the following tests may help arrive at a diagnosis in this case?

A. CA 125
B. Cytology of ascites fluid
C. Laparoscopy
D. B and C
E. A and B

149 A 23-year-old medical student reports "very embarrassing loud noises in the stomach" that are worse after eating. He has no abdominal pain, his appetite is good, and he feels well without any other symptoms. On questioning, he admits that he has lost about 12 pounds in the past six months, which he attributes to skipping meals because of a very busy schedule. He also reports an intermittent, sudden feeling of "warmth" and is concerned about his thyroid gland, especially because his mother had Graves disease. Physical examination reveals mild periumbilical tenderness and hyperactive bowel sounds. Rectal examination is normal, but he is heme occult positive. Laboratory testing that was performed elsewhere revealed all levels including thyroid-stimulating hormone to be normal, but the patient wonders if there was a laboratory error. What is the next indicated study?

A. Mesenteric angiography
B. Positron emission tomography
C. Upper GI radiographic examination with small bowel follow-through
D. Enteroclysis
E. None of the above

150 All of the following statements about the various purgatives used before colonoscopy are true *except*:

A. Polyethylene glycol solutions are very well tolerated because they do not cause fluid shifts during colonoscopy preparation.
B. Electrolyte abnormalities are common side effects of all purgatives currently given before colonoscopy.
C. Sodium phosphate should not be given to patients in renal failure.
D. Patients with severe diseases should be prepared for colonoscopy gradually over hours.

151 A 33-year-old patient with acute myelogenous leukemia who underwent an allostem cell transplantation five months earlier presents with dysphagia, poor appetite, some weight loss, retrosternal pain, and occasional aspiration of gastric contents. You perform an upper endoscopy. There is desquamation of squamous epithelium of the distal esophagus and diffuse mucosal edema and erythema in the gastric antrum. What is the most likely diagnosis?

A. CMV esophagitis
B. Graft-versus-host disease (GVHD)
C. Herpes simplex virus (HSV) esophagitis
D. Mucositis

152 A 48-year-old woman reports progressive swelling in her hands and feet, numbness in her hands and other symptoms of carpal tunnel syndrome, and intermittent galactorrhea. MRI of the head fails to reveal any pituitary abnormality, but there is a mass in the abdomen. What is the appropriate treatment for this patient?

A. Streptozocin
B. Doxorubicin
C. Octreotide
D. Surgical exploration
E. Bromocriptine

153 A 44-year-old woman presents with a two-month history of worsening watery diarrhea and cramps in the lower extremities. She describes passing large amounts of watery stool that is the color of diluted tea. Stool studies fail to reveal any WBCs or infection, but the stool osmolar gap is <50. A VIPoma is suspected. What other laboratory abnormalities would be expected if this diagnosis is correct?

A. Hyperglycemia
B. Hypochlorhydria
C. Hypokalemia
D. Hypercalcemia
E. All of the above

154 A 50-year-old woman five months post–kidney transplantation presents with anorexia, nausea, and vomiting. She is maintained on tacrolimus. The patient undergoes EGD (see figure). What is her most likely diagnosis?
A. HSV
B. CMV
C. *Candida* infection
D. GVHD

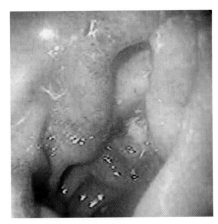

Figure for question **154**

155 Which of the following is the preferred treatment for diffuse large B cell lymphoma of the stomach?
A. Rituximab
B. Radiation alone
C. Surgery alone
D. Chemotherapy alone
E. **A**, **B**, and **D**

156 Which of the following techniques reduces the likelihood of radiation enteritis?
A. Using only anterior and posterior fields for pelvic radiation
B. Administering radiotherapy in the supine position
C. Maintaining an empty bladder during radiation therapy
D. Using misoprostol suppositories in patients undergoing radiation

157 The majority of gastric, and as many as 30% of esophageal, foreign bodies in children are asymptomatic, but symptoms that raise suspicion would include which of the following?
A. Failure to thrive
B. Choking
C. Drooling
D. Not wanting to eat
E. All the above

158 For the diagnosis of amyloidosis, it is advisable to biopsy all of the following sites *except*:

A. Stomach or duodenum
B. Liver
C. Colon
D. Subcutaneous abdominal fat pad

159 A 52-year-old man presents with four daily episodes of watery diarrhea for 18 months. There is no blood or mucus, abdominal pain, nausea, or vomiting. Symptoms have been accompanied by fatigue and a 15-pound weight loss. Laboratory test results reveal a hemoglobin of 11 with a mean corpuscular volume of 76 and a Ca^+ of 11. EGD demonstrates antral ulcers. All of the following laboratory tests could be used to confirm the diagnosis *except*:
A. Chromogranin A
B. Parathyroid hormone
C. Gastrin level
D. Serum protein electrophoresis
E. Neuron-specific enolase

160 All of the following statements about the adverse effects of imatinib are true *except*:
A. It has not been reported to cause myelotoxicity.
B. Diarrhea, myalgias, and skin rash reportedly occur in 30% to 45% of patients receiving the drug.
C. Its adverse effects tend to lessen with continued treatment.
D. GI hemorrhage from shrinking tumor masses has been noted in 5% of patients receiving this medication.

161 A 66-year-old woman presents with the symptoms of weight loss and a rash. On examination, there are several raised erythematous lesions with central blistering. They appear to be in several stages of healing with associated hyperpigmented areas and bullous crusted lesions. Laboratory test results reveal normocytic anemia, an elevated serum glucose, and a glucagon level of 1200. What is the diagnosis most likely to be?
A. Type 2 diabetes
B. Cirrhosis
C. Glucagonoma
D. Celiac disease
E. Hepatitis B

162 Gold therapy for rheumatoid arthritis has been associated with which of the following?
A. Diarrhea
B. Enterocolitis
C. Toxic megacolon
D. Death
E. All the above

163 Which of the following statements regarding bezoars is/are true?
A. They develop after surgery due to delayed gastric emptying, decreased gastric accommodation, and reduced acid-peptic activity.
B. They can cause gastric ulceration secondary to pressure necrosis.
C. Rapunzel syndrome can lead to pancreatitis/jaundice.
D. Trichobezoars typically require surgery more often than phytobezoars.
E. All of the above

164 A 37-year-old woman presents with episodic arthralgias, pleuritic chest pain, and vague abdominal pain. Her parents and one of her cousins experienced similar symptoms. Which of the following treatments should be initiated?
A. Diagnostic laparoscopy
B. Prednisone
C. Colchicine
D. Melphalan
E. No treatment

165 Metabolic derangements in glucagonoma patients include all of the following *except*:
A. Thromboembolic events
B. Anemia
C. Increased amino acid production
D. Hyperglycemia
E. Anorexia

166 Which of the following is the most common site of extranodal GI lymphoma in developed countries?
A. Colon
B. Small intestine
C. Prednisone
D. Stomach

167 A 48-year-old woman who is ten days post-HCT presents with nausea and vomiting for three days. Laboratory test results are significant for neutropenia and thrombocytopenia. Her symptoms have resolved with an antiemetic. However, she now reports severe retrosternal pain and painful swallowing. A barium swallow is shown in the figure. Given the findings, what is the most likely cause of her symptoms?
A. Esophageal malignancy
B. Intramural hematoma
C. Infectious esophagitis
D. Esophageal stricture

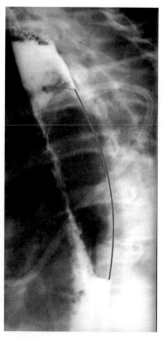

Figure for question **167**

168 Protein-losing enteropathy should be treated by
A. Replacing lost protein through albumin infusion
B. Aggressive protein nutritional resuscitation
C. Treating the underlying disease
D. H_2 receptor antagonists, anticholinergic agents, and octreotide

169 Which of the following is the most common site of gastrinoma?
A. The first portion of the duodenum
B. The third portion of the duodenum
C. Pancreatic tail
D. Pancreatic head
E. Jejunum

170 Which of the following statements about rectal carcinoid tumors is true?
A. The rectum is a very rare site of carcinoid tumors.
B. Rectal carcinoid tumors are more common in female than in male patients.
C. Carcinoid syndrome is a common feature of rectal carcinoid tumors.
D. Radical resection via a low anterior or abdominoperineal approach is the treatment of choice in cases of rectal carcinoid tumor.
E. The primary determinant of the prognosis for patients with rectal carcinoid tumor is the underlying tumor biology.

171 Which of the following statements about post-ERCP pancreatitis is false?
A. Pancreatitis is the most common complication of ERCP.
B. Risk factors for post-ERCP pancreatitis have been well defined and include both patient and procedural factors.
C. The only definitive way to minimize the complication rate is to avoid performing ERCP for diagnostic purposes.
D. Treatment of post-ERCP pancreatitis is supportive.
E. Using pure cutting current for sphincterotomy will decrease the risk of pancreatitis.

172 Which of the following statements regarding treatment of Zenker's diverticula is true?
A. All patients with Zenker's diverticula should be offered surgery regardless of the size of the diverticulum and symptoms.
B. An open surgical approach is not recommended for patients with large diverticula that extend into the thorax.
C. Compared with endoscopic techniques, there is a higher recurrence rate with open surgical procedures.
D. Compared with endoscopic techniques, there is a lower complication rate with open surgical procedures.
E. Upper esophageal sphincter myotomy should always be a part of the procedure.

173 A 23-year-old man with Crohn's disease is admitted with abdominal pain, increased WBC count, and fever. A CT scan of the abdomen and pelvis is shown in the figure. What is the next best step in his management?

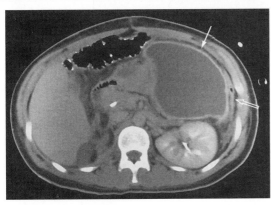

Figure for question **173**

A. Stat surgical consult
B. Intravenous antibiotics
C. Oral antibiotics
D. Antibiotics and percutaneous catheter aspiration/drainage

174 Factors predisposing to incisional hernias include all of the following *except*:
A. Obesity
B. History of aneurysm
C. Ascites
D. Smoking
E. Postoperative wound infection

175 The following statements about imatinib therapy are true *except*:
A. In patients with advanced disease, treatment is lifelong.
B. Increasing the dose from 400 to 800 mg/day will improve survival.
C. Positron emission tomography not only identifies tumor, but can predict the response to imatinib by the intensity of uptake.
D. Imatinib will work favorably in GISTs with a *KIT* mutation as well as in the 5% of GISTs with a *PDGFRA* mutation.

176 False-positive elevations of 5-HIAA levels in urine can result from ingestion of all of the following *except*:
A. Melatonin
B. Methyldopa
C. Walnuts
D. Rifampin
E. Isoniazid

177 A 54-year-old woman with a history of radiation therapy and chemotherapy for colon cancer reports that there is leakage of fluid from a small lesion on her abdominal wall. Although the leakage is small, it is continuous and causes her skin to become irritated. Imaging confirms a distal enterocutaneous fistula. She otherwise appears well nourished. What is the next best step to manage her symptoms?
A. Refer her for surgical management.
B. Place a wound vacuum-assisted closure over the fistula.
C. Provide assurance and ask her to continue enteral feeds.
D. Keep the patient on nothing by mouth and start total parenteral nutrition (TPN).

178 The sensitivity of free air on an upright chest x-ray in detecting a perforated viscous is
A. 60%
B. 10%
C. More than 90%
D. 35%
E. None of the above

179 The majority of patients with esophageal food impaction have an underlying predisposing esophageal pathology that might include all the following *except*:
A. Schatzki's ring
B. Eosinophilic esophagitis
C. *Candida* esophagitis
D. Altered surgical anatomy
E. Motility disorders

180 When evaluating GI symptoms in AIDS, all of the following are true *except*:
A. Because of HAART, GI symptoms are most often drug induced or nonopportunistic.
B. A CD4 count >200/mm favors common bacteria and other nonopportunistic infections.
C. A CD4 count <100/mm favors CMV, fungi, *Mycobacterium avium* complex (MAC), and unusual protozoa.
D. Chronic liver disease, most often due to hepatitis C, is a leading cause of illness requiring hospitalization and death.
E. Clinical signs and symptoms frequently suggest a specific diagnosis.

181 Which of the following is the treatment of choice for the management of food bolus impactions and foreign bodies?
A. Flexible endoscopy
B. Foley catheter extraction under fluoroscopy
C. Glucagon
D. Nifedipine
E. Gas-forming agents including sodium bicarbonate

182 Which of the following statements regarding radiation-induced enteritis is true?
A. Symptoms of radiation-induced enteritis may appear within a week of radiation therapy.
B. Younger patients are affected more than older patients.
C. Concurrent chemotherapy has not been shown to intensify the effects of radiation therapy.
D. Colonoscopy is the diagnostic test of choice for radiation enteritis.
E. Symptoms such as abdominal pain and diarrhea will not subside after discontinuation of radiation.

183 A 35-year-old white woman presents to the emergency department with right lower quadrant abdominal pain, anorexia, nausea, and vomiting. She has a temperature of 101°F. Based on her symptoms, physical examination findings, and abdominal CT scan findings, a diagnosis of acute appendicitis is made. The patient undergoes emergency appendectomy and is discharged home. Histopathologic examination of the appendix results in discovery of a 2.5-cm carcinoid tumor, and she is referred to a gastroenterologist. Which

of the following statements regarding this patient is true?
A. She had a carcinoid tumor of the appendix that was cured by appendectomy.
B. She may have metastatic disease and needs to undergo CT of the abdomen and pelvis every three months.
C. She is likely to have a recurrence of the tumor.
D. Her prognosis is poor; the five-year survival rate for patients with carcinoid tumor is 10%.
E. She should undergo right hemicolectomy.

184 Which of the following factors predict fibrosis and progression to cirrhosis in patients with hepatitis C who are also infected with HIV?
A. Higher ALT levels
B. Older age at infection
C. Higher inflammatory activity
D. Alcohol consumption of >50 g/day
E. All of the above

185 Anorexia, nausea, and intermittent vomiting develop one month after a 32-year-old woman has undergone a successful liver transplantation for primary biliary cirrhosis. Her immunosuppressant regimen includes tacrolimus and prednisone. What is the next best step?
A. Perform an endoscopy.
B. Reduce the tacrolimus dose.
C. Add a PPI.
D. Stop tacrolimus and add MMF.

186 All of the following statements regarding carcinoid syndrome are true *except*:
A. Atypical carcinoid syndrome is caused by foregut carcinoids.
B. Flushing and diarrhea are the first symptoms of carcinoid syndrome.
C. Typical carcinoid syndrome is caused by midgut carcinoids.
D. Patients with atypical carcinoid syndrome have normal serotonin levels.
E. Patients with typical carcinoid syndrome have increased rates of urine 5-HIAA excretion.

187 Polyarteritis nodosa, Churg-Strauss syndrome, and Henoch-Schönlein purpura are vasculitides. All three conditions can cause each of the following GI manifestations *except*:
A. Pancreatitis
B. Ischemic bowel
C. Cholecystitis
D. Appendicitis
E. Eosinophilic gastroenteritis

188 What is the most common group that unintentionally ingests foreign bodies?
A. Older adults
B. Children
C. College students playing "quarters"
D. Demented patients
E. Intoxicated patients

189 A 22-year-old man comes to the emergency department after ingesting an alkaline substance. He has no symptoms. Upper GI endoscopy reveals grade IIA injury. What should be done next?

A. Keep the patient on nothing by mouth and start TPN.
B. Keep the patient on nothing by mouth and insert a nasoenteral feeding tube.
C. Start him on a liquid diet and advance him to a regular diet in 24 to 48 hours.
D. Perform a barium swallow before allowing oral intake.
E. None of the above

190 There is an increased risk of esophageal cancer after alkaline caustic ingestion. All of the following statements are true *except*:
A. There is an increased risk of squamous cell cancer.
B. There is an increased risk of adenocarcinoma.
C. Lye ingestion leads to a 1000-fold increase in cancer risk.
D. There is an approximately 40-year lag time between ingestion and cancer onset.
E. Endoscopic surveillance every one to three years should begin 20 years after ingestion.

191 A 50-year-old woman with diverticulosis presents with lower left quadrant abdominal pain. A CAT scan of the abdomen reveals a 1- × 1.2-cm abscess in the lower left quadrant. What is the next best step in her management?
A. Perform CT-guided percutaneous catheter drainage.
B. Perform ultrasound-guided percutaneous catheter drainage.
C. Intravenous antibiotics
D. Surgery

192 All of the following are considered treatment options for insulinoma *except*:
A. Resection
B. Chemotherapy
C. Radiation therapy
D. Dietary control
E. Diazoxide

193 A 50-year-old man who has received a cadaveric kidney transplant for polycystic kidney disease presents to the emergency department reporting left lower quadrant crampy pain and a bloody bowel movement. He has a low-grade temperature and a WBC count of 15. Which of the following is the most likely diagnosis?
A. CMV colitis
B. Ischemic colitis
C. Infectious colitis
D. Diverticular bleeding

194 The best way to establish the malignant potential of GISTs is by which of the following criteria?
A. A diameter greater than 4 cm
B. The number of mitoses per high-power field
C. Irregular borders on endoscopic ultrasonography
D. The cystic area in the tumor by endoscopic ultrasonography
E. All of the above

195 A 53-year-old man received a liver transplant for hepatitis C–related liver disease. Approximately four months following the transplantation, he is

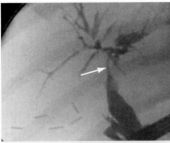
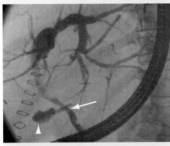
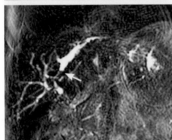

Figure for question **195**

admitted with cholangitis. ERCP findings are shown in the figure. Multiple biliary casts are seen as well. Which of the following should be performed?
A. Ultrasound scan to assess for hepatic artery patency
B. Surgical revision
C. Long-term antibiotic therapy
D. Repeat ERCP in two weeks

196 A 60-year-old diabetic man has had chronic renal failure for 10 years and has been on hemodialysis for three years. Recurrent bouts of melena have required continuous oral iron supplementation plus Epogen (epoetin alfa) every two weeks. Upper and lower endoscopy have not revealed a source for bleeding. What is the most likely source of bleeding?
A. Small bowel neoplasm
B. Angiodysplasia of small bowel
C. Meckel's diverticulum
D. Pyloric channel ulcer overlooked at endoscopy
E. Dieulafoy's lesion

197 Which solid organ transplant has the highest incidence of fungal infections?
A. Kidney and pancreas
B. Heart and lung
C. Liver
D. Intestinal

198 What is the main cause of mortality from GI fistulas?
A. Arrhythmias due to electrolyte imbalance
B. Underlying disease such as cancer

C. Sepsis with multiorgan failure
D. Complications of parenteral feeding

199 Match the following disorders of the oral cavity to the treatment:

Oral Cavity Condition	Treatment
1. Xerostomia	A. Topical tretinoin gel
2. Black hairy tongue	B. Topical anesthetics
3. Oral thrush	C. Oral acyclovir
4. Oral hairy leukoplakia (HL)	D. Oral mycostatin
5. Geographic tongue	E. Oral cevimeline

200 All of the following statements about resistance to imatinib are true *except*:
A. The incidence of resistance is <20%.
B. For patients intolerant or resistant, sunitinib 50 mg/day is available.
C. The response rate to sunitinib in these patients is only 6.8%.
D. These patients are beyond any further surgical help.

201 Hereditary syndromes with GISTs are associated with all of the other neoplasms listed *except*:
A. Pulmonary chondroma
B. Extra-adrenal paragangliomas
C. MEN-I syndrome
D. NF

202 Flushing is a symptom commonly associated with carcinoid syndrome. Other conditions in which flushing can occur include all of the following *except*:
A. Pheochromocytoma
B. VIPoma
C. Amyloidosis
D. Medullary carcinoma of the thyroid
E. Anaphylaxis

203 What is the optimal test to measure for intestinal protein loss?
A. Measurement of the fecal loss of radiolabeled, intravenously administered macromolecules such as 51Cr albumin.
B. Measurement of concentration of α_1-antitrypsin in the stool
C. Measure the clearance of α_1-antitrypsin from the plasma during a 72-hour stool collection
D. ^{99m}Tc-labeled dextran scintigraphy

204 All of the following statements about umbilical hernias are true *except*:
A. They should be repaired in the neonate to avoid the risk of incarceration.
B. They are more common in African-American children.
C. They may rupture in cirrhotic patients with ascites.
D. Strangulation may occasionally occur after rapid reduction in ascites.

205 A 32-year-old G2P1 at 37 weeks' gestation presents with intense pruritus for several weeks, which is worse at night and most severe over her palms and soles. She is without jaundice or rashes and states that she experienced itching during her last

pregnancy as well. She has no history of any other underlying liver disease. Which of the following interventions is most likely to result in the safe resolution of her symptoms?
A. Delivery of the baby
B. Cholestyramine
C. Steroids
D. Ursodeoxycholic acid
E. Phenobarbital

206 A 50-year-old woman presents to your office with 3 L of stool per day and hypochlorhydria and is requiring 200 mEq/day of potassium to maintain her electrolyte balance. Her symptoms persist without fasting, endoscopic evaluation findings are negative, and steatorrhea is absent. Which one of the following is the most likely medical therapy to help her condition?
A. Prednisone 60 mg/day
B. Clonidine
C. Indomethacin
D. Octreotide
E. Phenothiazine

207 Surgery should be considered in which of the following cases?
A. When a foreign body is sharp or pointed and fails to progress after three days
B. When ingested coupling magnets cannot be retrieved, to avoid fistula/perforation
C. When there is an esophageal perforation after ingestion of a caustic fluid
D. A and C
E. All of the above

208 A 56-year-old man with a recent diagnosis of glucagonoma presents with symptoms of diarrhea, weight loss, and new onset of shortness of breath. Which of the following conditions should be ruled out?
A. Steatorrhea
B. Metastatic disease
C. Pulmonary emboli
D. Anemia

209 Which of the following statements about hemolytic uremic syndrome (HUS) is true?
A. It includes renal failure, hemolytic anemia, and thrombocytosis.
B. Adriamycin is the chemotherapy most commonly implicated as a cause.
C. It usually leads to permanent dialysis.
D. It is associated with enteric pathogens such as *Salmonella, Shigella, Campylobacter, Yersinia,* and hemorrhagic 0157:H7 *E. coli.*
E. In adults, idiopathic and sporadic cases have been described.

210 In gastroparesis diabeticorum, the only symptom shown to be an independent predictor of delayed gastric emptying is which of the following?
A. Nausea
B. Vomiting
C. Abdominal bloating/fullness
D. Early satiety
E. Weight loss

211 A 56-year-old man with a history of alcoholism underwent OLT for cirrhosis complicated by hepatocellular carcinoma nine months earlier. He presents with mildly abnormal transaminase levels and multiple new hepatic masses seen on imaging. In addition, he is also found to have periportal lymphadenopathy, which appears stable in size when compared with previous imaging. What is his most likely diagnosis?
A. Hepatocellular carcinoma recurrence, multifocal
B. Focal nodular hyperplasia
C. Post-transplantation lymphoproliferative disorder of the liver
D. Post-transplantation lymphoproliferative disorder of the liver and periportal lymph nodes

212 Gastric antral vascular ectasia (GAVE), also called watermelon stomach, is a vascular lesion of the gastric antrum that can present as both an acute and chronic gastrointestinal bleed. All of the following statements about this condition are true *except*:
A. It is predominantly seen in females.
B. It is often associated with certain connective tissue diseases.
C. It is thought to be the result of accelerated gastric emptying, which is an associated phenomenon seen in this group of patients.
D. GAVE can be caused by hepatic venous occlusive disease.
E. Some believe that GAVE and portal hypertensive gastropathy are different manifestations of the same process.

213 Typical immunophenotype staging of gastric MALT lymphoma cells includes which of the following?
A. CD19
B. CD20
C. CD10
D. A and B only

214 A 36-year-old patient presents with symptoms of abdominal pain increasing in intensity in the right lower quadrant. She has associated nausea, vomiting, and fevers. Examination demonstrates rebound and guarding. Laboratory test results show leukocytosis. Which of the following is the recommended treatment for this patient?
A. Glucocorticoids
B. Fluid resuscitation and antibiotic therapy followed by urgent laparotomy or laparoscopy
C. Fluid resuscitation and antibiotic therapy
D. Vasopressors such as dopamine
E. None of the above

215 Long-term cyclosporine therapy may also lead to which of the following?
A. Thrombocytopenia
B. Congestive heart failure
C. Hyperlipidemia
D. Gallstones/biliary disease

216 A 24-year-old man is brought to the emergency department by the police because after his arrest for suspected drug dealing, he swallowed a few packets of white powder that were believed to contain cocaine. The patient is completely asymptomatic, and the results of his physical examination show no abnormalities. Abdominal radiographs show multiple sausage-shaped radiopaque areas in the small intestine. What is the next step in the management of this patient?

A. Emergency surgery
B. Emergency endoscopic removal of the foreign bodies in the intestine
C. Inpatient observation with a clear liquid diet
D. None of the above
E. All of the above

217 All of the following are techniques used to minimize GI side effects of radiation therapy *except*:
A. Early treatment with 5-hydroxytryptamine 3 antagonists
B. Concomitant chemotherapy
C. PPIs
D. Viscous lidocaine
E. Early treatment with dexamethasone

218 A 39-year-old woman reports progressive swelling in her hands and feet, numbness in her hands and other symptoms of carpal tunnel syndrome, and intermittent galactorrhea. MRI of the head fails to reveal any pituitary abnormality, but there is a mass in the abdomen. What is the appropriate treatment for this patient?
A. Streptozocin
B. Doxorubicin
C. Octreotide
D. Surgical exploration
E. Bromocriptine

219 A 42-year-old man presents one month after attempting suicide by drinking a caustic agent. He has been experiencing early satiety and progressive emesis that have resulted in a 5-pound weight loss. Upper endoscopy of the stomach is performed and reveals antral stenosis. What is the appropriate next step in the treatment of this patient?
A. Endoscopic dilation
B. Referral to a surgeon for antrectomy
C. Referral to a surgeon for vagotomy and antrectomy
D. Referral to a surgeon for pyloroplasty and gastroenterostomy
E. Referral to a surgeon for subtotal gastrectomy

220 A 62-year-old woman presents with dysphagia for solids for the past two weeks. Her medical history includes hypertension, diabetes, and hypothyroidism. She also underwent chemotherapy and radiation for lung cancer approximately six months ago. What is the most likely finding on barium swallow?
A. Esophageal stricture
B. Esophageal stenosis
C. Esophageal dysmotility
D. Esophageal ulceration

221 Which of the following best describes protein-losing enteropathy?
A. Excessive protein catabolism
B. Malabsorption of digested amino acids
C. Excessive leakage of plasma proteins into the lumen of the GI tract
D. Lack of pancreatic digestion of dietary proteins

222 Flushing is a distinctive feature of carcinoid syndrome and is present in 30% to 94% of patients with carcinoid syndrome at some time during the course of their illness. All of the following are incorrect statements about the proposed etiology of flushing *except*:

A. Flushing occurs due to the release of a number of polypeptide hormones.
B. Many studies have found a direct correlation between serotonin levels and degree of flushing.
C. Norepinephrine levels are not correlated with flushing episodes.
D. Flushing in carcinoid syndrome is not worsened by emotional or physical stress.

223 Ingested bread bag clips are associated with a high risk of GI tract complications. All of the following are true *except*:
A. Ingestion can result in bleeding, obstruction, and perforation.
B. The small bowel is the most common site of impaction.
C. The arms of the clip grasp the mucosa.
D. The clips are radiopaque and detected easily by conventional radiography.
E. Operative intervention is commonly required.

224 Factors that predispose to recurrent inguinal hernia include all of the following *except*:
A. Alcoholism
B. Smoking
C. Extension into the scrotum
D. Steroid therapy
E. Liver or renal failure

225 A 64-year-old man with a history of hypertension, diabetes mellitus, and prostate cancer, status post-radiation therapy six weeks earlier presents with diarrhea, bloating, belching, and a 10-pound weight loss. An appropriate approach to this patient's symptoms includes which of the following?
A. Lactose-free diet
B. Loperamide
C. Cholestyramine
D. Treatment for bacterial overgrowth
E. All of the above

226 A 23-year-old man with a history of Crohn's disease presents with increased diarrhea, abdominal pain, fever, and increased leukocyte count. He undergoes a CT scan of the abdomen that shows an intra-abdominal abscess. Subsequently, he undergoes percutaneous catheter drainage of the abscess. Four days later, he reports improvement in the diarrhea. Laboratory test results are significant for a decrease in the WBC count. However, he continues to have high output from the drain, which is his main symptom. What is the next best step to arrive at a diagnosis?
A. Repeat abdominal imaging
B. Removal of the drain
C. Perform a catheter study
D. Referral to a surgeon

227 Which of the following is the most common cause of death in celiac disease?
A. Ulcerative jejunitis
B. Lymphoma
C. Sepsis due to immunoglobulin deficiency
D. Malnutrition

228 All of the following are true about the association between DH and celiac disease *except*:
A. More than 80% of patients with celiac disease will have DH.

B. DH presents as papulovesicular lesions that are symmetrical and involve the extensor surfaces of the extremities, trunk, buttock, scalp, and neck.

C. Withdrawal of gluten reverses the condition in six to 12 months.

D. Although the exact pathogenesis of DH remains unclear, it is thought that antibodies to gluten that are formed in the small intestine are deposited at the dermoepidermal junction.

E. DH is rarely diagnosed in childhood.

229 All of the following statements about Behçet's disease are true *except*:

A. It should be in the differential diagnosis when patients present with Budd-Chiari syndrome.

B. Surgical intervention is highly successful.

C. As in Crohn's disease, the ileocecal region is the most commonly affected by ulceration.

D. GI involvement occurs in as many as 50% of cases.

E. "Punched-out" ulcerations are seen on colonoscopy.

230 A 40-year-old man who recently immigrated from India presents with increased abdominal girth and fevers for the past several weeks. An ultrasound scan of the abdomen reveals no evidence of cirrhosis and patent hepatic vasculature. Paracentesis reveals a protein count of 6.2 and a serum ascites albumin gradient of 0.5, as well as 568 WBCs with 87% lymphocytes. What would be the most appropriate next test to help determine the diagnosis?

A. CA 125

B. Cross-sectional imaging of the pelvis

C. Peritoneal fluid cytology

D. Peritoneal adenosine deaminase levels

E. Laparoscopy

231 Traction diverticula of the esophagus are often related to all of the following *except*:

A. Motility disorders

B. Enlarged mediastinal lymph nodes from lung malignancies

C. Achalasia

D. Inflammation associated with tuberculosis and histoplasmosis

E. Trauma

232 Which of the following statements regarding MAC in the GI tract is true?

A. MAC is the most commonly identified organism in patients with chronic diarrhea and low CD4 counts.

B. Many patients with MAC infection will have asymptomatic infection of the gut.

C. Duodenal involvement is common.

D. The diagnosis of MAC infection is best made by endoscopic biopsy.

E. All statements are true.

233 Regarding postpolypectomy bleed, all of the following statements are true *except*:

A. Patients taking warfarin are at increased risk of postpolypectomy bleeding.

B. Drugs such as aspirin, NSAIDs, ticlopidine, and clopidrogel have been clearly shown to increase the risk of postpolypectomy bleeding.

C. In patients with mechanical heart valves who are taking warfarin, low-molecular-weight heparin can be safely substituted for warfarin before and after the procedure.

D. This complication should always be discussed during the process of obtaining informed consent.

E. The incidence of bleeding postpolypectomy is 1.5% to 3% of all cases.

234 Abdominal pain, nausea, fevers, and chills develop at home in a 33-year-old woman with a history of Crohn's disease with ileal involvement and a history of recent fistula surgery (ileocolonic fistula). In the emergency department, her temperature is 101°F, her blood pressure is 110/80 mm Hg, and her heart rate is 100 beats per minute. On physical examination, she appears quite ill. Physical examination is notable for tenderness in the right lower quadrant with rebound. What is the most optimal study for this patient at this time?

A. MRI of the abdomen and pelvis

B. Abdominal ultrasound scan

C. Small bowel series

D. CAT scan of the abdomen/pelvis with intravenously and orally administered contrast medium

235 A 35-year-old obese woman had a Roux-en-Y gastric bypass two years ago. She has not been well since shortly after surgery, with recurrent bouts of mid-abdominal pain and vomiting every couple of weeks. A CT scan in the emergency department shows dilated loops of jejunum. What is the most likely diagnosis?

A. Anastomotic stenosis

B. Internal hernia

C. Marginal ulcer

D. Small bowel obstruction due to postoperative adhesions

236 In which of the following cases is gastric antral vascular ectasia (GAVE), also called watermelon stomach, least likely to be the diagnosis?

A. A 49-year-old white woman with iron deficiency anemia for five years and rheumatoid arthritis

B. A 50-year-old man with atrophic gastritis and heme-positive stools

C. A 47-year-old white man with cirrhosis secondary to hepatitis C, anemia, and possibly recurrent blood transfusions

D. A 65-year-old African-American man with a history of frequent NSAID use who presents with hematemesis and anemia

E. A 27-year-old white woman with systemic sclerosis and anemia for four years

237 Tumors that may stain positive for CD117 beside GISTs include which of the following?

A. Ewing's sarcoma

B. Small cell lung cancer

C. Melanoma

D. Seminoma

E. All of the above

238 All of the following are histologic characteristics of PETs *except*:

A. Homogeneity
B. Crypt distortion
C. Small round cells
D. Mitotic figures
E. Electron-dense granules

239 Analogous to the role of *H. pylori* in stimulating B cell activity in gastric MALT lymphoma, the following bacteria have been implicated in immunoproliferative small intestinal disease:
A. *E. coli*
B. *Bacteroides*
C. *C. jejuni*
D. *Yersinia enterocolitica*

240 A 30-year-old man with AIDS presents with a one-week history of progressive dysphagia and odynophagia that has resulted in a five-pound weight loss. On examination, he is afebrile, and there is no evidence of thrush or ulcers in the oropharynx, but his mucous membranes are dry. Which of the following is the most likely finding on endoscopy?
A. Extensive, deep ulcerations throughout the esophagus
B. Diffuse, shallow ulcerations with areas of vesicles
C. Friability and ulceration of the distal esophagus
D. Focal or diffuse white plaques in association with mucosal hyperemia and friability
E. A foreign body

241 All of the following are adaptive physiologic changes that occur in the GI system during pregnancy *except*:
A. An increase in maternal blood volume by 50%, resulting in a relative anemia
B. A decrease in plasma protein production
C. Alteration in bile acid composition, resulting in crystal/stone formation
D. An increase in the absorption of amino acids, calcium, and vitamins due to an increase in small bowel weight and villous height
E. A decrease in GI motility

242 Progressive systemic sclerosis (scleroderma) is characterized by vasculitis and fibrosis of multiple organs. All of the following are true *except*:
A. GI manifestations occur in approximately 90% of patients.
B. Esophagitis approaches 100% in patients with severe cutaneous involvement.
C. Esophageal dysmotility correlates with the development of interstitial lung disease.
D. Malabsorption is attributed only to bacterial overgrowth.
E. Calcific pancreatitis and ischemic pancreatic necrosis have been reported.

243 What is the percentage of cases of stage I MALT lymphomas responding completely to *H. pylori* eradication?
A. 90%
B. 75%
C. 60%
D. 50%

244 What is the rate of recurrence of hepatitis C virus in the allograft?

A. 60%
B. 75%
C. Nearly universal
D. 25%

245 Which of the following techniques is contraindicated in the endoscopic management of food impaction?
A. Forceful blinded pushing
B. Using forceps to disrupt and debulk the bolus
C. Insufflation and distention of the esophageal lumen
D. Use of an overtube
E. None of the above

246 When diagnosing foreign body ingestion, appropriate steps include all of the following *except*:
A. Thorough history and physical examination
B. Anteroposterior and lateral radiographs of the chest and abdomen
C. Endoscopy
D. Barium studies
E. CT scan

247 Which of the following is the least harmful to pregnant patients and their fetuses during an endoscopy?
A. Fluoroscopy
B. Meperidine
C. Morphine
D. Benadryl
E. Benzodiazepines

248 A 64-year-old man with a history of diverticulosis presents with left lower quadrant abdominal pain. His CAT scan reveals a 2- × 1.2-cm abscess. The patient is started on intravenous antibiotics. A repeat CT scan is performed four days later and reveals that the abscess is enlarging and now measures 4.0 × 4.2 cm. What is the next step in management of the patient?
A. Perform surgical resection and débridement.
B. Change antibiotics as he might have developed resistance to the existing ones.
C. Perform percutaneous drainage with catheter placement.
D. Perform colonoscopy to evaluate the colon.

249 What is the most common PET?
A. Gastrinoma
B. VIPoma
C. Somatostatinoma
D. Glucagonoma
E. GRFoma

250 All of the following modalities for treatment of advanced (stage II E) MALT lymphoma are advisable *except*:
A. Chemotherapy
B. Radiation therapy
C. Surgery
D. Immunotherapy with rituximab

251 The risk of cancer in long-lived transplant recipients is higher than in the general population for which of the following malignancies?
A. Lymphomas
B. Skin cancers

C. Anal cancers
D. Kaposi sarcoma
E. All of the above

252 Adverse effects of imatinib (Gleevec) include all the following *except*:
A. Edema (mostly periorbital)
B. Diarrhea
C. Myalgia
D. Myelotoxicity
E. Photophobia

253 Regarding Zenker's diverticula, all of the following are true *except*:
A. They are acquired.
B. The opening of the upper esophageal sphincter is impaired.
C. They generally present in the seventh or eighth decade of life.
D. Adenocarcinoma may develop in the diverticulum.
E. Aspiration of retained food may complicate induction of anesthesia.

254 Which of the following tumors may cause hypergastrinemia?
A. Ovarian cancer
B. Bronchogenic carcinoma
C. Acoustic neuroma
D. All of the above
E. None of the above

255 A 70-year-old man with a history of hypertension, diabetes mellitus, and coronary artery disease presents to the emergency department with two episodes of melena in the past 24 hours. He thinks that he may have had a dark, black stool two to three days ago but is unsure. He had dizziness earlier in the day but never lost consciousness. He feels fine now. He is accompanied by his wife who has a list of the medications that he is taking, which include oral hypoglycemic agents, an angiotensin-converting enzyme inhibitor, a β-adrenergic blocker, and NSAIDs for arthritis. His medical history includes an appendectomy several years ago, an abdominal aortic aneurysm repair 20 years ago, and a cardiac catheterization a year ago. He appears pale but is alert and oriented. His vital signs are pulse, 90 beats/minute; blood pressure, 105/80 mm Hg; respiratory rate, 22 to 24 breaths/minute; and temperature, 100.2°F. He does not have orthostatic hypotension, abdominal pain, nausea, vomiting, or hematemesis. During evaluation in the emergency department, he has another episode of melena. An intravenous infusion is started, and a blood sample is obtained in preparation for an upper endoscopy. His hemoglobin is 9.6 g% with a normal mean corpuscular volume; however, his bicarbonate level is 16 mEq/L. EGD performed in the emergency department shows a single, small, white-based ulcer in the duodenal bulb. There is no blood in the stomach or visualized portions of the duodenum. The patient now feels much better. Which of the following is the best approach at this point?
A. Stop NSAIDs, admit the patient, continue administration of intravenous fluids, and begin intravenous administration of a PPI.

B. Stop NSAIDs and discharge the patient with a prescription for an oral PPI medication twice daily.
C. Admit the patient, continue administration of intravenous fluids, start intravenous administration of a PPI medication, and repeat the EGD with a pediatric endoscope the next day.
D. Admit the patient, continue IV fluid administration, start IV administration of a PPI medication, and perform a CT scan of the abdomen stat.
E. None of the above.

256 Significant risk factors for the development of severe upper GI events in patients with rheumatoid arthritis include all of the following *except*:
A. Use of NSAIDs
B. Age older than 65 years
C. History of peptic ulcer disease
D. Severe rheumatoid arthritis
E. Use of cyclooxygenase-2 inhibitors

257 All of the following regarding food impaction are true *except*:
A. Food impaction is the most common ingested "foreign body" in the United States.
B. The increased risk of complication is proportional to the duration of the esophageal food impaction.
C. Endoscopic intervention should be achieved at the latest within 48 hours of onset of symptoms.
D. Success rates with the push method exceed 90%.
E. Eosinophilic esophagitis is increasingly associated with esophageal food impactions.

258 Acquired defects that allow internal hernias to occur develop after which of the following procedures?
A. Billroth II gastrectomy
B. Roux-en-Y gastric bypass
C. Colectomy/ileostomy
D. Tear in the sigmoid mesentery postcolonoscopy
E. All of the above

259 You are asked to provide a second opinion on a 45-year-old woman with an 11-year history of Crohn's disease. She tells you that she was found to have multiple enteroenteric fistulas during a recent workup for diarrhea. Her main symptom is voluminous nonbloody diarrhea. She has been treated with antibiotics without significant relief. She was placed on TPN but without significant improvement. Her gastroenterologist decides to start her on octreotide, and she wants to know why. You tell her that you agree with her primary gastroenterologist and explain to her that she is being started on octreotide for all the following reasons *except*:
A. Octreotide inhibits the release of gastrin, cholecystokinin, secretin, motilin, and other GI hormones.
B. Octreotide relaxes intestinal smooth muscle, thereby allowing for a greater intestinal capacity.
C. Octreotide increases intestinal water and electrolyte absorption.
D. Octreotide decreases abdominal distention and pain.

260 Mixed connective tissue disease shares all of the following similarities with scleroderma, systemic lupus erythematosus, and polymyositis *except*:
A. Abnormal esophageal motility
B. Impaired gastric emptying
C. Intestinal pseudo-obstruction
D. Pancreatitis
E. Abnormal esophageal motility improvement with the use of glucocorticoids

261 For each of the following circumstances, answer this statement with true or false: "Antibiotic prophylaxis should be given before this GI procedure."
A. A 57-year-old white man who is about to undergo esophageal stricture dilation had his left hip replaced two years ago.
B. A 49-year-old man with a history of alcohol abuse, recurrent pancreatitis, and pancreatic pseudocyst is about to undergo ERCP and possible pseudocyst drainage.
C. A 90-year-old nursing home patient transferred for percutaneous endoscopic gastrostomy (PEG) tube placement
D. A 45-year-old white woman with mitral valve prolapse and a 10-year history of ulcerative colitis who takes antibiotics before dental procedures and is about to undergo surveillance colonoscopy
E. A 50-year-old African-American man who had a defibrillator placed six months ago and is now admitted with painless obstructive jaundice and is about to undergo ERCP

262 A 45-year-old woman who underwent kidney transplantation three years ago has been experiencing fatigue and nonbloody, crampy diarrhea. Her stool studies are negative for *C. difficile*, but there are WBCs in the stool. Colonoscopy reveals mild patchy erythema throughout the transverse, descending, and sigmoid colon. Biopsy specimens reveal eosinophilic infiltrates. Which of the following medications is most likely responsible for the findings?
A. Tacrolimus and cyclosporine
B. MMF
C. Prednisone
D. Ganciclovir

263 True statements about the cutaneous manifestations of inflammatory bowel disease include all of the following *except*:
A. Cutaneous lesions are more common in people with Crohn's disease than in people with ulcerative colitis.
B. Erythema nodosum can occur in those with Crohn's disease or ulcerative colitis.
C. Treatment of the underlying disease usually improves the skin lesions.
D. Pyoderma gangrenosum presents as painless ulcers in 5% of patients with ulcerative colitis and 1% of patients with Crohn's disease.
E. Pyostomatitis vegetans may occur years before the onset of GI symptoms in those with irritable bowel disease (IBD).

264 A 40-year-old man presents with diarrhea, weight loss, and episodic blistery rash noted over his lower abdomen and buttocks. Which one of the following hormones will be produced by this lesion?
A. Somatostatin
B. Insulin
C. Glucagon
D. Vasoactive intestinal polypeptide

265 A 67-year-old man with a history of migraines treated with ergotamine preparations presents with symptoms of abdominal pain, nausea, vomiting, and abdominal distention. A CT scan demonstrates dilated loops of small bowel, air–fluid levels, inflammatory changes of the mesentery and retroperitoneum, and medial displacement of the ureters. A possible treatment option for this disorder includes which of the following?
A. Ureteral stenting
B. Steroids
C. Azathioprine
D. Decompressive nasogastric tube
E. All of the above

266 A 60-year-old obese woman who underwent surgical repair of a large incisional hernia a few hours previously is noted to be tachypneic and in respiratory distress. Her electrocardiogram shows no change from her preoperative electrocardiogram and a ventilation/perfusion scan of the lungs shows no embolism. What would be a likely mechanism for her symptoms?
A. Decreased venous return to the heart
B. Small undetected pulmonary embolism
C. Compression of the lungs due to increased abdominal volume and pressure postrepair
D. Previously undiagnosed chronic obstructive pulmonary disease
E. **A** and **C**

267 A 35-year-old woman has small bowel Crohn's disease for five years. She has recently gone from her usual four to five bowel movements per day to 10 to 15 episodes of voluminous diarrhea (>1 L output). She reports weakness and says that she frequently feels light-headed. What should be done next to evaluate her symptoms?
A. Small bowel series
B. CAT scan of the abdomen and pelvis
C. Colonoscopy
D. Capsule endoscopy

268 When compared with the general population, patients who survive more than 10 years following HCT have what risk for developing a new solid malignancy?
A. 20-fold
B. Twofold
C. Eightfold
D. No increase in risk

269 A 38-year-old woman who has undergone HCT has a history of chronic GVHD. She recently began tapering her immunosuppression medication. She now presents with nausea, fatigue, and an AST level of 3000 U/L. What is the next step?
A. Check the blood for viral hepatitis.
B. Perform a liver biopsy to exclude HSV, varicella-zoster virus, or viral hepatitis.

C. Perform a serum autoantibody test for CYP1A2.

D. All of the above

270 For adults with symptomatic esophageal food bolus impactions, which of the following is true?

A. Sialorrhea is uncommon.

B. Ingestion of a small sharp fish bone may cause odynophagia or persistent foreign body sensation due to a mucosal laceration.

C. A patient can accurately localize an ingested foreign body.

D. Dysphagia, odynophagia, and dysphoria have less than a 30% likelihood of suggesting partial obstruction.

E. If symptoms are restricted to retrosternal chest pain or pharyngeal pain, the foreign body is likely to still be there.

271 Regarding newly diagnosed metastatic carcinoid, all of the following statements are true *except*:

A. The patient should undergo cross-sectional imaging at the level of the tumor and liver.

B. Positron emission tomography is advantageous in these cases because it can identify disease throughout the body.

C. Identification of metastatic disease is more difficult than identification of a primary tumor.

D. Somatostatin scintigraphy is very helpful in these cases.

272 Which of the following is not indicated in the follow-up care of a patient who underwent successful endoscopic removal of a food impaction?

A. Education on methods of reducing further impactions

B. A repeat endoscopy within 48 hours

C. A 24-hour pH and/or manometry study

D. PPIs

E. All of the above

273 The husband of a 30-year-old white woman brings her to the physician because of multiple GI symptoms including postprandial abdominal pain, vomiting, and weight loss of 40 pounds in the past two months. The husband is extremely concerned that she may have an eating disorder. On examination, the patient is pale and asthenic, weighs 96 pounds, and is 5 feet 6 inches tall. She is tearful, very upset with her husband, and denies abuse of laxatives or any other symptoms of an eating disorder. On further questioning, she says that her weight loss began in the hospital as the result of "bad hospital food" when she was admitted for a spinal cord injury and had to be in a body cast, but the onset of vomiting is more recent. What should the physician do?

A. Perform a gastric emptying scan.

B. Initiate a nutrition consult with strict calorie counts.

C. Obtain an upper GI series of x-rays with small bowel follow-through.

D. Perform an upper endoscopy.

E. Start the patient on an antidepressant medication and obtain a psychiatry consult.

274 A 48-year-old man with a history of GERD presents at your office for the first time and is already taking a PPI prescribed by his primary care physician. An EGD is performed demonstrating a duodenal and several small gastric ulcers. He has no history of NSAID use. You obtain a gastrin level, which is 960. What is the most appropriate test for a definitive diagnosis?

A. Fasting gastrin

B. Repeat EGD with a gastric pH

C. Repeat gastrin off PPI therapy for one week

D. Serum *H. pylori* antibody

E. Secretin provocative test

275 What is the most common complication to develop during the first month after liver transplantation?

A. HSV

B. CMV

C. Fungal

D. Biliary sepsis

276 Which of the following can result from foreign body ingestion?

A. Pericarditis

B. Esophagoaortic fistula

C. Lung abscess

D. Mediastinitis

E. All of the above

277 Gastrinoma causes all of the following *except*:

A. Diarrhea

B. Atrophic enterochromaffin cells

C. Parietal cell hyperplasia

D. Large gastric folds

E. GERD

278 A 46-year-old, obese African-American woman is referred to a GI clinic for evaluation of recurrent abdominal pain and intermittently elevated transaminase levels. She has mild hypertension and asthma but is otherwise healthy. Her medical history is significant for two cesarean sections and cholecystectomy, performed six years ago. On examination, she appears comfortable, and her vital signs are stable. She is pain free at present, but states that she is tired of making recurrent visits to the emergency department and wants something done. She has heard about ERCP, but is afraid to undergo this procedure because two of her sisters with symptoms similar to hers had undergone ERCP and subsequently were hospitalized for a long time with more abdominal pain. Her medical record indicates that studies have been performed to rule out viral and other causes of hepatitis; an ultrasound scan of her abdomen and MRI with cholangiopancreatography show dilation of the bile duct lumen to 8 mm but no other abnormalities. Her AST and ALT levels are approximately two to 2.5 times normal. Sphincter of Oddi dysfunction is suspected. What is the best way to decrease the likelihood of complications in this patient?

A. Place her on ursodiol (Actigall, Urso) for three months and follow her clinically to see how she responds.

B. Proceed with ERCP but use only cutting current at the time of sphincterotomy to decrease the likelihood of pancreatitis.

C. Prescribe anticholinergics and follow her clinically.

D. Refer her to a surgeon for bile duct exploration.

E. Proceed with ERCP with placement of a temporary pancreatic stent to decrease the likelihood of post-ERCP pancreatitis.

279 Acrodermatitis enteropathica, a superficial scaling and blistering eruption of skin, is seen mainly in the perioral and groin area. It is a characteristic manifestation of which of the following?
A. Vitamin C deficiency
B. Zinc deficiency
C. Glucagon-secreting tumor of the pancreas
D. Whipple's disease
E. Tropical sprue

280 Which of the following is the most commonly identified pathogen in AIDS?
A. *Candida albicans*
B. CMV
C. HSV
D. *Mycobacterium avium-intracellulare*
E. Hepatitis C

281 A 40-year-old woman with ileal Crohn's disease presents with diffuse periumbilical pain and fevers to 101°F. A CAT scan of the abdomen and pelvis done in the emergency department reveals two enhancing collections, measuring between 1 and 2 cm within the mesentery of her small bowel, and thickening of the terminal ileum. What is the bacterium most likely to be associated with this pathology?
A. *E. coli* and *Enterococcus* species
B. *Bacteroides fragilis* and *Peptostreptococcus* species
C. *Enterococcus* species
D. *B. fragilis*
E. **A** and **B**

282 A 70-year-old white man is referred to a GI clinic for recent change in bowel habits and rectal bleeding. Change of bowel habits is characterized by a five- to six-month history of watery, nonmucousy, nonbloody diarrhea three to five times per day. In addition, he has noticed intermittent lower abdominal crampy pain accompanied by a small amount of bright red blood on the toilet paper after a bowel movement for the past three months. He has no history of fever, recent travel outside the country, unusual environmental exposures, or contact with ill individuals. On physical examination, he has mild lower abdominal tenderness without rebound and normal rectal sphincter tone with no palpable rectal masses. A stool sample is brown but tests heme positive. Laboratory test results are normal. A colonoscopy is performed to the terminal ileum without difficulty. Findings include pandiverticulosis, a normal-appearing terminal ileum, and a 3.5-cm yellow nodule in the rectum, which undergoes a biopsy. The histopathology report is carcinoid tumor. All of the following statements about this patient's condition are true *except*:
A. Rectal carcinoid tumors >2 cm in diameter pose a 60% to 80% risk of metastasis.
B. The incidence of rectal carcinoid tumors is three times higher in whites than in African Americans.
C. Carcinoid syndrome is an uncommon feature of rectal carcinoid tumors.

D. Invasion of the muscularis propria at diagnosis is a poor prognostic sign.
E. The overall survival rate for patients with rectal carcinoid tumors is 87%.

283 A 47-year-old white man is referred to a GI clinic with a history of recurrent heme-positive stools and normocytic anemia for two years. He has had two upper and lower endoscopies performed elsewhere, which showed no abnormality. He has yellow to orange redundant tissue on the side of his neck, which has been present for years. Recently, he noticed similar yellow lesions in the axillary region. He is very upset because a week ago he was in the emergency department with chest pain and was told that he had had a small "heart attack." He states "I don't know what I'm doing wrong; I eat healthy and exercise regularly." True statements about this patient's condition include which of the following?
A. GI bleeding develops in approximately 8% to 13% of patients with this condition.
B. This disorder occurs due to aberrant calcification of mature connective tissue.
C. The source of GI bleeding is often difficult to identify.
D. Biopsy of the skin will be diagnostic.
E. All of these statements are true.

284 Which of the following is/are the most common GI problems encountered in patients with rheumatoid arthritis?
A. Autoimmune hepatitis
B. Due to drug therapy with NSAIDs and disease-modifying antirheumatic drugs
C. Primary biliary cirrhosis
D. Hepatic amyloidosis
E. Ischemic cholecystitis secondary to rheumatic vasculitis

285 All of the following statements regarding the incidence of carcinoid tumors in the gut are true *except*:
A. Carcinoid tumors of the esophagus are rare.
B. The stomach is the most common foregut location for carcinoid tumors.
C. The appendix is the most common site in the gut for carcinoid tumors.
D. In the colon, carcinoid tumors are more likely to occur on the right side.
E. The incidence of rectal carcinoids is increasing.

286 The GI manifestations and associations of Sjögren syndrome include which of the following?
A. GAVE (watermelon stomach)
B. Duodenal ulcer disease
C. Dysphagia
D. Primary biliary cirrhosis
E. **A**, **C**, and **D**

287 A 64-year-old man is brought to the emergency department by his daughter because of midepigastric abdominal pain. He is found to have a fever of 102°F. On physical examination, he is tachycardic and hypotensive and is found to have an increasing oxygen requirement while he is in the emergency department. He undergoes an emergent CT scan of the chest and abdomen. Imaging results show bilateral patchy infiltrates in the lungs and pancreatic edema with phlegmon development surrounding the head and body. He is begun on broad-spectrum antibiotics. After 72 hours, he continues to have a fever. He undergoes a repeat CT scan of both the chest and the abdomen. There is no significant improvement in the size of the collection around the pancreas. The bacteria most likely contributing to his clinical condition include which of the following?

A. *Bacteroides* and *E. coli*
B. *Streptococcus* and *E. coli*
C. *Streptococcus* and *Bacteroides*
D. *Candida* and *Enterococcus*

288 Which of the following statements about Dieulafoy's lesion is false?

A. The most common site of bleeding from this lesion is 6 cm from the cardioesophageal junction.
B. These lesions are more common in men than in women.
C. The diagnosis is best made by early endoscopy.
D. These lesions were thought to represent the early stage of gastric ulcers.
E. These lesions cannot occur outside the GI tract.

289 Which of the following is the best treatment for immunoproliferative small intestinal disease (also called alpha heavy-chain disease)?

A. Surgery followed by radiation
B. Chemotherapy
C. Antibiotics followed by chemotherapy
D. Combined radiation and chemotherapy

290 A 28-year-old African-American woman with Crohn's disease complicated by multiple enteroenteral and enterocolonic fistulas, maintained on infliximab for five months, is seen in a GI clinic for follow-up. She was recently in the hospital for fever, abdominal pain, and worsening nonbloody diarrhea. Her condition temporarily improved with antibiotics, but symptoms returned when the antibiotics were stopped. However, she continues to have 8 to 10 watery bowel movements daily, up from her baseline of four soft bowel movements per day. She has been tried on octreotide and TPN in the past without significant relief. Small bowel x-rays continue to show unchanged fistulous disease. What is the next best step in her care?

A. Surgical therapy for resection of the involved bowel and restoration of intestinal continuity
B. Adding azathioprine to her current therapy
C. Discontinuing infliximab and starting adalimumab
D. Long-term course of ciprofloxacin and flagyl

291 A 52-year-old Asian man presents to the emergency department with cramping lower abdominal pain and a low-grade fever one day after colonoscopy. He has been passing flatus but has not had any bowel movements since the colonoscopy. His temperature is 100.6°F, but his other vital signs are normal. He has mild to moderate left lower quadrant abdominal tenderness. His WBC count is $12.6 \times 10^3/\mu L$ with a slight left shift. A plain film (scout film) of the abdomen obtained in the emergency department shows no free air. Review of

the colonoscopy records show that he had left-sided diverticulosis and a 4-mm polyp in the sigmoid colon, which was snared using electrocautery. The patient feels better in the emergency department after receiving pain medication and wants to go home. What is the next best step in his management?

A. Because the scout film shows no perforation, discharge him home with a prescription for pain medication and instructions to return if fever recurs.
B. He has probably developed diverticulitis, so he should be discharged home with a prescription for a 2-week course of an antibiotic.
C. Obtain stool cultures and then begin antibiotic therapy.
D. Admit the patient, begin antibiotic therapy, and perform CT scans of the abdomen and pelvis.

292 A 25-year-old woman with moderately severe ileal Crohn's disease requiring two previous small bowel resections and who is now stable on 6-mercaptopurine presents to your office after finding out that she is six weeks pregnant. How should she be advised regarding the treatment of her IBD during pregnancy?

A. Given the severity of her disease in the past and her clinical stability on 6-MP, she should continue on 6-MP but at a reduced dose.
B. Steroids are an acceptable treatment for flares of IBD during pregnancy.
C. Infliximab is generally not advised for use in the third trimester.
D. 5-Aminosalicylic acid agents are generally safe in pregnancy.
E. All of the above

293 Which is the most common cause of liver function test abnormalities in HIV-infected patients?

A. Acute hepatitis
B. CMV infection
C. HAART-induced injury
D. *Mycobacterium avium-intracellulare* complex infection
E. Chronic hepatitis C

294 Match the following disorders of the mouth and oral cavity to the disease with which they are associated.

Condition	Associated Disease
1. Glossodynia	A. Chronic smoking
2. Glossitis	B. Sjögren syndrome
3. Xerostomia	C. Psychiatric disease
4. Black hairy tongue	D. Magnesium deficiency
5. Dysgeusia	E. Pernicious anemia

295 All of the following comments about food protein–induced enterocolitis are true *except*:

A. Atopy patch testing has not had confirmation value in studies thus far.
B. Skin prick test and radioallergosorbent test are the basis for diagnosis.
C. Symptoms typically present in young children.
D. Cow's milk protein is the most frequent allergen.
E. Elimination diet provides the ultimate proof of causation.

296 Pellagra may occur as a result of any of the following conditions *except*:
- **A.** Inadequate intake of niacin
- **B.** VIPoma
- **C.** Carcinoid syndrome
- **D.** Prolonged treatment with isoniazid
- **E.** IBD

297 Diabetic autonomic neuropathy includes all of the following *except*:
- **A.** Esophageal dysmotility
- **B.** Gastroparesis diabeticorum
- **C.** Poor antral expulsion leading to bezoars
- **D.** Pylorospasm
- **E.** Decreased plasma levels of motilin

298 All of the following concerning hernias through the foramen of Bochdalek are true *except*:
- **A.** They occur predominantly in the left hemidiaphragm posteriorly.
- **B.** They are usually present at birth or in the neonatal period.
- **C.** Large congenital hernias can be associated with neonatal respiratory distress and hypoplasia of the left lung.
- **D.** The diagnosis can only be established after delivery when symptoms are noted.

299 Ingestion of disk batteries is a particular concern. All of the following are true *except*:
- **A.** Because the batteries contain alkaline solution, they can cause rapid liquefaction necrosis in the esophagus.
- **B.** Use of a retrieval net permits successful battery removal in close to 100% of cases.
- **C.** These batteries are ingested most commonly in children, and as many as 90% are symptomatic.
- **D.** Most pass through the GI tract in 72 hours.
- **E.** Once in the stomach or small intestine, they rarely cause clinical problems.

300 All of the following statements are correct *except*:
- **A.** At least half of patients with Felty syndrome have a liver enzyme abnormality.
- **B.** The degree of enzyme abnormality is unrelated to the histopathology in Felty syndrome.
- **C.** Portal hypertension and variceal bleeding rarely occur with Felty syndrome.
- **D.** Adult-onset Still's disease can present with hepatosplenomegaly and abnormal liver function test results.
- **E.** Acute liver failure is not a feature of Still's disease.

301 Most GI foreign bodies pass through the entire GI tract without difficulty. However, objects longer than 5 cm (2 inches), such as pens, pencils, or eating utensils, may not negotiate around/through which of the following?
- **A.** Pylorus
- **B.** Duodenal sweep
- **C.** Ligament of Treitz
- **D.** Ileocecal valve
- **E.** Valves of Houston

302 Patients with NF1 are at increased risk of developing which of the following disorders?

- **A.** Microscopic colitis
- **B.** Barrett's esophagus
- **C.** Carcinoid
- **D.** Melanoma
- **E.** GERD

303 As many as one third of patients with pancreatic growth hormone–releasing factor tumors also have which disorder?
- **A.** MEN-I
- **B.** Cushing syndrome
- **C.** ZES
- **D.** VIPoma
- **E.** Lymphoma

304 How is the liver affected in Hodgkin's disease?
- **A.** Diffuse lobular hepatitis
- **B.** Interface hepatitis
- **C.** Sclerosing cholangitis
- **D.** Idiopathic cholestatic hepatitis

305 A 55-year-old man presents with symptoms of dyspepsia, vomiting, and postprandial indigestion. He has a serum albumin level of 2.6 g/dL and a creatinine level of 0.8 mg/dL. He has noted increasing lower extremity edema. A CT scan of the abdomen reveals prominent and thick gastric folds. Which of the following medications should be prescribed for this patient?
- **A.** H_2 blockers
- **B.** Omeprazole
- **C.** Octreotide
- **D.** Antacids
- **E.** All of the above

306 The most appropriate initial therapy for radiation proctitis in a patient who presents with hematochezia includes which of the following?
- **A.** Short-chain fatty acids
- **B.** Argon plasma coagulation treatment of the telangiectasias
- **C.** Instillation of formalin in the rectum
- **D.** Sucralfate enemas
- **E.** Hyperbaric oxygen

307 Which one of the following is invariably increased in patients with carcinoid?
- **A.** Chromogranin C
- **B.** α Subunit of HCG
- **C.** Neuron-specific enolase
- **D.** Chromogranin A
- **E.** Synaptophysin

308 Regarding jejunal diverticula, all of the following are true *except*:
- **A.** They can be found by an upper GI x-ray with small bowel follow-through.
- **B.** They are commonly multiple and range in size from a few millimeters to 10 cm.
- **C.** They commonly occur on the antimesenteric border.
- **D.** Large enteroliths can form in the diverticula and lead to erosion with bleeding, diverticulitis, perforation, or intestinal obstruction.
- **E.** There is an association between small bowel diverticulosis and small bowel volvulus.

309 A 32-year-old G1P0 at 36 weeks' gestation presents with several weeks of mild proteinuria and hypertension. She now reports severe right upper quadrant pain, malaise, and dizziness. Her blood pressure is 100/60 with a heart rate of 119 Laboratory test results reveal a platelet count of 76,000, a hemoglobin level of 7.6, a total bilirubin level of 7.9, a direct bilirubin level of 6.6, an AST level 860 U/L, and an ALT level of 1090 U/L. What potential complication of her disorder must be ruled out?
A. Sepsis
B. Cholecystitis
C. Hepatic rupture
D. Fetal death
E. Hepatic infarct

310 All of the following statements about oral HL are true *except*:
A. It presents as black lesions along the lateral border of the tongue; hence, the name.
B. It is usually asymptomatic.
C. Development of HL in a person with HIV infection usually presages the development of AIDS in approximately 24 months.
D. This condition can occur in solid organ transplant recipients.
E. The epithelium of patients with this condition contains Epstein-Barr virus.

311 All of the following statements about spigelian hernias are true *except*:
A. They do not traverse the entire abdominal wall.
B. Twenty-five percent of all spigelian hernias are not diagnosed before surgery.
C. The pain can be mistaken for diverticulitis or appendicitis.
D. They occur in women older than the age of 40 and more often on the left.
E. They can be readily diagnosed as a bulge in the abdominal wall lateral to the rectus sheath and inferior to the umbilicus.

312 All of the following characteristics of the KIT-tyrosine kinase gene are accurate *except*:
A. It binds to ligand SCF (stem cell factor) to create the active kinase consisting of two KIT molecules facilitating cross-phosphorylation of tyrosine residues.
B. It signals cell proliferation and enhanced survival in the normal state.
C. It is normally found in most cells and interstitial cells of Cajal.
D. Its CD117 is found in 100% of GISTs.

313 A 24-year-old woman with no medical history presents with symptoms of right upper quadrant pain, fever, and abdominal distention. Her examination shows shifting dullness, right upper quadrant tenderness to palpation, and a hepatic friction rub. Ascitic fluid analysis reveals 400 WBCs with 90% neutrophils and a protein count of 9.6 g/dL. The abdominal ultrasound scan findings are normal. A laparoscopy is performed and "violin strings" are seen. Which of the following is the most appropriate treatment?
A. Ceftriaxone
B. Doxycycline

C. Lysis of adhesions
D. Rifampin
E. No therapy is needed

314 All of the following statements regarding diarrhea in AIDS are true *except*:
A. Cryptosporidiosis is self-limited in healthy hosts but is the most frequent protozoan in HIV patients worldwide.
B. The small bowel is the most common site of infection.
C. Cryptosporidiosis may be identified on small bowel or rectal biopsy specimens when stool test results are negative.
D. *Giardia lamblia* and *Entamoeba histolytica* are seen with increased frequency and virulence.
E. *Blastocystis hominis*, *Endolimax nana*, and *Entamoeba coli* are more common in men who have sex with men and occur with other protozoan parasites.

315 All of the following methods have been used in the treatment of recurrent aphthous ulcers in the oral cavity *except*:
A. Multivitamin supplementation
B. Metronidazole 500 mg orally twice daily for 14 days
C. Oral colchicine at a dose of 0.6 mg three times daily
D. Topical or systemic prednisone
E. Viscous lidocaine 2% with sucralfate

316 What is the first step in treating a lymphoma arising in an immunosuppressed patient following organ transplantation?
A. Exploratory laparotomy for staging
B. Chemotherapy with CHOP (cyclophosphamide, hydroxydaunomycin, Oncovin [vincristine], and prednisone)
C. Radiation therapy if no indication of disseminated disease
D. Stop the immunosuppressive drugs

317 All of the following statements regarding PEG tube placement are true *except*:
A. Administering antibiotic medications before the procedure has been shown to reduce the risk of local wound infection.
B. The most frequent complication of PEG tube placement is infection at the PEG tube entry site.
C. Buried bumper syndrome is a known complication.
D. The most common cause of aspiration pneumonia in patients fed via PEG tube is reflux of their enteral feedings.

318 The distinction of EE caused by chronic GERD can be difficult, but the resolution of all of the following issues can clarify the problem *except*:
A. Failure to perform a biopsy of normal mucosa
B. Failure to perform a biopsy of both the distal and midesophagus
C. Differential response to oral fluticasone
D. Failure to take an adequate history of atopy

319 A patient who has undergone HCT presents with nausea and a history of two episodes of hemateme-

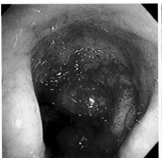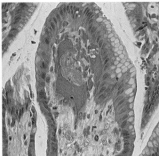

Figure for question **319**

sis. Upper endoscopy is performed (see figure). What is the best treatment for this patient?
A. Endoscopic laser therapy
B. Angiography with embolization
C. PPI drip
D. Surgery
E. None of the above

320 Dysphagia and the sense of esophageal obstruction along with chest pain develop in a 47-year-old man while eating a steak. What treatment is indicated for this patient?
A. A trial of sips of water
B. Esophagography using a water-soluble contrast
C. Intravenous glucagon administration
D. Urgent endoscopy using a rigid endoscope and intravenous sedation
E. Urgent endoscopy using a rigid endoscope and general anesthesia

321 Which of the following is the most common GI symptom in diabetics?
A. Diarrhea
B. Constipation
C. Nausea
D. Dysphagia
E. Acid reflux

322 Match the following cutaneous markers to the GI malignancy with which each has been historically associated.

Cutaneous Marker	GI Malignancy
1. Tylosis	A. Gastric cancer
2. Sweet's syndrome	B. Pancreatic cancer
3. Trousseau's syndrome	C. Lymphoma
4. Dermatomyositis	D. Esophageal cancer
5. Subcutaneous fat necrosis	E. Colorectal cancer

323 Although a CT scan is generally recommended as a first-line diagnostic tool for detecting PETs, the most sensitive study for their detection is
A. Ultrasonography
B. MRI
C. Positron emission tomography
D. Selective abdominal angiography
E. Somatostatin receptor scintigraphy

324 A 31-year-old African-American woman with perianal Crohn's disease presents to a GI clinic with symptoms of three months' duration of a draining perianal fistula. On examination, she is afebrile and without abdominal pain. She has a subcentimeter opening lateral to her anal orifice with mild erythema and no fluctuance or pain. Which treatment is most advisable for her condition to improve and facilitate healing and closure of the fistula?
A. Start ciprofloxacin and metronidazole
B. Start octreotide
C. Start infliximab
D. Start Rowasa enemas every night

325 What is the frequency with which granulomas are found on the liver biopsies of patients with sarcoidosis?
A. 10% to 20%
B. 30% to 40%
C. 50% to 60%
D. 80% to 90%

ANSWERS

80 E (S&F, ch32)
Patients who surreptitiously abuse insulin or sulfonylureas should have normal proinsulin and C-peptide levels because these are only produced during the endogenous production of insulin. They may have measurable amounts of sulfonylurea in the serum, and the plasma level of insulin to glucose should be low. An elevated ratio would suggest the presence of an insulinoma.

81 A (S&F, ch25)
Once in the esophagus, there are four areas of noted narrowing where food boluses and true foreign bodies become lodged, including all the areas listed except the area of a hiatal hernia. These areas are all true luminal narrowings. A careful history is important in eliciting risk factors for foreign body impaction. The results of physical examination tend to be unremarkable or nonspecific, but the examination must be carefully performed to recognize complications of foreign body ingestions such as perforation. Plain radiographs of the chest and abdomen can help determine the presence, type, and location of the foreign body. Radiographic contrast studies are relatively contraindicated in the evaluation of foreign body ingestions. Barium esophagography should not be performed because it may make the performance of subsequent therapeutic endoscopy more difficult if 23 mm or less.

82 C (S&F, ch28)
The loss of serum proteins in patients with protein-losing gastroenteropathy is independent of their molecular weight, and therefore the fraction of the intravascular pool degraded per day remains the same for various proteins, including albumin, IgG, IgA, IgM, and ceruloplasmin. Adaptive changes in endogenous protein catabolism may compensate for excessive enteric protein loss, resulting in unequal loss of specific proteins. For example, proteins such as insulin, clotting factors, and IgE have rapid catabolic turnover rates (short half-lives) and

as such are relatively unaffected by GI losses because rapid synthesis of these proteins ensues.

83 **D** (S&F, ch40)
Although the most feared complication of colonoscopy is perforation, cardiorespiratory complications arising from sedation are more common.

84 **A** (S&F, ch36)
This young woman has a condition called blue rubber bleb nevus syndrome, which is a rare disorder of the skin and GI tract. Its features include a constellation of cutaneous and GI tract malformations. In patients such as the woman described here, blue, compressible nodules develop subcutaneously. GI tract vascular malformations are very common, especially in the small intestine and colon, and GI bleeding is usually present. The malformations may be treated surgically or with photocoagulation.

85 **D** (S&F, ch27)
If eosinophilic infiltration involves mostly mucosa, there can be ulceration and GI bleeding. If it involves the muscularis propria, pyloric obstruction is a common complication. If it involves the serosa of the bowel, eosinophilic ascites can occur.

86 **B** (S&F, ch38)
Most women of childbearing age with chronic hepatitis B infection are healthy carriers of the virus with a very low risk of the development of complications of their disease during gestation. The importance of maternal hepatitis B infection during pregnancy is related to its role in the perpetuation of chronic infection through vertical transmission. Maternal-fetal transmission of hepatitis B virus is responsible for most cases of chronic hepatitis B infection worldwide. Mothers with a reactive serum test for hepatitis B e antigen have more circulating virus and higher rates of perinatal transmission than do mothers without detectable levels of serum hepatitis B e antigen or a reactive serum test for hepatitis B e antibody, although the latter individuals are still a source of neonatal infection. The infants of mothers with a reactive serum test for hepatitis B surface antigen should receive hepatitis B immunoglobulin at birth and also hepatitis B vaccine during the first day of life and at ages one and six months. Women with chronic hepatitis B are not treated with interferon during pregnancy. Therapy with the nucleoside analog lamivudine is safe in pregnant patients and has been reported to reduce the incidence of neonatal vaccination failure.

87 **E** (S&F, ch35)
Typhlitis (inflammation of the cecum) is associated with acute myelogenous leukemia and acute lymphocytic leukemia, and typically manifests after induction chemotherapy and is usually preceded by neutropenia. Cecal superinfecion with fungi and CMV has also been associated with typhlitis.

88 **B** (S&F, ch40)
Esophageal strictures do not need to be dilated to the size of uninvolved lumen but to a diameter that results in symptom resolution. The type of dilator used does not seem to affect the risk of perforation. Proximal esophageal strictures are the greatest risk.

89 **D** (S&F, ch29)
All three parameters are seen with MALT lymphoma. In addition, some large cells suggestive of different large B cell lymphomas may be present, but the disease may still respond to *H. pylori* eradication.

90 **B** (S&F, ch40)
Estimation of the suspected site or level of impaction by the patient is generally not reliable. The one area where patients may be able to accurately localize the object is at the cricopharyngeal muscle, but localization becomes progressively less accurate for distally impacted foreign bodies, with an accuracy of 30% to 40% for those in the esophagus and close to 0% for those in the stomach.

91 **E** (S&F, ch36)
The correct way to manage incidental telangiectasias of the colon, as in the case of this 54-year-old white man, is to do nothing.

92 **B** (S&F, ch34)
Giant gastric ulcers (>3 cm in diameter) may develop in liver transplant recipients despite routine use of acid suppression. These ulcers carry significant morbidity and mortality and are more often associated with bilateral lung transplantation, high-dose NSAID use after transplantation, acute rejection requiring high-dose glucocorticoids, and cyclosporine immunosuppression. For these reasons, some believe that NSAIDs should not be used in the post-transplantation setting.

93 **C** (S&F, ch35)
Involvement is not limited to skeletal muscle fibers. Perforations of the esophagus and duodenal diverticula are rare. Malabsorption, malnutrition, and pseudo-obstruction rarely occur. The pathology seems to result from vasculitis. Dermatomyositis and possibly polymyositis are associated with an increased prevalence of malignancy.

94 **A** (S&F, ch27)
Any esophageal dilation with EE carries a major risk of tear or even perforation. Medical treatment will improve the disease and probably avoid this risk. The usual diagnostic criterion for EE histologically is more than 15 eosinophils per high-power field. The white patches on the mucosa are clusters of eosinophils and will give a high yield on biopsy. Oral fluticasone is the treatment of choice, but recurrent symptoms can be expected within six months after treatment. Atopy is more frequently associated with EE in children than in adults, but the association is noted in adults as well.

95 **C** (S&F, ch38)
This patient has pemphigus vulgaris, which is a blistering disorder characterized by bullae and ulcers affecting the mucosa of the oral cavity, pharynx, esophagus, anus, conjunctiva, and skin. Half of these patients will present with oral ulcerations, and ulcerations will develop in virtually 100% during the course of the illness. Patients with IgG and IgA antibodies are more likely to respond

to treatment. Treatment consists of oral and topical glucocorticoids, sometimes in conjunction with immunosuppressant agents.

96   **C** (S&F, ch37)

Multifocal leiomyomas, also called leiomyomatosis peritonealis, is a rare disease that can mimic peritoneal carcinomatosis. The tumors may appear together with other leiomyomatous lesions or with endometriosis. These lesions consist of small, rubbery nodules, seem to be hormone sensitive, and develop during pregnancy or estrogen therapy. They can cause pain or gut bleeding and may regress with hormone withdrawal.

97   **E** (S&F, ch25)

Esophageal stricture will develop in as many as one third of caustic ingestion patients after initial recovery. Stricture formation occurs usually at two months after injury and occurs more commonly after IIB or III injuries. The primary treatment of esophageal strictures secondary to caustic ingestion is frequent dilation. As many as 10% to 50% of patients require surgical intervention.

98   **A** (S&F, ch38)

Severe persistent vomiting demanding medical intervention, or hyperemesis gravidarum, is less common, occurring in 2% or less of all pregnancies. Hyperemesis is associated with fluid, electrolyte, and acid-base imbalances, nutritional deficiency, and weight loss and is defined by the presence of ketonuria and a 5% decrease in prepregnancy weight. In as many as 20% of affected patients, however, vomiting persists until delivery. Pregnancy-related hormones, specifically HCG and estrogen, have been implicated as important causes of hyperemesis. Symptoms worsen during periods of peak HCG concentrations, and, in addition, conditions associated with higher serum HCG levels (e.g., multiple gestation, trophoblastic disease, and trisomy 21) are associated with an increased incidence of hyperemesis. Hospital admission for intravenous fluid and electrolyte replacement and sometimes nutritional support is indicated.

99   **B** (S&F, ch38)

Lifestyle modifications are suggested in the initial treatment of GERD, particularly in pregnant women. Liquid antacids and sucralfate (U.S. Food and Drug Administration category B) often are prescribed as first-line pharmacologic therapy. Ranitidine (U.S. Food and Drug Administration category B) remains the treatment of choice for patients who have persistent heartburn despite liquid antacid therapy. PPIs should be reserved for the most refractory cases, given their more recent introduction to the market. A recent meta-analysis found no significant risk of fetal malformations in infants exposed to PPIs in utero. Omeprazole is a pregnancy class C drug because it has caused fetal toxicity in animals; all other available PPIs are pregnancy category B drugs.

100   **A** (S&F, ch33)

Small bowel bacterial overgrowth is uncommon in AIDS patients, and its role in causing diarrhea seems limited. Infections by enteric bacteria are more frequent and more virulent in HIV-infected individuals compared with healthy hosts.

101   **E** (S&F, ch29)

MALT lymphoma does not take up [^{18}F]fluoro-2-deoxy-D-glucose on positron emission tomography. The upper airway is examined to rule out additional lymphoma in Waldeyer's ring (common with GI lymphomas). CT and bone marrow are commonly performed in staging for apparent reasons.

102   **B** (S&F, ch31)

Somatostatin and its analogs do block the effects of amines and peptides on target tissue. This results in decreased gut motility, blood flow, and both exocrine and endocrine function. They are most effective in the treatment of diarrhea and to some degree in the treatment of flushing, but they are not effective in the treatment of abdominal pain due to carcinoid tumor.

103   **D** (S&F, ch25)

Bezoars can be classified into four types: phytobezoars, composed of vegetable matter; trichobezoars, composed of hair or hair-like fibers; medication bezoars (pharmacobezoars), consisting of medications or medication vehicles; and lactobezoars, or milk curd bezoars, in infant formula reconstituted from powder. Gastroparesis is commonly seen in patients with bezoars. Patients with comorbid illnesses such as diabetes, end-stage renal disease on dialysis, or mechanical ventilation are at increased risk of bezoar formation. Of the numerous medications responsible for pharmacobezoars, cardiovascular medications such as nifedipine, procainamide, and verapamil are common.

104   **B** (S&F, ch34)

This patient is immunosuppressed and is not on antiviral prophylaxis. CMV is the predominant viral pathogen occurring within the first year after solid organ transplantation. The peak incidence is generally four to six months after transplantation. Either post-transplantation antiviral prophylaxis or preemptive therapy with either ganciclovir or valganciclovir significantly reduces the risk of CMV disease. Valganciclovir should not be used in the setting of liver transplantation, however, because there is a higher rate of tissue-invasive disease. In this setting, ganciclovir is recommended.

105   **B** (S&F, ch28)

The patient has allergic gastroenteropathy. This syndrome manifests by symptoms including abdominal pain, vomiting, and sporadic diarrhea; findings include hypoproteinemia, iron deficiency anemia, and peripheral eosinophilia. Serum levels of total protein and albumin, as well as IgA and IgG, will be markedly reduced, whereas levels of IgM and transferrin will be only moderately diminished. Characteristic histology of the small bowel in patients with this disorder includes a marked increase in the number of eosinophils in the lamina propria and may be found on stool examination.

106   **C** (S&F, ch36)

This patient most likely has Parkes Weber syndrome, which is a variant of Klippel-Trénaunay syndrome, differentiated from the latter by the fact that arteriovenous fistulas are common in the former. This syndrome consists of (1) vascular nevi of the lower limb, (2) varicose veins of the affected limb, (3) hypertrophy of all tissues including bone of the affected limb, and (4) arteriovenous fistulas. It usually manifests at birth; the results of the physical examination are almost always diagnostic.

107 **D** (S&F, ch38)
This woman has lichen planus, which is a common, chronic, inflammatory disorder involving the oral mucosa and skin. The white, lace-like oral lesions may occur with or without erythema and ulcerations. The disease usually begins in adulthood, and two thirds of all patients are women. Odynophagia or dysphagia may develop years after disease onset. Characteristic endoscopic findings include erythema, ulcerations, proximal esophageal web, and erosions at any location in the esophagus. Oral lichen planus is associated with an increased risk of squamous cell carcinoma, regardless of treatment.

108 **C** (S&F, ch24)
Obturator hernias are typically found on the right side in cachectic elderly women. Impingement of the hernia on the obturator nerve typically causes the pathognomic Howship-Romberg sign with medial thigh pain made worse by extension and internal rotation of the hip. Of these rare hernias, 88% present with intestinal obstruction.

109 **A** (S&F, ch28)
Giant hypertrophic gastropathy (Ménétrier's disease) is the most common gastric lesion causing severe protein loss.

110 **B** (S&F, ch35)
Hyperparathyroidism causes hypercalcemia, which in turn causes constipation. The mechanism of diarrhea in Addison's disease is unclear. The mechanism of diarrhea in **B**, **D**, and **E** is thought to be hormonal.

111 **E** (S&F, ch31)
Most physicians rely on the clinical features and the level of 5-HIAA in a 24-hour urine collection for the diagnosis of carcinoid syndrome. This test has its limitations; false-positive results may occur with dietary intake of foods that are high in serotonin and with certain medications. Excretion rates greater than 25 mg/day are diagnostic. Excretion rates of 5-HIAA correlate well with tumor mass and with symptoms. Midgut carcinoid tumors are associated with high rates of 5-HIAA excretion in the urine, whereas foregut carcinoid tumors may have normal rates of urinary excretion of 5-HIAA.

112 **D** (S&F, ch31)
The etiology of diarrhea in carcinoid syndrome is not very clear. It is thought to occur as a result of partial small bowel obstruction, accelerated small bowel and colonic transit, reduced colonic capacitance, and exaggerated postprandial colonic tone. However, unlike flushing, which does not respond to serotonin antagonists, diarrhea can be well controlled by these agents. This indicates a prominent role for serotonin in the pathogenesis of this feature of carcinoid syndrome. Glucocorticoids are given to a patient with carcinoid syndrome in whom hypotension develops.

113 **A** (S&F, ch25)
Within seconds of caustic exposure, necrosis develops. Twenty-four to 72 hours after the exposure, ulceration develops. Fibrosis can be seen after two to three weeks. Stricture takes weeks to years to develop. The most feared complication, carcinoma, takes decades to develop.

114 **B** (S&F, ch33)
Microsporidium has emerged as one of the most common intestinal infections in patients with AIDS. Intestinal and hepatobiliary disease may be caused by two species: *Enterocytozoon bieneusi* and *Encephalitozoon intestinalis*. Typical symptoms include watery, nonbloody diarrhea of mild to moderate severity, usually without associated crampy abdominal pain. Weight loss is common. Infection is associated with severe immunodeficiency with median CD4 counts less than 100/L.

115 **E** (S&F, ch35)
All of the conditions listed are more common in persons with systemic lupus erythematosus. Budd-Chiari syndrome is identified by the presence of anticardiolipin antibody or lupus anticoagulant. Mesenteric ischemia can be severe, causing bowel infarction. Pancreatitis is also due to ischemia. The peritonitis of polyserositis is well-known.

116 **A** (S&F, ch24)
Post-traumatic hernia can present with considerable delay (months to years) after the event as the positive intra-abdominal pressure and negative intrathoracic pressure create a constant gradient for herniation. Immediately after injury, symptoms of other injuries do obscure those of herniation, and pulmonary ventilation provides positive pressure in the chest that disappears on weaning from ventilation, making herniation more likely.

117 **D** (S&F, ch36)
This patient has hereditary hemorrhagic telangiectasia or Osler-Weber-Rendu disease. This is an autosomal dominant disorder characterized by telangiectasias of the skin and mucous membranes as well as recurrent GI bleeding. Telangiectasias can occur in the colon, but they occur more often in the stomach wall and the small intestines. Vascular involvement of the liver is not uncommon and may present as high-output heart failure due to right-to-left intrahepatic shunting, portal hypertension, and biliary tract disease. Giant hemangiomas in the liver are not a manifestation of hereditary hemorrhagic telangiectasia.

118 **A** (S&F, ch29)
H. pylori is seen histologically in 90% of biopsy specimens of MALT lymphoma. Serology is positive in 98% of these patients. There is also a correlation of incidence of MALT lymphoma in a geographic locale with the incidence of *H. pylori* infection.

119 **A** (S&F, ch35)

Only 21% of patients with amyloidosis have multiple myeloma. As with GI involvement by amyloidosis from other causes, bowel wall infiltration and dysmotility underlie most clinical symptoms.

120 **C** (S&F, ch32)

This patient likely has cholecystitis; therefore, a cholecystectomy would be warranted. All other options would either be nondiagnostic or too invasive.

121 **E** (S&F, ch22)

Cronkhite-Canada syndrome is a rare, sporadic syndrome of GI polyposis, mucocutaneous hyperpigmentation, alopecia, malabsorption, and nail dystrophy. Diarrhea, nail changes, abdominal pain, and weight loss are the most common symptoms. Alopecia occurs in more than 95% of patients and involves loss of both scalp and body hair. Hyperpigmentation occurs in 85% of patients and more commonly involves the upper extremities. Death can occur in approximately 50% of the patients as a result of malnutrition from the diarrhea. Aggressive nutritional support by TPN can lead to complete resolution of symptoms and treatment with the drug azathioprine (and 6-thioguanine).

122 **C** (S&F, ch24)

This is a classic presentation of an incarcerated femoral hernia. The inguinal nodule is frequently mistaken for a pathologic node and may even undergo biopsy, delaying simple surgery, which can cure the problem.

123 **B** (S&F, ch30)

GISTs become symptomatic when they become large enough to rupture (intraperitoneal), ulcerate (GI bleeding), or cause obstruction. They rarely spread through lymphatics, which is the mechanism for a Virchow's node.

124 **A** (S&F, ch32)

The main diagnostic challenge is differentiating the NF PET from a non-PET and also in determining whether the tumor is associated with a symptomatic tumor syndrome (e.g., insulinoma, glucagonoma, gastrinoma). Elevated plasma levels of pancreatic polypeptide do not establish the diagnosis of a PPoma even when a pancreatic mass is present. Plasma pancreatic polypeptide levels are reported to be elevated in 22% to 71% of patients with functional PETs in various studies as well as in nonpancreatic carcinoid tumors. The remainder of the statements are true.

125 **C** (S&F, ch39)

Radiation-induced liver disease is seen in approximately 5% of patients when the whole liver radiation dose reaches 30 to 35 Gy at 2 Gy per fraction. It is a clinical syndrome consisting of anicteric hepatomegaly, ascites, and elevated liver enzymes, particularly serum alkaline phosphatase, which may be elevated out of proportion to serum aminotransferase activity or serum bilirubin. Radiation-induced liver disease occurs typically between two weeks to four months after completion of radiation

therapy. Patients note fatigue, weight gain, increased abdominal girth, and occasionally right upper quadrant pain. Abdominal imaging with CT or MRI can be used in diagnosis. Radiation-induced liver disease can progress to a chronic phase, in which increasing fibrosis and liver failure can develop in patients.

126 **B** (S&F, ch32)

The somatostatin syndrome, seen in patients with somatostatinomas, is characterized by the following symptoms (93% of all patients with somatostatinomas have symptoms): abdominal pain (40%), weight loss (26%), jaundice (23%), diarrhea (18%), nausea/vomiting (16%), and hepatomegaly (22%).

127 **B** (S&F, ch29)

Diffuse large B cell lymphoma almost always involves the muscularis propria or a deeper layer when first diagnosed. Lower-grade MALT lymphoma in these tumors suggests a transition from a less aggressive to a more aggressive cell type. *TP53* and *P16* mutations may be additional factors that allow large B cells to escape their dependence on *H. pylori*, which is indicated by the response of early stages of these tumors to eradication of *H. pylori*.

128 **D** (S&F, ch35)

Although zinc deficiency is more common in patients with sickle cell disease due to renal loss of zinc, it is not a cause of acute liver damage, whereas the other diagnoses listed do cause damage. Zinc supplementation has been recommended for patients in sickle crisis in the past. Liver ischemia due to intrasinusoidal sickling can add to the toxicity of **B**, **C**, and **E**.

129 **B** (S&F, ch32)

PETs can be associated with four different inherited disorders: MEN-I, von Hippel-Lindau disease, tuberous sclerosis, and NF1 (von Recklinghausen's disease). These associations are important to recognize because family screening may be needed and because these PETs may have a different natural history. Osler-Weber-Rendu disease, otherwise known as hereditary hemorrhagic telangiectasia, has a variety of clinical manifestations (epistaxis, GI bleeding, and iron deficiency anemia), along with characteristic mucocutaneous telangiectasia and arteriovenous malformations. PETs are not common features of this disorder.

130 **A** (S&F, ch34)

CT, MRI, and endoscopic ultrasonography can give a clear view of the anatomy, particularly if there is pus present. When antibiotics covering both anaerobic and aerobic bacteria are given to patients with incipient perianal infection, far fewer patients require surgical drainage than in the past. Pain near the anal canal in a granulocytopenic patient is treated as if it were due to bacterial infection until proven otherwise. Extensive supralevator and intersphincteric abscesses may be present without being apparent on external examination. Perianal HSV infection may also lead to painful ulcerations. Perianal infections must be treated before HCT.

131　D (S&F, ch33)

The frequency of anorectal disease among homosexual AIDS patients is higher than in other AIDS patients. Anorectal squamous cell carcinomas are strikingly higher in homosexual men with AIDS. Cytologic specimens of the anal canal, similar to Papanicolaou smears, are increasingly used for screening and have high predictive value for dysplasia.

132　C (S&F, ch27)

Lymphoma is not associated with eosinophilic infiltrates, but association has been reported with the other choices. Medications reported with GI eosinophilia include carbamazine, interferon-α, tacrolimus, gemfibrozil, and enalapril. Additional diseases with GI eosinophilia include celiac disease, juvenile polyps, inflammatory fibroid polyps, and hypereosinophilic syndrome.

133　1-C, 2-D, 3-A, 4-B, 5-E (S&F, ch22)

DH is a very pruritic skin disorder characterized by vesicular or bullous lesions on the scalp, shoulders, elbows, knees, and buttocks. It is seen in association with celiac disease. Porphyria cutanea tarda is a metabolic disorder characterized by skin fragility, blisters, hypertrichosis, and hyperpigmentation in sun-exposed skin. It is associated with hepatitis C infection. Glucagonoma of the pancreas is associated with necrolytic migratory erythema of the skin, which is a rash seen around orifices, flexural regions, and the fingers. The rash is typically papulovesicular but may be in the form of erosions with fissures and crusting. Sister Mary Joseph's nodule is an umbilical metastasis of a GI carcinoma, most often a gastric cancer. Erythema nodosum appears as shiny, tender, deep, red nodules 1 cm or larger in diameter. They are seen typically in patients with IBD, in particular Crohn's disease. They are generally seen over the shins.

134　C (S&F, ch29)

Because the tumor is initiated by a response to bacterial antigen (*C. jejuni*) and diffusely involves the entire small bowel with mucosal lymphocytic proliferation (although wall thickness or mass is usually confined to the proximal bowel), the initial treatment is antibiotics for as long as six months and then chemotherapy, usually with CHOP (cyclophosphamide, hydroxydaunomycin, Oncovin [vincristine], and prednisone).

135　B (S&F, ch24)

He has acute gastric volvulus, likely associated with a hiatal hernia. The presentation of epigastric pain, unproductive retching, and inability to pass a nasogastric tube is known as Borchardt triad, typical of acute gastric volvulus. None of the other possibilities (myocardial infarction, severe GERD, cholecystitis, or intestinal obstruction) can account for these findings.

136　A (S&F, ch29)

Alpha heavy-chain lymphoma is considered to be an immune-stimulated disease from intestinal bacterial antigens. It is associated with poor hygienic living conditions in underdeveloped countries bordering the Mediterranean.

137　E (S&F, ch32)

The Whipple procedure can cure a high proportion of MEN-I/ZES patients. It is not generally recommended because of the excellent long-term prognosis of nonsurgically treated patients with small PETs (<2 cm) and because of the side effects of the Whipple procedure. Recent studies show that patients with PETs smaller than 2 cm with MEN-I1/ZES had a 100% survival rate at 15 years, which is similar to results in MEN-I patients with nonfunctional PETs smaller than 2 cm who had no increase in mortality compared with MEN-I patients without PETs. At present, the authors recommend surgical exploration only if lesions larger than 2 cm are imaged in MEN-I/ZES patients, and at surgery we do not recommend routine distal pancreatectomy, recognizing that this will rarely result in a cure but, because larger lesions are associated with more frequent liver metastases, it may decrease the liver metastasis rate. A small percentage of patients (10%-15%) with ZES develop limited metastatic disease in the liver, and a number of studies recommend surgical resection in these patients. Total gastrectomy, the only effective means to treat the gastric acid hypersecretion seen in ZES for many years, is now rarely used. It has been proposed that at the time of laparotomy for a possible cure, a parietal cell vagotomy should be performed to decrease antisecretory drug requirements in the 70% of patients who are not cured long term.

138　D (S&F, ch34)

It is important to recognize early the side effects of immunosuppressants. MMF causes watery diarrhea in as many as 30% of patients and may require dose reduction or discontinuation. The mechanism of MMF-induced diarrhea is unclear. Most cases of immunosuppressant-induced diarrhea can be managed with dose manipulation, but some are so severe that discontinuation of the immunosuppressant is required.

139　D (S&F, ch35)

The alpha heavy-chain immunoglobulin secreted is always monoclonal. As such, it can be detected by protein electrophoresis (it is located in the α_2 or β band) or by immunoelectrophoresis. The secretion of IgA is blocked by this process and allows infestation by *Giardia*. The association of Mediterranean lymphoma with living under conditions of poor sanitation suggests that the lymphoma develops due to chronic immunostimulation by overgrowth of intestinal bacteria.

140　A (S&F, ch28)

Hypoproteinemia and edema are the principal clinical manifestations of protein-losing gastroenteropathy. Dependent edema is frequently a clinically significant issue and results from diminished plasma oncotic pressure. Anasarca is rare in protein-losing gastroenteropathy. Despite a decrease in serum gamma globulin levels, increased susceptibility to infections is uncommon. Although clotting factors may be lost into the GI tract, the coagulation status typically remains unaffected.

141 **E** (S&F, ch35)

Bacterial overgrowth is often a result of impaired motility, especially in the small bowel, a feature that could be seen in any of these conditions.

142 **E** (S&F, ch32)

The key to establishing the diagnosis of insulinoma is suspecting by clinical history that the symptoms could be due to hypoglycemia and establishing the relationship of the symptoms to fasting. Organic hypoglycemia is generally defined as a fasting blood glucose level of less than 40 mg/dL. In healthy individuals, after an overnight fast, plasma glucose values usually do not decrease to less than 70 mg/dL. After an overnight fast, only 53% of patients with insulinoma have a blood glucose value less than 60 mg/dL and only 39% have a value less than 50 mg/dL. However, if a blood glucose determination is combined with a concomitant plasma insulin level, this insulin level will be inappropriately elevated in 65% of patients. C peptide and plasma proinsulin are released with the processing of insulin and so should be elevated.

143 **B** (S&F, ch23)

This patient has a Zenker's diverticulum. Presenting symptoms in patients with Zenker's diverticulum include dysphagia, regurgitation, halitosis, aspiration, voice changes, and weight loss. A barium swallow is the most useful diagnostic study. At endoscopy, it may be difficult to distinguish the lumen of the diverticula from the true lumen of the esophagus.

144 **C** (S&F, ch35)

This patient has cholestatic hepatitis related to severe extrahepatic infection/sepsis. This syndrome is frequently seen with pneumococcal infections. In the absence of ductal dilation or extrahepatic obstruction, liver function should become normal with clearing of the infection. Normalization of liver function usually occurs within several days but may take weeks if cholestasis is severe.

145 **A** (S&F, ch26)

The bacteria associated with intra-abdominal infections and abscesses in patients in the intensive care unit who have been subjected to broad-spectrum antimicrobial selection pressure are quite different from those in patients with abscesses that result from secondary bacterial peritonitis. Thus, the microbiological agents that cause tertiary peritonitis, defined as persistent intra-abdominal sepsis with or without a discrete focus of infection, generally after an operation for secondary peritonitis, are no longer *E. coli* and *B. fragilis* (see Chapter 37). Rather, nosocomial infections with resistant gram-negative organisms, *Enterococcus* species, and/or yeast are more common.

146 **E** (S&F, ch40)

All of these statements are true.

147 **D** (S&F, ch38)

Subclinical hepatitis associated with primary HSV infection is common. In pregnant or immuno-suppressed individuals, this virus may cause severe liver disease. Infection during pregnancy, particularly the third trimester, can result in fulminant hepatic failure. Affected individuals are obtunded and usually anicteric with elevated serum aminotransferase levels and coagulopathy. They may have subtle oropharyngeal or genital herpetic lesions. Encephalopathy may result from herpes encephalitis. The diagnosis of HSV infection can be confirmed by serologic testing. Liver biopsy specimens from affected patients usually demonstrate characteristic intracytoplasmic inclusion bodies and areas of focal hemorrhage. Treatment with acyclovir is effective and seems to prevent viral transmission to the fetus.

148 **C** (S&F, ch35)

This patient has tuberculous peritonitis, which can cause ascites in the absence of cirrhosis. The ascites fluid has a high protein content, low level of glucose, and low serum-to-albumin gradient. Patients with this condition usually have ascitic fluid, with an elevated WBC-count with lymphocyte predominance. The algorithm for evaluation of patients with high-lymphocyte-count ascites includes cytologic evaluation of the fluid and consideration of laparoscopy. Patients with lymphocytic ascites and fever, such as this patient, usually have tuberculosis, whereas afebrile patients usually have malignancy-related ascites. Laparoscopy is 100% sensitive in detecting tuberculous peritonitis. The level of CA 125 may be elevated in tuberculous peritonitis. Cytology is positive when peritoneal carcinomatosis is present.

149 **C** (S&F, ch31)

Periumbilical pain, borborygmi, and periumbilical tenderness all point to a disorder involving the small bowel. These symptoms, in association with weight loss, a sudden feeling of warmth, and heme-positive stools, make carcinoid tumor the most likely diagnosis. Therefore, the first best test for definitive diagnosis is an upper GI radiographic examination with small bowel follow-through. This young man is unlikely to have mesenteric angina. Although positron emission tomography may be useful if he has carcinoid tumor, that is not the next best test. Enteroclysis is a good test for the small bowel but is seldom performed today.

150 **A** (S&F, ch40)

Polyethylene glycol solutions, although considered safe for colonoscopy preparation, can cause fluid shifts in patients. All of the other statements are true.

151 **B** (S&F, ch34)

Some patients with chronic GVHD have esophageal desquamation, webs, submucosal fibrous rings, bullae, and long, narrow strictures in the upper and midesophagus. Although the most common symptom is dysphagia, some patients present with insidious weight loss, retrosternal pain, and aspiration of gastric contents. The diagnosis is made by barium contrast radiography and endoscopy, which should be done with caution because perforations have been reported.

152 C (S&F, ch32)

This patient has a tumor that is secreting growth hormone–releasing factor and causing acromegaly, as evidenced by enlargement of the hands and feet. Skin changes, headache, and peripheral nerve entrapment also occur with acromegaly. Hyperprolactinemia is observed in 70% of patients with tumors secreting growth hormone–releasing factor compared with 50% of patients with somatotroph adenomas. The diagnosis is established by demonstrating elevated plasma levels of growth hormone and insulin-like growth factor I. Octreotide is the agent of choice for treating patients with these tumors.

153 C (S&F, ch35)

This patient has secretory diarrhea as confirmed by the low osmolar gap. Some of the laboratory abnormalities seen in patients with VIPoma include hypercalcemia, hyperglycemia, hypokalemia, hypochlorhydria, and hypomagnesemia.

154 A (S&F, ch34)

This patient has a duodenal ulceration caused by HSV, showing a deep, irregular ulcer surrounded by edematous mucosa.

155 E (S&F, ch29)

Chemotherapy plus radiation gives survival rates as good as surgery plus radiation. Rituximab is a valuable adjunct to chemotherapy (monoclonal antibody that blocks the CD20 receptor on B cells).

156 D (S&F, ch39)

Prostaglandins have been investigated for their ability to protect patients from the side effects of radiation therapy. Misoprostol suppositories reduce symptoms of acute radiation enteritis in patients undergoing radiotherapy. Radiation therapy techniques play an important role in reducing the rate of complications. Use of only anterior and posterior fields should be avoided because of the high dose and large volume of bowel irradiated. Patients should be instructed to maintain a full bladder during irradiation of the pelvis because the full bladder mechanically displaces the small intestine out of the pelvis. Treatment in the prone position allows the small intestines to drop out of the radiation field.

157 E (S&F, ch25)

History obtained from children or noncommunicative adults is often unreliable. The majority of gastric and as many as 30% of esophageal foreign bodies in children are asymptomatic. As much as 40% of the time, there is no witness to the ingestion. Symptoms are thus often subtle in children, such as drooling, not wanting to eat, and failure to thrive.

158 B (S&F, ch35)

Increased risk of bleeding (as high as 4% in one report) after biopsy of a liver affected by amyloidosis has been reported. It is better to obtain tissue from other sites where bleeding can be controlled if it occurs.

159 D (S&F, ch32)

This patient has features consistent with gastrinoma or ZES, a type of PET. PETs frequently produce chromogranins or the α or β subunit of HCG, which can be localized by immunocytochemistry or by documenting elevated circulating levels. Plasma chromogranin A levels are elevated in more than 90% of patients with various PETs and carcinoid tumors. Neuron-specific enolase is also elevated in PETs. Elevated gastrin levels and parathyroid hormone support the diagnosis of ZES. MEN-I is present in 20% to 25% of patients with gastrinomas. Characteristically, hyperparathyroidism is the initial manifestation of MEN-I, usually presenting in the third decade of life, followed by the development of a PET in the fourth to fifth decades. It is important to recognize whether a patient has MEN-I because patients with and without MEN-I differ in their clinical presentation, in the possibility of surgical cure, and in the clinical and diagnostic approach to the tumor.

160 A (S&F, ch34)

Myelotoxicity is noted more frequently in patients being treated for chronic myelogenous leukemia, but it can occur in patients treated for GISTs.

161 C (S&F, ch32)

This clinical syndrome and rash are consistent with the presence of a glucagonoma. It is characterized by a specific dermatitis (migratory necrolytic erythema), weight loss, glucose intolerance, and anemia. Glucagonomas are usually suspected because of the skin rash, although occasionally the diagnosis is suspected in a patient with a pancreatic mass with weight loss or diabetes. The skin lesion is most frequently confused with pemphigus foliaceus, although a number of dermatologic lesions have also been misdiagnosed. The rash can be seen in myelodysplastic disorders, short bowel syndrome, hepatitis B infection, malnutrition, cirrhosis, celiac disease, other malignancies, malabsorptive syndromes, nutritional deficiencies, and IBD.

162 E (S&F, ch35)

The onset of gold colitis usually occurs within several weeks after the start of therapy and manifests with nausea, vomiting, diarrhea, and fever. Although it is most common in the colon, toxicity may affect the esophagus, stomach, and small bowel.

163 E (S&F, ch25)

Most patients with bezoars have a predisposing factor that decreases emptying of gastric contents. Previous gastric surgery is evident in as many as 70% to 94%. Bezoar-induced gastric ulcers can cause bleeding and gastric outlet obstruction. The Rapunzel syndrome describes trichobezoars located primarily in the stomach that extend past the pylorus into the duodenum, causing bowel obstruction or obstruction of the ampulla of Vater.

164 C (S&F, ch35)

This patient most likely has familial Mediterranean fever, which is an autosomal recessive disease. It could affect the peritoneum as well as other serous membranes. It is more frequently found in Ashkenazi Jews, Armenians, and Arabs. It is an aseptic form of recurrent peritonitis. Patients present with sporadic episodes of abdominal pain, fever, synovitis, and pleuritis. Treatment with colchicine appears to prevent attacks and can prevent fatal renal amyloidosis.

165 **C** (S&F, ch32)
All of these are characteristics of glucagonoma. Hypoaminoacidemia occurs in 26% to 100% of patients with glucagonoma, and essential fatty acid deficiencies have also been reported. Weight loss is a prominent feature; there was a mean weight loss of 20 kg in one study. The anemia is usually not severe and is usually normochromic and normocytic.

166 **D** (S&F, ch29)
Gastric lymphoma accounts for 5% of all GI neoplasms. In underdeveloped countries, the small intestine is the most common site.

167 **B** (S&F, ch34)
The abrupt onset of severe retrosternal pain, hematemesis, and painful swallowing suggests a hematoma in the wall of the esophagus, a result of retching when platelet counts are very low. Endoscopy is relatively contraindicated because many intramural hematomas represent contained perforations. The course of intramural hematomas is one of slow resolution over one to two weeks. (Refer back to the figure of the barium swallow shown with the question.)

168 **C** (S&F, ch28)
Because protein-losing gastroenteropathy is a syndrome and not a specific disease, treatment is directed at correction of the underlying disease. The goal of therapy in protein-losing gastroenteropathy is to identify the cause and direct dietary, medical, or surgical intervention, or a combination thereof, at the underlying disease. With reversal or control of the primary disease, a significant proportion of patients will have a partial or complete remission of enteric protein loss, edema, and other associated conditions.

169 **A** (S&F, ch32)
More than 50% of gastrinomas are located in the duodenum, and duodenal gastrinomas outnumber pancreatic gastrinomas by two- to fivefold in different series. Within the duodenum, gastrinomas are more frequent proximally (D1 [56%], D2 [32%], D3 [6%], and D4 [6%]). Within the pancreas, gastrinomas show a pancreatic head-to-body-to-tail ratio of approximately 1:1:2. The increased identification of duodenal gastrinomas accounts for the fact that 60% to 90% of gastrinomas are now found in the "gastrinoma triangle." This is an area formed by the junction of the cystic and bile ducts posteriorly, the junction of the second and third parts of the duodenum inferiorly, and the junction of the pancreatic neck and body medially. Gastrinomas originate in a nonduodenal/nonpancreatic abdominal location in 2% to 24% of patients in different series including in the ovary, liver and biliary tract, jejunum, mesentery, renal capsule, omentum, and pylorus.

170 **E** (S&F, ch31)
The rectum is a common site for carcinoids, and the incidence seems to be increasing. They usually appear at a younger age compared with other tumors of the colon, and the male-to-female ratio is approximately 1:1. There is a threefold higher incidence in African Americans compared with white Americans. Carcinoid syndrome due to rectal lesions is very uncommon despite the fact that low rectal carcinoids can secrete the hormones directly into the bloodstream. Rectal carcinoids can be treated in different ways: endoscopically by local excision or by low anterior or abdominoperineal resection. Because the primary determinant of outcome in patients with rectal carcinoid is the underlying tumor biology, radical surgery is not always indicated. The overall five-year survival rate is 87%.

171 **E** (S&F, ch40)
Use of cutting current during sphincterotomy has not been definitely shown to decrease the risk of post-ERCP pancreatitis. The other statements are true.

172 **E** (S&F, ch23)
Patients with large, symptomatic Zenker's diverticula should be offered surgical treatment, whereas those with small, asymptomatic or minimally symptomatic diverticula can be treated by observation alone because progressive enlargement is uncommon. Open surgical treatment may be considered in any symptomatic patient who has no contraindication to surgery. An open surgical approach is the safest alternative for patients with large (>5 cm) diverticula that extend into the thorax. Upper esophageal sphincter myotomy should always be part of the procedure. In general, compared with endoscopic techniques, open surgical procedures result in a lower recurrence rate and a greater proportion of patients obtaining symptom relief. However, the risk of complications is higher with open surgery than with endoscopic techniques.

173 **D** (S&F, ch26)
The CT diagnosis of abdominal abscess is suggested by identification of a loculated fluid density in an extraluminal location. Extraluminal gas within an abdominal mass is highly suggestive of an abscess, although necrotic tumors and resolving hematomas may occasionally exhibit this finding. Wall enhancement and adjacent inflammation favor the likelihood of infection in fluid collections. Percutaneous catheter development has allowed percutaneous aspiration drainage of abdominal abscesses combined with systemic antibiotic therapy to become the standard initial treatment of abdominal abscesses. Success rates for percutaneous aspiration drainage range from 70% to 93%. Most abdominal and pelvic abscesses can be safely accessed percutaneously.

174 **D** (S&F, ch24)
Smoking is not listed as predisposing for incisional hernias. Obesity, ascites, and aneurysm tend to increase abdominal pressure. Wound infection impairs healing of the incision.

175 **B** (S&F, ch30)
Large randomized controlled trials show no survival benefits of increasing the dose of imatinib, although there was a subtle benefit in duration of disease control with the larger dose. The intensity of [^{18}F]fluoro-2-deoxy-D-glucose uptake by the tumor on positron emission tomography is an indication of increased uptake of imatinib and favorable response to this drug. In patients in whom imatinib therapy was stopped after the initial response, there was a rapid progression, suggesting the need for lifelong therapy. The drug will inhibit the overactive kinase in the PDGFRA variant and therefore benefits this group.

176 **D** (S&F, ch31)
False-positive increases in urinary excretion of 5-HIAA can occur with dietary intake of foods that are rich in serotonin such as walnuts, pecans, bananas, and tomatoes; dietary supplements such as melatonin or serotonin; and medications such as guaifenesin, methyldopa, and isoniazid. Rifampin is not one of the medications that can cause false-positive increases in 5-HIAA in the urine.

177 **C** (S&F, ch26)
The patient has a low-output enterocutaneous fistula most likely due to radiation. Well-nourished patients without infectious complications are more likely to experience spontaneous closing. When spontaneous closure is likely, nutritional evaluation and support must be aggressively pursued. The decision to support the patient with a GI fistula with enteral or parenteral nutrition must be based on anatomic and physiologic considerations. If the fistula has a low output and is anatomically distal to the intestine, then a trial of enteral feedings should be pursued.

178 **A** (S&F, ch37)
Free air may be detected on upright chest radiograph or on upright or decubitus abdominal films, but this finding may be only 60% sensitive in detecting gut perforation. The absence of free air should not delay surgical intervention in an otherwise appropriate clinical setting. CT scan of the abdomen and pelvis, generally with both oral (occasionally rectal) and intravenous contrast, is increasingly preferred as the most sensitive and specific imaging modality for acute abdominal pain.

179 **C** (S&F, ch25)
Esophageal food impaction is the most common GI foreign body requiring medical attention in the United States. The vast majority occur in patients with an underlying predisposing esophageal pathology, most often peptic strictures, Schatzki's rings, and, increasingly, EE. Other contributing causes include altered surgical anatomy and motility disorders including achalasia and esophageal spasm.

180 **E** (S&F, ch33)
HAART decreases viral replication and, consequently, circulating HIV. There is substantial improvement in immune function that can be assessed by an increase in CD4 count, a decrease in opportunistic infections, and improved survival. The CD4 count can help predict what type of infection is more likely. Clinical signs and symptoms infrequently suggest a specific diagnosis.

181 **A** (S&F, ch25)
Although conservative management is effective in most cases of GI foreign body ingestion, it is more appropriate to perform selective endoscopy for treatment based on the location, size, and type of foreign body ingested. Medical therapies have been tried, but glucagon may cause nausea, vomiting, and distention. Nifedipine can lead to hypotension. Using a Foley catheter can be successful as much as 90% of the time, but a lack of control of the object, especially near the upper esophageal sphincter and hypopharynx, can be worrisome.

182 **A** (S&F, ch36)
Clinical symptoms of acute radiation enteritis usually appear during the third week of standard fractionated radiotherapy. Radiation-induced enteritis is rarely life-threatening except when chemotherapy is administered concurrently. Increased intestinal motility can lead to abdominal cramping, diarrhea, and nausea. These symptoms usually subside after the discontinuation of radiation. Malabsorption can occur due to the loss of intestinal crypt cells and decreased surface area for absorption. The diagnosis of acute radiation enteritis is based on the history, and no specific diagnostic tests are required. Colonoscopy should be avoided unless necessary because it poses a risk of perforation.

183 **E** (S&F, ch31)
Most appendiceal carcinoids are less than 1 cm in diameter, and very few are more than 2 cm. Most authors recommend simple appendectomy for tumors less than 1 cm and right hemicolectomy for carcinoid tumors of the appendix that are larger than 2 cm. Therefore, the correct answer is **E**. Appendiceal carcinoids have a good prognosis and have an overall 5-year survival rate of 71%. Distant metastasis is seen in 9.6% of cases at the time of diagnosis.

184 **E** (S&F, ch33)
Patients who are infected with both HIV and hepatitis C virus are more likely to be found to have active cirrhosis on biopsy and an accelerated course to clinical cirrhosis and liver failure. Factors that predict fibrosis and progression to cirrhosis in co-infected patients include older age at infection, higher ALT levels, higher levels of inflammatory activity, alcohol consumption of more than 50 g/day, and a CD4 count of less than 500 cells/mm^3. The mechanism for this rapid disease course is unknown, but it has been reported to occur in other patients who are immunocompromised.

185 **A** (S&F, ch34)
Anorexia, nausea, and/or vomiting are common after liver transplantation, particularly early in the post-transplantation course. These symptoms are often related to herpesvirus infections and medications, and thus endoscopic evaluation is necessary for diagnosis in most patients. Tacrolimus is a macrolide lactone that causes nausea, abdominal pain, and diarrhea. These side effects are dose dependent

and can be managed with a dose reduction or, more rarely, drug discontinuation. MMF has a similar side effect profile. Because HSV infection can be a serious complication, endoscopy should be performed before attributing the symptoms to a medication.

186 **B** (S&F, ch31)
Typical carcinoid syndrome is usually caused by metastatic midgut carcinoids. In typical carcinoid syndrome, tryptophan is converted to 5-hydroxy-tryptophan and then rapidly to 5-hydroxytryptamine (serotonin). Serotonin is then stored in granules or released into the circulation. Once in the circulation, the enzymes monoamine oxidase and aldehyde dehydrogenase convert serotonin to 5-HIAA, which is excreted in the urine. Therefore, patients with typical carcinoid syndrome will have elevated plasma and platelet serotonin levels and increased urinary excretion of 5-HIAA. On the other hand, atypical carcinoid syndrome is most often associated with foregut carcinoids. Patients with foregut carcinoids are deficient in the enzyme dopa decarboxylase, which is responsible for the conversion of 5-hydroxytryptophan to serotonin. Therefore, these patients have high plasma levels of 5-hydroxytryptophan and normal levels of serotonin. Urinary excretion of 5-HIAA may be normal or slightly elevated.

187 **E** (S&F, ch35)
Eosinophilic gastroenteritis is associated only with Churg-Strauss syndrome.

188 **B** (S&F, ch25)
The most common patient group that unintentionally ingests foreign bodies is children, particularly those between ages six months and three years. Accidental ingestion may also occur in adults with dental covers or dentures because of loss of tactile sensation during swallowing. Patients with altered mental status, including the very elderly, demented, or intoxicated, are at risk. Accidental coin ingestion has been noted in college-age adults who play a drinking game called "quarters," where the coin becomes lodged in the esophagus.

189 **C** (S&F, ch25)
The majority of patients with caustic ingestions can be safely started on oral liquids after 24 to 48 hours. Grade I or IIA injury is noncircumferential, and these patients can be safely fed a liquid diet after the endoscopy. In patients with grade IIB or III injuries, oral feedings may not be tolerated right away and if this is the case after 48 hours, a naso-enteric tube can be inserted.

190 **B** (S&F, ch25)
Alkaline caustic ingestion is associated with an increased risk of squamous cell cancer of the esophagus. Lye ingestion leads to a 1000-fold increased risk of esophageal cancer, so endoscopic surveillance should be performed routinely beginning at approximately 20 years after exposure.

191 **C** (S&F, ch26)
The patient has a diverticular abscess. Some small fluid collections, typically less than 3 cm, do not require catheter drainage and can be managed with percutaneous aspiration for diagnosis followed by antibiotic therapy.

192 **C** (S&F, ch32)
Treatment is directed at controlling the symptoms of hypoglycemia with diazoxide and then, after tumor localization studies, at a possible surgical cure. For the 5% to 13% of patients with metastatic insulinoma, chemotherapy or other therapies directed at the tumor itself may need to be considered. Dietary control can help improve hypoglycemic episodes by taking small frequent meals to avoid fasting. Radiation therapy is not considered a recommended treatment option.

193 **B** (S&F, ch34)
Kidney transplant recipients are at particular risk of the development of intestinal ischemia compared with other solid organ transplant recipients. However, the incidence is low (<5%) and the etiology is multifactorial. Intestinal ischemia and obstruction develop more often in recipients with polycystic kidney disease. Intestinal ischemia in this setting carries a high mortality rate. Ischemia should be considered in kidney transplant recipients with abdominal pain, particularly older patients (older than 40 years of age) who have received a cadaveric kidney.

194 **E** (S&F, ch30)
All four criteria have been validated by report. Cystic spaces are areas of tumor necrosis in the center of the larger mass. Needle biopsy is usually avoided to prevent tumor tracking if the primary decision is resection.

195 **A** (S&F, ch34)
The incidence of biliary cast syndrome has decreased to 5% to 20% and generally occurs within the first year post-OLT. Clinical factors associated with the development of biliary casts include hepatic ischemia and biliary strictures. Hepatic artery patency should be assessed by ultrasonography. Endoscopic and percutaneous therapies are successful in as many as 70%, but surgical intervention may be required, and the mortality rate is reported at 10% to 30%.

196 **B** (S&F, ch36)
Angiodysplasias are the most frequent cause of recurrent GI bleeding in patients on dialysis, especially when disease is long-standing. The first three conditions are not detectable by routine endoscopy and the last two are not infrequently missed at endoscopy.

197 **B** (S&F, ch34)
Heart and lung transplant recipients have the highest incidence of fungal infection in the solid organ transplantation setting in which *Aspergillus*, not *Candida* species, predominates.

198 **C** (S&F, ch26)
Early morbidity and mortality in the management of external fistulas result from initial fluid and electrolyte derangements that go unchecked. However, the major cause of mortality in patients with GI

fistulas is sepsis with multiple organ failure. In this setting, pooling of enteric contents occurs within the abdominal cavity and acts as a nidus where infection sets in.

199 **1-E, 2-A, 3-D, 4-C, 5-B** (S&F, ch22)

200 **S** (S&F, ch30)
Some suggestion has been made to resect areas of metastatic or bulky tumor as a source of new resistant clone formation, but continue imatinib to control the product of monoclones initially responsive. Although the improved response rate of sunitinib is low, it must be compared with 0% for the placebo group making it worthwhile.

201 **C** (S&F, ch30)
MEN-I is not associated with GIST. **A** and **B** are reported with smaller multifocal GISTs as found in the Carney triad. The *KIT* gene present with GISTs and NF is not mutated, and it is not clear whether it would respond to imatinib.

202 **C** (S&F, ch31)
The most distinctive feature of carcinoid syndrome is flushing, which is present in 30% to 94% of the patients at some time during the course of the disease. Flushing similar to carcinoid syndrome can be seen in all of the conditions listed except **C**.

203 **B** (S&F, ch28)
Enteric protein loss can be demonstrated by quantifying the concentration of α_1-antitrypsin in the stool or by measuring its clearance from the plasma; the latter is the more reliable indicator. Therefore, the optimal test is to measure the clearance of α_1-antitrypsin from the plasma during a 72-hour stool collection.

204 **A** (S&F, ch24)
Umbilical hernias will frequently resolve spontaneously, obviating surgery as long as four years postpartum. They are more common in African Americans (30%-40%) at birth. When an umbilical hernia ruptures in a cirrhotic patient, it is usually preceded by signs of maceration and ulceration, which should be an indication for repair. The occasional changes of strangulation after paracentesis mandate that the hernia be kept reduced during and after the procedure.

205 **A** (S&F, ch38)
This patient has cholestasis of pregnancy, which is a form of intrahepatic cholestasis associated with pruritus, elevated serum bile acid levels, and the findings of bland cholestasis on liver biopsy. It presents in the third trimester with intense pruritus of palms and soles and increases at night. Typically elevated serum bile acids are a feature. Improvement of symptoms and laboratory test results begins with delivery of the infant and usually, although not invariably, is prompt and complete. Cholestasis of pregnancy has serious implications for fetal well-being; therefore, prompt delivery after fetal lung maturity is recommended. Management of cholestasis of pregnancy is primarily palliative. Ursodeoxycholic acid is helpful in relieving symptoms, may reduce fetal complication rates, and is well tolerated by both the mother and fetus. Treatment with bile-acid binders such as cholestyramine and guar gum may also relieve symptoms, but it is important to keep in mind that therapy with these agents worsens steatorrhea and resultant fat-soluble vitamin deficiencies. Sedatives, such as phenobarbital, may relieve itching in cholestasis patients, but may adversely affect the fetus.

206 **D** (S&F, ch32)
The diagnosis of the VIPoma syndrome requires the demonstration of an elevated plasma concentration of VIP and the establishment of the presence of a large-volume secretory diarrhea. The volume of the diarrhea should suggest the diagnosis because in 70% to 85% of patients, the diarrhea is greater than 3 L/day and is never less than 700 mL/day. Long-acting somatostatin analogs such as octreotide and lanreotide are the agents of choice. Octreotide will control the diarrhea in both the short and long term in 78% to 100% of patients with VIPoma. In two reviews, octreotide completely abolished diarrhea in 10% of patients in one study and in 65% in the other, and it improved the diarrhea in 90% to 95% of patients. In the past, numerous drugs have been reported to control, to varying degrees, the diarrheal output in small numbers of VIPoma patients including prednisone (60-100 mg/day), clonidine, indomethacin, phenothiazines, lithium, propranolol, metoclopramide, loperamide, lidamidine, angiotensin II, and norepinephrine.

207 **E** (S&F, ch25)
Emergency surgery is required with esophagectomy or gastrectomy for perforation due to caustic ingestion. Colonic interposition is sometimes required. Because of the increased risk of perforation, ingestion of sharp objects should be followed by serial daily radiographs to ensure progression, which usually occurs without complication. If the object fails to progress over three days, surgery is usually in order. If multiple magnets are ingested, or if a magnet is ingested with other metal objects, magnetic attraction and coupling between interposed loops of bowel, with subsequent pressure necrosis, fistula formation, and bowel perforation can result.

208 **C** (S&F, ch34)
Thromboembolic phenomena were reported to have occurred in 13% to 35% of patients with glucagonoma in various series. In one series, venous thrombosis occurred in 24% of patients and pulmonary emboli in 12%. Because pulmonary embolus is life-threatening, it should be suspected in any patient with shortness of breath with glucagonoma. Weight loss is seen even in patients with small tumors without metastatic spread. Anemia, although common, is usually not severe enough to cause the symptoms listed.

209 **D** (S&F, ch35)
HUS consists of a triad of acute renal failure, microangiopathic hemolytic anemia, and thrombocytopenia. In children, idiopathic, sporadic, and epidemic cases have variously been described. In adults, HUS occurs in conjunction with complications during childbirth or chemotherapy, with mitomycin C being the most commonly implicated agent. Usually

adult HUS is preceded by a mild diarrheal illness. Enteric pathogens associated with HUS colitis include *Shigella*, *Salmonella*, *Yersinia*, *Campylobacter*, and the hemorrhagic 0157:H7 strain of *E. coli*. Because HUS is usually self-limited, therapy includes hemodialysis and supportive care.

210 **C** (S&F, ch35)
Only abdominal bloating or fullness has been shown to be an independent predictor of delayed gastric emptying. Although many diabetic patients have abnormal gastric emptying, overt clinical symptoms develop in few of them. Furthermore, an occasional patient may have symptoms suggestive of gastroparesis diabeticorum but little or no delay in gastric emptying.

211 **C** (S&F, ch34)
This patient's history is most consistent with post-transplantation lymphoproliferative disorder of the liver. Periportal nodes are likely reactive because they have not changed in size.

212 **C** (S&F, ch35)
All of the statements are correct except **C.** GAVE is actually thought to result from delayed gastric emptying. It has been proposed that recurrent gastric peristalsis causes prolapse of the loose antral mucosa with consequent elongation and ectasia of the mucosal vessels. It can be caused by portal hypertension and hepatic venous occlusive disease.

213 **D** (S&F, ch29)
CD19 and CD20 typically identify B cell antigens, which along with CD79a, CD5, CD10, and CD23, do not stain. These are used to identify the B cell population.

214 **B** (S&F, ch37)
Fluid resuscitation and antibiotic therapy followed by urgent laparotomy or laparoscopy are the mainstays of treatment for peritonitis. Glucocorticoids have been shown not to provide benefit for patients in septic shock. Vasopressor agents are generally to be avoided if possible. It should be recognized that a patient with cirrhosis may have spontaneous bacterial peritonitis, which is generally not a surgical disease.

215 **D** (S&F, ch34)
Long-term cyclosporine therapy may also lead to gallstone formation and biliary symptoms. There is a higher than expected incidence of gallstones and stone-related biliary problems after HCT than in an age-matched population, probably related to earlier formation of biliary sludge.

216 **C** (S&F, ch25)
Endoscopic removal of narcotic packets is absolutely contraindicated to avoid inadvertent rupture of the packages and release of the toxic contents. If the patient is asymptomatic, inpatient observation with a clear liquid diet is recommended. Whole-gut lavage and gentle purgatives have been reported to hasten the decontamination of the gut, but their use remains controversial because of the potential to promote package rupture. Surgery is the definitive

therapy for signs of intestinal obstruction, failure of packets to progress, and suspected rupture.

217 **C** (S&F, ch39)
Concomitant chemotherapy increases the likelihood that a patient receiving irradiation will have more side effects.

218 **C** (S&F, ch32)
The diagnosis of GRFoma should be suspected in any patient with acromegaly without a pituitary adenoma and yet associated with hyperprolactinemia, with a paradoxical growth hormone response to thyrotropin-releasing hormone or during an oral glucose tolerance test, or associated with an abdominal mass. Thus, the diagnosis should also be suspected in any patient with a pancreatic or intestinal tumor in whom clinical features of acromegaly develop.

219 **A** (S&F, ch25)
This patient presents with classic symptoms of antral stenosis, which has caused gastric outlet obstruction. Antral stenosis usually develops one to six weeks after ingestion but may not appear for several years. It seems to occur with equal frequency after acid and alkali ingestion. Endoscopic dilation has been used successfully and should be considered as an initial maneuver in patients with antral stenosis. Other options are reserved for refractory cases or patients with severe injury.

220 **A** (S&F, ch38)
The most common late complication of radiotherapy is esophageal stenosis or stricture, which appears four to six months after a course of radiotherapy. Esophageal dysmotility may be seen within four to 12 weeks after radiotherapy but may develop earlier in patients undergoing concurrent chemotherapy. A clinical syndrome of acute esophagitis with esophageal ulceration is often seen in the second or third week of standard fractionated thoracic radiotherapy. Patients often report dysphagia and odynophagia. Persistent chest pain unrelated to swallowing may develop in patients.

221 **C** (S&F, ch28)
Protein-losing enteropathy is the excessive leakage of plasma proteins into the lumen of the GI tract. Mechanisms for increased protein loss include increased mucosal permeability to protein secondary to cell damage or cell loss, mucosal erosions or ulcerations, and lymphatic obstruction. There is no evidence of maldigestion, malabsorption, or defect in protein or amino acid metabolism.

222 **A** (S&F, ch31)
The biochemical basis of flushing is not completely understood. The role of serotonin in flushing is unclear because elevated levels of serotonin have not been consistently associated with flushing. Flushing is, however, worsened with stress. Norepinephrine levels have been found to be elevated during flushing episodes. At present, the best explanation for flushing is that it is caused by the release of polypeptide hormones.

223 **D** (S&F, ch25)
Bread tabs or bread bag clips seem innocuous, but the arms can grasp mucosa, become impacted, and lead to serious complications. These clips are radiolucent and as such are not detected by conventional radiography.

224 **A** (S&F, ch24)
Alcoholism is not listed as one of the factors predisposing to recurrent inguinal hernia. Liver or renal failure, steroid therapy, and smoking are all associated with tissue deterioration. Scrotal hernia is associated with a more extensive repair.

225 **E** (S&F, ch39)
Radiation enteritis results in diarrhea, abdominal cramping, pain, nausea and vomiting, anorexia, and malaise. It occurs during the third week of a fractionated radiation course, at reported rates of 20% to 70%. Acute radiation enteropathy with diarrhea may be seen in some patients after delivery of doses of 18 to 22 Gy using conventional fractionation, and in most patients receiving doses of 40 Gy. Both the symptoms and pathologic findings typically subside and spontaneously disappear two to six weeks after completion of radiation therapy. However, there is growing evidence to suggest that patients who develop acute small intestine toxicity may be at higher risk of chronic effects. Other possibilities include bacterial overgrowth. Empirical treatment could be provided with antibiotics, loperamide, and cholestyramine.

226 **C** (S&F, ch26)
Persistently high catheter output in this scenario raises the suspicion of a fistula. A catheter study performed by instilling water-soluble contrast medium through the catheter under fluoroscopy is the best method to assess for an internal fistula as the cause of high drainage output. If a fistula is located, the catheter can be repositioned adjacent to the opening into the bowel for better control of bowel effluent. Poor clinical response can also be caused by catheter dislodgement from the major abscess cavity, undrained loculations, multiple abscesses, or new abscesses. Repeat CT can evaluate for these possible causes of poor clinical response and guide additional percutaneous interventions when appropriate. However, repeat CT scan is unlikely to be of further help and is not the best course of action in this patient.

227 **B** (S&F, ch29)
Lymphoma is the most common cause, although ulcerative jejunitis is also a known fatal complication. The diagnosis is usually made concomitantly with the diagnosis of celiac disease or shortly thereafter. It is rapidly progressive with a five-year survival rate of 20%. Observance of a gluten-free diet for more than five years reduces the risk.

228 **A** (S&F, ch22)
DH is an extremely pruritic skin disorder seen in early adulthood. All of the statements about DH are true except **A**. Less than 5% of patients with celiac disease will have DH. However, more than 80% of patients with DH have celiac disease. Gluten has been shown to be a dietary trigger of DH. Introduction of gluten to the diet of a patient with celiac disease who has been on a gluten-free diet will lead to reappearance of DH. Dapsone has been used to treat this condition.

229 **B** (S&F, ch35)
Differentiating Behçet's disease from Crohn's disease can be difficult because of similar symptoms, endoscopic findings, and extraintestinal manifestations. Surgical intervention is associated with a high rate of recurrence, with nearly 50% requiring repeat surgery.

230 **D** (S&F, ch37)
This patient likely has tuberculous ascites. Noncirrhotic patients with this form of peritonitis usually have ascites with a high protein content, low glucose concentration, and low serum-to-ascites albumin gradient of less than 1.1 g/dL. Patients almost always have an elevated ascitic fluid WBC count with a lymphocytic predominance. The algorithm in the evaluation of patients with high-lymphocyte-count ascites includes cytologic evaluation of the fluid and consideration of laparoscopy. Patients with lymphocytic ascites and fever usually have tuberculosis, whereas afebrile patients usually have malignancy-related ascites. Cancer is the cause of lymphocytic ascites approximately 10 times more frequently than is tuberculosis. If peritoneal carcinomatosis is present, the cytologic findings are positive more than 90% of the time, and laparoscopy can be avoided. If the cytology findings are negative, laparoscopy is performed and is nearly 100% sensitive in detecting tuberculous peritonitis. Tuberculous peritonitis may also appear in a miliary form or as a pelvic mass with high serum levels of CA125, making the diagnosis difficult to distinguish from metastatic ovarian cancer. Adenosine deaminase levels are typically elevated in the ascitic fluid in tuberculous ascites, and this finding can help differentiate tuberculous peritonitis from other causes of peritonitis and ascites.

231 **E** (S&F, ch23)
Diverticula located near the diaphragmatic hiatus are called epiphrenic diverticula. Congenital bronchopulmonary foregut malformations can communicate with the esophagus and present as esophageal diverticula. Traction diverticula are often related to mediastinal inflammation associated with tuberculosis and histoplasmosis. Enlarged mediastinal lymph nodes from lung malignancies can also lead to traction diverticula. Approximately 80% are associated with motility disorders such as achalasia, diffuse esophageal spasm, hypertensive lower esophageal sphincter, and nonspecific motilitiy disorders. Epiphrenic diverticula have been reported as a complication of obesity surgery.

232 **E** (S&F, ch35)
Mycobacterial involvement of the bowel by either *Mycobacterium tuberculosis* or MAC may lead to diarrhea, abdominal pain, and, rarely, obstruction or bleeding. In some series of patients, MAC was the most common organism identified in

patients with chronic diarrhea and low CD4 counts. Duodenal involvement is most common and may be suspected at endoscopy by the presence of yellow mucosal nodules, often in association with malabsorption, bacteremia, and systemic infection.

233 B (S&F, ch40)
Although it is a common practice to stop aspirin and NSAIDs 7 days before an elective endoscopic procedure, these drugs have never been shown clearly to increase the risk of bleeding during an endoscopic procedure. On the other hand, patients receiving an anticoagulant are at an increased risk of bleeding during procedures; to decrease the risk, warfarin, a long-acting anticoagulant, needs to be temporarily stopped and short-acting low-molecular-weight heparin should be substituted before endoscopy.

234 D (S&F, ch26)
The symptoms and signs of intra-abdominal abscess are nonspecific, and a high level of clinical suspicion and vigilance is needed to make the diagnosis. Fever and elevated leukocyte count are frequent but nonspecific findings. Abdominal pain, tenderness to palpation, distention, and a palpable mass are also common findings. Suspicion of the presence of an IAA warrants further diagnostic imaging. CAT with intravenous and oral contrast medium is the imaging modality of choice for the diagnosis of most abdominal abscesses.

235 B (S&F, ch24)
The intermittent nature of the symptoms and dilated bowel suggest small bowel obstruction. Internal hernia after Roux-en-Y gastric bypass occurs in as many as 4% of patients. The usual sites of herniation are the mesentery of the transverse colon adjacent to the Roux-en-Y limb, which is fashioned to penetrate that mesentery en route to a gastric anastomosis, and the area of jejunojejunostomy where the jejunum is divided to form the Roux loop. The jejunal mesentery should be closed after transection, but this does not always prevent herniation.

236 D (S&F, ch36)
GAVE or watermelon stomach is a vascular lesion of the gastric antrum that consists of tortuous, dilated vessels radiating outward from the pylorus like the spokes on a wheel and resembling the stripes on a watermelon. This lesion can cause both occult bleeding and acute hemorrhage. This condition is seen particularly in middle-aged or older women with achlorhydria, atrophic gastritis, or cirrhosis; with calcinosis cutis, Raynaud's phenomenon, esophageal dysfunction, sclerodactyly, and telangiectasia (CREST syndrome); or after bone marrow transplantation. This 65-year-old man presenting with hematemesis and a history of NSAID use does not fit the classic picture of a patient with GAVE.

237 E (S&F, ch30)
Additional tumors on the list include ovarian carcinoma, neuroblastoma, rare lymphoma, and acute myeloid leukemia. The presence of *KIT* (CD117)

staining does not imply that the gene is mutated or even causative in that tumor. It simply indicates that it is present.

238 B (S&F, ch32)
Ultrastructurally, the pancreatic endocrine cells often have electron-dense granules and produce multiple regulatory hormones and amines, neuron-specific enolase, synaptophysin, and chromogranin A or C. These cells are thought to give rise to carcinoid tumors, medullary carcinomas of the thyroid, melanomas, and pheochromocytomas, and there are marked similarities in the histology of these tumors and PETs. Histologically, PETs consist of a relatively homogeneous sheet of small round cells with uniform nuclei and cytoplasm. Mitotic figures are uncommon. Crypt distortion refers to colonic pathology.

239 C (S&F, ch29)
Although based on small studies, it has been suggested that *Campylobacter* is associated with immunoproliferative small intestinal disease (Mediterranean lymphoma). *Giardia* can be present, but is not thought to initiate the pathology.

240 D (S&F, ch33)
Patients with esophageal candidiasis generally report substernal dysphagia. Odynophagia, when present, is usually not severe. The definitive diagnosis is made by upper endoscopy findings of focal or diffuse plaques and biopsy findings of desquamated epithelial cells with typically appearing yeast forms. Although CMV is the pathogen most commonly identified with AIDS, *Candida* is more often associated with esophageal disease. CMV causes ulcerations that are large and deep. Biopsy allows demonstration of this viral cytopathic effect. Dysphagia is much less common than in patients with *Candida* esophagitis, and fever is often present. HSV esophagitis is uncommon in persons with AIDS. The disease follows a predictable sequence: discrete vesicles form and then shallow ulcers that coalesce into regions of diffuse shallow ulceration. Biopsy specimens are likely to show epithelial cell invasion and nuclear changes typical of herpes infections.

241 B (S&F, ch38)
During pregnancy, maternal blood volume increases progressively until, by the 30th week of gestation, it is 50% greater than normal, remaining so until confinement. This volume expansion, attributed to the effects of steroid hormones and elevated plasma levels of aldosterone and renin, is responsible for dilution of some blood constituents, such as red blood cells (physiologic anemia). Pregnancy causes an alteration in bile composition, including cholesterol supersaturation, decreased chenodeoxycholic acid and increased cholic acid concentrations, and an increase in the size of the bile acid pool. These changes are associated with greater residual gallbladder volumes in both the fasting and fed states. The absorptive capacity of the small intestine increases during pregnancy to meet the metabolic demands of the fetus; increased absorption of calcium, amino acids, and vitamins has been

demonstrated. Transit time of intestinal contents is prolonged during gestation; delayed small bowel transit is most pronounced during the third trimester and is associated with slowing of the migratory motor complex. Although the total serum protein concentration diminishes during pregnancy, there is actually a massive increase in the production of proteins during gestation.

242 **D** (S&F, ch35)
Malabsorption with steatorrhea is present in as many as one third of scleroderma patients and is due to bacterial overgrowth. Antibiotic therapy can be effective, but D-xylose malabsorption is often incompletely reversed, suggesting that collagen deposition may also contribute to malabsorption.

243 **B** (S&F, ch29)
The best response rate that one can expect with antibiotics for MALT lymphoma is 75%. The other 25% of cases are refractory because of the type of mutation in the tumor or more extensive disease (stage II E) involving transmural tumor or regional nodes. Those who respond to antibiotics have a 90% chance to remain in remission for three years.

244 **C** (S&F, ch34)
Recurrence of HCV in the liver allograft is nearly universal, with signs of liver damage developing in 75% of patients and 25% progressing to cirrhosis within five years, which leads to increased graft loss.

245 **A** (S&F, ch40)
The high association of underlying esophageal pathology accompanying food bolus impactions makes the practice of forceful blind pushing with the endoscope unacceptable. Esophageal muscular relaxation induced by sedation and expansion of the lumen with air insufflation may help food boluses pass with a gentle nudge forward with the tip of the endoscope, termed the push technique.

246 **C** (S&F, ch25)
A careful history is important in eliciting risk factors for foreign body impaction. Physical examination findings tend to be unremarkable or nonspecific, but the examination must be carefully performed to recognize complications of foreign body ingestions such as perforation. Plain radiographs of the chest and abdomen can help determine the presence, type, and location of the foreign body. Radiographic contrast studies are relatively contraindicated in the evaluation of foreign body ingestions. Barium esophagography should not be performed because it may make the performance of subsequent therapeutic endoscopy more difficult.

247 **B** (S&F, ch38)
Sedation with meperidine (pregnancy category B), which crosses the blood-brain barrier more slowly than fentanyl (pregnancy category C) and morphine (pregnancy category C), is preferred, although fentanyl may be superior during lactation because it is poorly excreted in breast milk. Sedation with benzodiazepines (pregnancy category D) should be avoided, especially during the first trimester, because diazepam has been reported to cause fetal malformations. Extensive experience with propofol

(pregnancy category B) is lacking, and its high lipid solubility is a reason for concern. The National Commission on Radiation Protection recommends limiting exposure to ionizing radiation during pregnancy to less than 5 cGy. The potential for radiation damage to the fetus is determined by dose and gestational age at the time of exposure.

248 **B** (S&F, ch26)
The patient has a diverticular abscess that did not resolve with intravenous antibiotics alone. The next step is percutaneous drainage. Catheter management is generally preferred for larger collections in most institutions; however, one-step percutaneous needle aspiration of abdominal and pelvic abscesses combined with systemic antibiotics has also been advocated as an alternative to catheter placement in larger abscesses.

249 **A** (S&F, ch32)
PETs account for 1% to 10% of tumors arising in the pancreas. The overall prevalence of functional PETs is low, reported to be approximately 10 per million population (or 1 per 100,000). In contrast, the prevalence of PETs in autopsy studies is higher at 0.5% to 1.5%. The annual incidence of PETs is reported at one to four cases per million per year. Nonfunctional PETs account for 14% to 30% of all PETs in most studies, but they are as high as 60% to 80% in some studies. Insulinomas and gastrinomas occur with an equal annual incidence of 0.5 to three cases per million population. VIPomas are one eighth as common and glucagonomas 1/17 as common as insulinomas and gastrinomas. Somatostatinomas are very rare, and the incidence of GRFomas, PETs secreting renin, erythropoietin, or leutenizing hormone or causing hypercalcemia is unknown.

250 **C** (S&F, ch29)
At this stage, lymphoma has invaded the serosa into adjacent structures or local lymph nodes. Surgery would consist of total gastrectomy with major symptomatic and nutritional effects. Chemoradiation with or without rituximab has shown equally effective results. Radiation is usually recommended (80% of patients survive five years disease free).

251 **E** (S&F, ch34)
The risk of cancer in long-lived transplant recipients is higher than in the general population, particularly for lymphomas; skin, colorectal, and anal cancers; and Kaposi sarcoma.

252 **E** (S&F, ch30)
Photophobia has not been reported. Myelotoxicity is much less common. Edema is the most common (74%). Diarrhea is seen in 45%.

253 **D** (S&F, ch23)
Zenker's diverticula are acquired and develop when abnormally high pressures occurring during swallowing lead to protrusion of mucosa through an area of anatomic weakness in the pharynx termed Killian's triangle. High pressures are generated when the opening of the upper esophageal sphincter is impaired. Squamous cell cancer may

develop in Zenker's diverticula. Bleeding may occur from ulcerated Zenker's diverticula, and medications may become lodged in a diverticulum. Squamous cell cancer may develop in Zenker's diverticula.

254 **A** (S&F, ch32)
Hypergastrinemia can be detected in 50% of patients with ovarian cancer. Gastric symptoms occur in some patients with bronchogenic carcinoma, acoustic neuroma, pheochromocytoma, or colorectal cancer; however, hypergastrinemia is not seen.

255 **D** (S&F, ch36)
It must be absolutely confirmed that this patient does not have an aortoenteric fistula, which usually is seen between the third and fourth portions of the duodenum. Although a clean-based duodenal bulb ulcer was found on upper endoscopy, the likelihood of this patient bleeding from that is small. That, together with the fact that he had a similar episode of melena two to three days earlier (which could have been a herald bleed from the aortoenteric fistula), suggests that CT of the abdomen is indicated and that the patient needs to be hospitalized. No test is diagnostic for an aortoenteric fistula; therefore, if CT of the abdomen fails to show any abnormality and he continues to have melena, surgical intervention is needed. Repeating EGD with a pediatric colonoscope to visualize the third part of the duodenum is acceptable practice but only when it is performed the same day.

256 **E** (S&F, ch35)
Significant risk factors associated with severe events are listed in the other options. Use of cyclooxygenase-2 inhibitors results in a lower incidence of GI complications than that seen with nonselective NSAIDs.

257 **C** (S&F, ch25)
Food impaction is the most common ingested foreign body in the United States. An increased risk of complications is thought to be proportional to the duration of esophageal food impaction. Endoscopic intervention should be achieved at the latest within 24 hours of onset of symptoms and more ideally within the first six to 12 hours. The primary method to treat food impaction is the push method, with success rates well over 90%. Eosinophilic esophagitis has increasingly been associated with esophageal food impactions.

258 **E** (S&F, ch24)
All of the procedures listed can create an opening in the mesentery of the large or small bowel that can permit internal herniation.

259 **D** (S&F, ch26)
A potential adjunct to TPN in the management of the patient with a GI fistula is the use of a long-acting somatostatin analog such as octreotide or lanreotide. Octreotide has been shown to decrease fistula output by three mechanisms. First, it inhibits the release of gastrin, cholecystokinin, secretin, motilin, and other GI hormones. This inhibition decreases secretion of bicarbonate, water, and

pancreatic enzymes into the intestine, subsequently decreasing intestinal volume. Second, octreotide relaxes intestinal smooth muscle, thereby allowing a greater intestinal capacity. Third, octreotide increases intestinal water and electrolyte absorption. At this time, the role of octreotide is limited to occasional use in high-output fistulas.

260 **E** (S&F, ch35)
All of the features listed can be seen in any of the three disorders. The important distinction is that, unlike scleroderma, the esophageal motility disturbances seen in mixed connective tissue disease seem to improve with administration of glucocorticoids.

261 **A**, false; **B**, true; **C**, true; **D**, false; **E**, true (S&F, ch40)

262 **A** (S&F, ch34)
Eosinophilic colitis with diarrhea has been reported with the use of both tacrolimus and cyclosporine. Histologically, this is characterized by eosinophilic colonic infiltrates and peripheral eosinophilia, or elevated serum IgE may be present in some patients.

263 **D** (S&F, ch22)
Cutaneous manifestations are more common and more specific in Crohn's disease than in ulcerative colitis. The most common cutaneous complication of Crohn's disease is granulomatous lesion of the skin, which can occur by direct extension of the underlying bowel disease. Pyostomatitis vegetans is characterized by pustules, erosions, and vegetations involving the buccal mucosa, gingival mucosa, and skin of the axilla, scalp, genitalia, and trunk. Diagnosis of pyostomatitis vegetans is by biopsy, and treatment is by local or systemic steroids. Pyoderma gangrenosum presents as painful ulcerations and is more common in those with ulcerative colitis than in those with Crohn's disease.

264 **A** (S&F, ch35)
Glucagonomas are glucagon-secreting tumors associated with hyperglucagonemia (necrolytic migratory erythema). The lesions wax and wane in a cycle of approximately 10 days, beginning with an erythematous patch that blisters centrally, erodes, and then crusts over and heals with hyperpigmentation. Hyperglucagonemia can be found as part of a polyfunctional endocrine tumor or an exclusively glucagon-producing tumor. The tumor may be part of a clinical syndrome (e.g., ZES). Although most glucagonomas appear to be sporadic, in approximately 3% of cases they occur in the setting of MEN-I.

265 **E** (S&F, ch37)
This patient likely has retroperitoneal fibrosis. Although many cases are idiopathic, a cause can be identified 30% of the time, including drugs, malignancy, trauma, and inflammation. Most of the reported cases have been drug induced (methysergide, ergotamine). The process of fibrosis may lead to ureteral or vascular obstruction. Successful treatment with immunosuppressive agents such as steroids and azathioprine has been reported.

266 E (S&F, ch24)

This syndrome is seen after repair of large incisional hernias. Respiratory motion of the diaphragm is weakened preoperatively because it does not contract against the pressure of a fixed abdominal volume but forces viscera out into the large hernia. Postoperatively, the weakened diaphragm and the increase in fixed abdominal volume increase pressure on the lungs causing decreased central venous return and pulmonary failure. Assisted ventilation is needed urgently.

267 A (S&F, ch26)

This patient has large-volume diarrhea suggestive of a fistula originating in the small bowel. Early management is directed at fluid and electrolyte replacement in these patients.

268 C (S&F, ch34)

The risk of hepatocellular carcinoma is particularly elevated after HCT. Transplantation survivors with risk factors for hepatocellular carcinoma (hepatitis C or B infection, obesity, diabetes, low platelet count) should be screened at yearly intervals. Chronic hepatitis C may also be a risk factor for the development of lymphoma and other lymphoproliferative disorders after transplantation.

269 D (S&F, ch34)

In patients presenting with acute hepatitis, blood sampling for viral DNA or RNA or liver biopsy is essential to exclude acute viral hepatitis due to herpesvirus (HSV or VZV) or hepatitis virus and to make a definitive diagnosis of hepatic GVHD. A serum autoantibody test may prove useful in the diagnosis of hepatic GVHD because this enzyme seems to be a target antigen in GVHD (see figure).

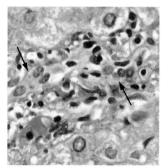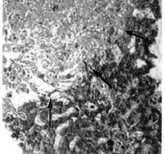

Figure for answer **269**

270 B (S&F, ch25)

Patients with esophageal food bolus impactions are symptomatic with complete or intermittent obstruction. They are unable to drink liquids or retain their own oral secretions. Sialorrhea is common. Ingestion of an unappreciated small sharp object including obscured fish or animal bones may cause odynophagia or a persistent foreign body sensation due to mucosal laceration. The type of symptoms can aid in determining whether an esophageal foreign object is still present. With dysphagia, odynophagia, or dysphonia, there is an 80% likelihood that a foreign body is present causing at least partial obstruction. If symptoms are restricted to

retrosternal chest pain or pharyngeal discomfort, less than 50% of patients will still have a foreign body present. Patient localization of an ingested foreign body is not accurate, with only 30% to 40% correct localization in the esophagus and essentially 0% accuracy in the stomach.

271 C (S&F, ch31)

Patients with a new diagnosis of carcinoid tumor should undergo cross-sectional imaging at the level of the tumor and liver, where metastatic disease is most likely to be located. Positron emission tomography is useful in these cases because it can identify disease throughout the body. Visualization of the primary tumor is more difficult than delineation of metastatic disease; therefore, **C** is an incorrect statement.

272 B (S&F, ch25)

Once the esophageal food impaction has been cleared, the presence of underlying esophageal pathology, reported in as many as 86% to 97% of patients, should be assessed. However, in the acute setting, there is usually considerable mural edema and mucosal erythema and abrasion, making it difficult to discriminate an acute from a chronic process. More than half of patients with this condition have abnormal results on a 24-hour pH study, and nearly half have esophageal dysmotility on manometry. A PPI may be prescribed and elective outpatient endoscopy scheduled after acute mural inflammation has had a chance to resolve. Patients should be educated about the methods to reduce the risk of food bolus impactions. Instructions include eating more slowly, chewing foods thoroughly, and avoiding troublesome foods.

273 C (S&F, ch36)

This patient has superior mesenteric artery syndrome, a condition in which the third part of the duodenum is compressed by the root of the superior mesenteric artery, leading to symptoms of intestinal obstruction. Typical symptoms include episodic epigastric distress, vomiting, and, in severe cases, weight loss. Diagnosis is by barium study, which typically shows an abrupt cutoff in the third part of the duodenum, with proximal dilation (particularly when the patient is supine). The syndrome has been associated with immobilization in a body cast, rapid growth in children, and marked rapid weight loss in adults. Treatment includes small feedings or a liquid diet; symptoms generally improve after body weight is gained. Surgery is rarely needed. Duodenojejunostomy has been performed laparoscopically.

274 E (S&F, ch32)

Because PPIs can elevate fasting serum gastrin levels as much as three- to fivefold, a range that overlaps with the gastrin levels in 60% of patients with ZES, it is difficult to diagnose ZES when the patient is taking PPIs. Therefore, if the fasting gastrin is elevated while taking a PPI, the fasting gastrin level testing should be performed after stopping the PPI for at least one week. However, abruptly stopping PPIs can lead to the rapid development of peptic complications in a small percentage of ZES patients. In patients with fasting serum gastrin levels less than 10-fold increased (i.e., usually <1000 pg/mL) and gastric pH of less than 2, which includes 60% of those with ZES, other conditions such as gastric outlet obstruction, *H. pylori* infection, renal failure (rarely), short bowel syndrome, antral G cell hyperfunction/hyperplasia, and retained gastric antrum syndrome can mimic ZES and need to be considered. In such patients, secretin and basal acid output tests should be performed.

275   **A** (S&F, ch34)
During the first month after OLT, infections include those present before transplantation (e.g., urinary tract infection), those related to technical complications of the procedure itself (e.g., biliary sepsis), and those transmitted with the allograft. Opportunistic viral, fungal, and parasitic infections are more likely to develop after the first month, with herpesvirus infections being the most common (see figure).

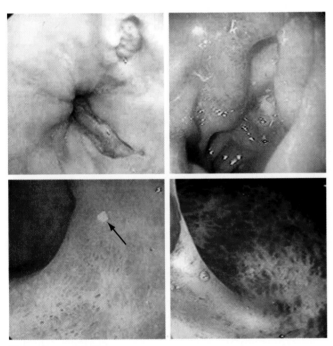

Figure for answer **275**

276   **E** (S&F, ch25)
Serious complications of esophageal foreign bodies include perforation, abscess, mediastinitis, pneumothorax, fistula formation, and cardiac tamponade.

277   **B** (S&F, ch32)
ZES is caused by ectopic secretion of gastrin by a PET (i.e., gastrinoma), which causes excessive gastric acid secretion, characteristically causing peptic disease (often severe), GERD, and diarrhea. High serum gastrin levels stimulate the growth of the gastric mucosa, resulting in large gastric folds with not only parietal cell hyperplasia but also proliferation of gastric enterochromaffin-like cells, which secrete histamine. The proliferation of enterochromaffin-like cells results in enterochromaffin-like cell hyperplasia, which can lead to the development of gastric carcinoid tumors (ECLomas), especially in patients with ZES and MEN-I.

278   **E** (S&F, ch40)
Acute pancreatitis is the most common and most feared complication of ERCP. The risk factors for ERCP include both patient and procedural factors. Young age, female sex, and suspected sphincter of Oddi dysfunction, all of which are present in this patient, put her at an increased risk of post-ERCP pancreatitis. Prescribing ursodiol (Actigall, Urso) or an anticholinergic agent is not going to affect her symptoms significantly. Use of cutting current for ERCP has not been shown definitely to reduce the risk of post-ERCP pancreatitis. Placing a temporary pancreatic duct stent at the time of ERCP has been shown to significantly reduce the risk of post-ERCP pancreatitis in high-risk patients such as this one. Sending her to a surgeon at this point for bile duct exploration would be inappropriate.

279   **B** (S&F, ch22)
Acrodermatitis enteropathica is a superficial scaling and blistering condition of the skin seen mainly in the groin area and periorally. It is often associated with alopecia. Replacement with zinc leads to rapid resolution of both alopecia and skin lesions. It is usually seen in patients with Crohn's disease, those on hyperalimentation, in children with congenital metabolic disorders, and in alcoholics with cirrhosis.

280   **B** (S&F, ch33)
CMV is the most commonly identified pathogen in AIDS. It causes mucosal ulceration, and co-infection with *Candida* is common.

281   **E** (S&F, ch26)
The typical abscess that forms as a complication of secondary bacterial peritonitis, defined as loss of integrity of the GI tract, is a mixed aerobic and anaerobic infection. Most abscesses contain mixed aerobic and anaerobic flora (60%-75%); a minority contains aerobic isolates only (10%-20%) or anaerobic isolates only (15%-20%). The number of anaerobic isolates has always been found to be greater than the number of aerobic isolates.

282   **B** (S&F, ch31)
The rectum is a common site for the occurrence of carcinoids and the incidence seems to be increasing. Rectal carcinoids appear at a younger age compared with other colon tumors. Men and women are equally affected, but the incidence in African Americans is three times that in whites. More than 80% of rectal carcinoids are still localized at the time of diagnosis. They can be treated endoscopically, by local excision, and by radical excision with either low anterior or abdominoperineal resection. Rectal carcinoids greater than 2 cm in diameter have a 60% to 80% chance of metastasis.

283   **E** (S&F, ch36)
This patient has pseudoxanthoma elasticum, which is a rare disorder characterized by aberrant calcification of mature elastic tissue. Skin lesions are usually the initial manifestation, appearing in the second decade as yellow to orange papules in the lateral neck ("plucked chicken skin"). Major complications of this condition such as retinal bleeding, intermittent claudication, premature onset of

coronary artery disease, and GI bleeding are the result of calcification of the elastic tissue of the arteries. GI bleeding occurs in 8% to 13% of the patients, and younger patients are more likely to be affected. GI bleeding is usually from the stomach, and often no specific bleeding site is found. Skin lesions may not be visible at the time of a GI bleed; therefore, a blind skin biopsy may be needed to make the diagnosis.

284 **B** (S&F, ch35)
The NSAIDs are most commonly associated with upper GI complications such as perforation, ulcers, and bleeding. Less commonly recognized complications include pill esophagitis, small bowel ulceration, strictures of the small and large intestine, and exacerbations of diverticular disease and inflammatory bowel disease.

285 **C** (S&F, ch31)
The most common site for carcinoid tumors is the ileum, not the appendix. It is true that carcinoid tumors of the esophagus are rare. The stomach is the most common location in the foregut for carcinoid tumors.

286 **E** (S&F, ch35)
The dysphagia common in persons with Sjögren syndrome is aggravated by xerostomia and frequently not associated with esophageal motility disturbance. GAVE is present in 25% of these patients. Among patients with primary biliary cirrhosis, Sjögren syndrome is common.

287 **D** (S&F, ch26)
The bacteria associated with intra-abdominal infections and abscesses in patients in the intensive care unit who have been subjected to broad-spectrum antimicrobial selection pressure are quite different from those in patients with abscesses that result from secondary bacterial peritonitis. The microbiological analysis of abscesses in severely ill patients (APACHE [Acute Physiology and Chronic Health Evaluation] II score >15) revealed that 38% had monomicrobial infections. The most common organisms were *Candida* (41%), *Enterococcus* (31%), and *Enterobacter* (21%) species and *Staphylococcus epidermidis* (21%); *E. coli* and *Bacteroides* species accounted for only 17% and 7%, respectively.

288 **E** (S&F, ch36)
Dieulafoy's lesion can result in a massive GI bleed, usually from the stomach, but the bleed can occur anywhere in the GI tract or even outside the GI tract (e.g. in the bronchus). The vascular abnormality consists of an artery of large caliber in the submucosa, and in some cases the mucosa, with a small overlying mucosal defect. These lesions are twice as common in men as in women and present at a mean age of 52 years. The diagnosis is best made by early endoscopy.

289 **C** (S&F, ch35)
Because bacterial infection is believed to be a major stimulant of the immune cells in this tumor, antibiotics should be tried first if the tumor is confined to the mucosa. Response rates range from 33% to 71%. If no response has been noted by six months after a course of antibiotic therapy or if the patient has advanced disease at presentation, chemotherapy with CHOP (cyclophosphamide, hydroxydaunomycin, Oncovin [vincristine], and prednisone) is preferred.

290 **A** (S&F, ch26)
Surgical therapy remains the mainstay of management of the complex fistula that either is not a candidate for conservative management or has had a prolonged course of conservative management (more than six weeks) without resolution of fistulous output. Indications for early surgery include inability to control the fistula without surgical drainage, sepsis or abscess formation, distal intestinal obstruction, bleeding, and persistence of fistulous output not responsive to conservative management.

291 **D** (S&F, ch40)
This patient most likely has postpolypectomy coagulation syndrome, which is characterized by a full-thickness electrocautery burn after polypectomy. Patients with this condition usually present, as in this case, with localized abdominal pain, fever, and leukocytosis without any evidence of free air on a scout film. In mild cases, the patient can be discharged home on antibiotics, but this patient needs to be observed in the hospital. It would only be by coincidence that diverticulitis would develop a day after a patient underwent colonoscopy, so this diagnosis is not likely.

292 **E** (S&F, ch38)
The majority of IBD patients require several medications to remain symptom free. Limited reliable safety data are available on the most commonly used IBD drugs; thus, it is important to carefully review the possible risks and known benefits of therapy with patients before conception. The 5-aminosalicylates (all pregnancy category B except osalazine, which is pregnancy category C) are widely used during pregnancy to treat mild IBD. A prospective study of pregnant patients treated with mesalamine, as well as a large case series, did not show any increased risk of teratogenicity from this therapy. Azathioprine and its metabolite 6-mercaptopurine (pregnancy category D) also are commonly used as maintenance treatments in patients with mild to moderate IBD. They both cross the placenta and are excreted in breast milk. However, data regarding the use of these agents in the transplantation setting have failed to confirm a study of pregnant IBD patients treated with 6-mercaptopurine that failed to demonstrate an increase in preterm delivery, spontaneous abortion, congenital abnormalities, or childhood neoplasia. Based on these data and extensive experience with this drug and its metabolites in pregnant women, experts concur that their discontinuation before or during pregnancy is not advisable. Instead, dose reduction and careful monitoring of metabolite levels in the mother are recommended. Glucocorticoids (pregnancy category C) have been used for decades to treat pregnant patients with moderate to severe IBD as well as other more common glucocorticoid-responsive diseases such as asthma. Experts have

suggested that therapy with antibodies against tumor necrosis factor-α be discontinued early in the third trimester to avoid significant fetal exposure until better data on the safety of these agents are available.

293 **C** (S&F, ch33)

Drug-induced liver injury has emerged as the most prevalent cause of abnormal findings on liver function tests in HIV-infected patients, largely due to the increasing array of antiretroviral medications used in their care. The protease inhibitors, especially ritonavir, are the most common causes of abnormal liver function test results in these patients. The major risk factors for drug-induced hepatotoxicity include coexistent viral hepatitis, older age, and greater increase in CD4 cells after HAART. The abnormalities usually follow a hepatocellular pattern.

294 **1-D, 2-E, 3-B, 4-A, 5-C** (S&F, ch22)

Glossodynia (burning sensation or pain in the tongue) may occur as a result of a deficiency of magnesium, vitamin B_{12}, or folate. In addition, it may also be found with anxiety or depression. Glossitis or inflammation of the tongue occurs in a heterogeneous group of disorders including ingestion of chemical irritants, nutritional deficiencies, iron deficiency, and pernicious anemia. Xerostomia or dry mouth is often seen in patients with Sjögren syndrome. Black hairy tongue is often seen in long-term smokers and occurs due to exogenous pigment trapped within the elongated keratin strands of the filiform papillae. Although dysgeusia may occur in association with glossitis, it is also seen in a variety of psychiatric disorders.

295 **B** (S&F, ch27)

Skin patch testing will demonstrate non–IgE-mediated allergy, but the predictive value is poor. Skin prick tests are dependent on the pure quality of the material used. Both skin prick and radioallergosorbent tests are only for IgE-mediated allergic reaction. Most food protein allergens are not IgE dependent, and these tests are not of value. Milk protein is the basis of allergy in most young children, although 50% are also allergic to soy. Elimination diet is the gold standard.

296 **B** (S&F, ch22)

Pellagra is characterized by symmetrical, brown-red blistering or scaling plaques, usually in sun-exposed areas of the body. It can occur with any of the conditions listed except VIPoma.

297 **E** (S&F, ch35)

The pathogenesis of diabetic autonomic neuropathy is related to hyperglycemia, neurovascular insufficiency, autoimmune damage, and neurohormonal growth factor deficiency. Motility disturbances are common in these patients, but do not correlate well with the presence or severity of symptoms. Gastric emptying, largely under the control of the vagus nerve, is grossly disturbed. Phase 3 contractions are frequently absent. The pathophysiology of these motor disturbances is unclear. High plasma levels of gut peptide motilin are reported in gastroparesis diabeticorum.

298 **D** (S&F, ch24)

The diagnosis of a Bochdalek hernia at birth can be a dire surgical emergency. Most of the large hernias with pulmonary hypoplasia can be detected in utero with fetal ultrasonography. The surgical team is then prepared at birth to artificially oxygenate the neonate before repairing the hernia.

299 **C** (S&F, ch25)

All the statements about disk batteries are true except that less than 10% of younger children will become symptomatic. Once in the stomach or small intestine, button batteries rarely cause clinical problems, with 85% passing within 72 hours.

300 **E** (S&F, ch35)

Acute liver failure occurs with adult Still's disease. It resembles autoimmune hepatitis and may respond to immunosuppressant drug therapy. It is the most common cause of death in patients with Still's disease, in contrast to the more benign disease seen in an uncomplicated case of rheumatoid arthritis.

301 **E** (S&F, ch25)

Once a GI foreign body passes through the esophagus, the majority will pass through the entire GI tract without further difficulty or complication. Exceptions are sharp, long, and large objects. Sharp or pointed objects may have a perforation rate as high as 35%. Large objects (>2.5 cm [1 inch] in diameter) may not pass through the pylorus. Long objects (>5 cm [2 inches] in length) such as pens, pencils, and eating utensils may not negotiate around the duodenal sweep. Objects may become obstructed at the ligament of Treitz or at the ileocecal valve.

302 **C** (S&F, ch32)

In various series, a carcinoid tumor develops in 0% to 10% of NF1 patients, usually in the periampullary region (54%) of the duodenum. Most of these duodenal carcinoids are somatostatinomas by immunocytochemistry, but they rarely produce the somatostatinoma syndrome. NF1 has rarely been associated with ZES and insulinomas. NF1 accounts for 48% of all duodenal somatostatinomas and approximately 25% of all ampullary carcinoid tumors.

303 **A** (S&F, ch32)

As many as 33% of patients with pancreatic GRFomas have MEN-I, 40% have Cushing syndrome due to an adrenocorticotropic hormone–producing pancreatic tumor, and 40% have ZES. Neither VIPomas nor lymphomas are associated with GFRomas to a large extent.

304 **D** (S&F, ch35)

While Hodgkin's disease may involve extrahepatic bile ducts or lymph nodes in the porta hepatis and cause extrahepatic obstruction, multiple reports describe an additional syndrome of *idiopathic intrahepatic cholestasis*. It appears unrelated to hepatic infiltration, extrahepatic obstruction, or other causes. The cholestasis is often out of proportion to the tumor burden. The cholestasis can resolve in response to systemic therapy, but in rare cases can result in fatal liver disease. Recent documentation suggests the stasis results from loss of small intrahepatic ducts either from tumor cell invasion of bile duct epithelial cells or the indirect effects of tumor cell cytokines.

305 **E** (S&F, ch28)
This patient has giant hypertrophic gastropathy (Ménétrier's disease), which is the most common gastric lesion causing severe protein loss. Patients usually have dyspepsia, postprandial nausea, emesis, edema, and weight loss. Prominent and thick gastric folds with protein-rich exudates are seen. In this disorder, tight junctions between cells are wider than those found in healthy subjects, and it is believed that proteins traverse the gastric mucosa through these widened spaces. Histamine receptor antagonists, anticholinergic agents, PPIs, and octreotide may be used to improve symptoms; however, most patients with persistent abdominal pain or severe protein loss require subtotal or total gastrectomy.

306 **B** (S&F, ch39)
This patient likely has radiation proctopathy complicated by rectal bleeding. An appropriate treatment includes argon plasma coagulation to cauterize the blood vessels.

307 **D** (S&F, ch32)
PETs frequently produce chromogranins or the α or β subunit of HCG. Plasma chromogranin A levels are found elevated in more than 90% of patients with various PETs and carcinoid tumors.

308 **C** (S&F, ch23)
Diverticula of the small bowel (apart from duodenal and Meckel's diverticula) are most commonly found in the proximal jejunum. They are commonly multiple and vary from a few millimeters to 10 cm in length. Jejunal diverticula are best diagnosed by upper GI x-rays with small bowel follow-through. They are most commonly found on the mesenteric border, in contrast to Meckel's diverticula, which occur on the antimesenteric border. Large enteroliths can lead to erosion with bleeding, diverticulitis, perforation, or intestinal obstruction. If a small bowel volvulus is found in an adult, small bowel diverticulosis should be considered because there is an association.

309 **C** (S&F, ch38)
Spontaneous rupture of the liver may complicate preeclampsia and HELLP (hemolysis, elevated liver enzymes, and low platelet count) syndrome, usually in the third trimester of pregnancy close to term or in the early postpartum period. Patients with this often fatal disorder present with abdominal distention and pain and cardiovascular collapse.

310 **A** (S&F, ch22)
Oral HL presents as corrugated white lesions on the lateral border of the tongue. Therefore, **A** is wrong. It is usually asymptomatic and may be an early sign of HIV infection. Although the severity of HL does not correlate with the severity of HIV, the presence of HL in an HIV-infected person has prognostic implications. It usually indicates that the time to development of AIDS is 24 months. It can also occur in kidney and other solid-organ transplant

recipients. Biopsy may be needed to confirm the diagnosis. Treatment is with oral acyclovir, topical retinoic acid, and podophyllum. HL recurs with the discontinuation of treatment.

311 **E** (S&F, ch24)
Spigelian hernias are difficult to palpate because they lie within the abdominal wall and are covered by the external oblique muscles. Only 75% are diagnosed preoperatively. The pain can be mistaken for acute intra-abdominal processes. Use of ultrasound and CT scanning assists the diagnosis.

312 **D** (S&F, ch30)
All the statements are correct except the fact that only 95% of GISTs have the CD117 molecules. The other 5% are attributed to other kinase activation such as platelet-derived growth factor receptor-α mutations. *KIT* or *PDGFRA* genes confer an increased activity of the kinase, which supports tumor growth.

313 **B** (S&F, ch37)
This patient likely has Fitz-Hugh-Curtis syndrome or perihepatitis from *Chlamydia*. It occurs only in women, owing to seeding of bacteria in the peritoneal cavity from the fallopian tubes. Symptoms presenting in these patients include inflammatory ascites, pain in the right upper abdominal quadrant, fever, and a hepatic friction rub. If there is enough ascitic fluid to be clinically detectable, it has an elevated WBC count with a predominance of neutrophils and a high protein content, even in excess of 9 g/dL. Laparoscopy is very helpful in confirming the diagnosis, revealing "violin strings" and "bridal veil" adhesions from the abdominal wall to the liver. Doxycycline is usually curative.

314 **D** (S&F, ch33)
In the era of HAART, diarrhea is less frequent and etiologically is now most often drug induced or is caused by disorders unrelated to HIV infection. Alterations in the mucosal immune system in AIDS that predispose to intestinal infections may lead to untreatable chronic infection by organisms that typically cause self-limited infection in healthy hosts. Protozoa account for the most prevalent class of diarrheal pathogens, largely because many of these infections can lead to chronic diarrhea and are refractory to treatment. The small bowel is the most common site of infection, although the organisms can be recovered in all regions of the gut. Although unclear, infections by the protozoa *G. lamblia* and *E. histolytica* are not consistently seen with increased frequency or virulence in AIDS.

315 **B** (S&F, ch22)
Aphthous ulcers, also called canker sores, are painful shallow ulcers that appear almost exclusively on unkeratinized oral mucosa. They are covered by yellowish-white or grayish-white exudate and surrounded by an erythematous margin. Rarely, they may occur in the esophagus, upper or lower GI tract, or anorectal mucosa. Management includes palliative and curative measures. All of the treatments listed have been used except **B**.

316 **D** (S&F, ch29)
Part of the pathogenesis can be proliferation of Epstein-Barr virus, which is reversed by stopping the immunosuppression. Other therapy if those options listed fail includes acyclovir and ganciclovir as an antiviral, interferon-α, surgery, chemotherapy, irradiation, and rituximab.

317 **D** (S&F, ch40)
Although aspiration pneumonia can occur in patients receiving enteral feedings from aspiration of either oropharyngeal contents or an enteral feeding, the former is more usual. Buried bumper syndrome is a condition in which the external bolster of the PEG tube is so tight that the internal bolster migrates into the gastric wall. The most common complication of PEG tube placement is local infection at the site of entry of the tube into the skin. The risk of this occurring can be reduced by preprocedure administration of an antibiotic medication.

318 **D** (S&F, ch27)
Items **A**, **B**, and **C** should provide a diagnosis of EE eventually. Although atopy is associated with EE in 50% to 80% of patients, the history cannot distinguish a patient with GERD who also has atopy. EE can respond to PPI therapy in the short term, but control of chronic symptoms by steroids strongly confirms EE.

319 **A** (S&F, ch34)
GAVE is also a cause of severe upper intestinal bleeding in HCT recipients. Diffuse areas of hemorrhage are seen in the gastric antrum and proximal duodenum, but the underlying mucosa is intact. Histopathologic findings or abnormal dilated capillaries, thromboses, and fibromuscular hyperplasia in the lamina propria are diagnostic. Endoscopic laser therapy is the treatment of choice to control bleeding, but multiple laser treatments may be required to obliterate ectatic lesions.

320 **C** (S&F, ch25)
In the United States, the foods that most often become impacted are larger pieces of beef, pork, chicken, and hot dog, which is why food impaction in the United States is often referred to as "steakhouse syndrome" or "backyard barbecue syndrome." During the evaluation of a patient with suspected food impaction, anteroposterior and lateral chest radiographs should be obtained to assess mediastinal or peritoneal free air and the presence of bones or other radiopaque foreign material in the food bolus. Urgent management is indicated when patients are in severe distress, excessively salivating, or unable to manage their secretions. This consists of flexible endoscopy, performed with the patient under intravenous sedation, rather than rigid endoscopy because flexible endoscopy has a high success rate, permits thorough examination, and is more safe, available, and cost-effective than rigid endoscopy. Food boluses may pass with intravenous administration of glucagon. Trial of sips of water should only be attempted when bolus passage is thought to have occurred.

321 **B** (S&F, ch35)
The most common GI symptom of diabetic patients is constipation, related in some cases to autonomic neuropathy. Occasionally, severe constipation with megacolon may be encountered. Complications of severe constipation include stercoral ulcer, perforation, volvulus, and anal overflow diarrhea.

322 **1-D, 2-C, 3-A, 4-E, 5-B** (S&F, ch22)

323 **E** (S&F, ch32)
The most sensitive and widely used study for confirming the presence of a PET is somatostatin receptor scintigraphy. CT and MRI localize less than 10% of PETs less than 1 cm in diameter, 30% to 40% of tumors 1 to 3 cm in diameter, and more than 50% of PETs greater than 3 cm in diameter. PETs are hypervascular tumors, and the ability to localize different PETs seems to be more influenced by tumor size and location than PET type. Selective arterial angiography identified as many as 60% of small insulinomas. Somatostatin receptor scintigraphy is becoming the study of choice for most PETs.

324 **C** (S&F, ch26)
A trial of an anti–tumor necrosis factor-α monoclonal antibody regimen should be considered in the initial management of fistulas in Crohn's disease and is supported by a recent Cochrane Database review. A prospective, randomized, double-blind, placebo-controlled study revealed the benefit of a maintenance infusion of infliximab given every eight weeks. The group that received maintenance therapy had significantly longer periods without fistula drainage compared with controls (>40 weeks vs. 14 weeks in controls), and at more than one year on maintenance infliximab infusions, 36% were fistula free compared with 19% of controls. This was associated with a decreased rate of subsequent hospitalization as well as both surgical and nonsurgical procedures. Subsequent data analyses from these and other trials have shown that the use of infliximab is associated with better outcomes for perianal than for abdominal wall fistulas.

325 **D** (S&F, ch35)
Granulomatous involvement of the liver is a very frequent occurrence with sarcoidosis, occurring in as many as 95% of patients in some studies. If the diagnosis is suspected, with or without overt systemic disease, it can be confirmed by liver biopsy.

CHAPTER
4

Esophagus

QUESTIONS

326 The pathogenesis of peptic esophagitis secondary to gastroesophageal reflux is most dependent on which of the following?
A. Gastric acidity
B. Pepsin
C. Gastric acid and pepsin
D. Gastric acid and bilirubin

327 Which of the following is the best-defined motor disorder of the esophagus?
A. Zenker's diverticulum
B. Gastroesophageal reflux disease (GERD)
C. Distal esophageal spasm
D. Achalasia
E. Dysphagia

328 A 36-year-old woman with acquired immunodeficiency syndrome reports persistent severe odynophagia despite a 10-day course of oral antifungal therapy. The most appropriate diagnostic test would be which of the following?
A. Barium swallow
B. Computed tomography of the chest
C. Endoscopy with brushings and biopsies
D. Cytomegalovirus titers

329 Which of the following is the most accurate statement regarding transient lower esophageal sphincter relaxation (TLESr)?
A. TLESr is a predominant mechanism of gastroesophageal reflux in patients with GERD, but not in those without this condition.
B. All TLESr episodes are accompanied by gastroesophageal reflux.
C. TLESr episodes are vagally mediated and occur in response to gastric distention.
D. TLESr episodes generally occur after swallowing and are usually accompanied by esophageal peristalsis.

330 A 27-year-old patient with herpes simplex infection is suspected of having esophageal involvement. Which of the following conditions may be found concurrent with this viral infection?
A. Gastrointestinal (GI) blood loss
B. Deep linear ulcerations
C. Esophageal stricture
D. Occasional dysphagia

331 Developmental abnormalities of the esophagus are relatively common. Which statement best characterizes esophageal atresia?
A. Long-term survival after surgery is limited because of high cancer risk.
B. After successful surgery, gastroesophageal reflux is common in adulthood.
C. Esophageal atresia is commonly associated with tracheal stenosis.
D. Tracheoesophageal fistula and esophageal atresia occur infrequently in the same patient.

332 Several conditions can predispose to GERD. Which of the following conditions is not related to GERD?
A. Post-Heller myotomy for achalasia
B. Pregnancy
C. Prolonged nasogastric tube intubation
D. Sickle cell disease

333 A 56-year-old man has biopsy-proven intestinal metaplasia at the gastric cardia. What should the treatment recommendation be?
A. Surveillance plus PPI medication
B. Surveillance alone
C. Evaluation for *Helicobacter pylori* infection and eradication if present
D. Coagulation of the site with an argon plasma laser

334 A 44-year-old man comes to your office with symptoms of occasional heartburn for several years and intermittent abdominal pain. He uses Tums

approximately once a week with excellent relief of his heartburn symptoms. Due to his abdominal pain and heartburn, you perform an endoscopy. He is found to have Barrett's esophagus by biopsy. What is the next step in management?
A. Begin H$_2$ blocker for acid suppression
B. Begin proton pump inhibitor (PPI) for acid suppression
C. Referral to a surgeon for fundoplication
D. Continue current therapy with Tums as needed for heartburn
E. No changes and repeat endoscopy in one month once the patient is no longer taking Tums

335 Congenital esophageal stricture or stenosis may occur, but is a rare anomaly. Which of the following comments is correct?
A. Stenosis is easily corrected with graded dilation.
B. Most stenosis presents with dysphagia and regurgitation in later childhood.
C. Many stenoses contain gastric remnants.
D. Esophageal stenosis in infancy is associated with maternal nonsteroidal anti-inflammatory drug (NSAID) use.

336 A 26-year-old man with a history of food impaction has had intermittent dysphagia for solids for five years. Barium swallow and esophageal manometry results are normal. Endoscopy reveals multiple rings throughout the length of the esophagus. Biopsy of the esophagus is likely to show which of the following conditions?
A. Active esophagitis with mucosal disruption
B. A dense infiltrate of lymphocytes
C. Eosinophilic infiltration
D. Columnar metaplasia with dysplasia
E. None of the above

337 Which of the following statements regarding the clinical course of GERD is most appropriate?
A. The clinical course is uncertain, and nonerosive disease tends to progress to erosive esophagitis over time.
B. Once effective treatment has been administered and healing has occurred, most patients will remain asymptomatic without the need for maintenance therapy.
C. GI bleeding is a common complication of reflux esophagitis.
D. Barrett's esophagus is predominantly a disease of middle-aged white men.

338 A 78-year-old man is recently diagnosed with adenocarcinoma of the esophagus. A computed axial tomography scan of the abdomen and pelvis reveals metastatic disease, with lesions in the liver and lung. He continues to have dysphagia with liquids and solids, along with a 50-pound weight loss. Endoscopic evaluation reveals a circumferential mass with significant narrowing of the lumen. There is also evidence of a tracheoesophageal fistula. What is the best therapeutic option for the patient?
A. Esophageal dilation
B. Esophageal dilation with rigid plastic stent placement
C. Covered self-expanding metal stent
D. Surgical resection

339 Which of the following statements regarding pill-induced esophagitis is true?
A. A bronchoesophageal fistula is a common complication of NSAID-induced esophageal ulceration.
B. Tetracycline or its derivatives cause pill-induced esophagitis by production of a caustic alkaline solution.
C. Antibiotics as a class are uncommon causes of medication-induced esophagitis.
D. Esophageal damage from a bisphosphonate medication, such as alendronate, can be minimized by ingestion of a full 8-oz glass of water taken in the upright position.
E. Chemotherapeutic agents are unlikely causes of pill-induced esophagitis.

340 Antireflux surgery for chronic GERD has been shown to have which one of the following benefits?
A. Reduction of the need for esophageal stricture dilation
B. Reduction of the risk of the development of esophageal adenocarcinoma in patients with Barrett's esophagus
C. Promotion of regression of Barrett's tissue in the esophagus
D. Allowance of step-down to an H$_2$ receptor antagonist medication

341 Which one of the following statements regarding Barrett's esophagus is most accurate?
A. Patients with Barrett's esophagus may have a 50-fold increased risk of the development of adenocarcinoma of the esophagus
B. The incidence of adenocarcinoma has increased rapidly over the past several years while the incidence of squamous cell carcinoma of the esophagus has decreased rapidly in the United States.
C. The risk of adenocarcinoma in patients with short-segment Barrett's esophagus is the same as the incidence in those with long-segment Barrett's esophagus.
D. Severe heartburn is seen in almost all patients with Barrett's esophagus.
E. Barrett's esophagus is diagnosed endoscopically by the appearance of salmon tongues above the esophagogastric junction.

342 The pharynx is critically involved in ingesting food. Its muscular components participate in swallowing and are densely innervated. Which of the following cranial nerves does not innervate pharyngeal muscles?
A. Trigeminal
B. Facial
C. Glossopharyngeal
D. Accessory
E. Hypoglossal

343 Which of the following statements best describes Barrett's esophagus?
A. Long-segment Barrett's esophagus is intestinal metaplasia more than 1 cm in length.
B. It is a malignant precursor lesion to squamous cell carcinoma of the esophagus.
C. It is columnar epithelium with gastric-type mucosa in the esophagus.

D. Specialized intestinal metaplasia is present with goblet cells on hematoxylin and eosin stain.

E. First diagnosed in 1950, it has slowly increased in frequency.

344 Achalasia is characterized by ganglion cell degeneration. Which of the following may contribute to cell loss?
A. Antibodies against myenteric neurons
B. Autoimmune process triggered by latent herpes simplex virus type 1 infection
C. Antibody formation in patients with HLA DQA1
D. T cell expansion in the myenteric plexus of the lower esophageal sphincter (LES)
E. All of the above

345 Which of the following statements regarding the treatment of esophageal cancer is true?
A. Transhiatal esophagectomy is performed on patients with widespread metastatic cancer for palliation.
B. Combined chemoradiotherapy can be definitive therapy in nonsurgical patients or as preoperative (neoadjuvant) therapy in early esophageal cancer.
C. Chemotherapy has no role in palliative treatment in patients with advanced esophageal cancer.
D. Esophageal dilation provides long-lasting palliation of malignant dysphagia.

346 A 78-year-old man with a history of hypertension and hyperlipidemia presents to your office with symptoms of progressive dysphagia to solids for one month. He has noticed that his pants are loose. He has an esophagogastroduodenoscopy (EGD), radiologic evaluation, and manometry testing. Which of the following is the most likely diagnosis?
A. Scleroderma
B. Pseudoachalasia from adenocarcinoma of the gastroesophageal junction
C. Eosinophilic esophagitis
D. Pseudoachalasia from sarcoidosis
E. Idiopathic achalasia

347 A 54-year-old man is referred by a radiologist because of suspected dysphagia lusoria. Which of the following best describes the suspected clinical abnormality?
A. Any esophageal obstruction related to muscular compression of the esophageal wall
B. A benign esophageal ring
C. Symptoms arising from vascular compression of the esophagus caused by an aberrant right subclavian artery
D. Difficulty in swallowing related to abnormal proximal esophageal spastic contractions

348 You have just completed a pneumatic dilation for Mrs. Smith, your patient with achalasia. Which of the following is the best predictor of efficacy after the dilation?
A. Ability to swallow a food bolus in the recovery area
B. Sphincter relaxation
C. Peristaltic function

D. Postdilation LES pressure <10 mm Hg
E. Postdilation LES pressure <25 mm Hg

349 A patient has been diagnosed with esophagitis. She has circumferential erosions in the distal esophagus. There are yellow exudates as well; however, no ulcers are identified. What is this patient's grade of esophagitis, according to the Savary-Miller classification?
A. 1
B. 2
C. 3
D. 4

350 Which of the following statements regarding testing for GERD is most accurate?
A. An empirical test of high-dose PPI therapy is a reliable test for suspected GERD.
B. Barium esophagography is helpful in detecting mild esophagitis.
C. Inspection of the esophagus at upper endoscopy is a reliable way to diagnose most cases of GERD.
D. Esophageal manometry is a valuable and important part of the evaluation of uncomplicated GERD.
E. Impedance testing is valuable in that it detects only nonacid gastroesophageal reflux.

351 Which of the following represents the molecular and histologic theory behind GERD causing metaplasia and Barrett's esophagus?
A. Multipotential stem cells in the basal layers are bathed in gastric juice, which stimulates abnormal differentiation into columnar cells.
B. Stem cells in ducts of esophageal submucosal glands may be the progenitor cells involved in metaplasia.
C. Reflux esophagitis up-regulates the expression of genes that play a role in squamous-to-columnar differentiation.
D. All of the above
E. None of the above

352 The vagus nerve innervates the esophagus. Which statement concerning this innervation is true?
A. The vagal nerves supply both motor and sensory innervation to the entire esophagus.
B. The vagal nerves regulate motor but not sensory activity.
C. The vagal nerves provide sensory pathways to the brain but not motor activity.
D. The vagus nerves provide innervation only to the smooth muscle, not the proximal skeletal muscle.

353 All of the following underlying diseases are known to increase the risk of the subsequent development of squamous cell cancer of the esophagus *except*:
A. Lye stricture
B. Achalasia
C. Plummer-Vinson syndrome
D. Partial gastrectomy

354 Which of the following statements are/is true regarding medication-induced esophageal injury?

A. Dysphagia and odynophagia are common clinical symptoms.
B. Double-contrast radiographic barium swallow is the preferred diagnostic modality.
C. An anatomic or motility disorder of the esophagus predisposes the patient to injury.
D. PPIs have been shown to be beneficial in altering the course of injury.
E. **A** and **C**
F. **A** and **B**
G. **B** and **D**
H. **B** and **C**
I. **A, B**, and **C**

355 A 58-year-old man with Barrett's esophagus has undergone an endoscopy with extensive biopsies. You have verified with a skilled pathologist the presence of low-grade dysplasia. This is his second endoscopy in the past 6 months to look for invasive cancer. You follow the American College of Gastroenterology recommendations on Barrett's esophagus, so you recommend which of the following?
A. Repeat surveillance endoscopy in three years and continue PPI therapy
B. Repeat endoscopy in one year and continue PPI therapy
C. Referral for radiofrequency ablation
D. Repeat endoscopy in six months and continue PPI therapy
E. Repeat endoscopy as soon as possible to exclude any high-grade dysplasia

356 A 46-year-old obese man reports reflux symptoms. He asks for more information on obesity and GERD. Which of the following statements is false with regard to obesity and GERD?
A. Obesity seems to be associated with the complications of GERD: Barrett's esophagus, adenocarcinoma, and erosive esophagitis.
B. The proposed mechanism is the increased incidence of sleep apnea in obese patients.
C. The proposed mechanism is the increased prevalence of hiatal hernia.
D. A possible contributing factor is increased activity of cytokines that affect the LES.
E. Central obesity (waist-to-hip ratio) is likely more important than body mass index.

357 Which of the following is the *least likely* primary malignancy to metastasize to the esophagus?
A. Breast
B. Melanoma
C. Small cell carcinoma
D. Renal cell carcinoma

358 The physiologic control governing striated and smooth esophageal musculature is distinct and complex. Experiments using nerve suture technique provided information about the innervation of the esophagus and the peristalsis. Which of the following statements regarding to innervation of the esophagus is true?
A. Contraction results from a sequential activation on motor units in the caudocranial sequence.
B. Primary peristalsis can be elicited in response to esophageal distention.

C. Deglutitive inhibition is the process by which a second swallow causes the rapid and complete inhibition of the previously induced contraction.
D. Deglutitive inhibition has a peripheral origin.
E. The esophagus usually exhibits spontaneous contractions.

359 Which of the following statements regarding infections of the esophagus is true?
A. Odynophagia is commonly seen in patients with human papillomavirus (HPV) infection of the esophagus.
B. The endoscopic appearance of herpes simplex esophagitis is characterized by diffuse friability and ulceration, mostly in the proximal esophagus.
C. Esophageal body manometric recordings in a patient with Chagas disease are identical to findings in achalasia.
D. The appearance of a "black esophagus" has been reported with *Mycobacterium tuberculosis* infection of the esophagus.

360 Esophageal rings are seen in humans. Both A and B rings have been characterized. Which comment is correct?
A. A rings are most common.
B. B rings are also called Schatzki rings.
C. B rings are mainly composed of muscular propria.
D. A and B rings are usually seen in conjunction with each other.

361 A 32-year-old man has an esophageal stricture on barium swallow. Dysphagia has been present since childhood. The stricture is suspected to be congenital. Which statement best characterizes this abnormality?
A. The stenotic segment varies in length, but is usually located within the middle or lower third of the esophagus.
B. The stenotic segment is usually short (<2 cm long).
C. The stenotic segment usually shows mucosal abnormalities.
D. Esophageal dilation is generally easily accomplished with through-the-endoscope balloons.
E. Congenital stenosis is often associated with congenital vascular abnormalities.

362 Your patient would like more information about the HALO ablation system. Which of the following statements is correct?
A. The system involves using a balloon-based array of closely spaced electrodes to deliver radiofrequency energy to ablate the mucosa.
B. Patients are given a dose of a light-activated chemical before the procedure.
C. This is a method in which the dysplastic area is injected with fluid after which the area is suctioned into a cap. A polypectomy snare is deployed over the area to remove it.
D. When used for high-grade dysplasia, the long-term benefit is very good, with only 10% to 15% of patients having high-grade dysplasia on repeat esophageal biopsy.

363 Oropharyngeal dysphagia occurs in neuromuscular disorders; 95% of patients with this disorder have demonstrable defects when evaluated videofluoroscopically with or without symptoms. What is the disorder?
A. Amyotrophic lateral sclerosis
B. Parkinson's disease
C. Poliomyelitis
D. Brain tumors
E. White matter cerebrovascular accident

364 Which statement regarding the pathogenesis of GERD is correct?
A. Hiatal hernia is not important in the pathogenesis of GERD.
B. Acid alone in the absence of pepsin causes severe esophageal damage.
C. Gastric acid output is normal in most patients with GERD.
D. *H. pylori* infection worsens GERD.

365 A 54-year-old man undergoes upper endoscopy for weight loss and dysphagia. Endoscopic evaluation reveals a 2-cm circumferential ulcerated mass in the distal esophagus. Biopsies of the mass are consistent with adenocarcinoma. A computed axial tomography scan of the abdomen and pelvis revealed no evidence of metastatic disease. What staging modality should be used next?
A. Magnetic resonance imaging of the chest
B. Positron emission tomography
C. Endoscopic ultrasonography
D. Laparoscopy

366 Zenker's diverticulum is the most common type of hypopharyngeal diverticulum. Where anatomically does it occur?
A. Lateral slit separating cricopharyngeus muscle from proximal esophagus
B. Penetration of the inferior thyroid artery into the hypopharynx
C. Midline posteriorly at Killian's dehiscence
D. Junction of the middle and inferior constrictor muscles

367 A 38-year-old engineer arrives at your office and reports feeling food getting stuck for the past several months. He has been struggling with intermittent dysphagia for a few years. He has recently immigrated to the United States from Brazil. Due to his symptoms and history, you are concerned that the patient has Chagas disease involving the esophagus. Which of the following statements regarding Chagas disease is true?
A. It is endemic to Brazil, Argentina, and Venezuela.
B. It is caused by the parasite *Trypanosoma cruzi*.
C. The GI organs most commonly affected are the esophagus, stomach, and liver.
D. Treatment of the infection improves symptoms.
E. All of the above
F. A and B only

368 All of the following medications cause direct injury to the esophageal mucosa because of their caustic nature *except*:
A. Ferrous sulfate
B. Bisphosphonates

C. Potassium chloride
D. Tetracycline
E. Calcium channel blockers

369 Which of the following factors has/have been demonstrated to alter LES pressure?
A. The migrating motor complex
B. Circulating of gut neuropeptides
C. Ingested foods
D. Intra-abdominal pressure
E. Respiration
F. All of the above
G. None of the above

370 With regard to mechanisms of reflux, which of the following accounts for nearly all reflux episodes in healthy subjects and 50% to 80% of episodes in GERD patients?
A. Hypotensive resting LES pressure
B. Transient LES relaxation
C. Swallow-induced LES relaxation
D. Vagal nerve dysfunction
E. Impaired fundic relaxation

371 Which of the following statements regarding squamous cell cancer of the esophagus is true?
A. It most commonly occurs in the proximal esophagus.
B. There can be invasion of local structures including the mediastinal pleura, trachea, bronchi, and aorta.
C. Chronic infections with herpes simplex or Epstein-Barr virus have been associated with squamous cell cancer of the esophagus.
D. It is the most common esophageal cancer in the United States.

372 A 54-year-old woman has been diagnosed with myasthenia gravis after presenting with dysphagia, fatigable chewing, and diplopia. Her esophageal manometry is most likely to show which of the following?
A. Deterioration in the amplitude of pharyngeal contractions with repeated swallows
B. Aperistalsis
C. Tertiary contractions
D. Disorganized contraction

373 The barium esophagogram and endoscopy demonstrate several complications of GERD. Which complication of GERD is not demonstrated on these images (see figure)?
A. Stricture
B. Perforation
C. Grade D esophagitis
D. Ulcerative esophagitis

374 A 36-year-old woman reports persistent severe odynophagia. Endoscopic evaluation reveals 3-mm vesicles in the mid to distal esophagus. What is the most appropriate therapy?
A. Fluconazole daily for 14 days
B. Nystatin, one to two troches four to five times daily
C. Acyclovir or valacyclovir daily for 7 to 10 days
D. No treatment is necessary.

375 A 42-year-old woman presents with dysphagia to solid food that has gradually worsened over the

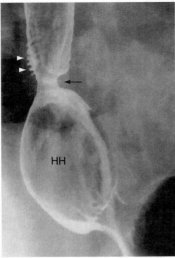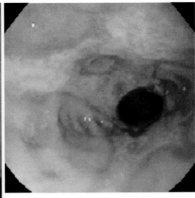

Figure for question **373**

past two years. After a thorough history and physical examination, you order further studies. Which of the following should be the first study to evaluate this patient's symptoms?
A. Upper endoscopy
B. Esophageal manometry
C. Trial of PPI once daily
D. Chest x-ray
E. Barium esophagography

376 A 74-year-old man has marked odynophagia. Endoscopy reveals white plaques along the entire esophagus. The oropharynx is normal in appearance. Which of the following statements best characterizes this condition?
A. *Candida tropicalis* is the fungal organism usually responsible for this clinical picture.
B. Topical administration of glucocorticoids has not been shown to be a risk factor.
C. Achalasia is an established risk factor for esophageal candidiasis.
D. Topical antifungal drugs are not effective therapy.

377 A 68-year-old man underwent cardiac radiofrequency ablation. He now presents to the emergency department with hematemesis and mental status changes. Which statement best characterizes the condition causing his symptoms?
A. It occurs 24 hours after radiofrequency ablation.
B. An echocardiogram reveals gas bubbles in the right atrium.
C. Symptoms are the result of air emboli to the brain from the esophagus through the fistula into the right heart.
D. It is generally fatal due to sepsis and upper GI hemorrhage.
E. All the above

378 Which of the following is not considered an alarm symptom of GERD?
A. Odynophagia
B. Dysphagia
C. Nocturnal symptoms
D. Weight loss
E. GI bleeding

379 An 81-year-old woman has recently been diagnosed with short-segment Barrett's esophagus with high-grade dysplasia. She has a history of moderate aortic stenosis; chronic obstructive pulmonary disease, for which she uses 2 L of oxygen continuously; hypertension; and hyperlipidemia. She spends most of her free time gardening and is interested in pursuing treatment for her Barrett's esophagus. Of the following treatment options, which would be the best one for this particular patient?
A. Esophagectomy
B. Photodynamic therapy
C. Repeat EGD in three months and continue PPI therapy
D. Radiofrequency ablation with endoscopic mucosal resection

380 A 47-year-old woman with prominent heartburn has been diagnosed with CREST syndrome (limited scleroderma). Esophageal manometry would be expected to show which of the following patterns?
A. Reduction in peristaltic contraction amplitude in the distal esophagus along with LES hypotension
B. Forceful esophageal contractions with impaired LES relaxation
C. Pharyngeal and upper esophageal hypomotility
D. LES hypotension with normal esophageal peristalsis

381 Which of the following statements regarding pill-induced esophagitis is/are true?
A. Dysphagia and odynophagia are common clinical symptoms.
B. Double-contrast radiographic barium swallow and endoscopy are the diagnostic modalities.
C. Substernal chest pain or heartburn after ingestion of small amounts of orange juice is a typical symptom.
D. Moderately severe erythema is the usual endoscopic finding.
E. A and C
F. B and D
G. A, B, and C
H. All of the above

382 An 86-year-old woman ingests tetracycline before going to sleep. The next morning, she has severe chest pain, odynophagia, and salivation. Which statement best characterizes the condition causing her symptoms?
A. The lesion is superficial and will heal within 48 hours.
B. The endoscopic appearance of this condition is pathognomonic.
C. Hematemesis is common.
D. The abnormality generally occurs at a site of an anatomic or physiologic narrowing or a stricture.

383 Which of the follow statements regarding esophageal injury is correct?
A. Routine endoscopy is suggested shortly after blunt trauma to the chest caused by an automobile accident.
B. Gastrograffin contrast studies are contraindicated in patients who have severe traumatic injuries.
C. Blunt trauma resulting in esophageal perforation most commonly occurs in the lower esophagus.
D. Cervical esophageal penetrating injuries are usually associated with concurrent tracheal, carotid, or spinal injury.

384 A 70-year-old woman presents to your office with symptoms of vomiting undigested food and halitosis. These symptoms have persisted for months. A barium swallow provides the likely diagnosis. She is otherwise healthy and takes only a multivitamin daily. You are confident in your diagnosis and discuss treatment options with the patient. Which of the following treatment options do you recommend?
A. Begin calcium channel blocker medication.
B. Eat pureed foods only.
C. Transcervical myotomy with diverticulectomy
D. Diverticulectomy
E. Dilation

385 One of your patients read on the Internet that the use of lozenges will improve reflux symptoms by increasing saliva production. Which of the following statements regarding saliva and acid clearance is false?
A. Saliva easily neutralizes a small amount of acid that remains in the esophagus after esophageal peristalsis.
B. Cigarette smokers have hyposalivation.
C. Oral lozenges increase salivation and therefore decrease acid clearance time.
D. Decrease in salivation during sleep does not seem to contribute to nocturnal reflux episodes.

386 Esophageal webs may be found in the proximal esophagus. Webs may cause dysphagia. Which statement best characterizes cervical webs?
A. Webs may be associated with an increased risk of adenocarcinoma of the mid esophagus.
B. Webs may be associated with iron deficiency anemia.
C. Webs are most common in men.
D. Webs are part of eosinophilic esophagitis syndrome.

387 Which of the following statements regarding GERD is correct?
A. Empirical trial of PPI is a reliable indicator for GERD.
B. Capsule endoscopy is an effective way to evaluate GERD.
C. EGD is a reliable study with which to diagnose GERD.
D. Esophageal manometry is a helpful evaluation for GERD.
E. Impedance testing is valuable in that it detects only nonacid gastroesophageal reflux.

388 A 76-year-old patient is referred for evaluation of dysphagia. Symptoms began after a cerebrovascular accident and have not progressed over the past three months. A barium swallow with video images was ordered by the speech therapy department. The barium swallow would be expected to show which of the following features?
A. Diffuse esophageal dilation with aperistalsis
B. A prominent cricopharyngeal muscular contraction with obstruction
C. Vallecular pooling with nasopharyngeal regurgitation
D. Asymmetrical cervical esophageal contractions opposite the side of the stroke

389 Which of the following statements regarding the routine use of endoscopy in patients with esophageal abnormalities is correct?
A. Endoscopy is important for the diagnosis of esophageal injury due to medications.
B. Routine endoscopy is suggested shortly after blunt trauma to the chest caused by an automobile accident.
C. Multiple "volcano-like" vesicles are characteristic of herpetic esophagitis.
D. Gastrograffin contrast studies are contraindicated in patients who have severe traumatic injuries.
E. All of the above

390 During endoscopy, a 61-year-old man is found to have an inlet patch of hypertrophic mucosa. The mucosa is gastric in type. Which step is now recommended?
A. Yearly surveillance with multiple biopsies
B. Argon plasma coagulation with high-dose PPI therapy
C. No further tests
D. pH monitoring with proximal electrode placement

391 A patient whom you have been following in the office asks for your advice on lifestyle modifications that may help with reflux symptoms. You mention all of the following except:
A. Elevate the head of the bed.
B. Stop smoking and restrict alcohol intake.
C. Avoid high-roughage foods.
D. Reduce meal size.
E. Avoid nighttime snacks.

392 A 56-year-old man presents for an endoscopy after experiencing heartburn for several years. You note patches of red mucosa in the distal esophagus that are approximately 3.5 cm. You obtain multiple

biopsy specimens from the area of concern. You suspect Barrett's esophagus. Which of the following will likely appear on pathologic testing to confirm your diagnosis?
A. Intestinal metaplasia with goblet cells
B. Specialized columnar epithelium
C. Squamous epithelium
D. Squamous epithelium with chronic inactive inflammation
E. A and B
F. B and D

393 A 45-year-old patient with dysphagia to liquids and solids and a prominent history of regurgitation over a six-month period is referred for evaluation. The barium swallow shows a minimally dilated esophagus with poor emptying in the supine position. The endoscope is easily passed into the stomach. Because of the minimal esophageal dilation, the diagnosis is questioned. Which study would be of greatest value?
A. A methacholine (Mecholyl) challenge
B. Serologic studies for scleroderma
C. An endoscopic ultrasound scan of the distal esophagus
D. Routine esophageal manometry
E. A 24-hour pH study

394 All of the following statements are more commonly associated with adenocarcinoma of the esophagus than with squamous cell carcinoma *except*:
A. It usually spreads to celiac and perihepatic lymph nodes.
B. It usually arises in the setting of Barrett's esophagus.
C. It can occur in the distal third of the esophagus, including the esophagogastric junction.
D. A strong association with alcohol and tobacco use is noted.

395 The pathogenesis of GERD may include which of the following?
A. Decreased LES pressure
B. Decreased acid clearance
C. Decreased esophageal mucosal resistance to acid
D. Peristaltic dysfunction
E. A and C
F. B and D
G. A, B, and C
H. All of the above

396 Which of the following statements regarding the effect of sclerotherapy on the esophagus is true?
A. Wall damage or neural effects may lead to abnormalities in esophageal motor function.
B. Strictures commonly occur as the result of sclerotherapy.
C. Ulcers occur at the site of sclerotherapy injection in a minority of patients.
D. H₂ receptor antagonist or PPI therapy may be effective in preventing esophageal damage from sclerotherapy.

397 Which of the following statements regarding the treatment of esophageal abnormalities is false?
A. Pill-induced esophagitis is most often treated by a surface coating agent such as sucralfate

suspension in conjunction with acid suppressive therapy.
B. *Candida* esophagitis is usually treated with a fluconazole or clotrimazole troche.
C. Severe herpetic esophagitis may be treated with orally administered acyclovir or valacyclovir.
D. Routine treatment of HPV involving the esophagus involves bleomycin or interferon.

398 A 52-year-old man with typical heartburn symptoms is referred for evaluation. His response to a standard dose of a PPI is excellent. Endoscopy reveals a 6-cm area of Barrett's esophagus without dysplasia. Which of the following recommendations should be made?
A. Endoscopic surveillance and continued maintenance PPI
B. Laser ablation plus fundoplication
C. Surveillance and step down to maintenance doses of H₂ receptor antagonists
D. Endoscopic surveillance only

399 Which of the following individuals is the most likely prototype for Barrett's esophagus?
A. A middle-aged obese white woman immigrant from India
B. A 47-year-old woman with recurrent heartburn during pregnancy
C. A middle-aged white American man
D. An older black male smoker with moderate to heavy ethyl alcohol use
E. A young *H. pylori*–positive black woman

400 A 58-year-old man has Barrett's esophagus without any current symptoms of heartburn. He had an endoscopy one year ago that did not show any signs of dysplasia. You performed an endoscopy last week and took biopsy samples of his esophagus. The pathology shows intestinal metaplasia with no signs of dysplasia. What do you recommend for this patient?
A. Stop PPI therapy and follow up in the office in six months.
B. Repeat endoscopy in three years and continue PPI therapy.
C. Repeat endoscopy in one year and continue PPI therapy.
D. Because the pathology is not consistent with Barrett's esophagus, he can stop PPI therapy and be followed clinically.
E. Confirm adequate acid suppression with pH monitor.

401 A 37-year-old woman is referred for evaluation of recurrent aspiration. She has frontal baldness, cataracts, and evidence of myotonia. Her mother had a similar illness. On manometry, she had markedly decreased contraction pressure of the pharynx and upper esophagus. What is the diagnosis?
A. Myotonia dystrophica
B. Amyotrophic lateral sclerosis
C. Oculopharyngeal dystrophy
D. Myasthenia gravis

402 Which of the following conditions is/are associated with esophagitis?
A. Scleroderma
B. Sjögren syndrome

C. Zollinger-Ellison syndrome
D. Pregnancy
E. **A** and **C**
F. **B** and **D**
G. **A**, **B**, and **C**
H. All of the above

403 Inlet patches of the esophagus are composed of heterotopic gastric mucosa. Which of the following statements is false?
A. Inlet patches are seen in approximately 10% of endoscopies.
B. Inlet patches are at high risk of adenocarcinoma, similar to Barrett's esophagus.
C. Inlet patches may be infected with *H. pylori*.
D. Inlet patches are generally asymptomatic.

404 Which of the following is the least common complication of esophagitis?
A. Stricture formation
B. Barrett's esophagus
C. Hemorrhage
D. Perforation

405 Which of the following actions predispose to Mallory-Weiss tears?
A. Forceful coughing
B. Transesophageal echocardiography
C. Cardiopulmonary resuscitation
D. Alcohol use
E. All of the above

406 Which statement regarding therapy for GERD is correct?
A. PPI therapy is effective because PPIs generally keep the pH above 4 for 24 hours.
B. Eight weeks of PPI therapy may lead to healing of ulcerative esophagitis in more than 80% of patients.
C. H_2 receptor antagonists are as effective as PPIs in healing esophagitis.
D. An H_2 receptor antagonist medication should not be taken at bedtime with a PPI drug.

407 A 37-year-old man with intermittent solid food dysphagia undergoes a barium swallow. The results show he has a ring-like narrowing at the distal esophagus. The diameter of the ring is 12 mm. Which of the following therapies is indicated at this time?

A. Careful food preparation with the avoidance of meat and bread
B. Endoscopy followed by bougie dilation
C. Laser ablation
D. PPI therapy
E. Observation only

408 A 40-year-old woman with acquired immunodeficiency syndrome presents to the emergency department with a one-month history of dysphagia and odynophagia. Before arriving, she had an episode of hematemesis. On physical examination, she has multiple dark pigmented lesions on her skin and in her mouth. What is the most likely diagnosis?
A. Lymphoma
B. Kaposi sarcoma
C. Adenocarcinoma
D. Squamous cell carcinoma

409 A 64-year-old man undergoes pneumatic balloon dilation for achalasia. The patient has severe chest pain and fever after the procedure. A gastrograffin swallow shows a small confined perforation with no contrast flowing into the pleural space. Management should consist of which of the following steps?
A. Intravenous antibiotics, parenteral alimentation, and observation
B. Intravenous antibiotics and placement of a removable stent
C. Intravenous antibiotics and immediate thoracotomy
D. Intravenous antibiotics and placement of a chest tube for drainage

410 A 64-year-old woman has been diagnosed with a hiatal hernia after undergoing an endoscopy for reflux symptoms. She asks for more information on hiatal hernia. Which of the following statements regarding hiatal hernia is true?
A. Reflux is worse in patients with a reducible hernia as opposed to a nonreducible hernia.
B. Hiatal hernia occurs in 10% to 15% of patients with reflux esophagitis.
C. Hiatal hernia occurs in 54% to 94% of patients with reflux esophagitis.
D. In patients with hiatal hernia, the esophageal junction opens at a higher pressure and remains patent for a longer duration, leading to an increase in air and liquid reflux.

ANSWERS

326 C (S&F, ch43)
Esophagitis requires that the esophageal mucosa be exposed to both gastric acid and pepsin.

327 D (S&F, ch42)
Achalasia is the most easily recognized and best defined motor disorder of the esophagus. Zenker's diverticulum is the most common anatomic etiology of oropharyngeal dysphagia. GERD is the most prevalent but likely multifactorial. Distal esophageal spasm is not as common nor easily

defined. The incidence of achalasia is 1/100,000 in the United States and Europe.

328 C (S&F, ch45)
Patients with acquired immunodeficiency syndrome who have persistent odynophagia after empirical antifungal therapy merit endoscopic evaluation to exclude cytomegalovirus infection, herpes simplex virus infection, other fungal diseases, and large esophageal ulcers.

329 C (S&F, ch43)
TLESr is the predominant form of gastroesophageal reflux in both patients with GERD and in

individuals without GERD. Not all TLESr episodes are accompanied by reflux. TLESr occurs independently of swallowing and is not accompanied by esophageal peristalsis.

330 **A** (S&F, chs41-46)
Herpes esophagitis generally presents with odynophagia, heartburn, or fever. Endoscopically, the condition is characterized by diffuse friability and ulceration of the mucosa and presence of exudates, usually in the distal esophagus. Discrete circumscribed ulcers with raised edges are usual, but not deep linear ulcers. Bleeding and perforation may occur, and dysphagia is persistent.

331 **B** (S&F, ch41)
Poor esophageal clearance due to abnormal esophageal motility leads to impaired acid clearance and GERD in adults. Successful surgery generally is associated with a prognosis. GERD is common, and an increase in Barrett's esophagus is noted in later life. Esophageal atresia and tracheoesophageal fistulas occur together in approximately 90% of cases.

332 **D** (S&F, ch43)
GERD-predisposing conditions including pregnancy, scleroderma, and the acid hypersecretory state of Zollinger-Ellison syndrome can predispose to GERD. After patients with achalasia have Heller myotomy, 10% to 20% will have GERD. Prolonged nasogastric tube intubation may cause reflux esophagitis by acid migration along the tube. Sickle cell disease is not a commonly recognized condition to predispose to GERD.

333 **C** (S&F, chs41-46)
Unlike intestinal metaplasia of the esophagus, this lesion is considered benign and not associated with an increased risk of cancer. *H. pylori* infection may play a role and should be eradicated if present.

334 **B** (S&F, ch44)
Initial and maintenance therapy with PPI should be provided to all patients with Barrett's esophagus, irrespective of symptoms. This is based on evidence that acid reflux promotes carcinogenesis in Barrett's metaplasia, and aggressive control of acid reflux may interfere with this process.

335 **B** (S&F, ch41)
Congenital stenosis usually presents when more solid food is ingested later in childhood. Graded esophageal dilation should be carefully performed but is often not successful, especially if the stenosis is caused by tracheobronchial remnants. Gastric remnants are generally not seen in esophageal stenosis, and no association with maternal NSAID use has been described.

336 **C** (S&F, ch42)
Eosinophilic esophagitis is a cause of solid food dysphagia. It is most common in young men. An allergic food diathesis is suspected.

337 **D** (S&F, ch43)
Barrett's esophagus is two to three times more common in men than women and is rare in African-American and Asian populations. As many as 85%

of patients with GERD will experience a relapse within six months after treatment stops. In most patients with nonerosive disease, the disease will not progress to erosive esophagitis. GI hemorrhage is a rare complication of reflux esophagitis and is generally associated with deep ulcers or severe esophagitis.

338 **C** (S&F, ch46)
Placement of a covered self-expanding metal stent is the only effective practical treatment available for management of malignant esophagorespiratory fistulas.

339 **D** (S&F, ch45)
Hemorrhage, which may be severe, is a common complication of NSAID-induced esophageal ulcers, especially when compared with other medication causes of esophagitis. Bronchoesophageal fistula is unlikely. Tetracycline causes direct esophageal toxicity. Toxicity from bisphosphonates or any pill-induced esophagitis can be minimized by taking the medication with copious liquid in an upright position. Both antibiotics and chemotherapeutic agents are frequent causes of pill-induced esophagitis.

340 **A** (S&F, chs41-46)
Stricture dilation is consistently reduced after fundoplication, but other changes are not consistently seen after this procedure.

341 **A** (S&F, ch44)
The risk of adenocarcinoma is much higher in patients with Barrett's esophagus than in the general population. The incidence of squamous cell carcinoma is steady. Barrett's esophagus has an increased risk of adenocarcinoma in long-segment rather than short-segment disease. Once Barrett's esophagus develops, 25% to 30% of patients may no longer experience heartburn symptoms. A biopsy of the esophagus is required to make the diagnosis of Barrett's esophagus.

342 **D** (S&F, ch41)
The pharyngeal muscles are innervated by motor fibers from the nuclei of trigeminal, facial, glossopharyngeal, and hypoglossal, as well as nucleus ambiguous and spinal segments C1-C3. The major pharyngeal muscles are innervated by trigeminal, facial, glossopharyngeal, vagus, and hypoglossal nerves. The accessory nerve controls muscles of the neck.

343 **D** (S&F, ch43)
Barrett's esophagus is specialized intestinal metaplasia and goblet cells. Short-segment Barrett's esophagus is, by definition, less than 3 cm in length. Barrett's esophagus has increased sixfold over the past 30 years and is a precursor lesion for adenocarcinoma of the esophagus.

344 **E** (S&F, ch42)
Although the etiology of ganglion cell degeneration in achalasia is not clear, increasing evidence points toward some of the listed theories. This may be an autoimmune process caused by a latent herpes simplex virus type 1 infection in patients with genetic susceptibility.

345 B (S&F, ch46)

Transhiatal esophagectomy is usually reserved for patients who have local disease. Palliative surgical procedures are no longer recommended. Chemotherapy plays a major role in advanced, unresectable esophageal cancer, particularly those with distant metastatic disease. Esophageal dilation may provide incomplete, temporary improvement in malignant dysphagia.

346 B (S&F, ch42)

Pseudoachalasia is more common in older age groups, in patients with recent onset of symptoms, and in those with weight loss. Eosinophilic esophagitis and sarcoidosis are not likely to present in this age group with recent onset of symptoms. Idiopathic achalasia is possible; however, it usually presents in patients at a younger age and with a more gradual onset of symptoms.

347 C (S&F, chs41-46)

Dysphagia lusoria is a specific disorder. It is caused by an aberrant right subclavian artery that arises from the left side of the aortic arch and crosses the esophagus, compressing the esophageal lumen. The result is a pencil-like indentation in the esophagus. Confirmation of this condition is made by seeing these anatomic aberrations on computed tomography or magnetic resonance arteriography.

348 D (S&F, ch42)

A postdilation pressure of less than 10 mm Hg is associated with prolonged remission. Dilation can be repeated with incrementally larger dilators. Return of sphincter relaxation or peristaltic function is not likely.

349 C (S&F, ch43)

Grade 3 esophagitis has circumferential erosions. Ulcers, stricture, and Barrett's esophagus are associated with higher grade system. Los Angeles classification uses grades A through D with a description of mucosal breaks. If this patient were to be evaluated using this classification, she would be grade D, circumferential mucosal break.

350 A (S&F, ch43)

A barium esophagogram is generally only useful in cases of severe reflux esophagitis. The results of upper endoscopy are generally normal in patients with GERD. A biopsy may assist in making the diagnosis, but inspection alone is not adequate. Impedance testing helps, both in cases with acid and those with nonacid reflux.

351 D (S&F, ch44)

The progenitor cells that give rise to metaplasia are not known. The hypothesis is that GERD damages the esophageal squamous epithelium, exposing multipotential stem cells in the basal layer to gastric juice; this then stimulates the abnormal differentiation into columnar cells. Other progenitor cell candidates are stem cells in ducts of submucosal glands and circulating bone marrow stem cells. Genes involved in metaplasia include *Cdx* genes, and the gene encoding bone morphogenetic protein 4.

352 A (S&F, ch41)

The proximal and distal esophagus receives both sensory and motor innervation from the vagus nerves.

353 D (S&F, ch46)

Adenocarcinoma of the stomach after partial gastrectomy is usually noted 10 to 20 years postoperatively. Lye strictures and achalasia have a well-established association with squamous cell cancers of the esophagus. A rare syndrome of iron deficiency anemia, dysphagia, and postcricoid esophageal web, known as Plummer-Vinson syndrome, has been reported to have an association with squamous cell cancers.

354 E (S&F, ch45)

Pill-induced esophagitis leads to disruption of the mucosal integrity of the esophagus, and dysphagia or odynophagia is commonly seen. Injury is predisposed by an anatomic or by a motility disorder of the esophagus or by medication taken incorrectly, in either case, allowing prolonged exposure of the medication to esophageal mucosa. Areas of normal hypomotility or extrinsic compression are the trough zone of the esophagus (where smooth and skeletal muscle overlap) or at the level of the aortic or left bronchial impression on the esophagus. Diagnosis is made with either double-contrast radiography or at endoscopy (the latter is the preferred). No specific treatments have been shown to be beneficial in altering the course of injury.

355 B (S&F, ch44)

According to recommendations, for a patient with low-grade dysplasia after extensive biopsy sampling, yearly surveillance is suggested. Repeat surveillance in 3 years is only recommended for those without dysplasia. If dysplasia is noted, another endoscopy should be performed to look for invasive cancer and should be interpreted by an expert pathologist. This is the second endoscopy for this patient, and the pathology has been confirmed by an expert pathologist, so there is no need to repeat an endoscopy any sooner than one year.

356 B (S&F, ch43)

The prevalence of GERD has been increasing in the Western population; one explanation may be the increase in obesity. A study from Kaiser Permanente found a relationship between abdominal diameter (waist-to-hip ratio) and reflux symptoms. Proposed mechanisms include increased prevalence of hiatal hernia, increased intragastric pressure, decreased LES pressure, and increased prevalence of esophageal motor disorder. Although obesity is related to sleep apnea, sleep apnea has not been proposed as a mechanism in the increase in GERD.

357 D (S&F, ch46)

The esophagus is the most common extrapulmonary site of small cell carcinoma. Melanoma and breast cancer are two cancers that are frequent causes of metastatic esophageal carcinoma.

358 C (S&F, chs41-46)

Deglutitive inhibition is the process by which a second swallow, if initiated while an earlier contraction is still progressing in the proximal esophagus, causes rapid and complete inhibition on the contraction induced by the first swallow. It is likely of central origin. The esophagus does not normally exhibit spontaneous contractions and when contractions occur they are craniocaudal. Primary peristalsis is initiated by a swallow; secondary peristalsis can be elicited by esophageal distention.

359   **C** (S&F, ch45)
Esophageal infections with HPV are typically asymptomatic. The endoscopic appearance of herpes esophagitis is characterized by diffuse friability, ulceration, and exudates, mostly in the distal esophagus. The appearance of a "black esophagus" has been reported with herpes and *Candida* esophagitis. Esophageal manometric recordings are identical to findings in achalasia, although the LES pressure is lower in Chagas disease.

360   **B** (S&F, ch41)
B rings are most common and may be found in 6% to 14% of patients and are called Schatzki rings, which are composed of mucosa and submucosa. The B rings occur at a squamocolumnar mucosal junction. A rings are muscular rings that correspond to the LES.

361   **A** (S&F, chs41-46)
Congenital stenosis of the esophagus is usually seen in the distal or middle third of the esophagus. The length of stenosis varies from 2 to 20 cm. The mucosa is usually normal. The wall may contain cartilaginous structures of tracheobronchial origin. Dilation may be difficult because mucosal tears are common.

362   **A** (S&F, ch44)
The system is one that delivers energy directed at the area of interest. Photodynamic therapy delivers light-activated chemical prior to the procedure. The suction method is used for endoscopic mucosal resection. Finally, although the HALO ablation system seems to have good results, there are very few data on long-term follow-up.

363   **B** (S&F, ch42)
Only 15% to 20% of patients with Parkinson's disease report swallowing problems. However, on videoscopic evaluation, most have a defect. Amyotrophic lateral sclerosis is a progressive neurologic disease, and only when cranial nerve nuclei are affected do swallowing difficulties begin. Medullary or vagal tumors can affect swallowing. Finally, cortical strokes are less likely to result in severe dysphagia than brainstem strokes.

364   **C** (S&F, ch43)
The presence of *H. pylori* infection may lessen the risk of GERD by decreasing hydrogen ion production by the gastric antrum. A hiatal hernia is, at the very least, a cofactor or promoter in the production of GERD. Pepsin, even in small amounts, is required for increasing the severity of gastroesophageal reflux on esophageal mucosa.

365   **C** (S&F, ch46)
Endoscopic ultrasonography is the cornerstone in the pretreatment staging evaluation of esophageal cancer. It is the best imaging modality for T staging, with an overall accuracy of as high as 85% to 90%.

366   **C** (S&F, ch42)
Hypopharyngeal diverticula occur at sites of potential weakness of the muscular lining of the hypopharynx through which the mucosa herniates, leading to a false diverticulum.

367   **F** (S&F, ch42)
Chagas disease can produce symptoms of achalasia. It is endemic in central Brazil, Venezuela, and northern Argentina. It is spread by the bite of reduviid bug that transmits *Trypanosoma cruzi*. The GI organs most commonly affected are the esophagus, colon, and duodenum. Megaesophagus and megacolon can occur. It also affects the heart and can cause cardiomyopathy, the most common cause of death. Treatment of the infection has limited efficacy.

368   **E** (S&F, ch45)
Calcium channel blockers are thought to facilitate injury of the esophagus by decreasing LES tone and increasing acid reflux in susceptible patients.

369   **F** (S&F, chs41-46)
LES pressure varies with many factors, including respiration, foods, and peptide hormones. The role of each of these factors in gastroesophageal reflux is unclear.

370   **B** (S&F, ch43)
TLESr accounts for nearly all reflux episodes in healthy subjects. In normal subjects, 40% to 60% of TLESr episodes are accompanied by reflux episodes. Five percent to 10% of reflux episodes occur during swallow-induced TLESr. Gastroesophageal reflux can occur with hypotensive LES by strain-induced reflux or free reflux. Vagal nerve dysfunction and fundic relaxation do not play a significant role in reflux.

371   **B** (S&F, ch46)
Squamous cell cancer of the esophagus most commonly occurs in the middle third of the esophagus. There is no association with herpes simplex virus or Epstein-Barr virus. However, there has been some association with HPV. Esophageal adenocarcinoma is now the predominant type of esophageal carcinoma in the United States. Invasion of local structures, such as mediastinal pleura, trachea, bronchi, and aorta as well as distant metastasis to liver, lung, and bone may be present in more than one third of patients at presentation.

372   **A** (S&F, ch42)
Myasthenia gravis is a progressive autoimmune disease. Dysphagia is prominent in more than one third of cases and can be the initial manifestation. Peristaltic amplitude recovers with rest or with administration of edrophonium chloride. Muscles of jaw closure are often involved and produce weakness with prolonged chewing (fatigue chewing).

373   **B** (S&F, ch43)
Pseudodiverticula, stricture, and hiatal hernia are all seen on the barium esophagogram. Ulcerative

and erosive esophagitis are evident on endoscopy, suggestive of grade D esophagitis. Perforation is a rare complication of reflux esophagitis and is not evident on these images.

374 C (S&F, ch45)

On endoscopic evaluation, the patient has herpes esophagitis. Treatment is the same as that for other herpes simplex infections in the immunocompetent host, such as prompt initiation of a 7- to 10-day course of orally administered acyclovir or valacyclovir. Treatment of fungal esophagitis is with oral fluconazole or a topical antifungal agent. Treatment of HPV is often not necessary, although large lesions have required endoscopic removal.

375 A (S&F, ch42)

Dysphagia should never be considered a functional symptom. The patient with dysphagia should first undergo endoscopy to detect most structural causes of dysphagia and biopsies, if needed. Manometry, chest x-ray, and barium esophagography may all be used in the workup of this patient, but EGD will be needed to rule out a carcinoma, stricture, or ring in the esophagus.

376 C (S&F, ch45)

Candida albicans accounts for the majority of infections. Topical glucocorticoids (i.e., inhalers) are a risk factor for esophageal candidiasis. It is seen with esophageal stasis in patients with scleroderma, achalasia, and other motility disorders. Topical and oral antifungal therapy can be effective.

377 D (S&F, ch45)

The condition described is atrial-esophageal fistula complicating radiofrequency ablation procedures. This serious and often fatal complication has been described to occur anywhere from 10 days to 5 weeks after ablation. The initial presentation includes fever and neurologic abnormalities, the latter as a result of air emboli to the brain from the esophagus through the fistula into the left heart. Laboratory studies may reveal leukocytosis and positive blood cultures. Imaging studies reveal gas bubbles in the left atrium.

378 C (S&F, ch43)

A patient who has an alarm symptom needs an endoscopic evaluation. If a patient does not have an alarm symptom, one can consider empirical therapy with PPI. Odynophagia suggests disruption of the esophageal mucosa and may indicate ulceration or carcinoma. Dysphagia is not seen in uncomplicated GERD but could suggest obstruction. Weight loss and GI bleeding are obvious alarm symptoms. Nocturnal symptoms occur in approximately 75% of GERD patients.

379 D (S&F, ch44)

Given the patient's age and comorbidities, an esophagectomy would likely not be the first therapeutic option to be considered. Photodynamic therapy carries with it a risk of serious complications, and cancer can still develop in these patients. Endoscopic mucosal resection followed by radiofrequency ablation with the HALO system would provide this patient with treatment with a relatively low risk.

380 A (S&F, chs41-46)

Patients with scleroderma have diminished esophageal contractions in the smooth muscle (distal) portion of the esophagus, along with LES hypotension. Similar changes are seen in patients with the generalized and limited (CREST) form of the disease.

381 G (S&F, ch45)

Pill-induced esophagitis leads to disruption of the mucosal integrity of the esophagus, and dysphagia (difficulty swallowing) or odynophagia (pain on swallowing) is commonly seen after ingestion of small amounts of even mildly caustic liquids such as citrus juice drinks or alcohol. Endoscopic findings include mucosal disruption; most commonly seen are ulcerations, single or multiple. These findings may be noted on double-contrast radiography or at endoscopy (the latter is the preferred evaluation technique).

382 D (S&F, chs41-46)

Pill-induced esophagitis may occur with many types of pills. Pain is the usual presentation. The endoscopic appearance varies from that of a discrete ulcer to that of a pseudomembrane to a tumor-like appearance.

383 D (S&F, ch45)

Routine endoscopy after blunt trauma to the chest is relatively contraindicated, but gastrograffin contrast studies may be quite useful as a noninvasive means of evaluating the esophagus after trauma. Blunt trauma of the esophagus resulting in perforation is rare; most cases have occurred in the cervical esophagus.

384 C (S&F, ch42)

This patient likely has Zenker's diverticulum. She is a good surgical candidate. The best treatment option according to current studies is transcervical myotomy with diverticulectomy. Good results are reported 80% to 100% of the time. Diverticulectomy alone carries a risk of recurrence. Calcium channel blockers, dilation, and a pureed diet will not change symptoms and are not treatment options for diverticula. In referral centers with trained endoscopists, there are reports of treatment options via either rigid or flexible endoscopy. The septum between the lumen of the diverticulum and the esophagus is divided with a monopolar argon plasma coagulator or needle-knife.

385 D (S&F, ch43)

Saliva is an essential factor that is required for normal esophageal acid clearance. It is a weak base but can easily neutralize the small amount of acid in the esophagus that occurs after normal peristalsis. Increased salivation occurs with use of lozenges, which decreases acid clearance time. Decreased salivation during sleep is a contributing cause of prolonged acid clearance in reflux patients. Cigarette smokers may have prolonged esophageal acid clearance times due to hyposalivation.

386 B (S&F, ch41)

Webs are seen mainly in women and may be associated with squamous cancer of the pharynx and esophagus. There is no association of eosinophilic esophagitis with esophageal webs.

387 **A** (S&F, ch43)
Barium esophagography is generally only useful in severe reflux esophagitis. The results of upper endoscopy are generally normal in patients with GERD, and inspection alone is inadequate. Impedance testing helps in both acid and nonacid reflux. Capsule endoscopy has not been shown to be effective for reflux symptoms.

388 **C** (S&F, chs41-46)
The classic radiographic features of oropharyngeal dysphagia after a stroke are vallecular pooling, tracheal aspiration, and nasopharyngeal aspiration.

389 **A** (S&F, ch45)
Endoscopic evaluation is considered the most effective means of evaluating suspected pill esophagitis in patients with odynophagia or dysphagia. Routine endoscopy after blunt trauma to the chest is relatively contraindicated, but gastrograffin contrast studies may be quite useful as a noninvasive means of evaluating the esophagus after such trauma. Herpetic esophagitis is characterized by multiple small vesicles in the esophagus.

390 **C** (S&F, chs41-46)
The inlet patch is composed of gastric fundic or antral mucosa. It is not Barrett's-type metaplastic tissue. The patch may secrete acid and is rarely associated with a web, stricture, or ulcer. It may be infected with *H. pylori*. There are no data to indicate that ablation therapy is needed.

391 **C** (S&F, ch43)
Lifestyle changes should be part of the initial management plan and can be highly effective in those with minimal symptoms. They can include elevating the head of the bed, avoiding tight fitting clothes, losing weight if overweight, decreasing alcohol use, stopping smoking, and avoiding bedtime snacks. Specific foods to avoid include fats, chocolate, citrus, spicy foods, tomato-based products, tea, and cola.

392 **E** (S&F, ch44)
Histology is necessary to confirm the diagnosis of Barrett's esophagus. The finding of intestinal-type epithelium with goblet cells, also called intestinal metaplasia, specialized intestinal metaplasia, or specialized columnar epithelium, provides clear evidence of metaplasia and confirms Barrett's esophagus.

393 **D** (S&F, chs41-46)
Routine esophageal manometry will show aperistalsis and a hypertensive, nonrelaxing LES. In early achalasia, the esophagus is only minimally dilated.

394 **D** (S&F, ch46)
Alcohol use and tobacco use are strong risk factors for esophageal squamous cell cancers. In general, smoking is considered a moderate risk factor for esophageal adenocarcinoma, whereas alcohol use has no association with esophageal adenocarcinoma. Barrett's esophagus is the major risk factor

for adenocarcinoma of the esophagus. Both tumors spread in a similar fashion.

395 **H** (S&F, ch43)
The pathogenesis of gastroesophageal reflux is complex and may involve each or all of the mechanisms listed.

396 **A** (S&F, ch45)
Esophageal motor function may be affected by sclerotherapy; the mechanism of damage may be vagal nerve damage or wall injury. Ulcerations appear within the first few days after sclerotherapy in virtually all patients. Strictures are uncommon, occurring in approximately 15% of patients. Only liquid sucralfate suspension has been shown to prevent or treat postsclerotherapy ulcerations. Acid suppression is generally not considered an effective form of therapy.

397 **D** (S&F, ch45)
Surface-acting agents are generally effective with acid suppression for pill-induced esophagitis. Effective therapy for other forms of infectious esophagitis are described. Infection with the HPV often does not require treatment; however, if the lesions are large, they may need to be removed by an endoscopic or even a surgical procedure. Routine medical treatments, including interferon and bleomycin administration, have not had consistently effective results and therefore are not commonly used.

398 **A** (S&F, chs41-46)
This patient has long-segment Barrett's esophagus and has an increased risk of esophageal adenocarcinoma. Treatment is with continuous acid-suppressive therapy. Discontinuation of acid suppression will result in recurrent esophagitis in the majority of patients. Endoscopic surveillance with biopsy to detect dysplasia is indicated every one to two years.

399 **C** (S&F, ch43)
H. pylori is thought to be somewhat protective for Barrett's esophagus through its urea-splitting effect, which causes an alkaline environment. *H. pylori* is still endemic in developing countries. Alcohol use and smoking are precursors for squamous cell carcinoma of the esophagus. Heartburn during the last trimester of pregnancy occurs in approximately 70% to 75% of women due to increasing fetal size and hormonal effects. Middle-aged white men, often obese, are classic Barrett's esophagus patients.

400 **B** (S&F, ch44)
According to the American College of Gastroenterology, patients with Barrett's esophagus should have a regular surveillance endoscopy. For patients with two consecutive endoscopies without dysplasia, the interval can be changed to every three years. The pathology is consistent with Barrett's esophagus. There is no need to monitor pH.

401 **A** (S&F, chs41-46)
The patient's history, physical examination, and manometry results are classic for individuals

with this dominantly inherited skeletal muscle condition.

402 **G** (S&F, ch43)

Pregnant women typically have GERD but rarely have histologically proven esophagitis. The two conditions are not the same. GERD encompasses all aspects of gastroesophageal reflux, whereas esophagitis specifically indicates mucosal injury. Esophagitis can complicate Sjögren syndrome because patients with this syndrome have xerostomia and therefore the inability of the saliva to neutralize normally refluxed acid. Patients with scleroderma have severe esophageal dysmotility with resultant poor acid clearance and consequent esophagitis. They may also have Sjögren syndrome, compounding the problem. Hypersecretory states of Zollinger-Ellison syndrome are often complicated by esophagitis.

403 **B** (S&F, ch41)

Inlet patches are common and are usually asymptomatic. Adenocarcinoma is possible but is quite rare.

404 **D** (S&F, ch43)

Spontaneous perforation secondary to esophagitis is quite rare. Strictures develop in 8% to 20% of patients with esophagitis. Barrett's metaplasia is seen in approximately 10% of patients with esophagitis. Significant GI hemorrhage complicates esophagitis in 2% to 5% of cases.

405 **E** (S&F, ch45)

Forceful coughing, straining, retching during endoscopy, transesophageal echocardiography, and cardiopulmonary resuscitation result in an abrupt increase in intra-abdominal pressure and gastric herniation, which can cause a Mallory-Weiss tear. Other factors that predispose to tearing include alcohol and aspirin use.

406 **B** (S&F, ch43)

Standard once-daily dosing with a PPI generally maintains pH levels above 4 for approximately 10 to 14 hours per day. Double doses or increased amounts of medication may further decrease acid production. H_2 receptor antagonists may be used, especially in the evening, for patients with nocturnal acid breakthrough as an additive form of therapy to decrease acid production. H_2 receptor antagonists are not as effective as PPIs in the treatment of esophagitis. PPI therapy will lead to healing after two months of therapy in more than 80% of patients.

407 **B** (S&F, chs41-46)

A Schatzki ring is a frequent cause of intermittent dysphagia for solids. The ring diameter is critical, with constriction to a diameter of 13 mm or less causing frequent symptoms. Dilation is effective, but repeat dilation may be required in approximately one third of cases.

408 **B** (S&F, ch46)

Kaposi's sarcoma has been reported in the esophagus, usually concomitant with oral and skin lesions in patients with AIDS. They can present with dysphagia, odynophagia, and rarely GI hemorrhage.

409 **A** (S&F, chs41-46)

Perforation after pneumatic dilation in patients with achalasia requires immediate surgery for closure of the perforation if the patient is febrile and if contrast extends into the pleural or peritoneal cavity. Limited or contained perforation can be managed conservatively.

410 **C** (S&F, ch43)

The contribution of hiatal hernia to GERD is unclear; however, a strikingly higher percentage of patients with reflux esophagitis have hiatal hernia (54% to 94%). Reflux is worse in patients with a nonreducible as opposed to a reducible hernia. Nonreducing hernias are those with gastric rugal folds above the diaphragm during swallows. An alteration of esophagogastric junction compliance occurs in GERD patients with hiatal hernia. For the same degree of intragastric pressure, the esophageal junction opens at a lower pressure. This change in compliance creates an increase in air and liquid reflux.

CHAPTER
5

Stomach and Duodenum

QUESTIONS

411 In a patient with early gastric cancer (EGC), which of the following is more likely to metastasize to the lymph nodes?
A. A tumor in the gastric cardia
B. A 1.5-cm sessile mass
C. A nodular raised mass >4.5 cm
D. None of the above

412 Which biopsy specimen is most suggestive of eosinophilic gastritis?

A.

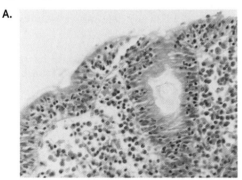

Figure for question **412A**

B.

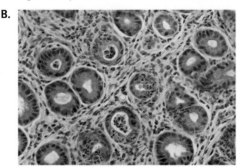

Figure for question **412B**

413 Mutations in the E-cadherin (*CDH1*) gene have been linked to the development of hereditary diffuse gastric cancer.
A. True
B. False

414 Which of the following statements regarding interstitial cells of Cajal (ICC) is false?
A. They originate from c-kit–positive mesenchymal cells.
B. Myenteric ICC are responsible for spontaneous generation of slow waves.
C. Intramuscular ICC facilitate propagation of slow waves in the stomach.
D. Intramuscular ICC in the cardia have a role in mechanoreception.
E. Loss of ICC in the antrum is associated with gastroparesis.

415 A mother brings her five-week-old infant to your office, reporting projectile vomiting, difficulty feeding, and weight loss. She states the infant was normal at birth with normal APGAR scores. Which of the following statements regarding this condition is false?
A. Fifty percent of identical twins are affected.
B. The incidence in the United States is 3 per 1000 live births.
C. It is more common in males.
D. An abdominal ultrasound scan may confirm the diagnosis.
E. None of the above

416 The most accurate method to stage gastric cancer is by which of the following studies?
A. Transabdominal ultrasonography
B. Magnetic resonance imaging
C. Helical computed tomography (CT) scan
D. Endoscopic ultrasonography (EUS)

417 True statements regarding nonsteroidal anti-inflammatory drug (NSAID) pathophysiology include all of the following *except*:
A. Cyclooxygenase (COX)-2 is the predominant COX in the stomach.
B. Prostaglandin concentration in the mucosa is reduced.
C. Gastric mucosal blood flow is decreased.
D. Injury may occur independent of the effect of decreased prostaglandin synthesis.

418 A 68-year-old black man residing in the United States was found to have a proximal adenocarcinoma of the stomach. After CT scan and EUS, the lesion was staged as T3N1M0. What is the appropriate five-year survival rate?
A. >80%
B. <5%
C. <20%
D. 50%

419 A patient with known cancer in the gastric antrum and no metastasis on CT undergoes EUS for staging. EUS (see figure) depicts a 2-cm hypoechoic mass. Based on this information, what is the most appropriate TNM classification of this tumor?
A. T2N1M0
B. T2N2M0
C. T2N3M0
D. T3N0M0
E. T3N2M0

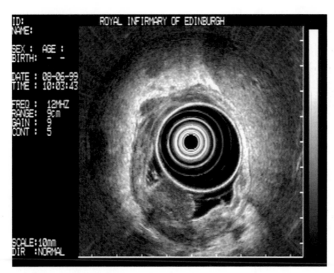

Figure for question **419**

420 Hyperglycemia is associated with all of the following *except*:
A. Antral hypermotility
B. Isolated pyloric contractions
C. Gastric dysrhythmias
D. Impaired action of prokinetic drugs

421 Which of the following regarding the cells lining the stomach is false?
A. Mucosal cells are simple columnar epithelial cells that secrete mucus for luminal cytoprotection.

B. Proton pumps in the parietal cells begin acid secretion 30 minutes after stimulation.
C. Parietal cells are the sites of intrinsic factor secretion.
D. Chief cells synthesize and secrete pepsinogen I and II.
E. Gastrin-secreting G cells secrete gastrin into the lumen of the stomach as well as the bloodstream.

422 Which of the following regarding diabetes mellitus (DM) gastroparesis is false?
A. Patients often have DM for >10 years.
B. Gastroparesis develops in 20% of patients with long-standing type 1 DM.
C. An important manifestation is erratic blood glucose control.
D. Patients may experience unexpected hypoglycemia in the postprandial periods.

423 All of the following paraneoplastic syndromes are associated with gastric cancer *except*:
A. Acanthosis nigrans
B. Disseminated intravascular coagulation
C. Thrombophlebitis (Trosseau's sign)
D. Pyoderma gangrenosum
E. Nephrotic syndrome

424 Anna, a 25-year-old woman born in Russia, has been diagnosed with a *Helicobacter pylori*–positive gastric ulcer. She is allergic to penicillin. What is the most appropriate treatment regimen?
A. PPI twice daily, 500 mg clarithromycin twice daily, and 1 g amoxicillin twice daily for 10 days
B. PPI twice daily, 500 mg clarithromycin twice daily, and 500 mg metronidazole twice daily for 10 days
C. PPI twice daily, 1 g amoxicillin twice daily for 5 days, then 250 mg levofloxacin twice daily for 5 days
D. PPI twice daily, 500 mg clarithromycin twice daily, and 525 mg bismuth subsalicylate four times daily for 10 days.

425 Clinically significant GI bleeding from stress-related mucosal injury can be decreased by which of the following methods?
A. Infusion of H_2 receptor antagonist
B. 1 g sucralfate every six hours via a nasogastric tube
C. PPI infusion
D. None of the above

426 Regarding gastric diverticula, which of the following is true?
A. Gastric diverticula are relatively common.
B. There is a risk of malignancy associated with a distal gastric diverticulum.
C. There is a risk of malignancy associated with a proximal gastric diverticulum.
D. A true congenital gastric diverticulum projects into but not through the muscle layer.
E. All of the above

427 Bile reflux gastropathy is least likely to occur in which of the following patients?
A. In patients with Billroth I or II anastomosis
B. In patients after truncal vagotomy and pyloroplasty for peptic ulcer disease

C. In patients after cholecystectomy and sphincteroplasty

D. In adult and pediatric patients who have not had surgery

428 All patients with the following conditions should undergo screening for gastric cancer *except*:
A. Those with hyperplastic/fundic gland polyps
B. Those with low-grade gastric dysplasia
C. Those with familial adenomatous polyposis (FAP)
D. Those with gastric adenoma

429 Which of the following statements regarding the duodenum is true?
A. The majority of it lies retroperitoneally.
B. It has circular folds known as plicae circulares.
C. Its arterial supply arises from the superior mesenteric artery and celiac axis.
D. All of the above

430 Which of the following regarding idiopathic gastroparesis is false?
A. It is usually preceded by an acute febrile illness.
B. Postviral gastroparesis may resolve completely over one to two years.
C. It accounts for >50% of cases of gastroparesis.
D. Viruses such as Norwalk, herpes simplex, and Epstein-Barr have been documented in a number of cases.

431 Which statement about pepsin is false?
A. It is produced in an inactive proenzyme form.
B. Activation of pepsin requires gastric acid.
C. Pepsin is produced in parietal cells.
D. It is inactivated at a pH of 5.

432 Potential chemoprotective agents for gastric cancer include all of the following *except*:
A. Antioxidants such as carotenoids and vitamins C and E
B. Aspirin
C. Green tea
D. High-fiber diet

433 A 45-year-old human immunodeficiency virus–positive man presents with severe epigastric pain, fever, and atypical lymphocytosis. An upper GI (UGI) tract radiographic study reveals a rigid and narrowed gastric antrum. An upper endoscopy is performed and the gastric biopsy reveals the following (see figure). The biopsy findings are suggestive of which of the following?
A. Herpes simplex gastritis
B. Gastric lymphoma
C. *H. pylori* gastritis
D. Cytomegalovirus gastritis
E. Gastric adenocarcinoma

434 Correct statements about peptic ulcer epidemiology in the developed world in the last decade of the 20th century include all of the following *except*:
A. Fewer patients require hospital care.
B. The mortality rate has decreased in all age groups.
C. Bleeding from peptic ulcer is less common.
D. Duodenal ulcers account for >80% of cases.

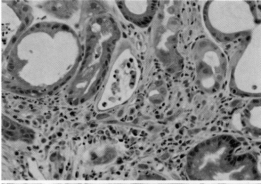
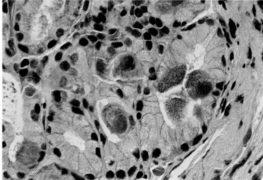

Figure for question **433**

435 All of the following tumors can metastasize to the stomach *except*:
A. Melanoma
B. Breast cancer
C. Prostate cancer
D. Colon cancer
E. None of the above

436 Which of the following statements regarding annular pancreas is true?
A. It usually presents in adulthood and rarely in infants.
B. The anomalous tissue is histologically abnormal.
C. Infant and childhood cases are commonly associated with other anomalies.
D. The anomalous tissue usually contains GI tissue.

437 A 65-year-old white man underwent upper endoscopy that revealed a 1-cm submucosal lesion in the gastric antrum. The lesion was removed by endoscopic mucosal resection (EMR). The gross and histologic specimens are seen in the figure (on p. 84). What is the diagnosis?
A. Gastric carcinoid
B. GI stromal tumor
C. Gastric lipoma
D. Schwannoma

438 A trial of empirical therapy with a PPI is indicated for which of the following patients with dyspepsia?
A. A 75-year-old attorney from Philadelphia
B. A 21-year-old college student who recently emigrated from Indonesia
C. A 50-year-old schoolteacher with weight loss
D. A 40-year-old electrician from New Jersey

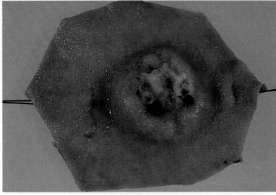

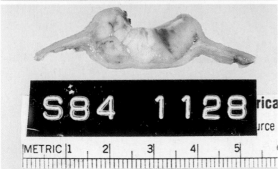

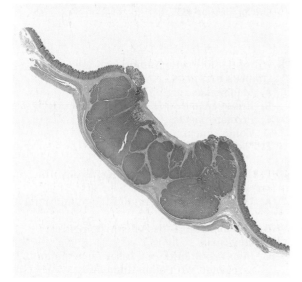

Figure for question **437**

439 Which is the least likely operation to cause chronic postsurgical gastroparesis?
A. Billroth I
B. Billroth II
C. Roux-en-Y gastrojejunostomy
D. Fundoplication
E. Vagotomy with pyloroplasty

440 Hydrochloric acid helps the absorption of which of the following?
A. Vitamin B_{12}
B. Calcium
C. Iron
D. Protein
E. All of the above

441 Clinical manifestations of chronic *H. pylori* infection include all of the following *except*:
A. Duodenal ulcers
B. Chronic gastritis
C. Adenocarcinoma of the stomach
D. Barrett's epithelium
E. Gastric ulcer

442 Lymphocytic gastritis has been associated with all of the following diseases *except*:
A. *H. pylori*
B. Gastric lymphoma
C. Splenic and mesenteric venous thrombosis
D. Celiac disease
E. None of the above

443 Indications for gastric biopsies include which of the following?
A. Gastric erosion or ulcer
B. Thick gastric fold(s)
C. Gastric polyp(s) or mass(es)
D. Diagnosis of *H. pylori* infection
E. All of the above

444 *H. pylori* infections in developing countries are characterized by all of the following *except*:
A. Acquisition before age 10 years
B. Can be spontaneously eliminated and reacquired
C. Rarely seen in adults older than age 50
D. More common in families with more siblings
E. Lack of hot or running water in household

445 Which of the following is the most common type of gastric lymphoma?
A. Non-Hodgkin's lymphoma
B. Mucosa-associated lymphoid tissue lymphoma
C. Hodgkin's lymphoma
D. None of the above

446 *H. pylori* infection can inhibit acid production by which mechanism?
A. Production of interleukin-1B
B. Tumor necrosis factor-α
C. Direct inhibition of parietal cells
D. All of the above

447 Duodenal ulcer pathophysiology is usually associated with which of the following?
A. Gastric acid hyposecretion
B. Elevated fasting serum gastrin levels
C. Pangastritis as the precursor lesion when caused by *H. pylori* infection
D. Increased duodenal bicarbonate production

448 A 53-year-old black woman undergoes upper endoscopy for evaluation of epigastric symptoms. Upper endoscopic findings reveal a 1.5-cm polypoid mass in the proximal stomach. Pathology reveals well-differentiated adenocarcinoma. Which of the following is the most appropriate next step?
A. Resection with snare polypectomy
B. EUS
C. CT scan of the abdomen
D. Positron emission tomography scan
E. Transabdominal ultrasonography

449 Acute severe epigastric pain develops in a 40-year-old man. In the emergency department, plain films

demonstrate pneumoperitoneum. Which of the following is correct?
- **A.** A perforated duodenal ulcer is much more likely than a gastric ulcer.
- **B.** Emergent surgery is indicated.
- **C.** Intra-abdominal abscess is unlikely because of the sterile nature of the UGI tract.
- **D.** At the time of surgery, a definitive ulcer operation should be done.

450 PPIs are very effective in acid peptic disease. Which of the following statements about PPIs is true?
- **A.** Hypergastrinemia due to profound acid suppression may lead to gastric carcinoid tumors.
- **B.** PPIs are maximally effective when most of the pumps are inactive.
- **C.** If long-term therapy is contemplated, a U.S. Food and Drug Administration advisory group recommends testing and treating for *H. pylori* first.
- **D.** Hepatic and renal insufficiency does not require dose adjustments.

451 Indications for testing for *H. pylori* include all of the following *except*:
- **A.** Duodenal ulcer
- **B.** Mucosa-associated lymphoid tissue lymphoma
- **C.** Gastric ulcer
- **D.** Gastroesophageal reflux disease
- **E.** Uninvestigated dyspepsia

452 Which patient diagnosed with EGC is most amenable to EMR?
- **A.** A 40-year-old white man with T2N0M0-stage gastric cancer
- **B.** A 75-year-old black man with a 4-cm mass in the gastric cardia with pathology revealing an intestinal type of gastric adenocarcinoma
- **C.** A 50-year-old black woman with a 2-cm T1N0M0-stage tumor along the lesser curvature, posterior mid body of the stomach associated with nodularity in the gastric antrum revealing a well-differentiated adenocarcinoma
- **D.** An 85-year-old white man with a 1.5-cm mass in the mid body greater curvature of the stomach of stage T1N0M0

453 The vagus nerve synapses with postganglionic neurons within the stomach wall. All of the following are postganglionic transmitters *except*:
- **A.** Acetylcholine
- **B.** Nitric oxide
- **C.** Vasoactive intestinal polypeptide
- **D.** Histamine

454 The ability of *H. pylori* to survive in the acid milieu of the stomach and to cause a chronic infection are due to all of the following factors *except*:
- **A.** Urease production
- **B.** Multiple unipolar flagellae
- **C.** Lewis antigens in host cells
- **D.** Presence of intestinal metaplasia in the stomach
- **E.** CAG pathogenicity island in the bacterial DNA

455 Which of the following medications and toxins are associated with reactive gastropathies?
- **A.** Aspirin (81 mg/day) and NSAIDs
- **B.** Oral iron
- **C.** Oral potassium
- **D.** Alcohol
- **E.** All of the above

456 What provides the strongest stimulus for satiety?
- **A.** Infusion of nutrients into the duodenum
- **B.** Infusion of nutrients into the stomach
- **C.** Nutrients taken by mouth
- **D.** Increase in plasma ghrelin levels

457 At the time of diagnosis, 75% of gastric adenocarcinomas are found to have metastasized to the lymph nodes. After surgical resection, which therapy provides the best adjuvant therapy?
- **A.** Chemotherapy alone
- **B.** Observation
- **C.** Radiation therapy alone
- **D.** Combined chemotherapy and radiation therapy

458 Among *H. pylori*–infected patients, the risk of peptic ulcer disease is increased by which of the following?
- **A.** Cigarette smoking
- **B.** NSAID use
- **C.** Alcohol use
- **D.** All of the above

459 The spread of *H. pylori* infection is attributed to which of the following?
- **A.** Contaminated water
- **B.** Exposure to vomitus in infected siblings
- **C.** Contact with infected cats
- **D.** Inadequately disinfected gastroscopes
- **E.** All of the above

460 Which of the following statements regarding gastric cancer is true?
- **A.** Patients younger than age 40 have a better prognosis.
- **B.** The depth of invasion is the primary prognostic indicator.
- **C.** Survival rates are worse for men than women.
- **D.** EGC is defined as penetration through the muscularis propria.
- **E.** Serum carcinoembryonic antigen levels >5 ng/mL are found in nearly 50% of patients with resectable gastric cancer.

461 All of the following are premalignant conditions related to gastric cancer *except*:
- **A.** Adenomatous gastric polyps
- **B.** Previous gastrectomy performed 25 years earlier
- **C.** History of gastric ulcer
- **D.** Ménétrier's disease
- **E.** None of the above

462 An 84-year-old man with a prosthetic cardiac valve needs treatment for a painful joint. He is diagnosed with osteoarthritis. He is also on low-dose aspirin and is receiving anticoagulation therapy with warfarin. The most correct advice for him is to
- **A.** Avoid NSAIDs altogether.
- **B.** Begin NSAIDs only after stopping the aspirin.
- **C.** Start a COX-2 inhibitor.
- **D.** Start a COX-2 inhibitor with a PPI.

463 A 70-year-old man presents with symptoms of midepigastric pain unresponsive to PPI therapy. Upper endoscopy is performed (see figure), and the pathology is consistent with high-grade dysplasia. What would the optimal management be?
A. Yearly surveillance endoscopy
B. EMR
C. Continue PPI therapy
D. Evaluate *H. pylori* status; if infection is present, treat and repeat endoscopy in three months.
E. Subtotal gastrectomy

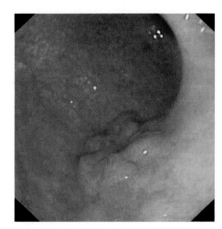

Figure for question **463**

464 PPI therapy is better than misoprostol or H_2 receptor antagonists in the treatment of NSAID-associated peptic ulcer disease (PUD).
A. True
B. False

465 Which of the following statements regarding *H. pylori* gastritis is false?
A. It is mainly seen in low and immigrant socioeconomic populations.
B. It is associated with an increased risk of gastric cancer.
C. In most cases, the gastric antrum appears normal to the endoscopist.

466 Histamine stimulates acid production by a variety of mechanisms, including which of the following?
A. Stimulation of parietal cells directly
B. Generation of cyclic adenosine monophosphate
C. Inhibition of somatostatin release
D. Binding to H_3 receptors
E. All of the above

467 Which of the following is the most likely to remain asymptomatic?
A. Annular pancreas
B. Gastric duplication
C. Gastric diverticulum
D. Duodenal duplication cyst

468 *H. pylori* infection localized to the gastric antrum is associated with which of the following?
A. Gastric ulcers
B. Duodenal ulcers

C. Gastric cancer
D. Atrophic gastritis

469 A 71-year-old white woman underwent upper endoscopy for dyspepsia and heme-positive stool. Upper endoscopy reveals a 1.5-cm sessile mass in the midbody greater curvature of the stomach. Biopsy specimens revealed adenomatous tissue with high-grade dysplasia. Initially, the mass was staged with CT of the abdomen and pelvis, the results of which were normal. Based on these findings and the results of EUS (see figure), what would be the most effective method to treat this patient?
A. Chemotherapy and radiation therapy
B. Photodynamic therapy
C. Subtotal gastrectomy
D. EMR

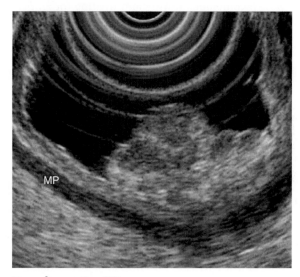

Figure for question **469**

470 PPI infusion in the treatment of bleeding PUD
A. Maintains the pH of 6 or greater in the stomach 99% of the time
B. Significantly reduces rebleeding when given after endoscopic therapy
C. May down-stage the stigmata of bleeding at the initial esophagogastroduodenoscopy (EGD)
D. Has not been shown to decrease mortality
E. All of the above

471 Which of the following forms of bacterial infectious gastritis is associated with draining sinus tracts demonstrated on UGI series, upper endoscopy, and gastric biopsy?
A. *H. pylori*
B. Mycobacteria
C. Actinomycosis
D. Syphilis

472 Formation of acid in parietal cells requires all of the following *except*:
A. Carbonic anhydrase
B. Apical K^+ channels
C. Basolateral HCO_3/Cl exchangers
D. High luminal pH

473 A 2-cm submucosal mass is identified in the fundus of the stomach. Based on the findings at endoscopy and EUS (see figure), what is the likely diagnosis?
A. Gastric adenocarcinoma
B. Gastric lipoma
C. Pancreatic rest
D. Gastric carcinoid
E. GI stromal tumor

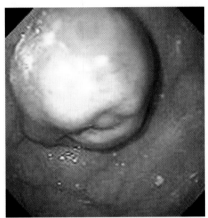

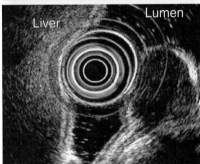

Figure for question **473**

474 All of the following stimulate cholinergic neurons in the enteric nervous system and acid production *except*:
A. Anticipation of the meal
B. Protein in the food
C. Mechanical distention of the stomach
D. Cholecystokinin

475 In the United States, at the time of diagnosis of gastric cancer, which region of the stomach is most likely involved?
A. Proximal third
B. Middle third
C. Distal third
D. Entire stomach

476 Which of the two forms of gastritis is associated with pernicious anemia?
A. Environmental metaplastic atrophic gastritis
B. Autoimmune metaplastic atrophic gastritis

477 According to the American Gastrointestinal Association guidelines, which of the following patients should undergo prompt upper endoscopy?
A. A 25-year-old black woman reporting a one-week history of midepigastric pain

B. A 45-year-old white man reporting midepigastric pain responsive to a two-week course of PPI therapy
C. A 70-year-old black man reporting a six-week history of midepigastric pain associated with a 10-pound weight loss, nausea, and vomiting
D. A 62-year-old asymptomatic white woman with normal hemoglobin, heme-positive stool, and normal colonoscopy findings

478 For patients with functional dyspepsia, which of the following statements is false?
A. They rarely present with nausea.
B. They have a normal endoscopy.
C. They have normal rates of gastric emptying the majority of the time.
D. Gastric dysrhythmias may be present.

479 A 20-year-old college student reports episodic midepigastric pain with a 5-pound weight loss over the past three months. His history reveals that he loves sushi and eats sushi two to three times per week. Which parasitic disease is he likely to have?
A. Anisakiasis
B. Cryptosporidiosis
C. Strongyloidiasis
D. Ascariasis
E. Hookworm infestation

480 Which group of patients is least likely to have a higher incidence of gastric cancer?
A. Those with FAP
B. Those with hereditary nonpolyposis cancer
C. Those with juvenile polyposis syndrome
D. Those with a family history of a second-degree relative with gastric cancer

481 Two months after her treatment regimen, Sophia was asymptomatic on a daily PPI. All of the following would be appropriate follow-up care *except*:
A. Do a breath test after the patient is off the PPI for two weeks.
B. Perform an endoscopy and obtain a biopsy specimen of the stomach to check for *H. pylori*.
C. Check a stool specimen for *H. pylori* antigen.
D. Do a serology test for *H. pylori* antibody.

482 Which of the following statements regarding graft-versus-host disease in the UGI tract is true?
A. It occurs more commonly in solid organ transplantation than allogeneic bone marrow transplantation.
B. Graft-versus-host disease is more common in the UGI tract than the lower GI tract.
C. Pathologic lesions consist of necrosis of single cells (apoptotic bodies) in the neck region of the gastric mucosa and the crypts of the large and small intestine.

483 Tolerance to the antisecretory effect can be seen with which of the following PPIs?
A. Omeprazole
B. Pantoprazole
C. Lansoprazole
D. All of the above
E. None of the above

484 Which of the following facts about gastric sarcoidosis is false?
- **A.** Gastric sarcoidosis can cause pyloric outlet obstruction, achlorhydria, and pernicious anemia.
- **B.** Least common section of the GI tract affected by sarcoidosis
- **C.** Glucocoticoid therapy is the cornerstone of treatment.
- **D.** Gastric biopsy specimens reveal noncaseating granulomas.

485 NSAID use or *H. pylori* infection is a predisposing factor in all peptic ulcerations of the stomach and duodenum.
- **A.** True
- **B.** False

486 All of the following statements regarding duodenal ulcer caused by *H. pylori* infection are true *except*:
- **A.** Compared with maintenance antisecretory therapy, *H. pylori* eradication has been shown to decrease the bleeding risk.
- **B.** After one to two weeks of therapy, additional antisecretory therapy is required.
- **C.** Noninvasive confirmation of eradication is advised for all complicated ulcers.
- **D.** Post-treatment maintenance with an antisecretory drug is not needed.

487 What is the most common genetic mutation found in gastric cancer?
- **A.** Adenomatous polyposis coli (*APC*)
- **B.** *FHIT* gene
- **C.** *TP53*
- **D.** K-*ras* and *Myc*

488 Hyperplastic gastropathy as seen in the figure is associated with all of the following conditions *except*:
- **A.** Pernicious anemia
- **B.** Zollinger-Ellison syndrome
- **C.** Ménétrier's disease
- **D.** Gastric neoplasm
- **E.** Gastric varices

489 Which of the following regarding histamine H_2 receptor antagonists is true?
- **A.** Tolerance is not seen with oral or intravenous dosing.
- **B.** They should not be used at all in liver failure.
- **C.** They have a side effect profile comparable to that of a placebo.
- **D.** They frequently result in clinically significant drug interactions.

490 Which environmental and/or dietary factor is least likely to trigger the multistep development of the intestinal type of gastric cancer?
- **A.** *H. pylori*
- **B.** High intake of fresh fruit and vegetables
- **C.** High intake of pickled foods, soy sauce, salted fish and meats
- **D.** Cigarette smoking
- **E.** Obesity

491 Which of the following statements regarding EGD for the evaluation of PUD symptoms is true?

- **A.** It should be done after UGI radiographic studies.
- **B.** Although more specific, it is less sensitive than UGI radiography.
- **C.** It should be done if weight loss or signs of bleeding are present.
- **D.** When malignant ulcer is excluded by pathology and cytology, a repeat EGD to confirm healing is not mandatory.

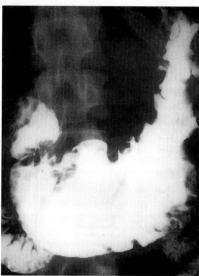

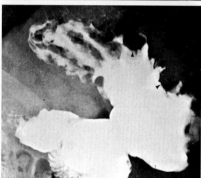

Figure for question **488**

492 Peptic ulcer is a common complication of NSAID treatment. Which statement regarding prophylactic therapy is correct?
- **A.** H_2 receptor antagonists do not lower the risk.
- **B.** Only high-dose misoprostol (800 μg/day) provides effective prophylaxis.
- **C.** *H. pylori*–infected patients should receive eradication therapy.
- **D.** Ulcer bleeding can be prevented in high-risk patients by omeprazole.

493 You are asked to evaluate and treat a patient with hematemesis. He is 34 years old, has no chronic medical illnesses, and presents with syncope soon after vomiting bright-red blood. In the emergency department, red hematemesis is documented. On examination, he is awake but agitated, with cool extremities and dry mucous membranes. His heart rate is 130 beats per minute and his supine blood pressure is 90/60 mm Hg. There is no scleral

icterus. The abdomen is soft and nontender without hepatomegaly, with black stool in the rectum that is flash positive for occult blood. Laboratory studies reveal a hemoglobin level of 11.0, BUN/creatinine levels of 40/0.9, normal prothrombin time/partial thromboplastin time, aspartate aminotransferase/alanine aminotransferase levels of 119/42, alcohol level of 280. What should be the first intervention for this patient?
A. Bolus and infusion of octreotide
B. Bolus and infusion of a PPI
C. Insertion of a nasogastric tube
D. Emergent upper endoscopy
E. Placement of large-bore intravenous lines for vigorous fluid resuscitation

494 During an endoscopy, active bleeding begins. What is the best course of treatment at this point?
A. Bolus and infusion of a proton pump inhibitor (PPI)
B. Epinephrine injection
C. Argon plasma coagulation
D. Contact thermal therapy (heater probe or multipolar electrocautery) or placement of hemoclips
E. Combination therapy with **B** and **D**

495 After endoscopic therapy, the bleeding stops and the patient stabilizes. He requires 3 units of packed erythrocytes to maintain a hemoglobin level at more than 10 g/dL. Three days later, on a clear liquid diet and taking a PPI twice daily, melena develops. His pulse increases to 100 beats per minute, but no orthostasis is noted. The hemoglobin level drops to 9 g/dL. What is the next best step?
A. Consult surgery for a definitive antiulcer operation.

B. Consult surgery for vagotomy and oversewing of the bleeding vessel.
C. Consult surgery to oversew the bleeding vessel.
D. Repeat EGD for possible endoscopic therapy.
E. Transfuse packed red blood cells and observe.

496 At urgent endoscopy, no active bleeding or old blood is seen. A few erosions are noted in the gastric antrum. Inspection of the duodenal bulb reveals a raised red protuberance in the center of an ulcer. The duodenal ulcer measures 15 mm in diameter. What is the approximate likelihood of rebleeding from this ulcer?
A. <10%
B. 20%
C. 40%
D. 80%

497 Compared with all patients with upper gastrointestinal (GI) bleeding, his mortality is higher than average.
A. True
B. False

498 Worldwide, which country has the greatest incidence of gastric cancer?
A. United States
B. Korea
C. Japan
D. Australia

499 Histamine receptor antagonists have never been shown to decrease the bleeding rate or mortality rate in patients with bleeding duodenal ulcer.
A. True
B. False

ANSWERS

411 **B** (S&F, ch54)
Studies have shown that gastric lesions smaller than 2 to 3 cm have a 3.5% chance of lymph node involvement. Lesions larger than 4.5 cm have a greater than 50% chance of spread into the submucosa and are associated with positive nodes.

412 **B** (S&F, ch51)
Features of gastric mucosal biopsy specimens suggestive of eosinophilic gastritis include marked eosinophilic infiltration, eosinophilic pit abscesses, necrosis with numerous neutrophils, and epithelial regeneration. Abnormal eosinophilic infiltration is defined as at least 20 eosinophils per high-power field, either diffusely or multifocally.

413 **A** (S&F, ch54)
Families with hereditary diffuse gastric cancer have been found to carry a germline mutation in the *CDH1* gene, all with diffuse-type cancer. Studies have shown that suppression of E-cadherin expression occurs in 51% of cancers, with a higher percentage found in diffuse-type cancers.

414 **D** (S&F, ch48)
ICC originate from c-kit–positive mesenchymal cell precursors. Myenteric ICC generate slow waves, whereas intramuscular ICC propagate slow waves. In addition, intramuscular ICC in the fundus act as sensory cells and play a role in mechanoreception, and loss of ICC in the antrum is associated with gastroparesis in patients with DM.

415 **E** (S&F, ch47)
The incidence of infantile hypertrophic pyloric stenosis in the United States is approximately 3 per 1000 live births. Males outnumber females by a ratio of 4:1 or 5:1; 50% of identical twins are affected. Noncontrast radiography demonstrates a distended stomach with paucity of gas beyond the stomach. Diagnosis is confirmed by abdominal ultrasonography of the pylorus, which has supplanted contrast radiography as the diagnostic study of choice for infantile hypertrophic pyloric stenosis.

416 **D** (S&F, ch54)
EUS is the best modality to stage gastric cancer. Imaging can provide one with T (depth of tumor invasion) and N (nodal status) with an accuracy of 80%. Helical CT and MRI can provide information regarding distant metastases.

417 **A** (S&F, ch52)
The COX isoform found in the stomach is COX-1. COX being the rate-limiting enzyme in prostaglandin synthesis, gastric mucosal concentrations are reduced by COX inhibition. Gastric mucosal blood flow, one of the main defense mechanisms, is compromised by NSAID-related decreases in prostaglandins. Increased leukotriene production caused by enzymatic shifts in arachidonic acid metabolism may lead to mucosal injury independent of prostaglandin inhibition.

418 **C** (S&F, ch54)
T3N1M0 adenocarcinoma of the stomach corresponds to stage IIIA disease. The five-year survival rate in the United States is less than 20% (see tables at end of chapter).

419 **D** (S&F, ch54)
The T stage signifies depth of tumor invasion; N, nodal status; and M, metastasis. The CT scan findings were negative for metastasis, making this an M0 tumor. The tumor extends beyond the serosa of the stomach, making this a T3 tumor, and there were no perigastric lymph nodes, making the nodal status N0. Thus, the tumor stage for this patient is T3N0M0.

420 **A** (S&F, ch48)
Hyperglycemia is associated with loss of ICC, antral hypomotility, isolated pyloric contractions, gastric dysrhythmias, and impaired prokinetic action of drugs like erythromycin.

421 **B** (S&F, ch47)
The gastric mucosal surface is composed primarily of columnar epithelial cells that secrete mucus for cytoprotection. Parietal cells begin acid secretion 5 to 10 minutes after stimulation and are also the sites of intrinsic factor secretion. Chief cells synthesize and secrete pepsinogen I and II into the gastric lumen. G cells secrete gastrin into the lumen as well as the bloodstream.

422 **B** (S&F, ch48)
Fifty percent of patients with long-standing type 1 DM will experience gastroparesis, usually after more than 10 years of having the disease. They experience erratic blood glucose control and postprandial hypoglycemia because of delayed gastric emptying.

423 **D** (S&F, ch54)
Acanthosis nigrans, disseminated intravascular coagulation, thrombophlebitis, and nephrotic syndrome can all be seen as paraneoplastic syndromes associated with gastric cancer. Pyoderma gangrenosum is most commonly associated with inflammatory bowel disease and more common in ulcerative colitis than in Crohn's disease.

424 **B** (S&F, ch50)
The treatment in **A** and **C** cannot be used because of penicillin allergy. The treatment in **D** is inadequate because a single antibiotic is a less effective regimen (see table at end of chapter).

425 **D** (S&F, ch53)
Although widely used in critically ill patients at risk of stress mucosal injury, H₂ blockers, PPIs, and sucralfate via a nasogastric tube have not been shown to prevent these ulcerations.

426 **B** (S&F, ch47)
A gastric diverticulum is the rarest type of GI diverticulum. The true congenital diverticulum contains all gastric tissue layers and is located on the posterior wall of the cardia. The intramural (or partial) diverticulum projects into but not through the muscular layer. In the case of an incidentally discovered proximal gastric diverticulum, treatment is unnecessary. Because of the risk of malignancy associated with distal gastric diverticula, surgical treatment by amputation, invagination, or segmental resection has been recommended.

427 **D** (S&F, ch51)
Bile reflux gastropathy least commonly occurs in adult and pediatric patients who have never had surgery. Bile reflux contributes to mucosal lesions in the stomach and may facilitate *H. pylori* colonization in the corpus region. Gastric atrophy may result in an increased risk of intestinal metaplasia and gastric cancer.

428 **A** (S&F, ch54)
The rate of malignant transformation of a hyperplastic/fundic gland polyp is less than 1%. Patients with gastric adenomas, FAP, and polyps with low-grade dysplasia have an approximately 11% risk of the development of carcinoma in situ within 4 years of follow-up.

429 **D** (S&F, ch47)
The first few centimeters of the duodenum are shrouded by anterior and posterior elements of the peritoneum. The remainder of the duodenum lies posterior to the peritoneum and thus is retroperitoneal. As is the case with the remainder of the small intestine, the luminal surface is lined with mucosa, forming circular folds known as the plicae circulares or valvulae conniventes. The branches of the celiac trunk supply the proximal duodenum, whereas the distal duodenum is supplied by branches of the superior mesenteric artery.

430 **C** (S&F, ch48)
One third of diagnosed cases of gastroparesis are idiopathic. Many of the cases are preceded by an acute febrile illness described as flu-like, and viruses such as herpes, Epstein-Barr, and Norwalk have been identified in some cases. Postviral gastroparesis may resolve completely over one to two years.

431 **C** (S&F, ch49)
Pepsin is produced in chief cells and mucus neck cells as a proenzyme. Pepsins are reversibly inactivated at a pH of 5 and are most active at a pH of 1.8 to 3.5.

432 **D** (S&F, ch54)
Carotenoids and vitamins C and E are antioxidants that seem to have a chemoprotective effect for gastric cancer. Aspirin inhibits COX and has been shown to potentially inhibit cell growth and apoptosis and increase angiogenesis. Green tea containing polyphenols has a variety of antitumor effects,

including antioxidant activity, induction of apoptosis, and inhibition of tumor cell proliferation.

433 **D** (S&F, ch51)
The biopsy specimen shown suggests cytomegalovirus colitis. The specimen reveals inflammatory debris, chronic active gastritis, and enlarged cell "owl-eye" intranuclear inclusions, which are the hallmarks of cytomegalovirus infection. Herpes simplex gastritis biopsy specimens show numerous single cells and clumps of cells, with ground-glass nuclei and eosinophilic intranuclear inclusion bodies surrounded by halos.

434 **B** (S&F, ch52)
The hospitalization rate decreased by 20% in the 1990s. The mortality rate also decreased by 22% in the same period, but not in elderly patients. In a Canadian study, the prevalence of bleeding from nonvariceal sources decreased by 31% over a similar period. In a Danish prospective peptic ulcer study, only 55% of cases were duodenal.

435 **C** (S&F, ch54)
Metastatic disease to the stomach can occur with melanoma and breast, lung, ovary, liver, colon, and testicular cancers, with breast cancer being the most common.

436 **C** (S&F, ch47)
The lesion may present in the neonatal period, childhood, or adulthood. It is the most common congenital anomaly of the pancreas presenting in children. Infant and childhood cases are associated with other congenital anomalies in an estimated 40% to 70% of cases. The anomalous tissue is histologically normal and contains a moderately sized pancreatic duct.

437 **A** (S&F, ch54)
Gastric carcinoid tumors account for 7% of all GI carcinoid tumors and 0.2% of all gastric neoplasms. In the stomach, the well-differentiated tumors are mainly of enterochromaffin-like cell origin, with a small minority being of endocrine cell types.

438 **D** (S&F, ch52)
Patients older than ages 50 to 55 years or those with alarm symptoms may have gastric cancer and should have an EGD before any empirical trial. Dyspeptic patients from areas of high *H. pylori* prevalence should have serologic testing before PPI therapy.

439 **E** (S&F, ch48)
Gastric neuromuscular dysfunction occurs in a subset of patients undergoing stomach operations. Vagotomy is associated with a number of gastric abnormalities that promote gastroparesis, and vagotomy performed during ulcer operations requires a pyloroplasty to reduce outflow resistance. Most patients recover from the effects of vagotomy, but in patients undergoing extensive resections of the antrum and corpus, as in Billroth I, Billroth II, or Roux-en-Y gastrojejunostomy, prolonged symptoms and chronic gastric neuromuscular dysfunction are likely.

440 **E** (S&F, ch49)
Acid facilitates the absorption of all options listed.

441 **D** (S&F, ch50)
Barrett's epithelium is inversely related to the presence of *H. pylori* infection.

442 **E** (S&F, ch51)
Lymphocytic gastritis is characterized by a dense lymphocytic infiltration of surface and pit gastric epithelium (see figure). This form of gastritis has been attributed to an atypical host immune response to *H. pylori*, gastric lymphoma, thrombosis of the confluence of the splenic and mesenteric veins, and celiac disease.

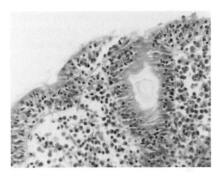

Figure for answer **442**

443 **E** (S&F, ch51)
Gastric biopsies provide an excellent opportunity for the clinician and pathologist to communicate to correlate clinic data, endoscopic findings, and pathologic findings. Biopsies allow the clinician to make an accurate diagnosis.

444 **C** (S&F, ch50)
Usually 80% of adults older than the age of 50 in developing countries have been infected.

445 **A** (S&F, ch54)
Gastric lymphomas comprise 3% of all gastric malignancies. More than 95% of gastric lymphomas are non-Hodgkin's lymphomas. Gastric lymphoma is the most common form of extranodal non-Hodgkin's lymphoma, accounting for more than 30% of all cases of primary non-Hodgkin's lymphoma.

446 **D** (S&F, ch49)
The mechanism is multifactorial. A constituent of the bacterium can directly inhibit parietal cells. Cytokines released in response to infection also inhibit parietal cells.

447 **B** (S&F, ch52)
Patients with duodenal ulcer are usually *hypersecreters* of acid. Serum gastrin levels are elevated. Pangastritis from *H. pylori* typically decreases acid secretion and is less likely to be associated with duodenal ulcers. Duodenal bicarbonate production is decreased in duodenal ulcers.

448 **C** (S&F, ch54)
Once the diagnosis of gastric adenocarcinoma is made, proper staging of the tumor should be performed before therapeutic intervention. The first test performed should be a computed axial

tomography scan of the abdomen with or without a positron emission tomography scan to exclude distant metastasis, and if findings are negative, EUS is used to obtain an accurate T (depth of tumor invasion) and N (nodal status) to stage the tumor. This will allow one to decide on endoscopic resection, surgical resection, or combined modality therapy.

449 **A** (S&F, ch53)
Approximately 80% of perforated ulcers are duodenal. In low-risk situations, medical therapy with nasogastric decompression, intravenously administered fluids, and pain control is appropriate. An intra-abdominal abscess may complicate a perforated ulcer when treated conservatively. When surgery is done to repair the perforation, a definitive antiulcer operation is not necessary in the era of antibiotics for *H. pylori* and potent antisecretory therapy.

450 **C** (S&F, ch53)
Carcinoid tumor of the stomach has never been observed in humans. The clinical effect of PPIs is maximized by administration before mealtimes to coincide with pump activation in the immediate postprandial state. PPI therapy in *H. pylori*–infected patients has been associated with gastric atrophy, but the U.S. Food and Drug Administration actually concluded that the data did not support routine testing for infection before initiation of long-term PPI treatment. PPIs are neither hepatotoxic nor nephrotoxic, and dose adjustment with liver and renal disease is not necessary.

451 **D** (S&F, ch50)
H. pylori does not cause GERD and should not be checked in acid reflux problems. It can cause all the other conditions listed (see table at end of chapter).

452 **D** (S&F, ch54)
Intramucosal tumors less than 2 to 3 cm in size are most amenable to endoscopic mucosal resection. In the cases listed, tumors described in answers **A**, **B**, and **C** were characterized as beyond the mucosa, larger than 2 to 3 cm, and having synchronous areas of tumor within the stomach.

453 **D** (S&F, ch49)
Histamine is not a postganglionic transmitter. It is a paracrine agent produced in enterochromaffin-like cells (see figure).

454 **D** (S&F, ch50)
H. pylori does not colonize metaplastic cells in the stomach. Urease produces ammonia to reduce acidity, and flagellae propel the organism through the mucus layer. Lewis antigens serve as a receptor on host cells for binding. CAG A provides proteins that help bacterial products to translocate into host cells.

455 **E** (S&F, ch51)
Aspirin, at any dose, NSAIDs, oral iron, oral potassium, bisphosphonates, hepatic arterial chemotherapy, ingestion of heavy metals (e.g., mercury sulfate), and alcohol have all been shown to cause reactive gastropathy manifested endoscopically by erythema, subepithelial hemorrhage, and erosions.

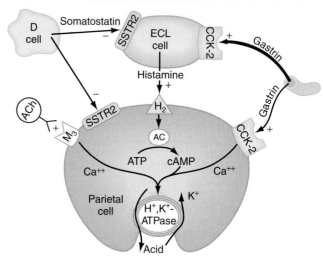

Figure for answer **453**

456 **C** (S&F, ch48)
The volume of food ingested suppresses hunger and stimulates a sense of fullness. Infusion of nutrients into the stomach induces a greater intensity of fullness than infusion into the duodenum, and the suppression of hunger is greater when nutrients are taken by mouth.

457 **D** (S&F, ch54)
Patients who were node positive after an attempt at curative resection have been found to have a local recurrence rate of 49%, peritoneal recurrence rate of 17%, locoregional disease 21%, and hematogenous spread of 17%. Combined modality therapy with combination chemotherapy consisting of a regimen of 5-fluorouracil, leucovorin, and radiation therapy had a mean increase in survival to 36 months compared with 27 months in a patient treated with surgery alone.

458 **D** (S&F, ch52)
Several studies indicate that smoking increases the risk of peptic ulcer only in *H. pylori*–infected individuals. Concomitant *H. pylori* infection and NSAID use increases the odds ratio for the development of peptic ulcer to 15.4. At least one study demonstrates an increased risk of peptic ulcer with regular alcohol use in *H. pylori*–positive patients.

459 **E** (S&F, ch50)
A and **B** are the most important sources of infection, but the others listed have been reported in a small number of cases.

460 **B** (S&F, ch54)
The most important prognostic indicator for gastric cancer is the depth of tumor invasion (T stage). The prognosis is worse in patients younger than age 40, equal among men and women, and high carcinoembryonic antigen levels seem to correlate with unresectablitiy. EGC is defined as tumor confined to the mucosa.

461 E (S&F, ch54)
Adenomatous gastric polyps undergo malignant transformation at a high rate, especially those polyps larger than 1 cm. Previous gastric resection performed before the age of 50 more than 20 years earlier carries a higher risk of gastric cancer on the gastric side of the surgical anastomosis. A history or the presence of a gastric ulcer is associated with a 1.8-fold increased risk of gastric cancer. Fifteen percent of cases of Ménétrier's disease are associated with gastric cancer.

462 A (S&F, ch53)
This patient is at high risk because of his age, comorbid illnesses, and concurrent therapy with aspirin and warfarin. GI bleeding would potentially be fatal, and NSAIDs should be avoided if at all possible. NSAIDs without prophylactic therapy would be risky. A COX-2 inhibitor with aspirin and without an antisecretory agent would be dangerous as well. COX-2 therapy with high-dose PPI is the next best option.

463 B (S&F, ch54)
EGC is defined as cancer that does not invade beyond the submucosa regardless of lymph node involvement. This can be confirmed by EUS. EGC of less than 2 cm can best be removed by EMR and spare the patient a subtotal or total gastrectomy. Candidates for EMR include those with mucosal involvement without lymph node involvement, maximum tumor size less than 2 cm, no evidence of multiple gastric cancers, and the intestinal type of gastric cancer.

464 A (S&F, ch53)
NSAID-associated peptic ulcers can be treated with misoprostol or H_2 receptor antagonists, but healing rates are higher with PPI therapy. PPIs are definitely superior if NSAID therapy must be continued.

465 B (S&F, ch51)
H. pylori gastritis is mainly seen in low socioeconomic and immigrant populations, and there is no increased risk of gastric cancer. Most patients are asymptomatic, and in most cases, the gastric antrum is normal endoscopically.

466 E (S&F, ch49)
Histamine stimulates acid production by binding to H_2 receptors. It indirectly stimulates acid by binding to H_3 receptors coupled to inhibition of somatostatin release.

467 C (S&F, ch47)
Most congenital gastric diverticula are asymptomatic and are incidental findings on radiography or endoscopy or at autopsy.

468 B (S&F, ch50)
Distal or antral infections lead to increased acid production because of decreased antral somatostatin content and increased gastrin secretion. The duodenal bulb becomes metaplastic and can then be colonized with *H. pylori* with subsequent ulceration.

469 D (S&F, ch54)
The EUS image corresponds to a T1 or tumor confined to the mucosa measuring less than 2 cm in diameter, making this lesion amenable to an attempt at EMR. Subtotal gastrectomy, chemotherapy, and radiation therapy can also be used as therapeutic options. Photodynamic therapy has yet to be adequately studied, and no definitive recommendations can be made.

470 E (S&F, ch53)
Highly effective at controlling gastric pH, PPI infusions have been shown to decrease rebleeding after endoscopic therapy. Early therapy with PPI infusion seems to decrease the incidence of high-risk stigmata (active bleeding or visible vessel) at the time of endoscopy. Mortality is not decreased by PPI infusion, according to a *Cochrane Database Systematic Review*.

471 C (S&F, ch51)
Actinomycosis is a rare, chronic, progressive, suppurative disease characterized by formation of multiple abscesses, draining sinuses, abundant granulation, and dense fibrous tissue. Mycobacteria and syphilis do not lead to sinus tracts; however, the differential for all forms of bacterial gastritis listed include benign ulcer disease, gastric carcinoma, gastric lymphoma, and Crohn's disease involving the stomach.

472 D (S&F, ch49)
H^+ is pumped out against a large concentration gradient by the H^+K^+-ATPase mechanism. The others are all essential features of H^+ production in the parietal cell.

473 E (S&F, ch54)
The endoscopic image reveals a submucosal mass with normal overlying mucosa. The endosonographic image reveals that the mucosa and submucosa are intact. The tumor arises from the muscularis propria and is well circumscribed. This would indicate that the lesion in the image shown would be most consistent with a GI stromal tumor. Adenocarcinoma of the stomach arises in the mucosa, and lipomas, pancreatic rests, and gastric carcinoids arise in the submucosa.

474 D (S&F, ch49)
Cholecystokinin stimulates somatostatin secretion, which decreases acid production.

475 A (S&F, ch54)
In the United States, the distribution of gastric cancer in the stomach is 39% in the proximal third, 17% in the middle third, 32% in the distal third, and 12% involving the entire stomach.

476 A (S&F, ch51)
Autoimmune metaplastic atrophic gastritis is relatively uncommon, accounting for less than 5% of all cases of chronic gastritis. Autoimmune metaplastic atrophic gastritis is the pathologic process in patients with pernicious anemia, an autoimmune disorder usually occurring in individuals of northern European or Scandinavian background. Environmental metaplastic atrophic gastritis is associated with *H. pylori* in 85% of cases. Environmental metaplastic atrophic gastritis intestinal metaplasia is a risk factor for dysplasia and gastric cancer, usually the intestinal type.

477   **C** (S&F, ch54)

American Gastrointestinal Association recommendations for prompt endoscopy include age older than 55 years with new-onset dyspepsia, age younger than 55 years with alarm symptoms (weight loss, recurrent vomiting, dysphagia, bleeding, anemia), and dyspeptic patients in whom empirical PPI therapy failed. Recommendations for upper endoscopy for an asymptomatic patient with a heme-positive stool and normal colonoscopy findings are less clear.

478   **A** (S&F, ch48)

Functional dyspepsia symptoms include epigastric discomfort, early satiety, fullness, nausea, and vomiting in the setting of a normal upper endoscopy. One of the dominant symptoms is unexplained nausea. The rate of gastric emptying is normal in the majority of patients; however, gastric dysrhythmias may be present.

479   **A** (S&F, ch51)

Anisakiasis may occur after the ingestion of raw marine fish containing nematode larvae of *Anisakis*. The parasite migrates into the wall of the stomach, small intestine, or colon, causing symptoms. Laboratory evaluation may reveal peripheral eosinophilia; radiographic studies may reveal notched-shadow defects; and endoscopy may reveal erosive hemorrhagic lesions or larvae.

480   **D** (S&F, ch54)

FAP has a 10-fold higher risk of the development of gastric cancer than the general population. Patients with hereditary nonpolyposis cancer have an 11% chance of the development of gastric cancer. Juvenile polyposis syndrome has a 12% to 20% incidence of gastric cancer. Those patients with a first-degree relative, but not a second-degree relative, with gastric cancer have a greater risk of the development of gastric cancer (see table at end of chapter).

481   **D** (S&F, ch50)

The serology test cannot distinguish an active from a previous infection. The other tests can detect a persistent *H. pylori* infection.

482   **C** (S&F, ch51)

Graft-versus-host disease is more common in allogeneic bone marrow transplantation rather than solid organ transplantation. Acute graft-versus-host disease (21 to 100 days post-transplantation) more commonly affects the small bowel and colon than the stomach. Pathology is noted in answer **C**, and necrosis that is identified consists of an intraepithelial vacuole filled with karyorrhectic debris and fragments of cytoplasm.

483   **D** (S&F, ch53)

Short-term studies have failed to demonstrate tolerance with any of the PPIs.

484   **B** (S&F, ch51)

GI manifestations of sarcoidosis are uncommon, but the stomach (usually the antrum) is the most common part of the GI tract affected in sarcoidosis and is involved in 10% of cases.

485   **B** (S&F, ch52)

Although *H. pylori* infection or NSAID use is present in most patients with PUD, an increasing number of patients have neither factor. Other drugs such as cocaine and the bisphosphonates may play a role in these cases.

486   **B** (S&F, ch53)

A meta-analysis showed a 1.6% rebleeding rate in the *H. pylori*–treated group compared with 5.6% in the medical therapy group. Combination therapy is associated with ulcer healing. In uncomplicated ulcers, additional antisecretory therapy is not clearly necessary. Complicated duodenal ulcers caused by *H. pylori* should be treated with antimicrobial therapy, and documentation of eradication is advised. After successful treatment of *H. pylori*, maintenance acid-lowering therapy is not needed.

487   **C** (S&F, ch54)

TP53 mutation is the most common genetic mutation found in patients with gastric cancer, with an incidence of 60% to 70%. The *FHIT* genetic mutation is found in 60% of cases, the *APC* genetic mutation in 50% of cases, and K-*ras*/*Myc* genetic mutations in 10% to 15% of cases of gastric cancer (see table at end of chapter).

488   **A** (S&F, ch51)

Hyperplastic gastropathy is a rare condition characterized by giant gastric folds associated with epithelial hyperplasia. The two clinical syndromes causing this are Zollinger-Ellison syndrome and Ménétrier's disease. Zollinger-Ellison syndrome is associated with or without increased or normal acid secretion, parietal and chief cell hyperplasia, with or without excessive gastric protein loss. Ménétrier's syndrome is associated with protein-losing gastropathy and hypochlorhydria.

489   **C** (S&F, ch53)

Tolerance rapidly develops within two or three days of intravenous administration of all H_2 receptor antagonists. Liver disease is not a contraindication to their use, and dose modifications are not needed. H_2 blockers are extremely safe, with a side effect profile similar to that of a placebo. Drug-drug interactions, though common, are rarely significant.

490   **B** (S&F, ch54)

H. pylori, pickled foods, soy sauce, salted fish and meats, cigarette smoking, and preserved foods high in nitrates have been clearly shown to be associated with an increased risk of the development of gastric cancer. Increased body mass index seems to be associated with a moderate risk of cardia cancer but not noncardia gastric cancer. Fresh fruits and vegetables containing antioxidants have been associated with a decreased risk of gastric cancer (see table for answer **480** at end of chapter).

491   **C** (S&F, ch52)

Expert UGI radiographic studies are not as available as they once were, and although not 100% sensitive, EGD is more sensitive and specific than UGI radiography. EGD is indicated when alarm symptoms of bleeding or weight loss are present. The false-negative rate for gastric cancer with EGD and biopsy may be as high as 4%.

492 **C** (S&F, ch53)

H$_2$ receptor blocker in high doses reduces NSAID-caused gastric ulcer. The prostaglandin analog misoprostol has been shown to reduce the ulcer risk with low-dose (400 µg/day) or high-dose regimens. Eradication of *H. pylori* lowers the risk of ulcer formation in patients who are planning long-term NSAID treatment. High-risk patients will ideally avoid NSAIDs altogether. The risk of bleeding in these patients cannot be eliminated even with high-dose PPIs.

493 **E** (S&F, ch53)

Fluid resuscitation is the most important intervention in this patient who is severely volume depleted from GI bleeding. Pharmacotherapy (with octreotide or PPI) is less urgent. With documentation of red emesis, nasogastric tube placement is not needed for diagnostic purposes; if there is ongoing vomiting, tube decompression will decrease the risk of aspiration. Emergent EGD should be performed after the volume depletion has been aggressively managed.

494 **E** (S&F, ch53)

Although high-dose PPI infusion may decrease rebleeding rates after endoscopic treatment, drug therapy alone is probably inadequate. Injected epinephrine is absorbed from the duodenal mucosa and provides only short-term hemostasis. Argon plasma coagulation lacks the mechanical component of therapy present in the contact-thermal modalities. Multiple trials have shown the most success with epinephrine injection, followed by the application of a contact-thermal device. Hemoclip placement seems to be equivalent to the thermal methods.

495 **D** (S&F, ch53)

The patient has rebled despite endoscopic and antisecretory medications. Although his surgical risks are probably low, repeating the endoscopy would confirm the clinical suspicion and allow a second endotherapy. If surgery is ultimately needed, the best option is vessel ligation and postoperative PPI therapy.

496 **C** (S&F, ch53)

The patient has a nonbleeding visible vessel in a duodenal ulcer. The rebleeding risk in most clinical trials is more than 40%.

497 **A** (S&F, ch53)

This patient presented with red hematemesis, which has been identified as an adverse clinical prognostic factor. In addition, he has signs of significant hemodynamic compromise, another adverse factor.

498 **C** (S&F, ch54)

The highest incidence rates for gastric cancer are in the Far East. Japan ranks first worldwide followed by Korea, South America, Costa Rica, and Ecuador. The lowest-risk areas include North America, Africa, South Africa, and Australia (see figure).

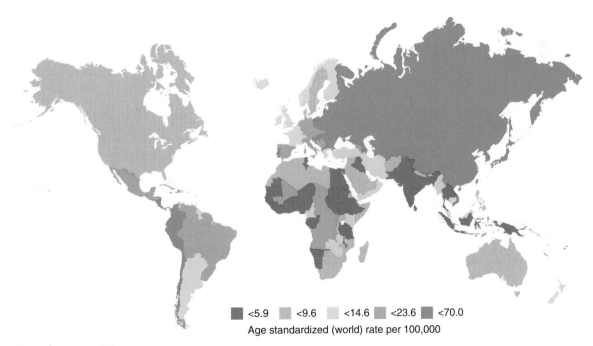

<5.9   <9.6   <14.6   <23.6   <70.0
Age standardized (world) rate per 100,000

Figure for answer **498**

499 **A** (S&F, ch53)

The clinical studies analyzing parenteral H$_2$ receptor antagonist in bleeding PUD demonstrate benefit in gastric ulcer alone. Tachyphylaxis to the effect of H$_2$ blockers may explain the absence of benefit in the typically increased acid state of duodenal ulcer disease.

Tables

Table 1 for answer 418 Clinical Staging of Gastric Cancer Based on the TNM Classification

	N0	N1	N2	N3	M1 (ANY N)
Tis	0	—	—	—	—
T1	IA	IB	II	IV	IV
T2	IB	II	IIIA	IV	IV
T3	II	IIIA	IIIB	IV	IV
T4	IIIA	IV	IV	IV	IV

is, in situ; M, metastases; N, node involvement; T, tumor.
From references 320 and 321. See text for further details.

Table 2 for answer 418 Five-Year Survival Rates (%) for Patients with Gastric Cancer Based on Clinical Staging

STAGE	UNITED STATES	JAPAN	GERMANY
IA	78	95	86
IB	58	75	72
II	34	46	47
IIIA	20	48	34
IIIB	8	18	25
IV	7	5	16

From Hundahl S, Philips J, Menck H. The National Cancer Data Base Report on poor survival of U.S. gastric carcinoma patients treated with gastrectomy: 5th ed. American Joint Committee on Cancer staging, proximal disease, and the "different disease" hypothesis. Cancer 200; 88:921-32.

Table for answer 424 First-Line Treatment of *Helicobacter pylori* Infection*

TREATMENT REGIMEN*	DURATION	ERADICATION RATE	COMMENTS
PPI†, clarithromycin 500 mg, amoxicillin 1000 mg (each twice daily)	10-14 days	70%-85%	Macrolide resistance affects eradication success; not appropriate for penicillin allergic individuals or those who have received a clarithromycin regimen in the past
PPI†, clarithromycin 500 mg, metronidazole 500 mg (each twice daily)	10-14 days	70%-85%	Appropriate for penicillin-allergic individuals who have not received a clarithromycin-containing regimen in the past
PPI†, amoxicillin 1000 mg (each twice daily) **followed by** PPI†, clarithromycin 500 mg, tinidazole 500 mg (each twice daily)	5 days 5 days	90%	Appears highly effective despite clarithromycin resistance; limited experience to date in the United States
Bismuth subsalicylate 525 mg, metronidazole 500 mg, tetracycline 500 mg (each four times daily) **plus** PPI† or H₂RA (twice daily)	10-14 days	75%-90%	Inexpensive but complicated regimen; consider in penicillin allergic individual or if clarithromycin resistance is suspected; can be used for retreatment (see Table 50-4)

*Note that not all of these regimens are currently approved by the U.S. Food and Drug Administration (FDA).
†Lansoprazole 30 mg, pantoprazole 40 mg, rabeprazole 20 mg, omeprazole 20 mg, or esomeprazole 40 mg (esomeprazole can be taken once daily).
H$_2$RA, histamine H$_2$-receptor antagonist; PPI, proton pump inhibitor.
Adapted from references 131, 150, and 151.

Table for answer 451 **Indications for Testing and Treatment of** *Helicobacter pylori* **Infection**

Supported by evidence
  Active peptic ulcer disease (gastric or duodenal ulcer)
  Confirmed history of peptic ulcer (not previously treated for *H. pylori* infection)
  Gastric MALT-lymphoma (low grade)
  Following endoscopic resection of early gastric cancer
  Uninvestigated dyspepsia (if *H. pylori* population prevalence high)
Controversial
  Functional dyspepsia
  GERD
  Persons using NSAIDs, especially when first initiating NSAID treatment
  Unexplained iron deficiency anemia or immune thrombocytopenic purpura
  Populations at higher risk of gastric cancer (e.g. Asians, Eastern Europeans, Mesoamericans)

GERD, gastroesophageal reflux disease; MALT, mucosa-associated lymphoid tissue; NSAIDs, nonsteroidal anti-inflammatory drugs. Adapted from references 129 and 131.

Table for answers 480 and 490 **Risk Factors Including Protective Factors for Gastric Adenocarcinoma**

Definite	*Helicobacter pylori* infection
	Chronic atrophic gastritis
	Intestinal metaplasia
	Dysplasia*
	Adenomatous gastric polyps*
	Cigarette smoking
	History of gastric surgery (esp. Billroth II)*
	Genetic factors
	Family history of gastric cancer (first-degree relative)*
	Familial adenomatous polyposis (fundic gland polyps)*
	Hereditary nonpolyposis colorectal cancer*
	Peutz-Jeghers syndrome*
	Juvenile polyposis*
Probable	High intake of salt
	Obesity (adenocarcinoma of cardia only)
	Snuff tobacco use
	History of gastric ulcer
	Pernicious anemia*
	Regular aspirin or NSAID use (protective)
Possible	Low socioeconomic status
	Ménétrier's disease
	High intake of fresh fruits and vegetables (protective)
	High ascorbate intake (protective)
Questionable	Hyperplastic and fundic gland polyps
	High intake of nitrates
	High intake of green tea (protective)

*Surveillance for cancer is suggested in patients with this risk factor.
NSAID, nonsteroidal anti-inflammatory drug.

Table for answer 487 **Genetic Abnormalities in Gastric Adenocarcinoma**

ABNORMALITIES	APPROXIMATE GENE FREQUENCY (%)
DNA aneuploidy	60-75
Microsatellite instability	15-50
Deletion/Suppression	
TP53 gene	60-70
Fragile histidine triad gene (*FHIT*)	60
Adenomatous polyposis coli (*APC*) gene LOH	50
Deleted in colorectal cancer (*DCC*) gene LOH	50
Decreased Expression Due to Hypermethylation	
p16	≈50
TFF1	≈50
p27	<50
MLH1	15-20
E-cadherin	50
Amplification/Overexpression	
Cyclooxygenase-2 (*COX-2*)	70
Hepatocyte growth factor (*HGF*)	60
Vascular endothelial growth factor (*VEGF*)	50
c-Met	50
Amplified in breast cancer-1 (*AIB-1*)	40
Beta-catenin	25
EGF/EGFR	15
Mutations	
PI3K	25
PTPRT	17

DNA, deoxyribonucleic acid; EGF, epidermal growth factor; EGFR, epidermal growth factor receptor; LOH, loss of heterozygosity; MLH1, human mutL homolog 1; PI3K, phosphatidylinositol 3-kinase; PTPRT, protein-tyrosine phosphatase receptor-type; TFF1, human trefoil factor 1.

CHAPTER
6

Pancreas

QUESTIONS

500 By definition, an episode of pancreatitis is considered chronic pancreatitis if
- A. It is a recurrent episode.
- B. It occurs in the face of alcohol use.
- C. There are radiographic findings of ductal irregularity and parenchymal fibrosis.
- D. It is associated with steatorrhea.
- E. A pseudocyst is present.

501 Which of the following is true in the pathogenesis of chronic pancreatitis?
- A. There is accumulation of damaging lipid granules in pancreatic stellate cells.
- B. Chronic alcohol use decreases protein content of pancreatic secretions.
- C. There is disorientation of acinar cell secretory function.
- D. There is migration of ductal cells into the acini.

502 A patient is admitted to the intensive care unit (ICU) for acute pancreatitis. Which of the following statements regarding the ICU management of acute pancreatitis is true?
- A. Nutrition should be provided by total parenteral nutrition (TPN) until the serum lipase is less than three times normal.
- B. Antibiotics should be initiated empirically.
- C. Oxygen by nasal cannula should be administered.
- D. Enterally administered probiotics should be initiated.

503 Which of the following is most accurate with regard to autoimmune pancreatitis?
- A. It is more common in women than in men.
- B. It is associated with sclerosis of extrapancreatic sites such as the salivary glands and retroperitoneum.

- C. It typically presents between the ages of 40 and 55.
- D. When sclerosing cholangitis occurs in association with autoimmune pancreatitis, it tends to be poorly responsive to corticosteroid treatment.

504 A patient is in the ICU with acute pancreatitis. The patient's condition has stabilized, and the issue of nutrition is being addressed. Which statement regarding the provision of nutrition in acute pancreatitis is true?
- A. When initiating a diet, a low-fat diet has been shown to be as safe as a clear liquid diet.
- B. Compared with nasojejunal feeding, TPN has been shown to decrease the length of stay.
- C. Studies have shown that nasoenteric tube feeding is better tolerated than nasogastric tube feeding.
- D. Although nasojejunal feedings reduce septic complications, the use of TPN is more cost-effective in the ICU setting.

505 What is the major mediator of pancreatic hydrogen ion–stimulated bicarbonate and water secretion?
- A. Cholecystokinin (CCK)
- B. Secretin
- C. Acetylcholine
- D. Gastrin
- E. Vasoactive intestinal polypeptide (VIP)

506 A 38-year-old woman presents to the emergency department with several hours of nausea and severe abdominal pain. The patient describes her pain as unrelenting midepigastric pain radiating to her back. On examination, the patient is in the fetal position and reluctant to move. She is tachycardic and has a low-grade fever. Orthostatic hypotension is noted. Laboratory study results are remarkable for an amylase level of 1100 and a lipase level of 1900. Which of the following tests is most appropriate for assessing the severity of her illness?

A. Abdominal radiograph (kidneys, ureter, bladder [KUB])
B. Abdominal ultrasonography (US)
C. Computed tomography (CT)
D. Magnetic resonance imaging (MRI)
E. Endoscopic retrograde cholangiopancreatography (ERCP)

507 In the patient from question 506, the other admission laboratories included white blood cell (WBC) count of 22,000, hemoglobin level of 15, total bilirubin level of 3.2 mg/dL, alkaline phosphatase level of 375 IU/L, aspartate aminotransferase (AST) level of 130 IU/L, alanine aminotransferase level of 170 IU/L, and PO_2 of 85. In this patient, which of the following laboratory studies is most indicative of severe disease?

A. Alkaline phosphatase
B. Amylase
C. AST level
D. WBC count
E. Bilirubin

508 A malnourished 10-year-old Sri Lankan boy with diabetes mellitus has been reluctant to eat because it exacerbates his severe abdominal pain. Evaluation with a CT scan demonstrated an atrophic pancreatic parenchyma with a dilated main pancreatic duct filled with stones. Which epidemiologic association is most reliably associated with this disease?

A. *SPINK1* mutation
B. Protein-calorie malnutrition
C. Cassava ingestion
D. Apolipoprotein (APO) C-II deficiency

509 Which of the following statements regarding populations at increased risk of developing pancreatic cancer is most correct?

A. Familial pancreatic cancer is transmitted in an autosomal dominant fashion.
B. Individuals with Peutz-Jeghers syndrome, although at increased risk of pancreatic cancer, need not undergo a screening regimen.
C. Patients with alcohol-induced chronic pancreatitis who concomitantly smoke have the greatest risk of the development of pancreatic cancer.
D. The *BRCA1* mutation carries with it an eightfold risk of pancreatic cancer.

510 Which is an accurate relationship between gallstones and pancreatitis?

A. Pancreatitis develops in approximately 5% of patients with gallstones.
B. Gallstones cause approximately 65% of all cases of acute pancreatitis.
C. Gallstone pancreatitis occurs with equal frequency in men and women.
D. Smoking increases the risk of gallstone pancreatitis.

511 The congenital anomaly seen on ERCP (see figure) is most likely a result of which of the following?

A. Failure of fusion of the dorsal and ventral pancreatic ducts

B. Failure of recanalization of the duodenal lumen during the third week of embryonic development
C. Isolated agenesis of the dorsal pancreas
D. Coalescence of pancreatic ductules
E. Right ventral pancreatic bud encircling the duodenum

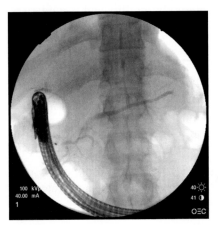

Figure for question **511**

512 A patient is admitted to the ICU with severe pancreatitis and systemic inflammatory response syndrome (SIRS). The patient has six Ranson criteria and an APACHE (Acute Physiology, Age, and Chronic Health Evaluation) II score of 11. A CT scan demonstrates more than 50% pancreatic necrosis. His WBC count is 26,000, and he is febrile to 103°F. Percutaneous needle aspiration of the necrotic area demonstrates gram-negative bacteria. Which of the following options for this patient's management is correct?

A. Early surgical débridement/necrosectomy is associated with improved survival.
B. Without surgical intervention, this patient has a nearly uniformly fatal outcome.
C. Compared with early surgical intervention, delaying surgical débridement beyond the fourth week is associated with a lower mortality rate.
D. Endoscopic transgastric necrosectomy can now be performed with an outcome equivalent to that with surgical necrosectomy.

513 What is the total daily volume of pancreatic secretions?

A. 0.5 L
B. 1.5 L
C. 2.5 L
D. 3.5 L

514 A 22-year-old graduate student, originally from India, is referred to you for concerns of abdominal pain and weight loss. When providing his history, he states that he eats three meals daily and experiences pain shortly after eating. You suspect tropical pancreatitis as the etiology of disease. Which of the following statements regarding this patient's disease is most accurate?

A. A CT scan will demonstrate an atrophic pancreas with diffuse punctate calcification and an attenuated pancreatic duct.

B. The etiology of disease is well defined and results from dietary intake of regional flora.
C. The greatest cause of mortality in an affected individual is due to the high prevalence of pancreatic carcinoma.
D. Both exocrine and endocrine pancreatic dysfunction is likely to develop in this patient.
E. This patient's weight loss is most likely due to enteric dysmotility and secondary bacterial overgrowth.

515 A 63-year-old woman presents with abdominal pain and painless jaundice. She states that she had been well until 2 months ago when she had onset of unexplained weight loss and has lost 12 pounds during this time. She has had mild midepigastric abdominal pain and no other symptoms. Laboratory studies reveal a total bilirubin level of 13.2 mg/dL with a direct fraction of 9.8 mg/dL, alkaline phosphatase level of 517 IU/L, AST level of 168 IU/L, and alanine aminotransferase level of 114 IU/L. A CT scan demonstrates a 1.4-cm mass in the head of the pancreas resulting in biliary obstruction. Which of the following statements regarding staging of pancreatic carcinoma for this patient is most correct?
A. Abdominal CT correctly predicts resectability only 50% to 75% of the time.
B. Abdominal MRI should be performed to better assess the primary tumor.
C. EUS-guided fine-needle aspiration (FNA) should be performed before surgery to exclude lymphoma.
D. Fluorodeoxyglucose-positron emission tomography (FDG-PET) scan is the appropriate next test for this patient.
E. Surgical laparoscopy should be performed to exclude occult metastases.

516 Which statement regarding markers of severity in acute pancreatitis is true?
A. Urinary trypsinogen activation peptide (TAP) is a surrogate marker of inflammation.
B. Multisystem organ failure is defined as two or more organs failing on the same day.
C. Percutaneous recovery of dark-colored peritoneal fluid predicts a poor prognosis only if the volume recovered is more than 60 mL.
D. The amount of elevation of the serum amylase and lipase correlates with severity.

517 A 7-year-old boy is on TPN in the ICU after undergoing partial small bowel resection for mesenteric ischemia. On day 10, the child develops increasing abdominal pain and is diagnosed with acute pancreatitis. Which study is most appropriate to help identify the etiology of the patient's pancreatitis?
A. Double-stranded DNA
B. *CFTR* gene analysis
C. Serum calcium
D. Epstein-Barr virus titer

518 Which of these is not usually a site of ectopic pancreatic tissue?
A. Stomach
B. Proximal jejunum
C. Meckel's diverticulum

D. Spleen
E. Duodenum

519 A 36-year-old woman presents to the hospital with her third episode of acute pancreatitis over a two-month period. Her initial episode was secondary to alcohol use, and she admits to long-standing alcohol abuse. She has not had any alcohol since her initial episode. On admission, her lipase level is 687 IU/L. After several days of bowel rest, she is clinically improved; however, on the day of discharge, her symptoms recur. A CT scan is performed demonstrating pancreaticolithiasis with upstream dilation of the pancreatic duct (see figure). What is the next appropriate step in the management of this patient?
A. ERCP with pancreatic sphincterotomy and stone removal
B. EUS-guided transgastric pancreatic duct decompression
C. Extracorporeal shockwave lithotripsy for stone dissolution
D. Lateral pancreaticojejunostomy (Puestow procedure)
E. TPN for 4 weeks

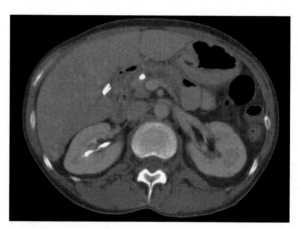

Figure for question **519**

520 A 2-year-old white boy, newly diagnosed with cystic fibrosis (CF), is referred to a neurologist for increased muscle weakness and difficulty in walking. On neurologic examination, the patient is found to have hyporeflexia, decreased proprioception, decreased vibratory sense, and distal muscle weakness. What is the etiology of the patient's neurologic impairment?
A. Demyelinating disease of the neurons
B. Calcium deficiency
C. Guillain-Barré syndrome
D. Vitamin E deficiency
E. Cerebral microinfarcts

521 A 12-year-old white boy with a history of CF that is confirmed by genetic testing and sweat chloride testing presents to his pediatrician with a two-month history of weight loss, foul-smelling bulky bowel movements, and inadequate growth velocity. He is clinically diagnosed as having pancreatic insufficiency and started on uncoated pancreatic enzyme supplements at a dose of 4000 units of

lipase with meals. Two weeks later, the patient's symptoms are essentially unchanged. What is the next best step for his treatment?
A. Increase the dose to 8000 units of lipase with meals.
B. Add a proton pump inhibitor.
C. Stop the pancreatic enzyme supplements and start metronidazole at 250 mg orally three times daily.
D. Obtain a CT scan of the pancreas.

522 Which of the following statements regarding the natural history of acute pancreatitis is correct?
A. Forty percent of patients have mild pancreatitis.
B. The overall mortality rate may be as high as 25%.
C. Twenty percent of patients have severe pancreatitis.
D. Most patients with acute pancreatitis have persistent morphologic and functional changes after recovery.

523 Which of the following statements regarding pancreas divisum is the most accurate?
A. Pancreas divisum is a rare anomaly found in less than 2% of the population.
B. Pancreas divisum is more commonly associated with acute recurrent pancreatitis than with chronic pancreatitis.
C. Pancreas divisum typically presents with diabetes as the initial manifestation.
D. Surgical ablation of the sphincter at the minor pancreatic papilla is the treatment of choice for those with abdominal pain thought to result from pancreas divisum.

524 A 39-year-old alcoholic individual is brought to the emergency department with pancreatitis. A CT scan is immediately performed with oral and intravenous contrast. There is pancreatic and peripancreatic inflammation extending into the right perinephric space. No perfusion defects within the pancreatic parenchyma are noted. The use of early intravenous contrast in this patient
A. Increases the risk of acute tubular necrosis
B. Excludes necrotizing pancreatitis
C. Increases the patient's risk of the development of pancreatic necrosis
D. Is required to obtain a Balthazar grade E

525 A 13-year-old white girl presents to the emergency department after having several hours of right upper quadrant pain that radiates to her back. Previous hospital records show that she has been admitted three times with a diagnosis of acute pancreatitis. The patient's mother has a history of systemic lupus erythematosus. A physical examination reveals a young girl in mild distress with a heart rate of 95 beats per minute, blood pressure of 135/65 mm Hg, and a temperature of 98.9°F. The patient has an amylase level of 456 IU/L (normal, 25 to 125 IU/L) and a lipase level of 340 IU/L (normal, 10 to 145 IU/L). The serum calcium level and lipid panel results are normal. The patient is admitted, started on intravenous hydration, and kept on nothing by mouth. An abdominal ultrasound scan performed in the emergency depart-

ment shows a normal gallbladder and bile duct with poor visualization of the pancreas. What test would most likely reveal the cause of the patient's clinical condition?
A. Abdominal CT scan
B. ERCP
C. Urine drug screen
D. Genetic testing for a mutation in the cationic trypsinogen gene (*PRSS1*)
E. Serum antinuclear antibody

526 A 40-year-old man has acute gallstone pancreatitis and is hospitalized for one week. Three weeks after discharge, a CT scan is performed that demonstrates a 9- × 12-cm pseudocyst adjacent to the stomach. The patient is tired but otherwise feels well. He is eating a low-fat diet without nausea or vomiting. His WBC count and total bilirubin, AST, alanine aminotransferase, amylase, and lipase levels are normal. His alkaline phosphatase level is minimally elevated. What is the recommended management for this patient?
A. Clinical and radiographic follow-up only
B. Endoscopic cystogastrostomy
C. Wait two weeks for the formation of an adequate cyst wall and then proceed with surgical cystogastrostomy.
D. Percutaneous drainage by interventional radiology
E. Administer octreotide (Sandostatin LAR) to decrease pancreatic secretion and promote resolution.

527 Which of the following genetic aberrations is not implicated in the pathogenesis of pancreatic carcinoma?
A. Mutation of the *p16* tumor suppressor gene
B. Mutation of the *TP53* tumor suppressor gene
C. Mutation of the K-*ras* proto-oncogene
D. Mutation of the *Rb* tumor suppressor gene
E. Loss of function of the *SMAD4* tumor suppressor gene

528 Acute pancreatitis develops in an 8-year-old male patient. Statistically, the most common etiology for his pancreatitis is which of the following?
A. Mutation of the cationic trypsinogen gene (*PRSS1*)
B. Mutation of the CF transmembrane conductance regulator (*CFTR*) gene
C. Trauma
D. Mumps
E. Pancreas divisum

529 A 72-year-old white woman was referred for the investigation of acute recurrent pancreatitis. She had been admitted to a district hospital through the emergency department four times in the previous two years for episodes of epigastric pain associated with nausea, vomiting, and markedly elevated serum lipase levels. In every episode, her transaminase levels had been elevated without an elevation of her alkaline phosphatase level. An abdominal sonogram revealed a dilated bile duct and diffuse swelling of the pancreas but no stones in the gallbladder. An ERCP revealed an anomalous pancreatobiliary ductal union associated with diffuse dilation of the bile duct and a diverticulum in the

proximal (upstream) bile duct. For which of the following conditions is this patient at increased risk?
A. Sclerosing cholangitis
B. Colon cancer
C. Cholangiocarcinoma
D. Colon polyposis syndrome
E. Pancreatic neuroendocrine tumor

530 A patient is admitted to the ICU with severe pancreatitis. A CT scan at 72 hours demonstrates marked pancreatic and peripancreatic edema and shows that 30% of the pancreas is necrotic. As a prolonged course is anticipated, what recommendations should be made regarding the patient's nutrition?
A. Fluid resuscitation should be provided this early in the patient's course, but nutrition should not be.
B. TPN without intralipids should be instituted to provide complete pancreas rest.
C. Nasojejunal feeding is the preferable route to provide nutrition in patients with severe acute pancreatitis.
D. Oral pancreaticolipase should be initiated before feeding via either the oral or gastric route.
E. Nutrition via any route should be initiated at no more than 250 kcal/day.

531 A 58-year-old woman presents with a skin rash to her dermatologist. A punch biopsy of the lesion is performed that demonstrates subcutaneous fat necrosis calcification and neutrophilic infiltrate consistent with pancreatic panniculitis. She is referred to you for further evaluation. She has no history of abdominal pain, liver disease, or pancreatitis, nor does she have risk factors for pancreatitis. She denies diabetes steatorrhea and weight loss. Laboratory test results demonstrate normal complete blood count, chemistries, and liver profile. There is elevation of the lipase level to 2410 IU/L and elevations of the amylase level to 1850 IU/L. An abdominal CT scan demonstrates a 2.3-cm mass in the head of the pancreas, upstream dilation of the pancreatic duct, and atrophy of the remainder of the gland. Which of the following statements regarding this patient's presentation is most correct?
A. This patient has a pancreatic polypeptide-secreting neuroendocrine tumor.
B. This patient has focal autoimmune pancreatitis.
C. This patient has pancreatic acinar carcinoma.
D. This patient has pancreatic ductal adenocarcinoma.
E. This patient has solid pseudopapillary neoplasm.

532 Which of the following regarding trypsin is true?
A. It is an exopeptidase.
B. It is produced by the action of trypsin on trypsinogen.
C. It converts prolipase to lipase.
D. It is produced by the action of enterokinase on trypsinogen.

533 A 52-year-old man presents with severe abdominal pain and is diagnosed with acute pancreatitis. Three days later, the patient is in the ICU with fever, leukocytosis, tachycardia, and hypotension requiring pressors. What is the pathophysiology most often associated with this picture at this point in time?
A. The presence of pancreatic necrosis
B. An infectious complication of acute pancreatitis
C. Systemic inflammatory response syndrome
D. The development of hemorrhagic pancreatitis.

534 A 37-year-old woman is admitted to the hospital with acute onset of midepigastric abdominal pain, nausea, and vomiting. She appears uncomfortable; her temperature is 100.8°F, blood pressure is 143/90 mm Hg, heart rate is 112 beats per minute, and respiratory rate is 16 breaths per minute. Laboratory studies reveal a WBC count of 17,300/mL, hematocrit of 51%, hemoglobin of 16 g/dL, total bilirubin of 2.4 mg/dL, direct bilirubin of 1.8 mg/dL, amylase of 1243 IU/mL, and lipase of 956 IU/mL. Aggressive intravenous fluids, analgesic medications, and antiemetics are initiated. An abdominal ultrasound reveals gallbladder sludge and small gallstones and a normal-caliber bile duct. The next day, her pain is better controlled; however, she appears to be clinically worsening. Her temperature is 101.9°F, blood pressure is 102/54 mm Hg, and heart rate is 116 beats per minute. You arrange for her to undergo ERCP based on what rationale?
A. ERCP is indicated to remove pancreaticolithiasis, particularly in those with severe pancreatitis.
B. ERCP is indicated to decompress an inflamed edematous pancreatic duct by pancreatic stent placement.
C. ERCP is indicated to manage obstructive cholangitis.
D. ERCP is the diagnostic and therapeutic modality of choice for those with presumed biliary pancreatitis.

535 What is the postulated sequence of events that is most characteristic of acute pancreatitis?
A. Acinar cell injury → expression of endothelial adhesion molecules → release of proinflammatory cytokines → release of anti-inflammatory cytokines → activation of hepatic Kupffer cells
B. Acinar cell injury → release of inflammatory mediators into the systemic circulation → translocation of bacteria into the systemic circulation → systemic inflammatory response syndrome
C. Bile reflux into the pancreatic duct → duct cell injury → increased intraductal secretion of calcium and protein → increased vascular permeability → release of tumor necrosis factor
D. Increased acinar cell glutathione → acinar cell injury → release of anti-inflammatory mediators → recruitment and activation of macrophages → release of reactive oxygen metabolites

536 Which of the following histologic features is most specific for chronic pancreatitis?
A. Acinar cell necrosis
B. Ductular plugging
C. Fat necrosis

D. Interlobular fibrosis
E. Parenchymal hemorrhage

537 A 45-year-old Asian woman is referred to a gastro-enterologist to have an upper endoscopy for surveillance of Barrett's esophagus. The patient has a 12-year history of heartburn that is well controlled with proton pump inhibitors. Her physical examination is unremarkable. The upper endoscopy shows an irregular, yellow mucosal nodule in the duodenum; the examination is otherwise unremarkable. A biopsy is performed on the nodule, and the pathologist reports that it is ectopic pancreatic tissue. What is the most appropriate management at this time?
A. EUS
B. Periodic surveillance esophagogastroduodenoscopy
C. Abdominal CT scan
D. No further evaluation
E. Colonoscopy

538 The initial step in the pathogenesis of acute pancreatitis is conversion of trypsinogen to trypsin within acinar cells in sufficient quantities to overwhelm normal mechanisms to remove active trypsin. Which is a mechanism that counteracts the intracellular conversion of trypsinogen to trypsin?
A. High intracellular calcium
B. Release of cathepsin B that in turn splits trypsin
C. Expression of endothelial adhesion molecules
D. Presence of pancreatic secretory trypsin inhibitor (SPINK1)

539 A 42-year-old man is admitted to the hospital with acute biliary pancreatitis manifesting as abdominal pain in the midepigastrium and left upper quadrant, fever, and hyperbilirubinemia. ERCP is performed and a biliary stent is placed. After a 12-day hospitalization, his symptoms have resolved and he is discharged home in stable condition. He returns to the hospital 3 weeks later with increased abdominal pain, marked early satiety, and recurrent vomiting. Liver-associated enzyme, amylase, and lipase levels are normal. A CT scan is performed (see figure). What is the next step for the appropriate management of this patient?

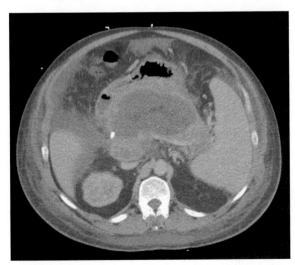

Figure for question **539**

A. Endoscopic transgastric drainage
B. EUS-guided aspiration
C. Percutaneous cyst access and intracystic antibiotic infusion
D. Surgical cystenterostomy

540 A 30-year-old woman was in a motocross accident and was impaled by her handlebar. She is brought to the emergency department. Which of the following provides a reliable indicator of pancreatic trauma?
A. Elevated serum amylase and lipase greater than three times normal
B. Magnetic resonance angiography
C. Elevated amylase levels within fluid obtained via paracentesis
D. CT scan showing enlargement of a portion of the gland and fluid within the anterior pararenal space

541 A deaf child is found to have growth retardation, pancreatic insufficiency, lipomatous transformation of the pancreas, and hypothyroidism. A core biopsy of the pancreas reveals preserved islets surrounded by connective tissue and a total absence of acini. What is the most likely diagnosis?
A. Shwachman-Diamond syndrome
B. Pearson marrow-pancreas syndrome
C. Johanson-Blizzard syndrome
D. Hereditary pancreatitis secondary to *N29I* mutation

542 A 57-year-old man presents at 2 AM with pain that had begun 2 hours earlier. The pain is severe and progressive. Abdominal examination reveals abdominal distention, absence of bowel sounds, and ecchymosis around the umbilicus. These physical findings are
A. Found in 10% of patients with acute pancreatitis
B. Associated with a poor prognosis
C. Diagnostic of necrotizing pancreatitis
D. Manifestations of severe vomiting associated with acute pancreatitis

543 Which of the following environmental risk factors contributes most to the pathogenesis of pancreatic cancer?
A. Alcohol use
B. Chronic steroid use
C. High dietary fat intake
D. Radon exposure
E. Tobacco use

544 On day 2 of life, an infant presents with intestinal obstruction. Dilated, firm, rubbery loops of bowel are palpable through the abdominal wall. What statement is true about this patient's clinical condition?
A. The patient can be treated with gastrograffin enemas.
B. The patient has a 50% infant mortality rate.
C. The patient must be treated with urgent surgery.
D. If this patient survives beyond 6 months of age, there remains a greater risk of complications than other CF patients might have.

545 In the patient in question 544, the CT scan shows inflammatory changes and subcapsular hematoma of the pancreatic body and fluid within the anterior pararenal space. What is the most important next step in this patient's care?
A. ERCP to diagnose and treat pancreatic duct disruption
B. Initiation of octreotide therapy
C. Laparoscopy for the diagnosis of pancreatic injury, pancreatic duct disruption, and surrounding organ injury.
D. Laparotomy for the diagnosis of pancreatic transaction, pancreatic duct disruption, and appropriate débridement.

546 Which of the following is not an inorganic component of exocrine pancreatic secretions?
A. Water
B. Sodium
C. Chloride
D. Potassium
E. Selenium

547 Which of the following is the main mediator of meal-stimulated enzyme secretion from the pancreas?
A. Secretin
B. VIP
C. CCK
D. Glucagon
E. Acetylcholine

548 A 48-year-old woman with severe chronic renal insufficiency reports nondescript abdominal discomfort to her family physician. A laboratory panel including serum amylase and lipase is performed. The serum amylase is fourfold greater than the upper limit of normal and the serum lipase is twofold greater than the upper limit of normal. When interpreting these findings it is important to consider which of the following?
A. Renal insufficiency does not affect the level of serum lipase.
B. The urinary amylase-to-creatinine clearance ratio (ACCR) can distinguish elevations of amylase due to renal insufficiency from other causes.
C. There is no clear relationship between creatinine clearance and serum amylase levels.
D. An elevated lipase level is only seen when there is disease of the pancreas.

549 Acinar cell protective mechanisms include all of the following *except*:
A. Presence of SPINK1
B. Sequestration of pancreatic enzymes within separate intracellular compartments
C. Presence of nonspecific antiproteases
D. High intracellular calcium concentration

550 The most common cause of hereditary pancreatitis is a mutation in the cationic trypsinogen gene (*PRSS1*). *PRSS1* mutation causes pancreatitis by
A. Altering the regulatory domains in trypsinogen controlled by calcium
B. Cleavage of TAP
C. Cyclic adenosine monophosphate activation of protein kinase A

D. Golgi apparatus stimulation to produce excessive trypsinogen

551 Which of the following regarding alcohol as a cause of chronic pancreatitis is most accurate?
A. Chronic pancreatitis will develop in almost half of those with regular alcohol use.
B. Chronic pancreatitis usually develops within the first 10 years of regular alcohol use.
C. Factors that contribute to the development of chronic pancreatitis in individuals who abuse alcohol include cigarette smoking, diets high in protein, and the pattern of alcohol use.
D. Chronic pancreatitis will ultimately develop in the majority of patients who present with acute alcohol-induced pancreatitis.

552 Which of the following cystic pancreatic masses does not require surgical resection?
A. Intraductal papillary mucinous neoplasm (IPMN)
B. Mucinous cystadenoma
C. Serous cystadenoma
D. Solid pseudopapillary neoplasm

553 Which of the following mechanisms most accurately describes the pathophysiologic mechanisms in chronic pancreatitis associated with genetic etiologies?
A. Altered function of the CFTR protein causes excess bicarbonate secretion and chronically elevated pancreatic duct pressures.
B. Genetic aberrations in the *SPINK1* gene lead to a fragile pepsinogen molecule that readily degrades, resulting in the release of an active pepsin.
C. *PRSS1* mutations cause constitutive activation of trypsin, resulting in lobular damage and local activation of additional digestive enzymes.
D. Mitochondrial DNA causes altered signaling in the exocytotic mechanisms of enzyme secretion and the premature release of active enzyme within the acinar cell itself.

554 A 60-year-old woman is taken to the hospital after an automobile accident in which she was an unbelted driver. During the accident, the patient experienced blunt trauma to the midabdomen when she was thrown against the steering wheel. What is the most accurate modality to diagnose pancreatic injury with pancreatic duct disruption?
A. ERCP
B. Elevated serum amylase
C. Fluid in the anterior pararenal space on CT scan
D. MRI with magnetic resonance cholangiopancreatography (MRCP)
E. Response to octreotide infusion

555 The histologic slide (see figure) is from a pancreatic biopsy in a child with chronic pancreatitis of unknown etiology. What is the most probable cause of the chronic pancreatitis?
A. Cystic fibrosis
B. Autoimmune fibrosis
C. α_1-Antitrypsin deficiency

D. Sarcoidosis
E. Drug induced

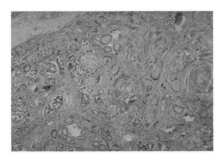

Figure for question **555**

556 A 45-year-old obese diabetic man presents to the hospital with crescendo-type midepigastric pain radiating to the back and associated with nausea. He denies alcohol use. On physical examination, his heart rate is 110 beats per minute. His vital signs are otherwise within normal ranges. His abdomen is remarkable for mild distention, decreased bowel sounds, and midepigastric tenderness without peritoneal signs. His serum amylase level is 370 U/L (normal limits <132 U/L) and serum lipase level is 2330 U/L (normal limits <52 U/L). Abdominal US reveals fatty infiltration of the liver, a normal gallbladder, and a normal biliary tree. Which of the following is the most likely etiology for this patient's pancreatitis?
A. Trauma
B. Gallstones
C. Hypertriglyceridemia
D. Medication induced
E. Autoimmune

557 A 64-year-old woman presents with a mass in the head of the pancreas and painless jaundice. She is palliated with an endoprosthesis, and EUS-guided FNA identifies a chronic inflammatory infiltrate and fibrosis. She is treated with 40 mg/day of prednisone. Interval MRI with MRCP at 4 weeks demonstrates resolution of pancreatic edema but a persistent mass in the head of the gland. Repeat ERCP is performed. There is a persistent biliary stricture. A repeat EUS-guided FNA is performed yielding fibrosis with little inflammation. Steroids are continued for an additional 6 weeks and repeat imaging is unchanged. What is the next appropriate step in managing this patient?
A. Combined FDG-PET scan
B. Pancreaticoduodenectomy
C. Placement of a covered metal endoprosthesis to allow for dilation of the biliary stricture
D. The addition of azathioprine to steroids and serial imaging

558 Which of the following statements about hypertriglyceridemia-induced pancreatitis in adults is most accurate?
A. It is most often associated with APO C-II deficiency.
B. It is exacerbated by the use of loop diuretics.
C. It is seen less frequently in diabetics.
D. It is responsible for approximately 5% of all cases of pancreatitis.

559 Shwachman-Diamond syndrome is the second most frequently recognized cause of pancreatic insufficiency in children after CF. Which of these features distinguishes Shwachman-Diamond syndrome from CF?
A. Shwachman-Diamond syndrome rarely has an onset within the first year of life.
B. Patients with Shwachman-Diamond syndrome have pancreatic insufficiency without reduced pancreatic bicarbonate secretion.
C. Patients with Shwachman-Diamond syndrome have decreased mucosal enterokinase activity.
D. In Shwachman-Diamond syndrome, infectious complications are less common.

560 Which of the following statements regarding surgical resection of pancreatic carcinoma is correct?
A. Attempts at surgical resection of pancreatic cancer are overused in the United States.
B. Outcomes are improved when surgery is performed at high-volume centers.
C. Total pancreatectomy improves mortality compared with less extensive resection for cancers of the body of the pancreas.
D. With recent improvement in techniques, the five-year survival rate approaches 45% for patients undergoing surgery.

561 A 31-year-old woman presents with a four-hour history of severe abdominal pain. On examination, she is in acute distress. Her blood pressure is 70/40 mm Hg and her heart rate is 130 beats per minute. Her abdomen is diffusely tender with no peritoneal signs, and her stool is negative for occult blood. Laboratory evaluation reveals a hematocrit of 20%, a serum amylase value twice the upper limit of normal, and normal liver enzymes. Serum lipase is normal. What is the most likely diagnosis?
A. Acute pancreatitis
B. Mesenteric ischemia
C. Perforated peptic ulcer
D. Ruptured ectopic pregnancy

562 Which statement regarding pancreatic secretory trypsin inhibitor is true?
A. *SPINK1* is categorized as a susceptibility gene in pancreatic disease.
B. *SPINK1* is synthesized by pancreatic duct cells.
C. *SPINK1* gene mutations are associated with tropical pancreatitis.
D. Serum concentrations of *SPINK1* decline with acute pancreatic inflammation.

563 Which of the following statements regarding congenital pancreatic cysts is true?
A. Congenital cysts are common and diagnosed at a young age.
B. These cysts are histologically indistinguishable from pancreatic pseudocysts.
C. Multiple congenital cysts are seen in patients with von Hippel-Lindau disease.
D. Congenital cysts are located more commonly in the head of the pancreas.
E. Congenital cysts require resection because of their malignant potential.

564 A 64-year-old man is seen in the office for concerns of abdominal pain. An abdominal CT scan demonstrates parenchymal pancreatic calcification, intraductal calculi, and two small cysts consistent with chronic pancreatitis. He reports drinking four to five glasses of scotch on most days and more on weekends and has been doing so for more than 25 years. He has been diagnosed with diabetes. He continues to abuse alcohol and cigarettes. He is unable to continue his work as a tollbooth attendant due to the pain. Clinically, his dominant symptom is abdominal pain located in the midepigastrium and radiating to his back. His pain is worse after meals. He reports marked fatigue and depression. Of the following factors, which is *least* likely to assist with improvement in his quality of life?
A. Alcohol cessation
B. Control of diarrhea
C. Increased physical activity
D. Improved blood glucose control
E. Pain management

565 Which of the following statements about *SPINK1* is true?
A. It protects the pancreatic acinar cell by inhibiting prematurely activated trypsin.
B. It regulates bicarbonate conductance.
C. It causes trypsin to be resistant to lysis by intracellular trypsin inhibitor.
D. It increases concentrations of TAP.

566 Which of the following statements regarding pancreatic cancer is most correct?
A. African-American men are disproportionately affected by pancreatic cancer.
B. Pancreatic cancer has an even distribution among men and women.
C. Pancreatic cancer is the second most common cause of cancer-related mortality in the United States.
D. The overall survival rate at five years approaches 25%.
E. The risk of developing pancreatic cancer increases sharply after age 60.

567 CT has become the standard for diagnosis and determining the severity of acute pancreatitis. The Balthazar grading system and CT severity index have been developed and validated. What statement regarding the use of CT in acute pancreatitis is true?
A. Balthazar grade D requires the presence of two or more peripancreatic fluid collections.
B. CT grading scores correlate better with the rate of local complications than with the mortality rate.
C. The CT severity index is more predictive of outcome than the Balthazar grade A through E score.
D. The Balthazar grading system requires a contrast-enhanced CT scan.

568 SPINK1 is a 56-amino-acid peptide that specifically inhibits trypsinogen activation by which of the following?
A. Inhibiting vagal stimulation
B. Decreasing secretion of CCK
C. Physically blocking its active site

D. Enzymatic cleavage of the trypsin
E. Stimulation of adenosine triphosphatase activity

569 A 64-year-old woman presents to your office for a second opinion. A laboratory panel drawn by another physician reveals an elevated serum amylase level. The patient has no abdominal pain. Further evaluation of this patient may include
A. Urinary amylase measurement and calculation of the ACCR
B. *CFTR* gene analysis
C. Fractionation of amylase into pancreatic and ovarian isoenzymes
D. Chest CT scan to assess for lung cancer

570 A 32-year-old woman presents to your office after having been diagnosed with her third episode of acute pancreatitis. She denies history of alcohol use and has no history of hypocalcemia or hypertriglyceridemia. There is no family history of pancreatitis. She is otherwise healthy. A CT scan is performed that demonstrates mild pancreatic ductal dilation and a cyst in the region of the head of the pancreas. ERCP is performed that demonstrates a saccular dilation with a central lucency communicating with the main pancreatic duct (see figure). Globules of clear viscous material were seen to extrude through the pancreatic os. Which of the following statements regarding this finding is most correct?
A. The next appropriate step for this patient would be EUS-guided FNA of the dilated segment.
B. The patient should be counseled that she has a premalignant lesion and should consider surgical resection.
C. This finding is diagnostic of a mucinous cystadenoma and requires resection.
D. This finding is diagnostic of a solid pseudopapillary tumor that may be observed radiographically.
E. This image demonstrates a pancreatic pseudocyst resulting from recurrent pancreatitis and can be managed with transpapillary drainage.

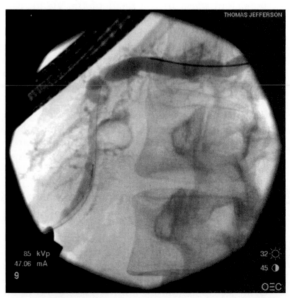

Figure for question **570**

571 Which congenital anomaly is not associated with annular pancreas?
A. Trisomy 21
B. Genitourinary defects
C. Tracheoesophageal fistula
D. Cardiac defects
E. Choledochal cysts

572 A 62-year-old man with a known history of dyslipidemia presents to the emergency department with acute pancreatitis. Physical examination is notable for fever, tachypnea, diffuse abdominal tenderness, and oliguria. Laboratory test results are significant for a WBC count of 22,000/mL, glucose level of 260 mg/dL, lactate dehydrogenase level of 500 IU/L, and PaO_2 of 82. A CT scan shows evidence of pancreatic necrosis and diffuse bilateral pulmonary infiltrates consistent with acute respiratory distress syndrome. Which of the following is a likely contributor to this patient's respiratory decompensation?
A. Surfactant degradation by phospholipase A_2
B. Infectious pneumonia
C. Elastase release from the injured pancreas
D. Increased intravascular fluid volume

573 A 25-year-old smoker presents with pancreatitis. He reports that he has had four other previous episodes of pancreatitis that were attributed to mild to moderate alcohol consumption. On further history, the patient is found to have a family history of pancreatitis and pancreatic cancer. What intervention is most important in this patient's management?
A. Genetic testing for *CFTR* mutations
B. Smoking cessation
C. Initiation of corticosteroid therapy
D. Initiation of pancreatic enzyme therapy

574 A patient starts a new medication. After 4 weeks, acute pancreatitis develops, which is thought to be secondary to the new medication. The medication is discontinued, and the pancreatitis resolves. Three months later, the same medication is reinitiated and pancreatitis develops within 8 hours. This temporal relationship between initiating the medication and the development of pancreatitis is most consistent with which pathogenetic mechanisms of drug-induced pancreatitis?
A. Intrinsic toxicity
B. Accumulation of toxic metabolite
C. Hypersensitivity reaction
D. Immunomodulatory up-regulation

575 Mutations of *CFTR* can cause or contribute to acute and chronic pancreatitis. Which statement regarding the CFTR molecule is true?
A. The CFTR molecule is the most important molecule for regulating pancreatic duct cell function.
B. The CFTR molecule is located on the basal side of the pancreatic duct cells.
C. The CFTR molecule is expressed on epithelial cells only in the respiratory tract and pancreas.
D. CFTR-associated secretion is inhibited by VIP acting on receptors that decrease intracellular cyclic adenosine monophosphate.

576 A 46-year-old woman is admitted to the hospital with abdominal pain and jaundice. An abdominal MRI with MRCP was performed and demonstrated two 1.7-cm masses in the pancreas, one located in the head and the other in the body. The mass in the head of the pancreas was causing biliary obstruction. ERCP was performed and an endoprosthesis was placed for biliary decompression. EUS-guided FNA of the lesions was performed on two occasions yielding nondiagnostic results. Exploratory laparotomy was performed with biopsy of the masses that confirmed non-Hodgkin's lymphoma. Which of the following statements regarding this diagnosis is true?
A. The cure rate for primary pancreatic lymphoma is 30%.
B. Primary pancreatic lymphoma accounts for 5% of pancreatic malignancies.
C. Primary pancreatic lymphoma is a subset of Hodgkin's disease.
D. The next appropriate management step would be to resect the mass in the head of the pancreas.

577 Death in patients with severe pancreatitis
A. Most often occurs in the first 24 hours
B. Is most often associated with hemorrhagic pancreatitis
C. Is frequently associated with infection
D. Is not influenced by patient age

578 A 47-year-old woman is diagnosed with chronic pancreatitis secondary to long-standing pancreatic duct stricture in the body that is related to a severe bout of biliary pancreatitis. She describes four bulky, foul-smelling stools daily with oil droplets within the stool. On laboratory testing, her HbA1c is elevated at 8.2%. Which of the following is most accurate with regard to this patient?
A. Destruction of the islet cells occurs early in chronic pancreatitis because they are more sensitive to destruction than other cellular components of the pancreas.
B. Her diabetes is a result of disruption of the production of insulin and glucagon.
C. Presenting simultaneously with exocrine and endocrine insufficiency is uncommon in patients with chronic obstructive pancreatitis.
D. She will almost assuredly require lifelong insulin therapy to manage her diabetes.

579 A 40-year-old man who admits to heavy alcohol consumption presents with acute pancreatitis. What pancreatic abnormality is most likely to be present?
A. Activation of pancreatic stellate cells
B. Increased acinar cell GP2 protein
C. Acinar cell cytoplasmic lipid accumulation
D. Expression of endothelial adhesion molecules

580 What percentage of patients with pancreas divisum and acute pancreatitis will have symptomatic relief after dorsal duct stent placement?
A. 5% to 10%
B. 20% to 40%
C. 50% to 60%
D. 70% to 90%

581 A patient presents with acute pancreatitis with the development of a 5-cm asymptomatic pseudocyst. Four weeks later, abdominal pain develops. Her CT scan reveals a 16-cm pseudocyst (see figure). What aspect of this pseudocyst would prompt pseudocyst drainage?
- **A.** The location of the pseudocyst is near the tail of the pancreas.
- **B.** The pseudocyst has a homogeneous, low-attenuation, fluid-filled appearance.
- **C.** The pseudocyst is 16 cm.
- **D.** The pseudocyst has increased in size.

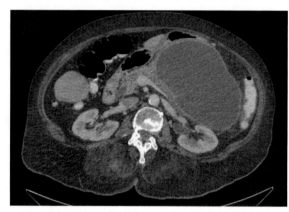

Figure for question **581**

582 A 45-year-old man was admitted to the ICU 10 days ago with severe gallstone pancreatitis. You are asked to see him because of a decrease in hemoglobin from 13.6 to 8.2 g/dL. He is tachycardic, and his nasogastric aspirate consists of fresh blood. Upper endoscopy reveals small esophageal and large gastric varices. In addition to his pancreatitis, which of the following conditions is most likely to be present?
- **A.** Chronic viral hepatitis
- **B.** Alcohol abuse
- **C.** Cavernous transformation of the portal vein
- **D.** Splenic vein thrombosis
- **E.** Hemosuccus pancreaticus

583 Maldigestion and malabsorption do not occur until the residual functional capacity of the pancreas is reduced to
- **A.** 5% to 10%
- **B.** 15% to 20%
- **C.** 25% to 30%
- **D.** 35% to 40%
- **E.** 45% to 50%

584 Which of the following patients is least likely to be associated with changes of chronic pancreatitis on imaging studies?
- **A.** An 87-year-old woman with hypertension and peripheral vascular disease
- **B.** A 49-year-old man on hemodialysis for six years for glomerulosclerosis
- **C.** A 32-year-old man with α_1-antitrypsin disease
- **D.** A 71-year-old woman with type 2 diabetes mellitus

585 Trypsin is recognized as the critical molecule in pancreatitis because it is the master enzyme that controls activation of the other digestive enzymes inside the pancreas. Most factors that increase susceptibility to pancreatitis disrupt a mechanism protecting the pancreas from trypsin-associated injury. Which is a true statement about trypsin activation?
- **A.** Fifty percent of trypsinogen is anionic trypsinogen.
- **B.** Decreased cellular calcium facilitates activation.
- **C.** Three mutations have been identified in *PRSS1* that increase susceptibility to recurrent acute pancreatitis.
- **D.** TAP maintains trypsinogen as inactive.

586 A 46-year-old man presents to the emergency department with 12 hours of severe midepigastric pain that radiates to his back and is associated with fever, nausea, vomiting, and light-headedness. He has a medical history significant for chronic low back pain, for which he takes nonsteroidal anti-inflammatory drugs. His wife reports that he works as a mechanic and has one or two drinks on the weekends. On examination, he looks acutely ill, has orthostatic hypotension, decreased bowel sounds, and diffuse abdominal tenderness. Laboratory tests are notable for leukocytosis, elevation of serum amylase, and mild cholestatic abnormalities of liver chemistries. CT of the abdomen shows cholelithiasis and evidence of acute edematous pancreatitis. Which of the following is the most likely cause of his acute presentation?
- **A.** Alcohol
- **B.** Gallstones
- **C.** Helminthic infection
- **D.** Nonsteroidal anti-inflammatory drugs
- **E.** Pancreas divisum

587 What is the currently favored way to determine the severity of acute pancreatitis?
- **A.** Use of Ranson criteria and CT severity index
- **B.** The Marshall scoring system for organ failure
- **C.** The presence of SIRS, organ failure, and anatomic complications on a CT scan
- **D.** Admission vital signs and APACHE II score

588 A 34-year-old white woman presents to her primary care doctor reporting a four-month history of abdominal pain and episodes of vomiting. She is otherwise healthy. Routine laboratory test results, including amylase, lipase, and CA 19.9 tests, are normal. The patient undergoes an abdominal CT scan that demonstrates a 2-cm cyst in the pancreatic head. On the primary physician's recommendations, the patient is sent for EUS. EUS findings show a 2-cm smooth-walled anechoic cystic lesion in the pancreatic head without any debris, septations, or papillary projections. Dilation of the pancreatic duct upstream from the cyst was present. What would be the appropriate recommendation for the patient?
- **A.** Observe patient and repeat EUS in 6 months
- **B.** Surgical resection of the cyst
- **C.** CT-guided FNA of the cyst
- **D.** Genetic testing for a mutation in the cationic trypsinogen gene (*PRSS1*) to evaluate for congenital pancreatitis as a cause of the patient's cyst
- **E.** MRI/MRCP to evaluate the pancreatic cyst

589 A patient with a body mass index of 30 has had 3 weeks of colicky right upper quadrant pain. Today, severe abdominal pain developed, and the patient presented to the emergency department. His pulse is 120 beats per minute and his respiratory rate is 24 breaths per minute. Laboratory studies demonstrate an amylase of 2200 U/L. When compared with nonobese patients, which statement about obese patients with pancreatitis is true?
A. Obese patients have a tendency to present with higher levels of amylase and lipase.
B. Obese patients often have the severity of their disease underestimated by CT scan.
C. Obese patients have an increased risk of dying of sterile pancreatic necrosis.
D. Obese patients with pancreatitis have a lower incidence of local complications.

590 In contrast to other forms of pancreatic insufficiency, patients with CF in whom pancreatic dysfunction develops have
A. A significantly higher duodenal pH
B. A significantly lower duodenal pH
C. Decreased secretory IgA
D. Elevated gastric pH
E. Lower gastric pH

591 A 45-year-old man who admits to heavy alcohol consumption and who uses an angiotensin-converting enzyme inhibitor presents to the hospital with midepigastric pain. His amylase level is three times normal and his lipase level is five times normal. His serum triglyceride level is 1700 mg/dL. An important aspect about this patient's evaluation and care should include
A. Seeking lipoprotein lipase deficiency
B. Discontinuing angiotensin-converting enzyme inhibitor therapy
C. Performing lipoprotein electrophoresis
D. A delay in initiating therapy for hyperlipidemia

592 A 40-year-old man with long-standing alcohol abuse and a history of chronic pancreatitis is admitted to the hospital with mild right upper quadrant abdominal pain and jaundice for one week. His total bilirubin level is 12.2 mg/dL, direct bilirubin is 9.9 mg/dL, and alkaline phosphatase is 377 IU/L. MRI was performed and demonstrated a stricture of the distal bile duct with proximal dilation, a 1.6-cm ill-defined mass in the head of the pancreas with dilation of the upstream pancreatic duct, a lobular contour to the liver, and prominent perigastric and paraesophageal venous collaterals. What is the next appropriate step in the management of this patient?
A. EUS and FNA of the pancreatic mass
B. ERCP for placement of a biliary endoprosthesis
C. Lateral pancreaticojejunostomy (Puestow procedure)
D. Pancreaticoduodenectomy (Whipple procedure)
E. Percutaneous transhepatic biliary drain placement

593 A 60-year-old man with mild underlying coronary artery disease is admitted to the hospital with acute pancreatitis. During the first 48 hours, he is found to have six Ranson criteria and the Grey Turner sign. In the ICU, management should include

A. Gentle fluid resuscitation
B. Swan-Ganz catheterization so that intravascular volume can be maintained without precipitation of congestive heart failure
C. Correction of low serum calcium level
D. Broad-spectrum antibiotics
E. Nasogastric suctioning

594 A 62-year-old man presents with sudden-onset mid-epigastric pain and nausea. The patient is diagnosed with mild acute edematous pancreatitis and is hospitalized for five days. Which test result or outcome best defines mild acute edematous pancreatitis?
A. The presence of an ileus on obstruction series
B. Amylase three times normal and lipase four times normal
C. Bright appearance of pancreatic parenchyma on a contrast-enhanced CT scan
D. Five-day length of stay
E. Fewer than six Ranson criteria

595 Which of the following is the best statement about how to perform a standard pancreatic hormone stimulation test?
A. A catheter is placed in the pancreatic duct to collect secretions.
B. After CCK stimulation, pancreatic bicarbonate is measured.
C. Pancreatic secretions are collected over two hours.
D. Serum lipase is measured simultaneously with pancreatic secretions.

596 Which of the following statements regarding direct tests used for diagnosing chronic pancreatitis is most correct?
A. ERCP is the most sensitive diagnostic test for chronic pancreatitis.
B. Secretin-stimulated measures of pancreatic secretion are most accurate in those with structural pancreatic abnormalities.
C. The reproduction of pancreatic pain with pancreatic stimulation is diagnostic of chronic pancreatitis.
D. ERCP is the gold standard for the diagnosis of chronic pancreatitis.
E. Direct collection of pancreatic juice collected from within the pancreatic duct is more sensitive than tests collecting duodenal aspirate.

597 Which of the following statements regarding serum amylase in the diagnosis of acute pancreatitis is most accurate?
A. Serum amylase increases within two hours after the onset of symptoms.
B. Serum amylase has a half-life of 20 hours.
C. Serum amylase is primarily excreted by the kidneys.
D. Serum amylase remains elevated for approximately 7 to 10 days.
E. Serum amylase may be normal in severe pancreatitis.

598 What is the estimated cumulative lifetime risk for the development of pancreatic cancer in patients with hereditary pancreatitis?
A. 5%
B. 10%

C. 20%
D. 40%
E. 60%

599 A patient undergoes ERCP for suspected choledocholithiasis. A pancreaticogram and cholangiogram were obtained and a biliary sphincterotomy was performed. Balloon biliary clearance did not produce a stone. Which of the following statements regarding this patient's condition is true?
A. The patient has a 45% risk of the development of asymptomatic hyperamylasemia.
B. The patient has a 20% risk of the development of procedure-related acute pancreatitis.
C. The patient should be started on gabexate mesylate to reduce the risk of post-ERCP pancreatitis.
D. The patient would have had a reduced risk of pancreatitis if, instead of biliary sphincterotomy, balloon sphincteroplasty was performed.
E. The patient would have had a reduced risk of pancreatitis if nonionic contrast had been used to obtain the pancreatogram.

600 Which of the following statements regarding pancreatic exocrine insufficiency in chronic pancreatitis is most accurate?
A. Decreased pancreatic bicarbonate secretion contributes to the destruction of pancreatic enzyme by failing to buffer acidic gastric secretions.
B. Fat malabsorption occurs relatively early in pancreatitis when pancreatic lipase levels are less than 30%.
C. Protein maldigestion typically precedes fat malabsorption as gastric lipase hydrolyzes a significant fraction of dietary fat.
D. The median time for exocrine insufficiency to develop in chronic pancreatitis is relatively uniform despite varying etiologies.
E. Weight loss is the hallmark of pancreatic exocrine insufficiency.

601 A patient presents with acute gallstone pancreatitis. The CT scan reveals severe edematous pancreatitis. What features on the CT scan are consistent with this diagnosis?
A. More than 30% of the gland is not perfused, with low attenuation
B. Peripancreatic fluid collection
C. The presence of parenchymal calcifications
D. The presence of walled-off pancreatic necrosis

602 An 18-year-old man who recently migrated from India presented to his physician with history of periumbilical pain since age 6. The pain was intermittent and radiated to his back. The patient noticed increased weight loss and diarrhea during the past 5 months. He did not have any family history of similar symptoms. On examination, he was of a very lean build with gross pallor. Abdominal examination revealed localized rigidity in the epigastrium but no tenderness or distention. Laboratory tests showed a blood glucose level of 297 mg/dL and an amylase level of 560 IU/L. An x-ray of the abdomen revealed a radiopaque shadow in the region of the pancreas and the left kidney. ERCP was performed that showed ductal obstruction, and a CT scan performed later showed marked dilation of the pancreatic duct. What is the mostly likely diagnosis for this patient?
A. Hereditary pancreatitis
B. Tropical pancreatitis
C. Cystic fibrosis
D. Shwachman-Diamond syndrome
E. Gallstone pancreatitis

603 In the emergency department, a serum amylase test is most frequently ordered to assess patients with abdominal pain and diagnose acute pancreatitis because it can be measured quickly and inexpensively. What is an accurate limitation of the use of serum amylase in the diagnosis of acute pancreatitis?
A. Serum amylase may be artificially increased in hypertriglyceridemia-induced pancreatitis.
B. The sensitivity of serum amylase for the diagnosis of acute pancreatitis is 60%.
C. Serum amylase may be normal in acute pancreatitis.
D. Only 75% of patients with an elevated serum amylase have pancreatic disease.

604 A 49-year-old woman is referred to you for evaluation of a pancreatic cyst. Recently, she had been diagnosed with pyelonephritis and while in the hospital underwent an abdominal CT scan. On the CT scan, an incidental 4-cm cyst was identified in the tail of the pancreas. This cyst contains multiple thick-walled septations, and enhancement of the cyst wall with intravenous contrast is seen. What is the most appropriate recommendation at this time?
A. Endoscopic cystogastrostomy
B. EUS to better characterize the morphology of the lesion
C. MRI with MRCP to identify the relationship of the cyst with the pancreatic duct
D. Pancreatic enzyme replacement
E. Surgical consultation for distal pancreatectomy

605 Cystic fibrosis is the most common lethal genetic defect of white populations. Which other statement about CF is true?
A. Approximately 40% of CF cases are diagnosed within the first year of life.
B. Forty percent of patients with CF present with evidence of exocrine pancreatic dysfunction.
C. The median survival of patients with CF is more than 40 years.
D. Exocrine pancreatic insufficiency presents when the secretion of lipase and trypsin decreases to less than 30% of normal.

606 An eight-year-old, previously healthy, Hispanic girl presents to the emergency department with a three-day history of diarrhea. The patient had a one-week history of an upper respiratory illness for which her pediatrician had prescribed amoxicillin. Her parents report that the patient initially had loose watery bowel movements, but on the day of presentation, the patient had two episodes of bloody diarrhea. The patient reports having severe right upper quadrant and epigastric pain for one day. The patient has a temperature of 99.7°F, a pulse of 113 beats per minute, respiratory rate of 15 breaths per minute, and a blood pressure of 82/45 mm Hg. On physical examination, the patient has epigastric tenderness with voluntary guarding. Poor bowel sounds are heard. A rectal examination reveals bright red blood per rectum. Laboratory test results are hemoglobin 10.2 g/dL; platelet count 60,000/mL; serum creatinine 3.2 mg/dL; amylase 840 IU/L; lipase 1200 IU/L; total bilirubin 3.9 mg/dL; and indirect bilirubin 2.5 mg/dL. The prothrombin time, activated partial thromboplastin time, D-dimer, and fibrinogen are normal. Peripheral blood smear shows the presence of schistocytes. A CT scan of the abdomen reveals colon wall thickening, normal bile ducts, and pancreatic parenchymal edema with stranding. What is the most likely cause of the patient's pancreatitis?

A. Sepsis
B. Acute gallstone pancreatitis
C. Cystic fibrosis
D. *Clostridium difficile* colitis
E. Hemolytic-uremic syndrome

607 What are the most common types of genetically inherited hyperlipidemia associated with the development of pancreatitis in adults?

A. Types I and III
B. Types II and IV
C. Types I and V
D. Types II and V

608 A 64-year-old man has idiopathic chronic pancreatitis that is complicated by progressive abdominal pain. MRI with MRCP demonstrates an atrophic and fibrotic appearance of the pancreatic parenchyma. The main pancreatic duct measures 3 mm. There is a small 1.2-cm pseudocyst in the tail. Which of the following options would be an appropriate therapy for this patient?

A. Endoscopic cystogastrostomy
B. ERCP with pancreatic duct decompression
C. EUS-guided celiac plexus neurolysis
D. Lateral pancreaticojejunostomy
E. Subtotal pancreatectomy

609 An 18-year-old African-American boy presents to the emergency department with a five-day history of periumbilical pain, early satiety, persistence of nausea, and several episodes of projectile vomiting of foul-smelling copious material. An abdominal CT scan in the emergency department reveals findings suspicious of an annular pancreas. What would be the definitive management of the patient?

A. Conservative management with antibiotic and intravenous fluid administration
B. An abdominal MRI and MRCP to confirm the diagnosis of an annular pancreas
C. Proceed to endosonography to evaluate for pancreatic malignancy mimicking annular pancreas.
D. Surgical resection of the pancreatic tissue causing duodenal obstruction
E. Surgical bypass of the duodenum

610 A previously healthy five-year-old girl with acute-onset abdominal pain is brought to the emergency department by her father. Her vital signs are normal.

Her abdomen is tender to percussion and palpation. Her bowel sounds are decreased. There is subtle periumbilical ecchymoses. Laboratory studies reveal an elevated amylase and lipase, and the child is diagnosed with acute pancreatitis. What is the most likely etiology of pancreatitis in this patient?

A. Hereditary pancreatitis
B. Trauma
C. Hyperlipidemia
D. Gallstones/microlithiasis

611 You are asked to consult on a 51-year-old man for concerns of painless jaundice and a mass in the head of the pancreas. He is otherwise healthy. He has experienced an unintentional 12-pound weight loss. He has not had abdominal pain, fevers, or chills. MRI is performed (see figure). ERCP demonstrates a distal bile duct stricture and dilation of the extrahepatic biliary tree. What is the next appropriate step in managing this patient?

A. EUS with FNA
B. Initiate 40 mg/day of prednisone.
C. Obtain a serum IgG4 level.
D. Placement of a metal biliary endoprosthesis
E. Surgical referral for pancreaticoduodenectomy

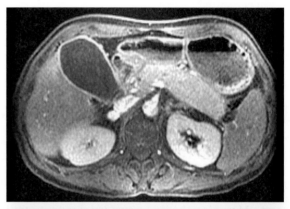

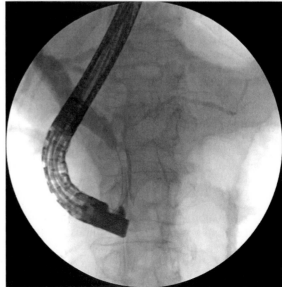

Figure for question **611**

612 Which of the following is the gold standard test for pancreatic function?
A. Lundh test meal
B. Collection of pancreatic secretions after CCK administration
C. Fecal fat
D. Fecal chymotrypsin
E. Bentiromide test

613 A 69-year-old man with chronic alcoholic pancreatitis is experiencing persistent abdominal pain. He describes the pain as unrelenting, located in the midepigastrium, and radiating to his back. He was given oxycodone by his primary care doctor, which resulted in incomplete pain relief. Which of the following statements regarding this patient's pain syndrome is most accurate?
A. Chronic inflammatory mediators stimulate pancreatic blood flow, resulting in increased parenchymal pancreatic pressures.
B. His pain is caused by pancreatic ischemia, which in turn results in tissue necrosis and decreased pancreatic duct pressures.
C. Intrapancreatic neural elements are central to the transmission of pain in this individual.
D. The pain is likely to persist in quality and severity in the future.

614 What is the initial pathophysiologic event in acute pancreatitis?
A. Intra-acinar cell conversion of trypsinogen to trypsin
B. Release of phospholipase A
C. Increased capillary permeability
D. Fat necrosis
E. Decrease in cell membrane protein GP2

615 A 68-year-old man presents with nausea and severe abdominal pain. Evaluation demonstrates an amylase level of 2400 IU/L and a lipase level of more than 6000 IU/L. The CT scan reveals pancreatic and peripancreatic inflammation with a Balthazar grade C. Which is a true statement about this patient's management?
A. Morphine should be avoided due to its ability to increase sphincter of Oddi tone.
B. A nasogastric tube should be placed to treat vomiting and reduce nausea and the possible risk of aspiration.
C. Proton pump inhibitors should be initiated in all patients with acute pancreatitis.
D. Isotonic saline should be administered at a rate of at least 250 to 300 mL/hr for the first 48 hours.

616 A three-year-old African-American boy has frequent foul-smelling stools and is found to have an abnormal nasal bioelectric response. What other finding would be expected?
A. Pancreatic parenchymal calcifications on CT scan
B. Findings of pancreatic inflammation
C. Diabetes mellitus
D. Two severe *CFTR* mutations

617 In patients with chronic pancreatitis, which of the following comorbidities most affects long-term survival?
A. Alcohol use
B. Coronary artery disease
C. Diabetes
D. Malabsorption
E. Abdominal pain

618 A 17-year-old boy was brought to the hospital by ambulance after being in a motor vehicle accident. He was the driver and was restrained with a seat belt. His dominant symptom is midepigastric abdominal pain. Laboratory studies reveal a normal complete blood count, metabolic panel, and liver-associated enzymes. The amylase level is 601 IU/mL and lipase level is 527 IU/mL. A CT scan is performed the following day and demonstrates a laceration of the pancreatic neck with fluid tracking along the pancreatic bed and mild pelvic ascites. Two days later, his pain persists and a repeat CT demonstrates an increase in the amount of ascites. The ascites is sampled and is found to have an amylase level of 7200 IU/mL. What is the next appropriate step in the management of this patient?
A. Endoscopic transgastric drainage of the pancreatic fluid collection
B. ERCP to bridge the site of pancreatic duct disruption
C. Initiation of octreotide infusion
D. Surgical laparotomy with planned pancreaticojejunostomy

619 What is the most common mechanism of drug-induced pancreatitis?
A. Accumulation of a toxic metabolite
B. Hypersensitivity reaction
C. Alteration of acinar cell membrane permeability
D. Alterations in trypsin inhibitor
E. Induction of hypertriglyceridemia

620 A stricture in the ascending colon develops in a six-year-old boy with CF, exocrine pancreatic dysfunction, and malabsorption. His outpatient medications include corticosteroids, antibiotics, 6000 U/kg/day of lipase, and an H_2 receptor antagonist. Colonoscopy with biopsy shows ischemic ulceration with mucosal and submucosal fibrosis. What course of action should be followed?
A. Provide vitamins A, E, K, and D.
B. Stop antibiotics.
C. Decrease the dose of pancreatic enzymes.
D. Initiate *N*-acetylcysteine therapy.

621 You are caring for a 59-year-old woman with a history of familial hypertriglyceridemia and diabetes. She has experienced recurrent hypertriglyceridemic pancreatitis, and pancreatic duct stricture developed that has evolved into chronic pancreatitis. Diabetes and steatorrhea develop. You are able to manage her steatorrhea with pancreatic enzyme replacement. Which of the following statements regarding the management of her diabetes is most correct?
A. She will not respond to an oral hypoglycemic, and there is no utility in attempting to use one.
B. She requires very aggressive glucose control to improve her ability to control her triglycerides.
C. Aggressive glucose control will result in medication-induced hypoglycemia due to

glucagon insufficiency and is contraindicated for this patient.

D. Managing her hypertriglyceridemia with a statin will facilitate better control of her steatorrhea.

E. Her diabetes is likely to resolve with management of the pancreatic ductal obstruction.

622 Which of the following is an accepted definition of severe pancreatitis?

A. APACHE II score >5

B. C-reactive protein >100

C. Three or more Ranson criteria

D. Respiratory rate >30 breaths per minute

E. Hematocrit <50%

ANSWERS

500 **C** (S&F, ch58)

Chronic pancreatitis is a persistent or progressive disorder in which changes in pancreatic structure and function usually precede symptoms and always persist even after the precipitating cause of pancreatitis has been corrected. The only way to confirm that an attack of pancreatitis can be categorized as chronic pancreatitis is to demonstrate the findings consistent with chronic pancreatitis including ductal irregularity and parenchymal fibrosis. Acute pancreatitis may be recurrent and may occur in the face of alcohol use and steatorrhea. Pseudocysts can be seen in both acute and chronic pancreatitis.

501 **C** (S&F, ch59)

Among the hypothesized pathophysiologic mechanisms in chronic pancreatitis, the secretion of pancreatic enzyme precursors is altered such that the enzymes are secreted at the basolateral membrane of the acinar cells rather than at the apical location. This secretion in turn causes local damage and acinar cell necrosis. Pancreatic secretions in chronic pancreatitis are protein rich and lack adequate bicarbonate, causing increased viscosity and obstruction of the ducts. Stellate cells become activated, lose their lipid granules, and propagate a fibrotic response. Pancreatic ductal cells may also be damaged and exhibit degrees of metaplasia and fibrosis.

502 **C** (S&F, ch58)

Although refeeding pancreatitis occurs more frequently if the serum lipase is more than threefold elevated, nasojejunal feedings are preferred over TPN. The use of empirical antibiotics is not recommended. Convincing evidence that probiotics decrease infectious complications in acute pancreatitis is scarce. Due to the common and indolent nature of hypoxemia affecting patients with acute pancreatitis, current guidelines recommend the initial routine use of nasal cannula oxygen for all patients with acute pancreatitis.

503 **B** (S&F, ch59)

Autoimmune pancreatitis is most commonly diagnosed in men (2:1) older than age 50. In addition to fibrosis in the pancreas, other sites may be affected including the bile ducts, salivary and lacrimal glands, retroperitoneum, and kidneys. The disease tends to be steroid responsive with resolution of abnormalities in both the pancreatic and extrapancreatic locations.

504 **A** (S&F, ch58)

Once refeeding is begun, a low-fat diet seems to be comparable to a clear liquid diet as the initial meal. Nasojejunal tube feeds have been shown to normalize blood glucose levels, decrease septic complications, decrease total complications, improve acute phase response markers, improve disease severity scores, and decrease costs compared with the administration of TPN. Nasojejunal tube feeds have not been reliably shown to be better tolerated than nasogastric tube feeds.

505 **B** (S&F, ch56)

The major mediator of hydrogen ion–stimulated bicarbonate and water secretion is secretin. The quantity of secretin released, as well as the volume of pancreatic secretion, is dependent on the load of titratable acid delivered to the duodenum. Secretin-induced bicarbonate secretion is augmented by CCK when both agents are infused to reproduce concentrations observed during a meal. CCK alone causes no bicarbonate secretion. The bicarbonate response to secretin is also dependent on cholinergic input because atropine partially inhibits the response stimulated by exogenous secretin. Thus, the complete meal-stimulated response results from a combination of mediators. The mediators of the enzyme secretory response from intestinal stimuli are both neural and humoral. Truncal vagotomy and atropine markedly inhibit the enzyme (and bicarbonate) responses to low intestinal loads of amino acids and fatty acids. These results suggest a vagovagal enteropancreatic reflex that mediates enzyme secretion and augments bicarbonate secretion stimulated by secretin.

506 **C** (S&F, ch58)

CT is the modality of choice to assess the severity of acute pancreatitis and the presence of associated complications. More specifically, CT with dynamic intravenous contrast injection can determine the presence and extent of pancreatic necrosis, which remains the primary determinant of length of hospitalization and mortality. Although a KUB can rule out other etiologies for abdominal pain, it does not directly image the pancreas. Imaging by transabdominal US is severely limited by poor transmission of ultrasound waves through bowel gas that normally surrounds the pancreas. MRI is not superior to CT for imaging in acute pancreatitis and is both less available and more expensive. ERCP is contraindicated in acute pancreatitis unless there is evidence of concurrent cholangitis.

507 **D** (S&F, ch58)

In acute pancreatitis, the Ranson criteria have been time-tested indicators of disease severity and prognosis. Ranson criteria include five admission criteria: (1) age older than 55, (2) WBC count greater than 16,000, (3) glucose level greater than 200, (4) lactate dehydrogenase level greater than 350, (5) AST level greater than 250, and five criteria determined at 48 hours: (1) hematocrit decrease more than 10, (2) BUN increase more than 5, (3) calcium less than 8, (4) PO_2 less than 60, (5) base deficit more than 4. Amylase and lipase levels are not good predictors of disease severity or prognosis.

508 **A** (S&F, ch57)

The child in the question has tropical pancreatitis. Tropical pancreatitis is associated with *SPINK1* mutations. There is no strong association with protein-calorie malnutrition or cassava ingestion and no association with APO C-II deficiency.

509 **A** (S&F, ch60)

Populations at risk of the development of pancreatic cancer include those with hereditary chronic pancreatitis, nonhereditary pancreatitis, kindreds with familial pancreatic cancer, familial atypical mole-malignant melanoma syndrome, *BRCA2* mutations, and multiple first-degree relatives affected by the disease. Familial pancreatic cancer is inherited in an autosomal-dominant fashion. The likelihood of people with nonhereditary forms of chronic pancreatitis developing pancreatic cancer is 2% per decade. For those affected by Peutz-Jeghers syndrome, the risk of developing pancreatic cancer is 132 times that of the general population. Although screening for pancreatic cancer is controversial, expert opinion is that individuals who are at increased risk should be screened with a combination of cross-sectional imaging and EUS as the initial tests.

510 **A** (S&F, ch58)

Gallstones cause approximately 40% of cases of acute pancreatitis, although pancreatitis develops in only 3% to 7% of patients with gallstones. Gallstone pancreatitis is more common in women than men because gallstones are more frequent in women. Smoking increases the risk of alcoholic and idiopathic pancreatitis, but not gallstone pancreatitis.

511 **A** (S&F, ch55)

Pancreas divisum occurs in approximately 7% of patients undergoing ERCP for diagnosis of non-pancreatic diseases. It results because the embryologic dorsal and ventral pancreas fail to fuse. Whether pancreas divisum is related to pancreatitis or abdominal pain is controversial. Pancreatitis in individuals with pancreas divisum develops in adulthood, not in childhood. With ERCP in pancreas divisum, contrast injection after cannulation of the ampulla of Vater demonstrates a small pancreatic duct of Wirsung, which drains the pancreatic head, and cannulation of the minor ampulla demonstrates filling of a separate larger duct of Santorini, which drains the entire pancreatic body and tail.

512 **C** (S&F, ch58)

Although in the past, infected pancreatic necrosis mandated surgical débridement because otherwise it was considered uniformly fatal, nonsurgical management is now the standard of care. In one study, 14 of 28 patients with infected necrosis were successfully treated with no surgical, endoscopic, or radiologic drainage. If surgery is entertained, delaying surgery beyond the fourth week to allow for walled-off pancreatic necrosis is associated with a lower mortality rate. Although less invasive methods of débridement are being successfully performed, there have been no prospective trials with comparisons of surgical management.

513 **C** (S&F, ch56)

Pancreatic secretion, composed largely of bicarbonate, enzymes, and electrolytes in a healthy pancreas, is approximately 2.5 L/day.

514 **D** (S&F, ch59)

Tropical pancreatitis is a disease of young individuals stemming from endemic regions such as southern India and portions of South America. Affected individuals most commonly present with profound weight loss and malnutrition, often accompanied by abdominal pain. The cause of malnutrition is typically pancreatic exocrine dysfunction and is the dominant cause of mortality in endemic areas. Endocrine deficiency with difficult-to-control diabetes ensues in the majority of affected individuals. Secondary complications of diabetes are common. Imaging demonstrates pancreatic fibrosis, a dilated pancreatic duct with large intraductal calcifications. The pathogenesis of disease is poorly defined but has been linked to ingestion of local fruits (e.g., cassava), although more reliably to genetic factors such as SPINK-1.

515 **A** (S&F, ch60)

A contrast-enhanced abdominal CT scan is the most common method of staging pancreatic cancer. The initial goal of staging is to determine whether a cancer can be resected. This determination requires a detailed assessment of involvement of the peripancreatic vasculature and evaluation for metastasis. A contrast-enhanced abdominal CT with pancreatic cancer protocol can demonstrate exquisite anatomic detail, particularly when coupled with three-dimensional vascular reconstructed images. The addition of abdominal MRI will add little useful information. In the setting of a resectable mass, EUS-guided sampling of the mass is not required to exclude a benign etiology because the likelihood of malignancy is high, and an aspirate that was negative for malignancy would not preclude surgery. EUS-guided FNA may diagnose lymphoma or autoimmune pancreatitis, which would alter the patient's treatment course. FDG-PET is not part of the standard staging before pancreatic cancer. Surgical laparoscopy can identify occult intra-abdominal metastases, although for a 1.4-cm mass, the likelihood of this occurrence is low. The use of laparoscopy is controversial, and given the size of the primary tumor, laparoscopy would not be indicated for this patient.

516 **B** (S&F, ch58)
Multisystem organ failure is defined as two or more organs failing on the same day. Urinary TAP is not a surrogate marker of inflammation. Premature intrapancreatic activation during acute pancreatitis results in the release of TAP. The degree of pancreatic necrosis and systemic inflammatory response/sepsis is directly related to TAP concentration. Percutaneous recovery of any volume of peritoneal fluid with a dark color or recovery of at least 20 mL of free intraperitoneal fluid of dark color portends a significant mortality. Amylase and lipase do not correlate with severity.

517 **C** (S&F, ch58)
Hypercalcemia during parenteral nutrition can lead to pancreatitis. Although systemic lupus erythematosus, *CFTR* gene mutation, and Epstein-Barr virus are associated with pancreatitis, they are unlikely to be causes in this patient.

518 **D** (S&F, ch55)
Ectopic (or heterotopic) pancreatic tissue, also called a pancreatic rest, occurs in 0.5% to 14% of the population. The most common sites are the stomach, duodenum, proximal jejunum, and ileum. Less commonly they are seen in the umbilicus, bile duct, gallbladder, and Meckel's diverticulum. Pancreatic rests have been associated with ulceration, bleeding, and intussusception, and rarely pancreatic adenocarcinoma may result. Treatment is surgical resection if the patient is symptomatic.

519 **A** (S&F, ch61)
This patient is exhibiting episodes of recurrent pancreatitis in the setting of a pancreatic duct stone obstructing the main pancreatic duct. Endoscopic therapy at ERCP is the preferred management strategy with pancreatic sphincterotomy and attempted stone removal. Should that be unsuccessful, alternative modalities such as extracorporeal shockwave lithotripsy and transgastric decompression of the pancreatic duct may be considered. In patients with significant duct dilation and recurrent stones, particularly those who have responded to endotherapy, a lateral pancreaticojejunostomy may be appropriate. Although complete bowel rest with TPN may alleviate acute symptoms, it will not address the duct obstruction, and pancreatitis will recur.

520 **D** (S&F, ch57)
Vitamin deficiencies may develop as a consequence of fat maldigestion and malabsorption, and therefore patients with CF are at risk. Nearly half of all newly diagnosed CF patients have a deficiency of vitamins A, D, and/or E. Chronic vitamin E deficiency is associated with hemolytic anemia (usually in infants) and neuroaxonal dystrophy with prominent neuromuscular symptoms, although these clinical symptoms seem to be rare. Supplementation with pancreatic enzymes, a multivitamin preparation, and additional vitamin E is usually associated with rapid normalization of serum albumin, retinol, and 25-hydroxyvitamin D. However, frequent and serial monitoring of the serum concentrations of fat-soluble vitamins is essential in children with CF because deficiencies may occur during therapy, especially with vitamin E.

521 **B** (S&F, ch56)
Fat and protein maldigestion with fecal losses are the primary manifestations of pancreatic involvement in CF. Numerous pancreatic preparations are available commercially, but enzyme activities vary considerably from one product to another, and reduced activity of lipase remains a problem for some patients. The use of histamine H_2 receptor blockers or proton pump inhibitors along with uncoated or enteric-coated pancreatic enzyme supplements should also be considered in patients with CF. Enteric-coated microspheres are now the preferred form of replacement because they protect the digestive enzymes from destruction by gastric acid (pH <4) and are effective in treating steatorrhea. Initial therapy for pancreatic exocrine insufficiency in CF includes pancreatic enzyme replacement at doses ranging from 500 to 2000 units of lipase activity per kilogram of body weight per meal, given just before a meal and with snacks.

522 **C** (S&F, ch58)
Eighty percent of pancreatitis attacks are mild, and normal pancreatic morphology and function are the rule after recovery. Twenty percent of patients have severe pancreatitis that is accompanied by pancreatic necrosis and organ failure. Of this group, the disease-related mortality rate is 25% to 35% but the overall mortality rate is 2% to 10%.

523 **B** (S&F, ch59)
Pancreas divisum is a relatively common anomaly of the pancreas occurring in 4% to 11% of individuals. Pancreas divisum is most often diagnosed incidentally when abdominal imaging is performed for indications other than chronic pancreatitis. When symptomatic, the more common clinical presentation is acute recurrent pancreatitis rather than chronic obstructive pancreatitis. Should therapy directed at the minor papilla be required, this is best achieved endoscopically at ERCP. Surgery is reserved for those with initial responses to endoscopic therapy in need of a more durable intervention.

524 **A** (S&F, ch58)
Pancreatitis is associated with severe dehydration. The use of intravenous contrast before adequate hydration increases the risk of radiographic contrast-mediated acute renal failure. On the other hand, it has not been proven that intravenous contrast can increase the development of pancreatic necrosis in humans. Intravenous contrast is not required to attain a Balthazar score. Perfusion defects associated with necrotizing pancreatitis may not show up for 72 hours after the onset of symptoms. Therefore, an early CT scan with intravenous contrast that does not show perfusion defects does not definitively exclude necrotizing pancreatitis.

525 **D** (S&F, ch57)
Hereditary pancreatitis is recognized as an autosomal-dominant disorder caused by a genetic defect

identified in the members of a family affected with pancreatitis. Several large kindreds were identified during the past 50 years, demonstrating that disease susceptibility is transmitted in an autosomal-dominant pattern, with high penetrance (80% of gene mutation carriers affected) and variable expression. These large kindreds all proved to have a pancreatitis disease gene locus on chromosome 7. The disease gene was identified as the cationic trypsinogen gene (*PRSS1*). Several common mutations in the cationic trypsinogen gene are now known to be associated with hereditary pancreatitis. In addition, mutations in the *SPINK1/PSTI* gene have recently been associated with familial pancreatitis and with idiopathic chronic pancreatitis. Growing experience with genetic testing reveals that family history alone is not an accurate predictor of detecting or excluding specific genes or mutations that predispose to pancreatitis. Thus, family history serves as an important clue to a genetic predisposition, but the final determination continues to require genetic testing.

526 **A** (S&F, ch58)
Regardless of size, an asymptomatic pseudocyst does not require treatment. Therefore, intervention by any route (answers **B**, **C**, and **D**) should not be entertained, and periodic clinical and radiographic assessment is the recommended management. There is no evidence that octreotide (Sandostatin LAR) is beneficial in a patient with a pancreatic pseudocyst.

527 **D** (S&F, ch60)
Numerous molecular abnormalities have been identified in patients with pancreatic cancer. The most commonly detected mutation is the K-*ras* proto-oncogene. Mutations are detected in more than 90% of pancreatic ductal adenocarcinomas. Other genetic sites known to contribute to carcinogenesis include *p16 SMAD4* and *TP53* tumor suppressor genes. The *Rb* tumor suppressor gene is implicated in retinoblastoma.

528 **C** (S&F, ch58)
Statistically, the most common etiology of acute pancreatitis in children is blunt trauma to the abdomen, often secondary to child abuse. All the other answers are less common causes of acute pancreatitis in children.

529 **C** (S&F, ch55)
Anomalous pancreaticobiliary union is a congenital malformation of the confluence of the pancreatic and bile ducts. A common channel for the bile and pancreatic fluid is formed by the absence of a septum between the ducts. This malunion is associated with pancreatitis, choledochal cysts, and proliferative abnormalities that manifest in adults. Choledochal cysts are frequently associated with this abnormality (94%-100% in two series). Malunions were seen in the following percentages in adults with the following diseases: gallbladder cancer, 62.5%; gallbladder adenomyomatosis, 50%; bile duct cancer, 33.3%; and pancreatitis, 13.4%. Considering the cancer risks associated with a pancreaticobiliary malunion, consideration of cholecystectomy, resection of the bile duct, and hepaticojejunostomy may be advised. Diverting the bile duct from the

pancreatic duct by a choledochal cyst excision prevents the recurrence of pancreatitis in most cases.

530 **C** (S&F, ch58)
Nutrition should be instituted early in the course of a patient with severe acute pancreatitis. Although the standard of care had been TPN, several recent studies demonstrated this route to have more complications and no benefit with regard to length of stay when compared with nasojejunal feeding. Nasojejunal feeding is therefore the preferred route for providing nutrition in this group of patients. If TPN is provided, however, there is no additional risk to providing intralipids, although in this case, serum triglycerides should be monitored.

531 **C** (S&F, ch60)
Pancreatic panniculitis is a form of subcutaneous fat necrosis that occurs in the setting of a number of pancreatic diseases. Pancreatic panniculitis occurs in both acute and chronic pancreatitis, particularly in those with very high level of circulating pancreatic enzymes. This presentation is also seen in patients with pancreatic acinar cell carcinoma, a subset of pancreatic cancer that accounts for less than 5% of pancreatic malignancies. These tumors elaborate enzymes including lipase, and the high circulating levels induce the subcutaneous fat necrosis. The findings of a mass with pancreatic duct dilation and gland atrophy are more supportive of neoplasm or focal chronic pancreatitis rather than of autoimmune pancreatitis. The latter presents with a diffusely edematous pancreas and attenuated pancreatic duct.

532 **D** (S&F, ch56)
Enterokinase, secreted by duodenal mucosal cells, serves to activate trypsinogen.

533 **C** (S&F, ch58)
The first phase of acute pancreatitis usually lasts a week. During this phase, fever, tachycardia, hypotension, respiratory distress, and leukocytosis are typically related to SIRS elicited by acinar cell injury. Infectious complications are uncommon at this time. Multiple cytokines are involved, including platelet-activating factor, tumor necrosis factor-α, and various interleukins. These symptoms and signs may develop independently of pancreatic necrosis.

534 **C** (S&F, ch61)
ERCP early in the course of acute pancreatitis is limited to biliary decompression in the setting of acute cholangitis. This patient has fever, hyperbilirubinemia, and progressive hemodynamic compromise secondary to acute cholangitis. The most recent data suggest that ERCP for pancreatic duct decompression is not indicated, even for those with severe acute pancreatic, and does not improve the mortality rate. The risks of ERCP should not be undertaken for diagnostic purposes in the setting of acute pancreatitis.

535 **A** (S&F, ch58)
Acute pancreatitis is felt to result from an initial acinar cell injury causing expression of endothelial adhesion molecules, followed by cytokine release and Kupffer cell activation.

536 D (S&F, ch59)

Fat necrosis and acinar cell necrosis are hallmarks of acute pancreatitis and may be seen in those with chronic pancreatitis. Lobular hemorrhage also occurs commonly in acute pancreatic injury. Ductular plugs may be seen in CF and chronic pancreatitis. Fibrotic changes to the lobules and parenchymal atrophy are features of chronic pancreatitis.

537 D (S&F, ch55)

Heterotopic, ectopic, or aberrant pancreatic tissue, or pancreatic rest, is defined as the presence of pancreatic tissue that lacks anatomic and vascular continuity with the main body of the pancreas. Focal expression of pancreatic cells outside of the pancreatic gland seems to be relatively common in humans and is observed on careful histologic examination of 1% to 14% of autopsy cases. It is rarely of clinical significance. Heterotopic pancreatic tissue is usually seen in the stomach, duodenum, and jejunum. Heterotopic pancreatic tissue usually appears as discrete, firm, yellow submucosal nodules from 2 mm to 4 cm in diameter. The management of heterotopic pancreatic tissue has been controversial because it is usually of no clinical significance. When complications occur, surgical excision is curative. Surgical excision should be considered if there is doubt about the diagnosis or if the lesion is large.

538 D (S&F, ch58)

SPINK1 binds and inactivates approximately 20% of the trypsin activity. Other mechanisms for removing trypsin involve mesotrypsin, enzyme Y, and trypsin itself, which splits and inactivates trypsin. The pancreas also contains nonspecific antiproteases such as α_1-antitrypsin and α_2-macroglobulin. Additional protective mechanisms are the sequestration of pancreatic enzymes within intracellular compartments of the acinar cell during synthesis and transport and the separation of digestive enzymes from lysosomal hydrolases as they pass through the Golgi apparatus, which is important because cathepsin B activates trypsin from trypsinogen. Low intra-acinar calcium concentrations also prevent further autoactivation of trypsin.

539 A (S&F, ch61)

The CT image demonstrates a collection of fluid compressing the distal stomach and duodenum with debris in the collection, consistent with walled-off pancreatic necrosis. The patient is one month from his initial insult, and a well-defined fluid collection has developed. This patient is best treated by endoscopic cystogastrostomy, either by a transduodenal or transgastric route. Although there is a risk of inducing infectious complications due to the presence of internal debris, the symptoms of gastric outlet obstruction are an indication for decompression. Endoscopic decompression is preferred over the percutaneous route because a percutaneous route may result in a persistent pancreaticocutaneous fistula. Surgical drainage may be reserved should less invasive means be unsuccessful.

540 D (S&F, ch58)

The diagnosis of traumatic pancreatitis is difficult and requires a high degree of suspicion. CT and MRI are the most reliable indicators of pancreatic trauma, although a normal imaging study within the first 48 hours does not exclude pancreatic trauma. Serum and ascitic fluid amylase and lipase activity may be increased in abdominal trauma, whether or not the pancreas has been injured. Magnetic resonance angiography is not used to diagnose pancreatic trauma.

541 C (S&F, ch57)

This child has the classic features of Johanson-Blizzard syndrome. Johanson-Blizzard syndrome is a rare autosomal recessive syndrome linked to a mutation in the *UBR1* gene. Johanson-Blizzard syndrome is characterized by nasal alar hypoplasia, hypothyroidism, pancreatic achylia, and congenital deafness syndrome. It can be distinguished from Shwachman-Diamond syndrome and Pearson marrow-pancreas syndrome by the presence of deafness and the absence of hematologic and skeletal abnormalities.

542 B (S&F, ch58)

The patient has an ileus manifesting as the absence of bowel sounds and abdominal distention and periumbilical ecchymosis (Cullen sign), which is a result of hemorrhagic pancreatitis. The Cullen sign is seen in less than 1% of all cases of acute pancreatitis and is associated with a poor prognosis. The Cullen sign is not caused by vomiting and is not a reliable indicator of necrotizing pancreatitis.

543 E (S&F, ch60)

Of environmental carcinogens contributing to pancreatic cancer, tobacco use has the strongest association. Although alcohol use may predispose to chronic pancreatitis, which carries an increased risk of the development of pancreatic cancer, a direct association between alcohol and pancreatic cancer is less well established. Diets high in fat are also implicated as a risk factor for pancreatic malignancy, although to a lesser degree than smoking. Radon exposure and chronic steroid use are not risk factors for pancreatic cancer.

544 A (S&F, ch57)

This infant has meconium ileus. Until 1948, meconium ileus was uniformly fatal. Now the long-term survival rate approaches 90% for uncomplicated meconium ileus. Patients may be treated with *N*-acetylcysteine (Mucomyst) and polysorbate (Tween 80), a mild industrial detergent and preservative. Nonoperative relief of obstruction with gastrografin enemas is also possible. Infants with CF and meconium ileus who survive beyond 6 months of age have the same prognosis as any patient with CF and do not tend to have more severe disease.

545 B (S&F, ch58)

In blunt trauma, it is important to preoperatively determine whether there is injury to the pancreas. When the CT scan shows an abnormality, ERCP is required to define whether there is pancreatic duct injury. Laparoscopy cannot definitively diagnose pancreatic duct disruption. If the pancreatic duct is intact at the time of ERCP and there are no other significant intra-abdominal injuries, surgery is not required. If ERCP reveals duct transection with extravasation of pancreatic fluid and there are no other intra-abdominal injuries, placement of a pancreatic duct stent is indicated. The use of octreotide in pancreatic trauma is not of proven benefit.

546 E (S&F, ch55)
Pancreatic juice is composed of a number of organic and inorganic compounds. Organic compounds include active and inactive enzymatic forms such as amylase, lipase, trypsinogen, trypsin, chemotrypsinogen, chemotrypsin, enterokinase, procarboxypeptidase, and carboxypeptidase. The remainder of the juice is mostly water, bicarbonate, and chloride, with lesser concentrations of other compounds such as calcium and zinc. The principal inorganic components of pancreatic secretions are water, sodium, potassium, chloride, and bicarbonate.

547 C (S&F, ch56)
CCK is the major humoral mediator of meal-stimulated pancreatic enzyme secretion. The circulating concentration of CCK increases with a meal. Experiments using highly specific CCK receptor antagonists have demonstrated that pancreatic enzyme secretion with a meal is largely mediated by CCK. CCK is released from the upper small intestinal mucosa by digestion products of fat and protein and, to a small extent, by starch digestion products. Experimental data suggest that CCK activates afferent neurons in the duodenal mucosa. These afferent neurons mediate an enteropancreatic reflex that causes pancreatic enzyme secretion.

548 C (S&F, ch58)
There is no clear relationship between creatinine clearance and serum amylase levels. Renal insufficiency can increase serum amylase as much as fivefold more than the upper limit of normal and serum lipase as much as twofold more than the upper limit of normal. On the other hand, 30% of patients with renal insufficiency still have a normal serum amylase. The ACCR can only be used to diagnose macroamylasemia and cannot be used to distinguish elevations of amylase due to renal insufficiency from other causes. An elevated serum lipase level is not 100% specific for pancreatic disorders.

549 D (S&F, ch58)
SPINK1 binds and inactivates approximately 20% of trypsin activity. Other mechanisms involve mesotrypsin, enzyme Y, trypsin itself, and nonspecific proteases such as α_2-antitrypsin and α_2-macroglobulin. Additional protective mechanisms are the sequestration of pancreatic enzymes within intracellular compartments of the acinar cell during synthesis and transport and the separation of digestive enzymes from lysosomal hydrolases such as cathepsin B as they pass through the Golgi apparatus. Low intracellular concentrations of calcium prevent further autoactivation of trypsin.

550 A (S&F, ch57)
Hereditary pancreatitis is a syndrome of recurrent acute pancreatitis that develops in an individual from a family in which the pancreatitis phenotype seems to be inherited through a disease-causing gene mutation expressed in an autosomal-dominant pattern. The most common cause is a mutation in the cationic trypsinogen gene (*PRSS1*) that seems to cause a gain of function through altering the regulatory domains in trypsinogen usually controlled by calcium. In two large studies, 19% and 35% of pancreatitis-affected patients from hereditary pancreatitis families had no identifiable *PRSS1* mutations, suggesting that other genes or factors may be responsible for the high risk of pancreatitis.

551 C (S&F, ch59)
Chronic pancreatitis develops in a small minority (15% or fewer) of individuals who drink regularly. When it does occur in one who regularly consumes alcohol, the usual time course is in excess of 10 years of drinking before the development of clinical disease. Most of those (as many as 40%) with acute pancreatitis secondary to alcohol do not progress to chronic pancreatitis. Of those in whom chronic pancreatitis does develop, there are factors that appear linked to the development of disease. These include smoking, a diet high in fat and protein, and drinking in excess of five drinks per day.

552 C (S&F, ch60)
Mucinous cystadenoma, IPMN, and solid pseudopapillary neoplasm all have the potential to behave in a malignant fashion. Serous cystadenoma is considered a benign entity; there have only been isolated reports of a serous cystadenoma behaving in an aggressive fashion and invading local regional structures. The diagnosis of a serous cystadenoma does not require surgical removal of the lesion.

553 C (S&F, ch59)
Genetic causes of chronic pancreatitis are best described in association with altered function of the *CFTR*, *PRSS1*, and *SPINK1*. Mutations in the *CFTR* gene result in a decrement in bicarbonate secretion resulting in viscous pancreatic secretions that promote ductular plugs and obstruction. *SPINK1* mutations are associated with a sentinel acute pancreatitis event. This initial episode of acute pancreatitis then stimulates a cascade of inflammatory responses including stimulation of immune and stellate cells that, in conjunction with environmental insults (i.e., alcohol and/or tobacco), leads to chronic pancreatitis. *PRSS1* mutations cause constitutive activation of trypsin that is resistant to degradation. Trypsin in turn activates other digestive enzymes as well as causes local tissue damage.

554 A (S&F, ch58)
After blunt trauma to the abdomen, the most reliable way to diagnose and treat a pancreatic duct disruption is ERCP. Serum amylase may be elevated secondary to pancreatic contusion or injury to other intra-abdominal organs. Pancreatic or peripancreatic inflammatory changes may suggest pancreatic duct disruption but are not diagnostic. The CT scan may also appear normal. MRI with MRCP is not significantly better than CT for the diagnosis of pancreatic duct disruption.

555 A (S&F, ch57)
Pancreatic abnormalities are present in approximately 85% to 90% of patients with CF. In the mild

cases, there may be only accumulations of mucus in the small ducts, causing dilation of the exocrine glands. In advanced cases, usually seen in older children or adolescents, the ducts are completely plugged, causing atrophy of the exocrine glands and progressive fibrosis.

556 C (S&F, ch58)
This is the most common presentation of pancreatitis secondary to hypertriglyceridemia in adults; that is, the poorly controlled obese diabetic individual with underlying hyperlipidemia. Other common scenarios are the alcoholic patient with hyperlipidemia and the patient with drug- or diet-induced hypertriglyceridemia. In pancreatitis due to hypertriglyceridemia, serum amylase may not be substantially elevated.

557 B (S&F, ch59)
An important concept in managing suspected autoimmune pancreatitis is to exclude malignancy. This patient did have histologically confirmed inflammation and imaging consistent with autoimmune pancreatic disease. However, despite a prolonged course of steroids, there was a persistent mass in the head of the pancreas. To ensure that no occult malignancy exists, of the choices provided, the correct next step would be surgical exploration and resection of the mass. Azathioprine is typically used as a steroid-sparing agent in those requiring prolonged therapy; the protracted onset of clinical efficacy with azathioprine would preclude the timely diagnosis of cancer should it be present. FDG-PET scan cannot reliably distinguish between inflammatory pancreatitis and pancreatic malignancy.

558 D (S&F, ch58)
Hypertriglyceridemia may cause as many as 5% of cases of acute pancreatitis. Hypertriglyceridemia-induced pancreatitis in adults is most commonly seen in patients with a mild form of genetically inherited type I or V hyperlipoproteinemia. APO C-II deficiency is a rare disorder that presents with acute pancreatitis in childhood. Thiazide diuretics, not loop diuretics, elevate serum triglycerides, and hypertriglyceridemia-induced pancreatitis is seen more commonly in diabetic patients.

559 B (S&F, ch57)
In Shwachman-Diamond syndrome, duodenal and pancreatic bicarbonate secretion is spared. The clinical features of Shwachman-Diamond syndrome, including severe pancreatic insufficiency, steatorrhea, and failure to thrive, usually become evident in the first year of life. Because of the characteristic cyclic neutropenia, patients with Shwachman-Diamond syndrome often have more infectious complications than patients with CF. Patients with Shwachman-Diamond syndrome have normal mucosal enterokinase activity.

560 B (S&F, ch60)
Surgical resection for pancreatic cancer is the only means for potential cure. At high-volume centers of excellence, surgical complication rates are lower than in other settings; however, even in these situations, the five-year survival rate is only 25% to 30%. Total pancreatectomy is no longer considered a standard of care for management of pancreatic cancer. Pancreaticoduodenectomy (Whipple procedure) is the most commonly performed surgery because tumors are most frequently located in the head of the pancreas.

561 D (S&F, ch58)
All the conditions listed may result in an elevated serum amylase. In this young woman, the abrupt onset of abdominal pain, shock, and severe anemia is best explained by a ruptured ectopic pregnancy.

562 C (S&F, ch57)
Pancreatitis associated with SPINK1 gene mutations is associated with early-onset recurrent acute and chronic pancreatitis in children, familial pancreatitis, and tropical pancreatitis and is often a feature of the polygenic pancreatitis-associated genotype. SPINK1 is categorized as a modifier gene and is synthesized in the acinar cell. SPINK1 is an acute phase reactant, and concentrations in serum increase markedly with inflammation.

563 C (S&F, ch55)
Multiple pancreatic cysts tend to occur in patients with associated anomalies and may be seen in systemic disorders such as von Hippel-Lindau disease and polycystic kidney disease. Congenital cysts of the pancreas are rare, can be diagnosed at any age, may be single or multiple, and can be distinguished from pancreatic pseudocysts by the presence of an epithelial lining. Cysts are more often located in the body and tail of the pancreas and are thought to be benign, without malignant potential.

564 C (S&F, ch59)
The diagnosis of chronic pancreatitis is associated with decreased quality of life. A number of independent predictors have been associated with decreased quality of life in the setting of chronic pancreatitis. Factors that have been independently associated with chronic pancreatitis include ongoing alcohol use, uncontrolled diarrhea, poorly controlled diabetes, and chronic abdominal pain. Other factors include low body weight, persistent tobacco abuse, and depression.

565 A (S&F, ch58)
SPINK1 protects the pancreatic acinar cell by inhibiting prematurely activated trypsin. Mutation of the SPINK1 gene results in pancreatitis by limiting the activity of this protein. Heterozygous mutations of the CFTR gene change bicarbonate conductance and mutations to the trypsin gene cause hereditary pancreatitis by making trypsin resistant to lysis. Trypsinogen activation peptide is a marker for acute pancreatitis.

566 A (S&F, ch60)
Although it is the second most common gastrointestinal malignancy in the United States, pancreatic cancer is the fourth leading cause of cancer-related mortality in both men and women. Men are disproportionately affected, with the highest incidence in African Americans, in whom the incidence is almost twice that of the general population.

The risk of the development of pancreatic cancer increases sharply after age 45 and continues to increase with advancing age. The five-year survival rate for all individuals diagnosed with pancreatic cancer is 5%.

567 B (S&F, ch58)
The Balthazar grading system is based on a nonenhanced CT scan. The Balthazar grading system correlates better with local complications than with mortality. The CT severity index is not more predictive of outcome than the Balthazar grade A through E score. Grade D is defined as the presence of one peripancreatic fluid collection, whereas grade E is the presence of two or more peripancreatic fluid collections or gas in the pancreas or retroperitoneum.

568 C (S&F, ch56)
SPINK1 is a 56-amino-acid peptide that specifically inhibits trypsin by physically blocking its active site. SPINK1 is synthesized by pancreatic acinar cells along with trypsinogen, and it colocalizes with trypsinogen in the zymogen granules. In the mechanistic models of pancreatic acinar cell protection, SPINK1 acts as the first line of defense against prematurely activated trypsinogen in the acinar cell. However, because of a 1:5 stoichiometric disequilibrium between SPINK1 and trypsinogen, SPINK1 is capable of inhibiting only approximately 20% of potential trypsin. Thus, in the pancreas, SPINK1 seems to act as a limited first line of defense against prematurely activated trypsinogen.

569 A (S&F, ch58)
Elevations of serum amylase may occur in many nonpancreatic conditions. Amylase may be elevated in pathologic processes in organs (salivary glands, fallopian tubes, ovary, and lung) that normally produce amylase. Mass lesions such as papillary cystadenocarcinoma of the ovary, benign ovarian cyst, and carcinoma of the lung cause hyperamylasemia because they produce and secrete salivary type–isoamylase. Transmural leakage of pancreatic-type isoamylase and peritoneal absorption can occur in some patients with small bowel mucosal diseases including Crohn's disease and radiation enteritis. Amylase can be fractionated into pancreatic and salivary isoenzymes, but there are no ovarian isoenzymes. Renal failure increases serum amylase as many as four to five times the upper limit of normal due to decreased renal clearance of this enzyme. Chronic elevations of serum amylase occur in macroamylasemia. In this condition, normal serum amylase is bound to an immunoglobulin or abnormal serum protein to form a complex that is too large to be filtered by renal glomeruli and thus has a prolonged serum half-life. Macroamylasemia can be diagnosed with a low ACCR.

570 B (S&F, ch60)
This pancreatogram demonstrates a saccular dilation communicating with the main pancreatic duct. A central lucency is seen within the dilated duct segment. These findings, coupled with the presence of mucin extruding through the pancreatic os, are

diagnostic of an IPMN. Because IPMN is a premalignant lesion, it should be considered for surgical resection in this healthy young individual. EUS-guided FNA is unlikely to yield additional valuable information. A mucinous cystadenoma does not communicate with the main pancreatic duct and is more commonly found in the tail of the pancreas. Solid pseudopapillary tumors are commonly found in young women, although they do not communicate with the main pancreatic duct. Although a pancreatic pseudocyst is a consideration, the presence of a central lucency within the cyst and mucin seen to extrude from the pancreatic os are diagnostic of IPMN.

571 E (S&F, ch55)
Annular pancreas is a congenital anomaly in which a portion of the pancreas forms a thin band around the preampullary portion of the duodenum, leading to complete or partial obstruction. It has been associated with trisomy 21, cardiac defects, malrotation, genitourinary anomalies, and tracheoesophageal fistula. Annular pancreas may present with poor feeding in infancy due to duodenal obstruction, although its diagnosis may not be made until later in life. Patients typically present with symptoms of gastric outlet obstruction, although acute recurrent pancreatitis may occur.

572 A (S&F, ch58)
The injured pancreas releases many systemically active substances. The release of phospholipase A_2 into the systemic circulation degrades surfactant and contributes to the development of adult respiratory distress syndrome. Elastase is also released by the injured pancreas but primarily affects blood vessels. Patients with acute pancreatitis have decreased intravascular fluid volume, and infectious pneumonia is a rare complication of acute pancreatitis.

573 B (S&F, ch57)
This patient likely has hereditary pancreatitis based on a *PRSS1* mutation. Smoking cessation is most important because smoking doubles the patient's already high risk of the development of pancreatic cancer. Smoking can also increase the severity of acute attacks of pancreatitis. In this patient, genetic testing should be entertained. Genetic testing, however, must be discussed at length with the patient and, if available, with a young adult such as this, a genetic counselor should be involved. Genetic testing in this patient would include tests for *PRSS1*, *SPINK1*, and *CFTR*. At this juncture, there is no clinical indication for the initiation of pancreatic enzyme therapy, and the initiation of corticosteroid therapy is incorrect.

574 C (S&F, ch58)
The question describes the classic pattern of a hypersensitivity reaction, which is the most common mechanism for drug-induced pancreatitis. Drugs that operate through this mechanism include 6-mercaptopurine/azathioprine, aminosalicylates, metronidazole, and tetracycline. Accumulation of a toxic metabolite and intrinsic toxicity often occur after a longer duration of initial drug use and do not occur as quickly with reinitiation.

Immunomodulatory up-regulation is not a pathogenetic mechanism of drug-induced pancreatitis.

575 **A** (S&F, ch57)
CFTR is the most important molecule for regulating pancreatic duct cell function. The CFTR molecule is located on the apical side of the pancreatic duct cells. The CFTR molecule forms a regulated ion channel expressed on epithelial cells in the respiratory system, sweat glands, digestive tract mucosa, biliary epithelium, pancreatic duct cells, and other locations. CFTR-associated secretion is stimulated when the duct cell is stimulated by secretin or VIP acting on receptors that increase intracellular cyclic adenosine monophosphate.

576 **A** (S&F, ch60)
Primary pancreatic lymphoma is an uncommon form of non-Hodgkin's lymphoma, representing less than 1% of all cases of extranodal non-Hodgkin's lymphoma and 1% to 2% of pancreatic malignancies. Cure is achieved in approximately one third of patients, mostly through the administration of chemotherapy. Management is typically nonsurgical.

577 **C** (S&F, ch58)
In patients with severe acute pancreatitis, the mortality rate is 25% to 35%. There are two time peaks for mortality. Death can be very rapid, with a significant fraction of patients dying within the first 48 hours. After the second week of disease, the majority of patients die of pancreatic infection in association with multisystem organ failure. Patients who are older and have comorbid illnesses have a substantially higher rate of mortality than younger patients. Hemorrhagic pancreatitis does not independently factor into the risk of dying of pancreatitis.

578 **B** (S&F, ch59)
Diabetes is common in long-standing chronic pancreatitis and seems to occur with an incidence similar to that of exocrine insufficiency. The simultaneous diagnosis of both exocrine and endocrine failure is not uncommon in patients with chronic pancreatitis. The disease results from disruption of insulin and glucagon secretion from pancreatic islet cells. The islet cells appear relatively resistant to destruction in chronic pancreatitis, which may be one factor accounting for the long duration from onset of inflammation to the development of endocrine failure. Approximately half of those with diabetes due to chronic pancreatitis will require insulin.

579 **D** (S&F, ch58)
Many mechanisms for alcohol-induced pancreatitis have been proposed. Although theories include the activation of pancreatic stellate cells, a decrease in GP2, and acinar cell cytoplasmic lipid accumulation, these mechanisms have not been proven in humans and may not be present in all cases of pancreatitis in patients who consume alcohol. The expression of endothelial adhesion molecules, however, is an early step in the pathophysiology of all cases of acute pancreatitis.

580 **D** (S&F, ch55)
Symptoms develop in only a minority of patients with pancreas divisum; however, those in whom they do develop can benefit from endoscopic therapy. Studies have reported 90% and 73% rates of symptomatic improvement in patients with pancreas divisum and acute pancreatitis who have undergone stent placement or sphincterotomy. Clinical improvement was much less likely in patients with pancreatic-type pain absent pancreatic enzyme elevations rather than true acute pancreatitis.

581 **D** (S&F, ch58)
It is not necessary to drain pseudocysts, no matter how large, unless they are enlarging or precipitating symptoms. Although the ability to drain a pseudocyst is influenced by its location, the location of the pseudocyst in the tail does not make drainage any more essential. The appearance of a homogeneous low-attenuation, fluid-filled appearance does not exclude the pseudocyst containing necrotic debris.

582 **D** (S&F, ch58)
Acute pancreatitis may result in splenic vein thrombosis due to the peripancreatic inflammation. Splenic vein thrombosis, in turn, leads to gastric varices and the potential for gastrointestinal hemorrhage. Cavernous transformation of the portal vein may develop in the face of chronic portal vein thrombosis, but not within 10 days from the onset of acute pancreatitis. Hemosuccus pancreaticus is bleeding from the pancreatic duct into the duodenum. It is often secondary to erosion of a pseudocyst or pseudoaneurysm into the peripancreatic vasculature. It is a rare cause of gastrointestinal hemorrhage related to pancreatitis. In this patient, there is no basis to suspect viral hepatitis or alcohol abuse.

583 **A** (S&F, ch56)
Exocrine and endocrine pancreatic insufficiency occurs in patients in whom pancreatic function is reduced by more than 90%. Thus, pancreatic insufficiency tends to occur with long-standing chronic pancreatitis, most commonly in the United States secondary to alcohol abuse.

584 **C** (S&F, ch59)
Features of chronic pancreatitis may be seen on imaging including gland atrophy and lobularity, heterogeneic echotecture, and pancreatic calcifications. The presence of these findings does not denote clinical disease absent physiologic sequelae such as endocrine and exocrine pancreatic dysfunction. In fact, these findings are not uncommon in subsets of the population including those of advanced age, those with chronic renal failure, and those with diabetes.

585 **D** (S&F, ch57)
An eight-amino-acid extension of the enzyme, TAP, maintains the enzyme as inactive trypsinogen until it is cleaved by enterokinase or another trypsin molecule (autoactivation). Cleavage of TAP allows a conformation change that activates trypsin. Cationic trypsinogen is the major form of trypsinogen

(~65%) followed by anionic trypsinogen (PRSS2, ~30%) and mesotrypsin (PRSS3, ~5%). Regulation of trypsin activity is determined by cellular calcium, with increased cellular calcium facilitating activation, preventing inactivation and low cellular calcium levels, limiting activation, and permitting autolysis. More than 20 mutations have been identified in *PRSS1* that increase susceptibility to recurrent acute pancreatitis.

586 B (S&F, ch58)
In the presence of gallstones and abnormal liver tests, gallstone pancreatitis is the most likely diagnosis. Although alcohol is a common cause of acute pancreatitis, it is not as common a cause as gallstones and most often is associated with heavy alcohol use. The other listed causes are far less common and need not be implicated in this case.

587 C (S&F, ch58)
The APACHE II score, Ranson criteria, and Glasgow Outcome Score are cumbersome tools with multiple measurements that are not accurate until 48 hours after presentation. In general, they are no longer used clinically. The Marshall scoring system for organ failure is commonly used by intensivists for patients admitted to an ICU. Data have not yet been generated using this system to prognosticate mortality in acute pancreatitis. The presence of SIRS, organ failure, and anatomic complications on CT scan are the currently favored mechanisms with which to assess severity in acute pancreatitis.

588 B (S&F, ch55)
Congenital cysts of the pancreas are rare and are distinguished from pseudocysts by the presence of an epithelial lining. It is believed that these cysts are caused by anomalous development of the pancreatic ductal system in which sequestered segments of a primitive ductal system give rise to microscopic or macroscopic cystic lesions. Clinical presentations can include an asymptomatic mass, abdominal distention, vomiting, and jaundice from biliary obstruction. Symptomatic pancreatic cysts should be surgically removed whenever possible.

589 C (S&F, ch58)
Obese patients with pancreatitis have a higher incidence of local complications, respiratory failure, severe acute pancreatitis, and death from sterile necrosis than do nonobese patients. There is no evidence that there is a difference in the levels of amylase or lipase between obese and nonobese patients and, providing that CT imaging can be performed, there is no difference in the ability of CT to estimate the severity of disease.

590 B (S&F, ch57)
In contrast with other forms of pancreatic insufficiency, the bicarbonate secretion within the duodenum and biliary tree is impaired to a greater degree in CF. Decreased duodenal bicarbonate results in a more acidic duodenum (i.e., lower duodenal pH).

591 C (S&F, ch58)
In adults, hypertriglyceridemia-induced pancreatitis is most commonly seen in patients with a mild form of genetically inherited type I or V

hyperlipoproteinemia, and this should be formally assessed by performing lipoprotein electrophoresis. Lipoprotein lipase deficiency is a disorder that presents as acute pancreatitis in early childhood. Angiotensin-converting enzyme inhibitors are not one of the classes of medications that can increase serum triglycerides and trigger hypertriglyceridemia-induced pancreatitis. Therapy for hyperlipidemia in these patients should be started as soon as the patient has recovered from pancreatitis.

592 B (S&F, ch61)
This patient presents with biliary and pancreatic duct obstruction in the setting of chronic alcoholic pancreatitis. The next appropriate step would be ERCP with placement of an endoprosthesis for biliary decompression. The differential diagnosis of the etiology of the mass is focal chronic pancreatitis versus pancreatic adenocarcinoma arising in a setting of chronic pancreatitis. This may be distinguished at EUS-guided FNA, although the jaundice should be addressed first. Surgical intervention with either a Whipple or Puestow procedure would be relatively contraindicated in this patient, who has evidence of cirrhosis and portal hypertension.

593 B (S&F, ch58)
With six Ranson criteria, this patient has a 60% mortality rate. The presence of a Grey Turner sign is a manifestation of hemorrhagic pancreatitis. In most patients with underlying heart disease and severe acute pancreatitis, a Swan-Ganz catheter is recommended so that aggressive fluid resuscitation can be provided without inducing congestive heart failure. Fluid resuscitation in acute pancreatitis should almost never be gentle. Hypocalcemia is often a manifestation of hypoalbuminemia and does not need to be corrected or of hypomagnesemia, which should be corrected first. Nasogastric suctioning is recommended only in the face of intestinal ileus or intractable vomiting. Antibiotic therapy remains controversial and should not be used routinely. If used, antibiotics should be used for clinical evidence of infection or in patients with necrotizing disease.

594 C (S&F, ch58)
The presence of a well-perfused gland on CT excludes necrotizing pancreas and therefore defines edematous pancreatitis. The presence of an ileus can occur with both mild edematous and necrotizing pancreatitis. The levels of amylase and lipase have no prognostic value, and more than three Ranson criteria may be associated with severe disease.

595 C (S&F, ch56)
The pancreatic hormone stimulation test is performed by placing a tube into the third portion of the duodenum under fluoroscopic guidance, administering a secretagogue, and measuring the resultant pancreatic secretion. With CCK stimulation, pancreatic lipase secretion is measured; with secretin stimulation, bicarbonate secretion is measured. Collection requires two hours. The test is generally performed in specialized laboratories that have established reference values so that test results can be clearly interpreted as normal or abnormal.

Another test that can be performed is the intraductal secretin test. For this test, a catheter is placed in the pancreatic duct, and output is measured over 15 minutes. However, this test does not add any useful diagnostic information to that obtained from the pancreatic hormone stimulation test, and the intraductal secretin test alone is likely to be less accurate for diagnostic purposes than the pancreatic hormone stimulation test.

596 **B** (S&F, ch59)
Diagnostic tests for chronic pancreatitis, whether by pancreatography or functional assessment of pancreatic secretion, are most accurate late in the disease when structural changes are present. Secretagogue-stimulated testing with duodenal collections over one hour seems to be the most sensitive and specific testing modality. The gold standard for diagnosis is histologic changes of chronic pancreatitis, which are difficult to obtain and are variable in extent throughout the gland. Attempts at direct intraductal collection of pancreatic juice have not yielded results superior to those with more conventional strategies.

597 **E** (S&F, ch58)
Serum amylase is not 100% sensitive and actually may be normal or minimally elevated in fatal pancreatitis, mild to moderate pancreatitis, or an attack superimposed on chronic pancreatitis. Serum amylase increases within 6 to 12 hours, has a half-life of 10 hours, and remains elevated for three to five days. It is likely that only 25% of serum amylase is removed by the kidneys, although other routes of excretion have not been elucidated.

598 **D** (S&F, ch57)
The reason for this high incidence of pancreatic cancer is unknown. The recurrent pancreatic injury caused by unregulated trypsinogen activation and subsequent inflammation seems to provide an environment that promotes oncogenesis. The *PRSS1* gene does not seem to play a role in sporadic pancreatic cancer.

599 **A** (S&F, ch58)
There is no difference in the rate of post-ERCP pancreatitis between those studies performed with ionic contrast agents and nonionic contrast agents. Balloon sphincteroplasty has a greater risk of post-ERCP pancreatitis than sphincterotomy. Randomized, controlled trials show no difference in post-ERCP pancreatitis in patients receiving gabexate versus patients not receiving gabexate. This patient has a 5% to 7% risk of the development of post-ERCP pancreatitis and a 35% to 70% risk of the development of asymptomatic hyperamylasemia.

600 **A** (S&F, ch59)
Pancreatic exocrine dysfunction ensues when secretion of pancreatic enzymes decreases to less than 10% of normal physiologic levels. Fat malabsorption precedes protein maldigestion due to decreased secretion and increased destruction of pancreatic lipase compared with other pancreatic enzymes. Among these mechanisms is a decrease in bicarbonate secretion resulting in destruction of pancreatic lipase by gastric acid. Exocrine insufficiency

typically develops in those with long-standing chronic pancreatitis, although there is significant variability depending on the cause and age at onset of pancreatitis. Weight loss is uncommon in those with exocrine insufficiency alone but may be a sign of a secondary complication such as small bowel overgrowth or pancreatic carcinoma.

601 **B** (S&F, ch58)
Thirty percent to 50% of cases of acute pancreatitis are associated with an acute peripancreatic fluid collection. The presence of greater than 30% necrosis and walled-off pancreatic necrosis are evidence of necrotizing pancreatitis. Parenchymal calcifications are diagnostic of chronic pancreatitis, and their presence does not influence the diagnosis of edematous pancreatitis.

602 **B** (S&F, ch57)
Tropical pancreatitis is the most common form of chronic pancreatitis in regions of India and Asia. The disease typically presents at a young age with abdominal pain, severe malnutrition, and exocrine or endocrine insufficiency. Clinical steatorrhea is rare owing to a very low dietary fat intake. Endocrine insufficiency is an inevitable consequence of tropical chronic pancreatitis and is often classified as a specific cause of diabetes called fibrocalculous pancreatic diabetes. Pancreatic calculi develop in more than 90% of these patients. The pathophysiology of tropical pancreatitis is unknown. Protein-calorie malnutrition is present in the majority of these patients. This disease is treated similarly to other forms of chronic pancreatitis.

603 **C** (S&F, ch58)
The sensitivity of amylase in the diagnosis of acute pancreatitis is 85%. Serum amylase may be normal in acute pancreatitis and is frequently normal in patients with acute-on-chronic pancreatitis. Serum amylase may also be falsely normal in hypertriglyceridemia-associated pancreatitis because an amylase inhibitor may be associated with triglyceride elevations. Hyperamylasemia is not specific for pancreatitis because it occurs in many conditions other than acute pancreatitis. In fact, one half of all patients with elevated serum amylase may not have pancreatic disease.

604 **E** (S&F, ch60)
A multiseptated cyst in the tail of the pancreas in a middle-aged woman is strongly suggestive of a mucinous cystadenoma. Because this is a premalignant lesion, distal pancreatectomy would be the appropriate next step. EUS may more accurately define the morphology; however, EUS alone would not alter the clinical decision making. Similarly, the results of an aspirate are unlikely to affect decision making. The absence of a previous diagnosis of pancreatitis makes pseudocyst unlikely, and this lesion has features worrisome for transformation to malignancy, specifically thick-walled septation. MRI with MRCP may better delineate whether this lesion is an IPMN or mucinous cystadenoma due to the detail of ductal anatomy; in either case, surgical excision of the cyst would be appropriate.

605 C (S&F, ch57)

The median survival of patients with CF is more than 40 years. Seventy percent of CF cases are diagnosed within the first year of life, and 85% of patients with CF present with evidence of exocrine pancreatic dysfunction. Exocrine pancreatic insufficiency presents when the secretion of lipase and trypsin decreases to less than 10% of normal.

606 E (S&F, ch58)

Hemolytic-uremic syndrome is the most common cause of acute pancreatitis of the systemic diseases listed. Acute hemorrhagic colitis, which was first recognized in two separate outbreaks in Michigan and Oregon in 1982, has been associated mainly with a specific serotype of *Escherichia coli* O157:H7. This organism is estimated to be responsible for 0.6% to 2.4% of all cases of diarrhea and 15% to 36% of cases of hemorrhagic colitis in Canada, the United Kingdom, and the United States. The spectrum of disease associated with *E. coli* O157:H7 includes bloody diarrhea, which is seen in as many as 95% of patients, nonbloody diarrhea, hemolytic-uremic syndrome, acute renal insufficiency, and thrombotic thrombocytopenic purpura.

607 C (S&F, ch58)

Types I and V are the types of inherited hyperlipidemia most commonly associated with the development of pancreatitis in adults. Type II hyperlipidemia is also associated with pancreatitis but to a lesser extent.

608 B (S&F, ch59)

Endoscopic treatments for chronic pancreatitis are widely used and include duct decompression via pancreatic sphincterotomy or stent placement, stone extraction, and celiac plexus neurolysis. In this patient, who does not have a dilated pancreatic duct, decompression will not yield clinical benefit, whether performed endoscopically or surgically. A lateral pancreaticojejunostomy is not feasible for a 3-mm pancreatic duct, and subtotal pancreatectomy would be an extreme measure when other options remain available. EUS-guided celiac plexus neurolysis may afford benefit to the patient, although experience and success are greater for pancreatic cancer than for chronic pancreatitis.

609 E (S&F, ch55)

Annular pancreas is a band of pancreatic tissue encircling the second part of the duodenum and is of ventral pancreas origin. Annular pancreas has a bimodal presentation, with peaks in neonates and in adults in the fourth and fifth decades. This entity is a common anomaly obstructing the duodenum in infancy and usually involves growth of pancreatic tissue into the wall of the duodenum. Adult presentations include duodenal stenosis, peptic ulceration, or chronic pancreatitis, or it may be an incidental finding. The most common symptom in adults is upper abdominal pain. Biliary obstruction is a rare complication. Because pancreatic tissue often extends into the duodenal wall and because the annular tissue may contain a large pancreatic duct, symptomatic cases are best treated by surgical bypass rather than by surgical resection.

610 B (S&F, ch58)

In the United States, the most common causes of acute pancreatitis in children are idiopathic (22.2%), association with systemic disease (20.8%), trauma (18.6%), structural (e.g., pancreas divisum) (10.6%), and medications (10.2%). Gallstones, hereditary disorders, hypercalcemia, hyperlipidemia, and "other" causes made up the remaining etiologies. In a patient who was previously well, currently has no other manifestations of systemic disease, and has periumbilical ecchymoses, trauma (and specifically child abuse) is the most likely etiology for pancreatitis.

611 A (S&F, ch59)

The MRI demonstrates a diffusely enlarged, edematous, sausage-like pancreas gland. ERCP images identify a biliary stricture with an irregular, attenuated pancreas duct. These are more typical findings of autoimmune pancreatitis than pancreatic carcinoma. The next most important step in this patient in whom autoimmune pancreatitis is suspected is to exclude pancreatic malignancy. EUS-guided FNA should be performed to exclude carcinoma in the head of the pancreas. If the aspirate does not identify cancer, a course of steroids may be initiated with the intent to reimage the pancreas in two to four weeks and assess for resolution of the identified abnormalities. An elevation of the IgG4 level would be supportive of an autoimmune pancreatitis but is inadequate to exclude cancer as a cause of painless jaundice. Biliary obstruction is best alleviated by the placement of a plastic biliary endoprosthesis, which is readily removed and less likely to cause chronic alteration of the biliary anatomy compared with metal stents.

612 B (S&F, ch56)

Direct tests are considered the gold standard for the measurement of pancreatic function. Classically, juice is collected from the duodenum to minimize contamination of the pancreatic secretions by gastric output. Secretin, CCK, or both, injected intravenously, are used to stimulate pancreatic secretion. The Lundh test meal stimulates pancreatic secretion through oral ingestion of a stimulatory meal rather than through intravenous injection of a secretagogue. Results of pancreatic stimulation are more variable and somewhat less accurate compared with intravenous stimulation studies.

613 C (S&F, ch59)

Abdominal pain in chronic pancreatitis is common and a major cause of disease-related morbidity. The pain tends to vary in intensity and character, and some studies show a decrease in pain over time. The etiology of pain is multifactorial, caused by a complex interaction of physiologic mechanisms. These include pancreatic ductal hypertension, pancreatic ischemia, decreased pancreatic blood flow, and neuropathic alterations. Intrapancreatic neural anatomy is distorted, as is physiologic function of these neurons, and plays an important role in the pathogenesis of pancreatic pain. The specific interactions between these factors are complex and vary both within specific individuals and among differing populations of those with chronic pancreatic pain.

614 A (S&F, ch58)
The initial step in the pathogenesis of acute pancreatitis is the conversion of trypsinogen to typsin within acinar cells in sufficient quantities to overwhelm normal mechanisms to remove active trypsin. Release of phospholipase A_2, increased capillary permeability, and fat necrosis are all subsequent steps. A decrease in GP2 is one postulated mechanism for direct alcohol-induced acinar cell cytotoxicity in the development of chronic pancreatitis.

615 D (S&F, ch58)
Although morphine has been reported to increase sphincter of Oddi tone, its use to treat the pain of pancreatitis has not been shown to adversely affect outcome. Nasogastric intubation is used only to treat ileus or intractable vomiting. Proton pump inhibitors or H_2 receptor blocking agents have not been shown to be beneficial. Early vigorous intravenous hydration for the purpose of intravascular resuscitation is of foremost importance. Too often patients with acute pancreatitis are given suboptimal intravenous hydration. Ranson and colleagues found that a sequestration of more than 6 L of fluids during the first 48 hours was an independent predictor of disease severity in nongallstone pancreatitis. If this amount of fluid (6 L) is added to the minimal intravenous fluid requirements of a 70-kg person during the first 48 hours, intravenous hydration should be at least 250 to 300 mL/hr for 48 hours.

616 D (S&F, ch57)
A diagnosis of CF can be made by the presence of one or more characteristic clinical features, a history of CF in a sibling, or a positive newborn screening test result with confirmation by laboratory evidence of CFTR dysfunction. Either the sweat chloride or nasal bioelectrical responses should be abnormal on two separate days. Genetic testing confirms the clinical diagnosis if two severe mutations are identified. Histologically, hyperplasia and eventual necrosis of ductular and centroacinar cells, together with inspissated secretions, lead to blockage of pancreatic ductules and subsequently encroach on acini, causing flattening and atrophy of the epithelium. Cystic spaces are filled with calcium-rich, eosinophilic concretions. Calcifications are rare. Over a 30-year follow-up, the incidence of pancreatitis in patients with typical CF is less than 2% and tends to be more problematic in older patients. Only 10% of young patients have clinically significant diabetes mellitus.

617 A (S&F, ch59)
Chronic pancreatitis is associated with increased mortality. Causes of death include complications related to the disease such as pancreatic cancer and malnutrition as well as complications of associated diseases such as coronary artery disease and diabetes. Postoperative complications are also a common cause of morbidity and mortality. The factor that most strongly influences mortality is ongoing alcohol use, particularly in those with alcohol-induced pancreatitis.

618 B (S&F, ch61)
This patient is presenting with pancreatic duct disruption secondary to a motor vehicle accident. The location of disruption is at the neck of the pancreas secondary to the deceleration injury. Initial attempts at management of pancreatic duct disruption are via ERCP with the goal of reestablishing continuity of the duct with placement of a pancreatic stent. Intravenous octreotide infusion may be used as an adjuvant therapy but will not address the site of disruption. Should ERCP fail, pancreaticojejunostomy may be required.

619 B (S&F, ch58)
The most common mechanism for drug-induced pancreatitis is a hypersensitivity reaction. Examples of drugs that act by this mechanism include 6-mercaptopurine, aminosalicylates, and metronidazole. Accumulation of a toxic metabolite and induction of hypertriglyceridemia are less common mechanisms of drug-induced pancreatitis. Alteration of acinar cell membrane permeability and alteration in trypsin inhibitor are not mechanisms of drug-induced pancreatitis.

620 C (S&F, ch57)
The pathologic changes described are characteristic of fibrosing colopathy associated with high-dose formulations of pancreatic enzymes, particularly in patients taking more than 5000 U/kg/day. Patients with CF also have vitamin deficiencies, but the described pathology is a consequence of these deficiencies. *N*-acetylcysteine is administered for meconium ileus and distal intestinal obstruction syndrome, not fibrosing colopathy.

621 B (S&F, ch59)
In the majority of patients with diabetes associated with chronic pancreatitis, management of the blood sugar should not be done aggressively to prevent medication-induced hypoglycemia. The lack of glucagon and insulin together result in very severe glucose dysregulation, and the results of medication-induced hypoglycemia can be life-threatening. Accordingly, an oral hypoglycemic agent is often a reasonable choice for these individuals. However, for those with hypertriglyceridemic pancreatitis, tight glucose control is required to facilitate regulation of the triglycerides and prevent further attacks of pancreatitis. For those with very high triglyceride levels, the initial medication treatment consists of fibrates, niacin, and fish oil. Bypass of her pancreatic duct will not reverse the diabetes.

622 C (S&F, ch58)
It is important to distinguish mild from acute pancreatitis because severe pancreatitis is associated with a high disease-related mortality rate. There are several physiologic parameters and scoring systems that have been developed to define severe pancreatitis. Three or more Ranson criteria correctly define severe pancreatitis. An APACHE II score of more than 8, C-reactive protein greater than 200, and hematocrit greater than 50% would also be correct. Tachypnea is one physiologic parameter of severe pancreatitis, but alone it is insufficient.

CHAPTER

7

Biliary Tract

QUESTIONS

623 Which of the following is the most correct statement regarding complications from endoscopic retrograde cholangiopancreatography (ERCP)?
A. Retroperitoneal air identified after ERCP does not always require surgical intervention and can be managed conservatively in the asymptomatic patient.
B. Retroperitoneal air identified after ERCP with concomitant postprocedure pancreatitis is an indication for urgent surgical intervention.
C. Perforation of a bile duct occurs in 5% of all ERCP procedures.
D. Sphincter of Oddi manometry is associated with a 50% likelihood of the development of pancreatitis.

624 What is the best first diagnostic test to perform when biliary colic is suspected?
A. CT scan
B. Magnetic resonance imaging (MRI) and magnetic resonance cholangiopancreatography (MRCP)
C. Endoscopic ultrasonography (EUS)
D. ERCP
E. Transabdominal ultrasonography

625 A 20-day-old infant girl is referred for evaluation of jaundice. The infant was born at 40 weeks' gestation and weighed 7 lb, 10 oz at birth. The mother had no complications during the pregnancy. In the postnatal period, weight gain has been normal. Upon examination, the infant is notably jaundiced. The liver is palpable at 4 cm below the right costal margin. No splenomegaly or ascites is noted. Laboratory studies demonstrate a total bilirubin concentration of 10 mg/dL and a direct bilirubin concentration of 7.5 mg/dL. Aspartate aminotransferase (AST) and alanine aminotransferase (ALT) levels are 50 U/L and 62 U/L, respectively, and the alkaline phosphatase concentration is 155 mU/L. Based on the appearance of a liver biopsy specimen (see figure), what is the likely cause of this infant's jaundice?
A. Alagille syndrome
B. Caroli syndrome
C. Choledochal cyst
D. Extrahepatic biliary atresia
E. Neonatal sclerosing cholangitis

626 A 34-year-old white man with known primary sclerosing cholangitis (PSC) for 10 years is having periodic evaluation to detect the presence of cholangiocarcinoma. Which of the following statements is most correct?
A. Brush cytology of dominant strictures in the biliary tree is 80% to 90% sensitive for the detection of cholangiocarcinoma.
B. Elevated CA19-9 is highly specific for the presence of cholangiocarcinoma.
C. EUS with fine-needle aspiration is not indicated in the screening of patients for cholangiocarcinoma.
D. The most common locations for cholangiocarcinoma in patients with PSC are the common hepatic duct and biliary hilum.

627 A 47-year-old woman is referred to you for recurrent episodes of biliary colic, occurring approximately once per month. She has been seen in the emergency department four times in the past year but has never been admitted. She has never had acute cholecystitis. Abdominal ultrasonography has demonstrated gallbladder sludge and possibly a few small stones. You refer the patient to a surgeon, who performs a laparoscopic cholecystectomy. Which histologic changes are most likely to be found on pathologic examination?
A. Eosinophilia of the gallbladder wall
B. Intramural diverticula (Rokitansky-Aschoff sinuses)

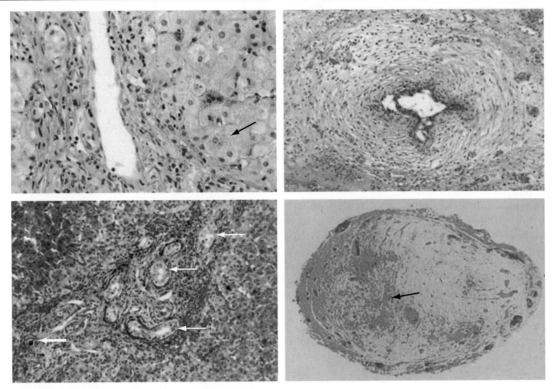

Figure for question **625**

C. Normal gallbladder and mucosa with the exception of intraluminal sludge/stones

D. Predominantly neutrophilic infiltrate with caseating granulomas

---

628 A 40-year-old woman presents to your office for a routine history and physical examination. During your interview, she reports an episode that occurred approximately 3 months ago of diffuse abdominal pain after a fatty and greasy meal. The episode lasted approximately 2 hours and later that night she had diarrhea. She states one week after this episode, her gynecologist ordered an abdominal ultrasound scan that showed gallstones. She has had no further episodes. Which of the following patients would be least likely to benefit from cholecystectomy?

A. A patient who is of Native American heritage

B. A morbidly obese patient

C. A patient who has previously undergone a heart-lung transplantation

D. A patient who has previously undergone a kidney transplantation

E. A patient whose ultrasound scan shows a heavily calcified gallbladder wall

629 Which of the following statements regarding malignant biliary obstruction is most correct?

A. The placement of an uncovered self-expanding metal stent (SEMS) in a patient with a malignant biliary stricture before surgery is contraindicated.

B. Placement of a SEMS is cost-effective only if the patient survives longer than six months.

C. Uncovered SEMSs are associated with a higher migration rate compared with covered SEMSs.

D. Occlusion of an uncovered SEMS in the distal bile duct for malignant biliary obstruction requires percutaneous biliary drainage.

630 A six-week-old boy is brought for evaluation of jaundice and increasing abdominal girth. At birth, the infant was healthy and weighed 8 lb, 1 oz. The mother's pregnancy was uncomplicated, as was the birth. The infant was healthy until one week ago when he started to vomit and his appetite decreased. The parents also report noticing a gradual increase in abdominal girth during the past week and that the baby's stools are clay colored and his urine dark. Laboratory studies demonstrate a total bilirubin concentration of 4 mg/dL and a direct bilirubin concentration of 3 mg/dL. An ultrasound scan confirms the presence of fluid in the abdomen. A sample obtained by paracentesis is bile stained but sterile. Based on these findings, bile duct perforation is suspected. What is the most likely location of this perforation?

A. At the junction of the cystic and bile ducts

B. At the junction of the left and right hepatic ducts and common hepatic duct

C. In the cystic duct

D. In the distal bile duct

E. In the gallbladder

631 An 82-year-old man undergoes coronary artery bypass graft surgery and has a prolonged postoperative course in the intensive care unit with respiratory failure. He receives nutrition by total parenteral nutrition. During his course, fever and leukocytosis develop. His abdominal examination reveals diminished bowel sounds. A CT scan demonstrates a thickened gallbladder wall and

pericholecystic fluid. What is the most likely etiology for this finding?
A. Chemical and ischemic injury to the gallbladder epithelium
B. Engorgement of the gallbladder vascular system due to hyperdynamic circulation
C. Gallstones obstructing the cystic duct
D. Ischemic hepatitis with secondary inflammation of the gallbladder
E. Normal gallbladder variant on CT

632 Which of the following patients is the best candidate for oral dissolution therapy with ursodeoxycholic acid?
A. A 22-year-old woman with sickle cell disease and gallstones
B. A 35-year-old woman who is admitted to the hospital with a mild episode of gallstone pancreatitis and discharged two days later
C. A 40-year-old woman with gallstones who has mild biliary colic three times yearly that has never resulted in an emergency department visit
D. A 55-year-old man with known cholelithiasis who has weekly episodes of severe right upper quadrant abdominal pain after eating that lasts several hours
E. A 70-year-old healthy man with right upper quadrant abdominal pain and an abdominal ultrasound scan showing two 1.5-cm gallstones

633 Which of the following statements about indeterminate biliary strictures is most correct?
A. A definitive diagnosis is requisite before surgery for indeterminate strictures to determine the appropriate surgery.
B. Injection of corticosteroids into an indeterminate biliary stricture has been associated with a 40% resolution of these cases.
C. Photodynamic therapy for an indeterminate stricture is associated with resolution in more than 75% of patients.
D. Choledochoscopy, with or without biopsy, should be considered as a diagnostic option in these patients.

634 What is the volume of fluid that the gallbladder can accommodate?
A. 10 mL to 30 mL
B. 30 mL to 50 mL
C. 50 mL to 70 mL
D. 70 mL to 100 mL

635 A 70-year-old man is admitted to the hospital with three hours of right upper quadrant abdominal pain without fever or chills. The pain improves spontaneously. He has a history of coronary artery disease and a permanent cardiac pacemaker. On initial evaluation in the emergency department, his total bilirubin is 4.2 mg/dL, direct bilirubin is 3.1 mg/dL, alkaline phosphatase is 250 IU/L, AST is 155 IU/L, and ALT is 185 IU/L. Transabdominal ultrasonography demonstrates stones in the gallbladder, prominent intrahepatic ducts, and a bile duct diameter of 1.1 cm. There is no bile duct stone visualized. The next day, the patient's laboratory studies are repeated and show that his total

bilirubin is 5.1 mg/dL, direct bilirubin is 4 mg/dL, alkaline phosphatase is 275 IU/L, AST is 175 IU/L, and ALT is 198 IU/L. Which of the following diagnostic tests should be performed?
A. CT of the abdomen and pelvis
B. ERCP
C. EUS
D. Laparoscopic cholecystectomy with intraoperative cholangiography
E. MRCP

636 A 90-year-old male nursing home resident presents with abdominal distention, abdominal pain, nausea, and coffee-ground emesis. There is no fever, and liver function tests are normal. A CT scan (see figure) shows a markedly distended stomach, air in the biliary tree, and a thickened gallbladder containing two large gallstones. What is the most likely site of obstruction?
A. Cecum
B. Duodenum
C. Ileum
D. Jejunum
E. Rectum

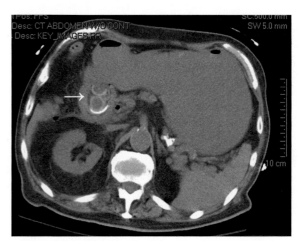

Figure for question **636**

637 A five-year-old boy with a history of Kawasaki's disease presents with acute onset of crampy abdominal pain, nausea, and vomiting. On examination, he is afebrile. There is abdominal tenderness with a palpable gallbladder. A complete blood count reveals a normal white blood cell count. Ultrasonography demonstrates enlargement and distention of the gallbladder but no evidence of stones, sludge, a thickened wall, or pericholecystic fluid. What is the most likely diagnosis?
A. Acalculous cholecystitis
B. Acute cholecystitis
C. Acute hydrops of the gallbladder
D. Biliary dyskinesia
E. Mesenteric ischemia

638 Which of the following is *not* a well-documented risk factor for cholangiocarcinoma?
A. Caroli disease
B. Choledochal cysts
C. PSC
D. Tobacco smoking

639 Regarding transplantation in patients with PSC, which of the following statements is most correct?
- **A.** An endoscopic cholangiogram is necessary as part of the pretransplantation evaluation.
- **B.** Patients with ulcerative colitis and PSC undergo simultaneous colectomy at the time of liver transplantation.
- **C.** Recurrent cholangitis refractory to medical or endoscopic management is an indication for liver transplantation.
- **D.** Survival rates for patients undergoing liver transplantation for PSC have similar survival rates compared with those who undergo transplantation for viral hepatitis.

640 A 79-year-old man with multiple medical problems presents with right upper quadrant pain, fever, and an elevated white blood cell count. A transabdominal ultrasound scan demonstrates a fluid-filled gallbladder with a thickened wall and fluid surrounding the gallbladder. A hepatobiliary iminodiacetic acid (HIDA) scan demonstrates no uptake into the gallbladder fossa, consistent with acute cholecystitis. The patient is considered a poor surgical candidate. Which of the following statements is most true regarding this patient?
- **A.** A cholecystostomy tube is indicated to acutely manage this patient.
- **B.** ERCP with sphincterotomy is indicated to alleviate biliary obstruction.
- **C.** ERCP with cannulation and stenting of the cystic duct is indicated to decompress the gallbladder.
- **D.** EUS-guided transgastric puncture of the gallbladder will decrease the risk of spontaneous perforation of the gallbladder by 80%.

641 A 37-year-old woman is referred for evaluation of classic biliary colic. She has had laboratory testing revealing normal ALT, alkaline phosphatase, total bilirubin, amylase, and lipase. A right upper quadrant ultrasound scan with a cholecystokinin (CCK) injection did not find gallstones but did reveal a delay in gallbladder emptying. What is your treatment recommendation for the patient?
- **A.** Cholecystectomy
- **B.** ERCP
- **C.** MRCP
- **D.** Bile acid testing
- **E.** Oral analgesia and reassurance

642 A 28-year-old patient with chronic hepatitis B infection acquired by vertical transmission undergoes routine abdominal ultrasonography for hepatocellular carcinoma screening. The patient is otherwise healthy and has no signs or symptoms of cirrhosis. Abdominal ultrasonography demonstrates no liver lesions, but a 21-mm solitary pedunculated polyp is seen in the gallbladder fundus. What are the best management course and justification?
- **A.** The lesion is likely a metastatic deposit from a small hepatocellular carcinoma, and the patient should therefore be referred for orthotopic liver transplantation.
- **B.** The lesion should be removed because it frequently detaches and causes pancreatitis.
- **C.** The patient likely has adenomyomatosis, and therefore no treatment is needed.
- **D.** The polyp is likely an adenoma, and the patient should undergo cholecystectomy.
- **E.** The polyp is likely an adenoma; however, no surgery is recommended at this time because it is smaller than 2.5 cm.

643 Which portion of the gut is responsible for the reabsorption of the majority of secreted bile salt molecules, and what percentage of these molecules are reabsorbed in the healthy individual?
- **A.** Colon, 95%
- **B.** Distal ileum, 75%
- **C.** Distal ileum, 95%
- **D.** Proximal jejunum, 75%
- **E.** Proximal jejunum, 95%

644 A one-year-old boy is brought in for evaluation of jaundice and intense pruritus. In addition to generalized jaundice, he has xanthomata on the extensor surfaces of the fingers and in the creases of his palms and hepatosplenomegaly. He has a broad forehead, deeply set and widely spaced eyes, a pointed mandible, a flattened malar eminence, and prominent ears. Laboratory tests demonstrate a total bilirubin level of 7.2 mg/dL and a direct bilirubin level of 5.8 mg/dL. Serum alkaline phosphatase is 500 U/L. The findings suggest Alagille syndrome. What findings on examination of a liver biopsy specimen would be diagnostic of this condition?
- **A.** Concentric periductal fibrosis ("onion skin" appearance)
- **B.** Expanded portal tract with portal fibrosis, bile duct proliferation, and bile plugs within the bile duct
- **C.** Paucity of interlobular bile ducts
- **D.** Portal tract edema and fibrosis

645 Which of the following antibiotics has been known to promote biliary sludge formation?
- **A.** Ceftriaxone
- **B.** Erythromycin
- **C.** Gentamicin
- **D.** Metronidazole
- **E.** Vancomycin

646 Cholesterolosis of the gallbladder is
- **A.** Frequently present in individuals with cholesterol stones
- **B.** Highly prevalent in certain ethnic groups
- **C.** More common in women
- **D.** Often symptomatic
- **E.** Rare, found in fewer than 1% of autopsy specimens

647 Regarding signs and symptoms of PSC, which of the following statements is most accurate?
- **A.** Fatigue and abdominal pain are the most frequent symptoms in patients with PSC.
- **B.** More than one third of patients have ascites at the time of diagnosis.
- **C.** Splenomegaly is seen in the majority of patients at the time of diagnosis.
- **D.** Weight loss is frequent and may be life-threatening for the majority of patients with PSC.

648 Which of the following statements regarding sphincter of Oddi dysfunction (SOD) is correct?
A. There is a male preponderance of 60% to 70%.
B. There is an increased frequency in patients with achalasia.
C. Of affected patients, 70% have abnormal liver biochemical test results.
D. The modified Milwaukee classification system is partly based on the presence of bile duct dilation to a diameter of more than 10 mm.

649 Which of the following conditions is not an important factor in the pathophysiology of common gallstone formation?
A. Cholesterol nucleation
B. Dietary calcium intake
C. Gallbladder hypomotility
D. Genetic factors such as *LITH* genes
E. Hepatic hypersecretion

650 Regarding the diagnosis of PSC, which of the following statements is most true?
A. Gallbladder disease occurs in less than 5% of patients with PSC.
B. The diagnosis relies on serum protein electrophoresis demonstrating decreased IgG_2 subclass deficiency.
C. The presence of extrahepatic biliary disease distinguishes PSC from primary biliary cirrhosis.
D. At the time of diagnosis of PSC, liver test results are usually normal.

651 A 44-year-old woman presents with abdominal pain and jaundice 3 months after an uncomplicated cholecystectomy. She is afebrile and her vital signs are normal. Alkaline phosphatase and bilirubin levels are significantly elevated and AST and ALT levels are slightly elevated. ERCP is performed (see figure). Based on the ERCP findings, what is the best long-term management strategy in this case?
A. Endoscopic dilation
B. Endoscopic metal stent placement
C. No treatment is required.
D. Percutaneous drainage
E. Surgery

652 Paucity of bile ducts in children has been associated with all of the following except:
A. Noonan syndrome
B. Congenital rubella infection
C. Toxoplasmosis infection
D. α_1-Antitrypsin deficiency
E. Inborn errors of bile acid metabolism

653 Regarding bile duct injuries related to laparoscopic cholecystectomy, which of the following statements is most correct?
A. To prevent bile duct injuries, it is recommended that patients routinely undergo preoperative retrograde cholangiography or MRCP to define the biliary anatomy.
B. Most bile duct injuries are related to anatomic variation in the left side of the biliary tree or inadequate exposure of the bile duct during dissection at the time of surgery.
C. Bile duct and right segmental injuries are the most common bile duct injuries during laparoscopic cholecystectomy.
D. Most bile duct injuries lead to segmental hepatectomy.

654 Regarding the association between PSC and inflammatory bowel disease, which of the following statements is most correct?
A. More than 75% of patients with PSC have inflammatory bowel disease.
B. Patients with Crohn's disease and PSC have a higher likelihood of having more severe disease than a patient with ulcerative colitis and PSC.
C. PSC is present in approximately 20% of patients with ulcerative colitis or Crohn's disease.
D. The two diseases often progress together.

655 Which of the following statements regarding intestinal bile acid malabsorption is true?
A. It occurs when the proximal 50 cm of ileum is resected.
B. Colonic bile acids induce fat absorption through the colonic lymphatics.
C. It decreases renal oxalate excretion, protecting against kidney stones.
D. It is common after cholecystectomy.

656 A 40-year-old woman has had two episodes of right upper quadrant pain in the six months since undergoing laparoscopic cholecystectomy. Each episode lasted between 30 and 60 minutes, and a serum sample obtained during each episode showed an ALT level 2.5 to 3 times the upper limit of normal. An ultrasound examination revealed that the diameter of the bile duct is 13 mm, and MRCP shows no evidence of a stricture or filling defect within the biliary tree. What is the recommended next step?

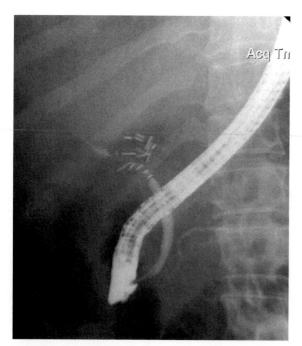

Figure for question **651**

A. A trial of nitrates or a calcium channel blocker
B. Biliary manometry
C. Endoscopic sphincterotomy
D. Initiation of treatment with an anticholinergic medication
E. Noninvasive testing

657 Which of the following complications of gallstone disease is most rapidly fatal?
A. Biliary colic
B. Cholangitis
C. Cholecystitis
D. Gallstone ileus
E. Pancreatitis

658 A 12-year-old boy is brought in for outpatient evaluation of chronic abdominal pain. According to the parents, episodes of abdominal pain of varying degree have occurred for two years. On several occasions, the patient has had fever and mild jaundice associated with the pain. All episodes resolved spontaneously. The physical examination reveals hepatosplenomegaly. The results of laboratory tests, including total and direct bilirubin, alkaline phosphatase, and aminotransferase levels, are within normal limits. An ultrasound scan demonstrates multiple bilateral renal cysts and cystic dilation of the intrahepatic ducts. What is the most likely diagnosis in this case?
A. Alagille syndrome
B. Caroli disease
C. Choledochal cyst
D. Extrahepatic biliary atresia
E. PSC

659 Which of the following statements regarding malignant biliary obstruction is most correct?
A. Most patients with hilar obstruction will be adequately palliated with unilateral biliary decompression.
B. SEMS placement results in higher rates of complications, including obstruction, bleeding, and perforation, than plastic stents for the palliation of malignant obstruction of the biliary hilum.
C. Unresectable hilar obstruction palliated via a percutaneous approach is associated with fewer complications than the endoscopic approach.
D. In patients with malignant hilar tumors, drainage of an atrophied lobe is important to prevent future cholangitis.

660 A 24-year-old woman presents to her primary care physician with three weeks of recurrent right upper quadrant pain. An abdominal ultrasound scan demonstrates a 2.5-mm gallbladder polyp. Which type of polyp is most likely in this patient?
A. Adenoma
B. Adenomyoma
C. Cholesterol polyp
D. Inflammatory polyp
E. Lipoma

661 A 53-year-old man with a 20-year history of ulcerative colitis involving the entire colon has had PSC for 15 years. He asks you about his risk of the development of colon cancer. Which of the following statements is most correct?
A. His risk of colon cancer is increased to more than that of those with ulcerative colitis without PSC.
B. He can decrease the risk of the development of colon cancer by 60% with oral administration of ursodeoxycholic acid.
C. He requires screening with colonoscopy for colorectal cancer as well as duodenoscopy for ampullary carcinoma.
D. Liver transplantation would decrease his risk of colon cancer such that he could have colonoscopy at three- to five-year intervals.

662 For which of the following is biliary manometry most necessary before sphincterotomy?
A. Type I SOD
B. Type II SOD
C. Type III SOD
D. Type IV SOD

663 Which of the following statements regarding bile storage in patients without a gallbladder (postcholecystectomy) is true?
A. Bile acids are stored in the distal small intestine.
B. Bile acids are stored in the proximal small intestine.
C. Bile acids are stored in the biliary tree.
D. Bile acids are not stored in the gastrointestinal tract.

664 Which of the following is not a common risk factor for bile plug syndrome?
A. Prolonged total parenteral nutrition
B. Premature infants
C. Multiple comorbidities
D. Massive hemolysis
E. Biliary strictures

665 An eight-year-old girl with a history of sickle cell disease was discovered to have gallstones when a CT scan of her chest was performed to evaluate shortness of breath and chest pain. An ultrasound scan confirmed the presence of several gallstones. What is the composition of the stones (see figure)?
A. Calcium bilirubinate
B. Calcium oxalate
C. Cholesterol
D. Free hemoglobin
E. Urate

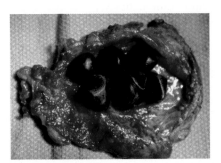

Figure for question **665**

666 A 24-year-old swimsuit model with biliary colic and gallstones demands treatment with extracorporeal shock wave lithotripsy to avoid scars. If your patient undergoes this treatment, what is the approximate, cumulative five-year recurrence rate?
A. 5%
B. 20%
C. 40%
D. 60%
E. 80%

667 Which of the following is the rate-limiting step in the hepatic transport of bile acids from blood into bile?
A. Intestinal absorption
B. Gallbladder contraction
C. Sinusoidal bile acid uptake
D. Canalicular secretion

668 A 24-year-old white man with known primary sclerosing cholangitis presents for evaluation and management of worsening jaundice. On ERCP, a dominant stricture is identified involving the mid bile duct, 2 cm in length. There is slight bilateral multifocal stricturing of the intrahepatic ducts. Cytology is collected from the stricture, and a plastic stent is inserted. A liver biopsy specimen demonstrates no cirrhosis. His albumin and prothrombin time are normal, and a CT scan demonstrates no other abnormalities. Which of the following statements regarding treatment is most correct?
A. Definitive chemotherapy combined with adjuvant radiation should be initiated.
B. Intraductal photodynamic therapy should be initiated.
C. Primary resection of the lesion with a pancreatoduodenectomy is appropriate.
D. This patient should be evaluated for liver transplantation.

669 A 70-year-old man with a history of coronary artery disease and a depressed left ventricular ejection fraction is admitted to the intensive care unit with septic shock and multiorgan failure, requiring vasopressor support and mechanical ventilation. Two days later, abdominal distention and tenderness on palpation in the right upper quadrant develop. A transabdominal ultrasound scan demonstrates a markedly distended gallbladder with wall thickening and pericholecystic fluid. Which of the following statements regarding the treatment of this condition is true?
A. Cholecystectomy should be performed in this patient.
B. Endoscopic cholecystoduodenostomy and stent placement are safe, widely accepted treatment for this condition.
C. Intravenous antibiotics alone will resolve this condition in nearly all patients.
D. Percutaneous cholecystostomy in combination with intravenous antibiotics is successful in 95% to 100% of patients.
E. Ursodeoxycholic acid should be initiated because this condition was likely precipitated by cholelithiasis.

670 A patient presents to you having had PSC for at least 10 years. Her liver function test results have been normal, and she has been taking 13 to 15 mg/kg/day of ursodeoxycholic acid during that time. Which of the following statements is most correct?
A. Normal liver function test results correlate with the absence of histologic progression to cirrhosis.
B. She should discontinue ursodeoxycholic acid because it may increase the risk of colon cancer.
C. She should have regular surveillance for early detection of cholangiocarcinoma.
D. Tacrolimus would be an appropriate drug in this circumstance to slow the histologic progression of her PSC.

671 In what percentage of individuals do the bile and pancreatic ducts open separately into the duodenum?
A. 1% to 5%
B. 10% to 15%
C. 20% to 25%
D. 30% to 35%

672 Which of the following genes likely plays a role in the etiology of the findings presented in the figure?
A. ABC B4 (ATP-binding cassette transporter B4; formerly multidrug resistant-3 gene)
B. CCK-1R (CCK-1 receptor)
C. CYP7A1 (variant of cholesterol 7 alpha-hydroxylase)
D. All of the above

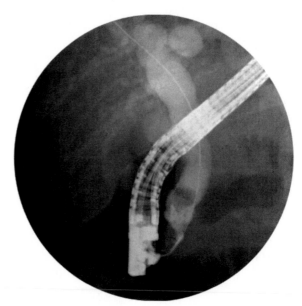

Figure for question **672**

673 The daily volume of bile secreted by the liver ranges from
A. 50 to 100 mL
B. 250 to 300 mL
C. 500 to 600 mL
D. 900 to 1000 mL

674 A 56-year-old patient undergoes liver transplantation for PSC. The explant is identified as harboring a small focal cholangiocarcinoma. Which of the following statements is most correct?

A. A living relative is the preferred donor for patients with PSC.

B. Aggressive endoscopic surveillance is 80% sensitive in detecting cholangiocarcinoma in patients with PSC.

C. If this patient had a known cholangiocarcinoma, it would not have precluded liver transplantation.

D. The three-year survival rate in this patient is less than 10%.

675 Which of the following is *not* a common cause of benign biliary strictures?
A. Chronic pancreatitis
B. PSC
C. Postcholecystectomy biliary injury
D. Anastomotic stricture after liver transplantation
E. Congenital hepatic fibrosis

676 A 47-year-old woman presents to your office because of recurrent epigastric and right upper quadrant abdominal pain that is sometimes worse after meals. She has had an extensive workup for gallstone disease, including a detailed examination of her gallbladder and biliary system by EUS, which was normal. Which of the following should be considered a cause of the patient's symptoms?
A. Angina pectoris
B. Gastroesophageal reflux disease
C. Irritable bowel syndrome
D. Peptic ulcer disease
E. All of the above

677 Which statement regarding the etiology and pathogenesis of PSC is most correct?
A. Biliary epithelial cells have been shown to aberrantly express major histocompatibility complex class II antigens.
B. The absence of IgG-4 staining in the biliary epithelium is a hallmark of PSC.
C. Perinuclear anti-neutrophilic cytoplasmic antibody is rare, occurring in less than 15% of patients with PSC.
D. Serum IgG_4 levels are elevated in patients with PSC.

678 A 32-year-old Taiwanese man presents with abdominal pain, fever, and jaundice. An ultrasound scan shows dilation of the biliary tree, more prominent on the left, and numerous intrahepatic filling defects are present. An ERCP scan is performed (see figure). Which of the following statements regarding the etiology of this patient's disease is most correct?
A. A CCK-stimulated HIDA scan demonstrates a markedly diminished gallbladder ejection fraction.
B. Brown intrahepatic stones harboring the ova of enteric parasites occur in patients with this disorder.
C. A history of total parenteral nutrition is common in these patients.
D. Numerous antibodies are present that cross-react with the colon and bile duct.
E. Patients have a genetic deficiency of bacterial glucuronidase.

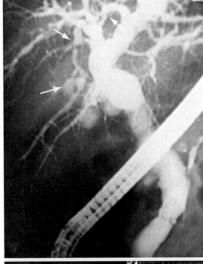

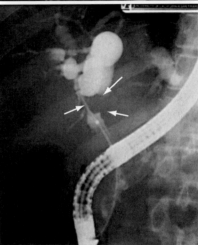

Figure for question **678**

679 Which of the following statements regarding pancreaticobiliary anatomy of the major papilla is most accurate?
A. The bile duct and pancreatic duct enter the duodenum together in half of individuals.
B. The sphincter choledochus is absent in 30% of individuals.
C. Pancreatic secretion is partly regulated by fasciculi longitudinales whose contraction impedes flow into the duodenum.
D. Contraction of the sphincter ampullae prevents reflux of duodenal content into the pancreaticobiliary ducts.

680 Bile acid transporter gene mutations have been identified in all of the following *except*:
A. Primary bile acid malabsorption
B. Intrahepatic cholestasis of pregnancy
C. Primary biliary cirrhosis
D. Progressive familial intrahepatic cholestasis
E. Dubin-Johnson syndrome

681 All of the following are true of patients with acalculous biliary pain *except*:
A. The majority will have a depressed gallbladder ejection fraction when tested with CCK-stimulated cholescintigraphy.

B. When a depressed gallbladder ejection fraction is present, approximately two thirds of patients will obtain symptom relief after cholecystectomy.

C. Most patients are young women.

D. One half of patients with acalculous biliary pain may actually have microscopic cholelithiasis in resected gallbladder specimens.

E. Acalculous biliary pain is listed as a functional gastrointestinal disorder in the Rome III criteria.

682 A patient presents with a history of acute recurrent episodes of pancreatitis. The patient's status is post-cholecystectomy with normal liver enzymes. There is no history of hypercalcemia or hypertriglyceridemia. MRCP findings are normal. Which of the following statements regarding the clinical management of this patient is most accurate?

A. Cholangioscopy is the appropriate next diagnostic procedure.

B. CCK analog–stimulated ERCP will exclude microlithiasis as a cause of recurrent pancreatitis.

C. Empirical placement of a biliary stent will reduce the recurrence of pancreatitis by 30%.

D. Sphincter of Oddi manometry may be performed to determine the cause of recurrent pancreatitis.

683 A 25-year-old woman is pregnant and experiencing frequent episodes of right upper quadrant abdominal pain, nausea, and vomiting. Her symptoms have been increasing in severity and frequency during the past two weeks. She is unable to tolerate oral intake. An ultrasound scan demonstrates several small gallstones but no evidence of acute cholecystitis. When is the ideal time to perform a cholecystectomy?

A. First trimester

B. Second trimester

C. Third trimester

D. Postpartum

E. None of the above

684 A 35-year-old woman is diagnosed with PSC after an episode of right upper quadrant pain, fever, and abnormal liver chemistries. Which of the following statements is most correct?

A. An annual liver biopsy for the first three years of the diagnosis is important to establish the natural history of the disease in this patient.

B. Budesonide is standard therapy for patients at the initial diagnosis of PSC.

C. Standard-dose ursodeoxycholic acid has been established to increase time to transplantation, decrease histologic progression, and decrease the death rate in patients with this disease.

D. No medical treatment has been shown clearly to alter the course of PSC.

685 A 46-year-old woman arrives at the emergency department reporting acute-onset right upper quadrant pain that radiates to her back. After 2 hours and 2 mg of morphine, the pain resolves. She is afebrile. Laboratory studies show a normal white blood cell count, total bilirubin of 2.8 mg/dL, alkaline phosphatase of 248 IU/L, AST of 120 U/L, and ALT of 165 U/L. A transcutaneous abdominal ultrasound scan shows multiple stones in the gallbladder and a bile duct that measures 10 mm in diameter. Which of the following is the least invasive procedure that accurately identifies choledocholithiasis?

A. CT

B. Endoscopic retrograde cholangiography

C. EUS

D. MRCP

E. Repeat transabdominal ultrasound scan with dedicated bile duct protocol

686 An 11-year-old boy with recently diagnosed ulcerative colitis is brought for outpatient evaluation of fatigue and jaundice. The patient has been having intermittent abdominal pain for the past 8 weeks and has been jaundiced for the past 3 days. There is no family history of liver disease. The patient has not been exposed to any hepatotoxic chemicals. The family denies any recent travel or contact with sick individuals. The physical examination reveals the presence of scleral icterus and mild hepatosplenomegaly. Laboratory studies show a total bilirubin level of 4 mg/dL with a direct fraction of 3.2 mg/dL. The alkaline phosphatase level is 420 IU/L. On ERCP, alternating areas of intrahepatic stricture and dilation are seen (see figure). The diagnosis is PSC. Which of the following statements is correct with regard to PSC in children?

A. There are no reported cases of hepatocellular carcinoma in children with PSC.

B. Liver biopsy is often diagnostic.

C. Inflammatory bowel disease always precedes the diagnosis of PSC in the pediatric population.

D. Recurrent PSC often occurs in those who have received a liver transplant.

E. There have been no reported cases of cholangiocarcinoma in children with PSC.

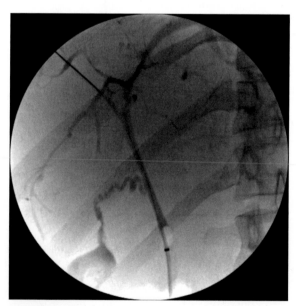

Figure for question **686**

687 A 45-year-old diabetic patient presents for outpatient evaluation of gallstones that were detected on a CT scan performed for follow-up of a lung nodule. Two 5-mm nonobstructing gallstones are seen. The patient has no history of abdominal pain, nausea, vomiting, or fever. What is the most appropriate management at this time?

A. Perform a transabdominal ultrasound scan for further evaluation.

B. Observe without intervening at this time.

C. Perform an HIDA scan of the gallbladder.

D. Schedule the patient for elective laparoscopic cholecystectomy.

E. Schedule the patient for elective open cholecystectomy and intraoperative cholangiography.

688 Which of the following statements regarding biliary strictures in an individual after liver transplantation is most correct?

A. Ischemic strictures after liver transplantation are predisposed to focal necrosis and spontaneous rupture.

B. In patients with a hepaticojejunostomy between the donor liver and the recipient jejunum after liver transplantation, percutaneous management is a first-line option for management of biliary strictures.

C. Stricture of the choledochocholedochal anastomosis after liver transplantation is often inaccessible by ERCP.

D. Anastomotic strictures after liver transplantation typically require surgical reconstruction because they are managed successfully without surgery in only 20% of cases.

689 Regarding hilar cholangiocarcinoma, which of the following is most correct?

A. Cholangioscopy is performed to determine the extent of disease.

B. Liver transplantation is indicated and has led to five-year survival rates exceeding 70%.

C. Fluorodeoxyglucose–positron emission tomography is indicated to assess regional lymph node involvement and evaluate for distant metastases.

D. EUS is the most accurate means of regional tumor staging.

690 Bile formation is essential for all of the following *except*:

A. Intestinal lipid digestion

B. Cholesterol homeostasis

C. Excretion of drug metabolites

D. Excretion of heavy metals

E. Enterohepatic circulation of short-chain fatty acids

691 A seven-week-old girl is brought in for evaluation of increased irritability, vomiting, poor appetite, a one-week history of worsening jaundice, and the development of clay-colored stools. On physical examination, there is moderate hepatomegaly and a palpable abdominal mass. Laboratory studies demonstrate a total bilirubin concentration of 8.3 mg/dL and a direct bilirubin concentration of 6.7 mg/dL. Alkaline phosphatase and aminotransferase levels are only mildly elevated. An ultra-

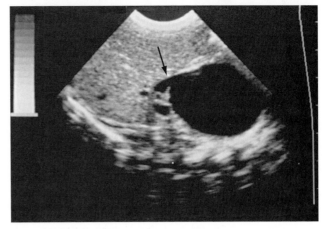

Figure for question **691**

sound examination is performed (see figure). What is the most likely diagnosis?

A. Alagille syndrome

B. Bile plug syndrome

C. Biliary atresia

D. Choledochal cyst

E. PSC

692 Defective bile acid conjugation can cause which of the following?

A. Fluid overload

B. Ascites

C. Fat-soluble vitamin deficiency

D. Vitamin B_{12} deficiency

693 A 21-year-old woman is brought to the emergency department by her roommate. She is mildly disoriented and reports several hours of severe right upper quadrant pain, nausea, vomiting, and shaking chills. She has a temperature of 102.5°F, a heart rate of 105 beats per minute, and a blood pressure of 100/60 mm Hg. She has a positive Murphy's sign but no peritoneal signs. Her white blood cell count is 15,000 cells/mm^3. An ultrasound scan demonstrates multiple gallstones, a thickened gallbladder wall, and pericholecystic fluid. Which antibiotic regimen is most appropriate for this patient in the emergency department?

A. Intravenous cefotoxin

B. Intravenous ciprofloxacin

C. Intravenous metronidazole

D. Intravenous piperacillin-tazobactam

E. Intravenous vancomycin

694 A 33-year-old woman presents with right upper quadrant pain that is intermittent, lasts 45 minutes, is associated with meals, and radiates into her back. She has had a cholecystectomy. Laboratory evaluation reveals ALT and AST values approximately three times normal, with a slightly elevated alkaline phosphatase level. Her bile duct is dilated to 9 mm on MRCP. No other abnormality is seen. She has no fever, weight loss, or other constitutional symptoms. Which of the following statements regarding this patient is most correct?

A. A biliary manometry would be the most appropriate first step for this patient.

B. An ERCP with evaluation for choledocholithiasis and empirical biliary sphincterotomy would be appropriate management.
C. This patient requires an evaluation for chronic liver disease.
D. This patient would classify as having type III SOD.

695 A 65-year-old white woman presents to her primary care physician with melenic stools of three days' duration. She had no abdominal pain, no fevers, and no other symptoms. She is referred for an upper endoscopy that reveals a 2-cm exophytic friable mass on the major papilla. Biopsy specimens of the mass are obtained, and the pathology results indicate adenocarcinoma of the ampulla. A CT scan is performed that demonstrates no additional abnormalities. Of the options provided, which of the following is correct?
A. EUS would be the next most appropriate step in the management of this patient.
B. Neoadjuvant chemoradiation should be performed and then surgical resection.
C. Photodynamic therapy as definitive treatment would be the next best option.
D. The patient should be referred for surgical consultation for planned resection.

696 Which of the following statements regarding PSC is most correct?
A. Celiac disease, Sjögren syndrome, Peyronie disease, and rheumatoid arthritis can each be associated with PSC.
B. Crohn's disease is not associated with the diagnosis of PSC.
C. Patients with PSC should be routinely screened for proteinuria to exclude concomitant renal disease.
D. Smoking is a risk factor for the development of PSC.

697 A 36-year-old woman with a history of biliary colic and gallstone disease presents with nausea, vomiting, and right upper quadrant abdominal pain and tenderness on examination. There is no fever, and vital signs are stable. The white blood cell count is normal, and liver function test results are slightly elevated. A transabdominal ultrasound scan demonstrates multiple gallstones, and an MRCP demonstrates choledocholithiasis. Which of the following statements is correct?
A. Percutaneous cholangiography with stone removal is indicated to prevent complications of pancreatitis.
B. Endoscopic retrograde cholangiography and stone retrieval followed by laparoscopic cholecystectomy are appropriate.
C. Laparoscopic cholecystectomy with bile duct exploration via either a transcystic or transcholedochal approach increases mortality compared with a preoperative ERCP.
D. No biliary intervention is required because small biliary stones are likely to pass spontaneously.

698 Which of the following statements regarding choledocholithiasis is most correct?

A. Transabdominal ultrasonography for choledocholithiasis has a sensitivity of greater than 80%.
B. EUS has a sensitivity that is similar to that of ERCP.
C. MRI/MRCP has a sensitivity of less than 50% for detecting choledocholithiasis.
D. Multidetector CT is not useful in the detection of bile duct strictures or bile duct stones.

699 A 36-year-old woman is referred to you for two episodes of self-limited right upper quadrant abdominal pain after a fatty meal. An outpatient abdominal ultrasound scan demonstrates two 5-mm gallstones in the gallbladder. The patient is currently asymptomatic. What are the patient's chances (per year) of the development of another episode of biliary colic and/or a more serious complication of gallstone disease, respectively?
A. 10% and 1%
B. 20% and 10%
C. 45% and 1%
D. 80% and 2%
E. 85% and 12%

700 A 46-year-old man is admitted to the hospital with his first episode of pancreatitis. He has no significant medical history and does not drink alcohol. Based on the results of his gallbladder ultrasound scan (see figure) and assuming no complications develop, what surgery would be recommended for this patient?
A. Cholecystectomy after the pancreatitis resolves before discharge
B. Cholecystectomy four to eight weeks after discharge
C. Immediate cholecystectomy
D. No surgery is indicated unless the patient has a repeat episode of pancreatitis.
E. Pylorus-sparing pancreaticoduodenectomy (Whipple procedure)

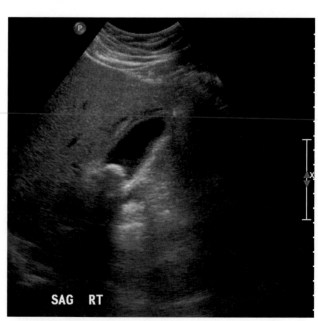

Figure for question **700**

701 Which of the following statements regarding recurrent pyogenic cholangitis (RPC) is most correct?
- **A.** Infection with *Clonorchis sinensis, Opisthorchis* species, and *Ascaris lumbricoides* is endemic to the same geographic region where RPC is prevalent.
- **B.** Patients often have associated urinary seeding at the time of clinical presentation.
- **C.** Patients with RPC are at increased risk of the development of duodenal carcinoma.
- **D.** The majority of patients will present with biliary colic secondary to extrahepatic biliary stones.

702 A 65-year-old woman is brought to the emergency department after a motor vehicle accident and reports midepigastric and left-sided abdominal pain. She was wearing a seat belt in the passenger seat. A portable transabdominal ultrasound scan is performed while the patient is waiting for a CT scan that shows diffuse thickening of the gallbladder wall in association with intramural diverticula (seen as round, anechoic foci). What are the diagnosis and treatment most appropriate for this patient's findings?
- **A.** Adenomyomatosis: laparoscopic cholecystectomy should be performed.
- **B.** Adenomyomatosis: no treatment is needed.
- **C.** Emphysematous cholecystitis: urgent cholecystectomy should be performed.
- **D.** Ruptured gallbladder; open cholecystectomy should be performed.
- **E.** Ruptured gallbladder: a percutaneous cholecystostomy tube should be placed.

703 A 30-year-old woman comes to your office and is concerned about two small gallstones found incidentally on a CT scan performed for a kidney stone. She is asymptomatic. What are the chances that symptoms from her gallstones will develop over the next 5 years?
- **A.** 4%
- **B.** 10%
- **C.** 30%
- **D.** 50%
- **E.** 75%

704 Which of the following is not a component of bile?
- **A.** Water
- **B.** Lipase
- **C.** Phosphatidylcholine
- **D.** Cholesterol
- **E.** Bile pigments

705 A hilar tumor that starts below the confluence of the left and right hepatic ducts and reaches the confluence has a Bismuth-Corlette classification of what type?
- **A.** Type I
- **B.** Type II
- **C.** Type IIIa
- **D.** Type IV

706 Which of the following statements regarding percutaneous transhepatic cholangiography (PTC) is most correct?
- **A.** Access to the biliary tree can be either from the left hepatic duct or right hepatic duct.
- **B.** Hemobilia is a frequent and usually fatal complication.
- **C.** An advantage of percutaneous drainage of the biliary tree includes the life span of a percutaneous biliary catheter of more than one year.
- **D.** PTC provides an excellent option for patients with SOD who wish to avoid pancreatitis.

707 A 65-year-old white man with a history of hypertension and non–insulin-dependent diabetes mellitus presents with painless jaundice. MRI with MRCP is performed that reveals a stricture of the biliary hilum. At ERCP, a complex stricture involving the common hepatic duct, bifurcation, and left and right main ducts is identified. Cytology brushings and biliary biopsy specimens yield cholangiocarcinoma. Which of the following is a true statement?
- **A.** EUS-guided injection of oxaliplatin into the mass should be considered to improve biliary patency.
- **B.** Photodynamic therapy in conjunction with stenting in this setting is a therapeutic option and may improve the quality of life.
- **C.** The placement of an SEMS into each of the right and left main hepatic ducts is indicated for increasing survival and decreasing hospitalization time.
- **D.** Transcutaneous drainage of the left and right systems is more lasting and associated with less expense compared with SEMS placement.

708 A 19-year-old woman presents with right upper quadrant pain, abnormal liver function test results, a slightly elevated white blood cell count, and fever. An ultrasound scan is performed that demonstrates dilation of the bile duct to 8 mm and multiple stones in the gallbladder but no evidence of cholecystitis. The patient is placed on antibiotics and ERCP is performed (findings can be seen in the two figures). Which of the following statements regarding this patient is most correct?
- **A.** This patient will need a biliary endoprosthesis placed until she has an elective cholecystectomy.
- **B.** This patient has a greater than 50% chance of the development of pancreatitis after her ERCP.

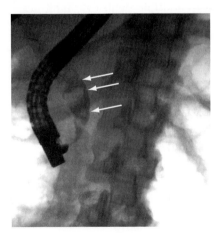

Figure 1 for question **708**

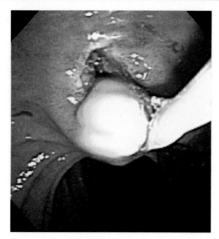

Figure 2 for question **708**

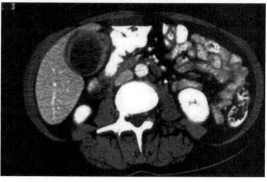

Figure for question **711**

C. This patient has an anatomic variant that will require surveillance every two to three years by EUS.

D. This patient should proceed to cholecystectomy without placement of a biliary stent.

709 A 39-year-old woman with primary biliary cirrhosis, jaundice, diarrhea, and pruritus is started on a bile acid sequestrant. Which of the following would be the mechanism by which the bile acid sequestrant improves the patient's diarrhea?

A. Slowing of colonic peristalsis

B. Direct inhibition of colonic secretion

C. Decreased concentration of free bile acids in the colon

D. Reduced bile acids in the systemic circulation

E. Improved enterohepatic circulation

710 Which of the following statements regarding the endoscopic management of benign biliary strictures is most correct?

A. A single stent provides a similar rate of stricture resolution compared with multiple, simultaneously placed stents.

B. Uncovered SEMSs may have a role in the management of benign biliary strictures.

C. Endoscopic management of benign strictures with multiple stents over multiple sessions leads to resolution in approximately 60% of patients.

D. Biliary strictures secondary to chronic pancreatitis should be managed surgically because of the poor outcomes associated with endoscopic management.

711 A 45-year-old man known to have gallstones presents with painless jaundice. Which feature of this patient's presentation is most commonly associated with the CT findings (see figure)?

A. Age of 45

B. Gallstones

C. Male sex

D. Painless jaundice

E. None of the above

712 Of the following, which medication is most likely to increase the basal sphincter of Oddi pressure?

A. Diazepam

B. Morphine

C. Midazolam

D. Meperidine

E. Verapamil

713 Which of the following statements regarding percutaneous biliary access is most correct?

A. T-tube removal is safe two weeks after placement and may be performed at the bedside.

B. The presence of ascites increases the risk of bile leakage with percutaneous access of the gallbladder or bile ducts.

C. Percutaneous biliary cholangiography is the diagnostic and therapeutic modality of choice for imaging bile duct stones larger than 1.5 cm.

D. Permanent biliary stent placement for malignant biliary obstruction should be performed by ERCP even if percutaneous biliary drainage has been achieved.

714 A healthy 44-year-old man presents with right upper quadrant abdominal pain and jaundice that began two days ago. He has a low-grade fever but otherwise normal vital signs. His laboratory tests reveal a total bilirubin concentration of 6 mg/dL, direct bilirubin concentration of 4.5 mg/dL, alkaline phosphatase of 250 IU/L, AST of 180 IU/L, and ALT of 240 IU/L. An abdominal ultrasound scan is performed and demonstrates bilateral intrahepatic biliary ductal dilation, a proximal common hepatic duct measuring 12 mm in diameter, and a nondilated bile duct measuring 7 mm in diameter. The gallbladder is contracted and contains stones. MRI and MRCP do not show a pancreatic mass. An early ERCP image is shown (see figure). Which of the following is the most likely cause of the patient's condition?

A. Gallbladder carcinoma

B. Hepatic artery thrombosis with resulting biliary necrosis

C. Impaction of a gallstone in the neck of the gallbladder or cystic duct, causing extrinsic compression of the common hepatic duct

D. Pancreatic cancer with extrinsic compression of the distal common bile duct

E. None of the above

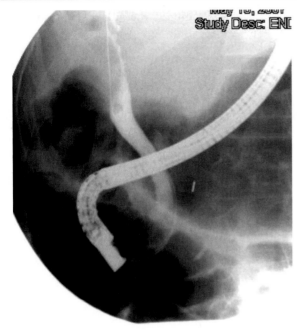

Figure for question **714**

---

715 A 16-day-old girl is admitted to the hospital for evaluation of persistent hyperbilirubinemia. Initial evaluation demonstrates a total bilirubin concentration of 9.3 mg/dL and a direct bilirubin concentration of 6.1 mg/dL. Serum aminotransferase and alkaline phosphatase levels are slightly elevated. Based on a suspicion of biliary atresia, an ultrasound scan is ordered. What ultrasound findings would be most suggestive of this diagnosis?
A. A cone-shaped fibrotic mass, cranial to the portal vein
B. Gallbladder length of 2.5 cm
C. Large cystic mass in the right upper quadrant
D. Massive hepatosplenomegaly

716 A 45-year-old woman presents with jaundice. She has a total bilirubin concentration of 6 mg/dL and a direct bilirubin concentration of 4.1 mg/dL. Eight months earlier, she had laparoscopic cholecystectomy for biliary colic. MRCP demonstrates bile duct dilation. What is the most likely site of stricture formation in this scenario?
A. Bile duct
B. Common hepatic duct
C. Cystic duct
D. Left hepatic duct
E. Right hepatic duct

717 Which of the following statements regarding EUS is true?
A. EUS is more sensitive than ERCP, CT, and MRI in detecting pancreatic tumors.
B. EUS has a sensitivity of 70% in the detection of common bile duct stones.
C. EUS can detect SOD in as many as 40% of patients.
D. EUS has a sensitivity of detecting lesions in the right lobe of the liver of approximately 75%.

718 Which of the following statements regarding RPC is most correct?

A. Ampullary papillitis and SOD have been described in these patients.
B. Ova and parasites are often found within the stones of patients with RPC.
C. Cholangiocarcinoma develops in more than 30% of patients with RPC.
D. RPC is associated with immunoglobulin deficiencies, particularly IgA deficiency.

719 Adenomyomatosis of the gallbladder
A. Carries a significant risk of malignancy that increases when a villous component is present
B. Is characterized by excessive proliferation of surface epithelium with invaginations into a thickened muscularis
C. Is characterized by multiple small (<3 mm) adenomas lining the lumen of the gallbladder
D. Often is a cause of biliary colic in patients with gallstones
E. Should be treated with cholecystectomy

720 A 23-year-old Hispanic woman presents with right upper quadrant pain and fever five days after an uneventful laparoscopic cholecystectomy for symptomatic gallstone disease. A transabdominal ultrasound scan detects a 4- × 3-cm fluid collection in the gallbladder fossa. A HIDA scan demonstrates tracer in the same region as the fluid collection. Which of the following statements is most correct?
A. It is likely that this patient will need a surgical procedure to correct the problem.
B. The patient should be placed on antibiotics and, with time, has a 90% chance that this issue will resolve.
C. Endoscopic retrograde cholangiography with stenting is necessary and has a greater than 80% chance of resolving the problem.
D. The fluid collection must be drained percutaneously before any other interventions are considered.

721 Which of the following statements regarding ampullary carcinoma is most correct?
A. Ampullectomy is indicated for those with carcinoma limited to the duodenal wall.
B. Endoscopic biopsies are usually insufficient to make the diagnosis of ampullary carcinoma when a mass is endoscopically identified.
C. Pancreatitis is the most common presentation for patients with ampullary malignancies.
D. Transduodenal resection of ampullary carcinomas is associated with an inferior survival outcome compared with pancreaticoduodenectomy.

722 A 74-year-old man presents to the emergency department with right upper quadrant abdominal pain for three days, a fever as high as 103°F, blood pressure of 95/55 mm Hg, and a heart rate of 110 beats per minute. Laboratory studies are notable for a white blood cell count of 22,000/mm^3, a total bilirubin concentration of 1.2 mg/dL, and an ALT level of 100 IU/L. A CT scan is performed (see figure on p. 140). Given the CT findings, which answer is most correct?
A. Cholecystectomy should be delayed to decrease the amount of inflammation surrounding the gallbladder and decrease the surgical risks.

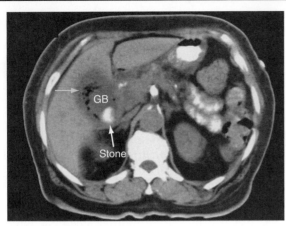

Figure for question **722**

C. Balloon dilation of the biliary sphincter carries a risk of pancreatitis similar to that of sphincterotomy.
D. A balloon is always indicated as a first tool for the removal of a stone given that it is safer and less traumatic than a basket.

725 An 80-year-old man admitted with septic shock from a urinary tract infection has a cardiac arrest and is resuscitated after 20 minutes. Two days later, his white blood cell count doubles and there is abdominal tenderness on examination. A portable abdominal ultrasound scan is performed. In addition to a positive Murphy's sign, the following ultrasound image is obtained (see figure). What is the most likely diagnosis?
A. Acalculous cholecystitis
B. Ascending cholangitis
C. Calculous cholecystitis
D. Emphysematous cholecystitis
E. Secondary sclerosing cholangitis

B. The patient has a typical case of uncomplicated acute cholecystitis.
C. This is a common complication of acute cholecystitis.
D. The risk of gallbladder perforation is high.
E. This condition is typically more common in young women.

723 On routine laparoscopic cholecystectomy, a patient is found to have a T1a gallbladder adenocarcinoma on the pathologic specimen. Which of the following statements is most correct?
A. Adjuvant chemotherapy is indicated to improve long-term survival.
B. The five-year survival rate is 85% to 100%, and no further treatment is necessary.
C. Exploratory laparotomy and lymph node dissection is necessary to complete staging.
D. Pancreaticoduodenectomy should be performed with the intent to remove all possible malignant tissue.

724 Which of the following statements regarding choledocholithiasis is most correct?
A. The success rate of mechanical lithotripsy is 80% to 90%.
B. Extracorporeal shock wave lithotripsy is inappropriate for patients with large common duct stones.

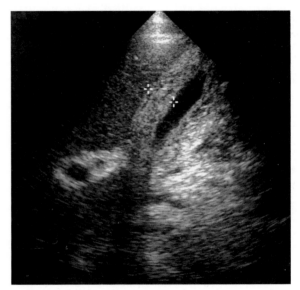

Figure for question **725**

ANSWERS

623 **A** (S&F, ch70)
Retroperitoneal air does not always require surgical intervention and can often be managed conservatively. Pancreatitis does not necessarily change that. Perforation of the bile duct is a rare occurrence during ERCP, and SOD is associated with a rate of pancreatitis of approximately 7% to 25%, but not 50%.

624 **E** (S&F, ch65)
In patients with suspected biliary colic, transabdominal ultrasonography is generally the first imaging study performed because it is noninvasive and inexpensive relative to the other choices. Transabdominal ultrasonography is 95% sensitive for gallstones larger than 2 mm and 95% specific for gallstones that produce acoustic shadowing.

625 **D** (S&F, ch62)
Biliary atresia is characterized by the complete obstruction of bile flow as a result of the destruction or absence of all or a portion of the extrahepatic bile ducts. Laboratory studies initially reveal evidence of cholestasis, with a serum bilirubin level of 6 to 12 mg/dL, at least 50% of which is conjugated. Serum aminotransferase and alkaline

phosphatase levels are moderately elevated. Serum γ-glutamyl transpeptidase and 5´-nucleotidase levels also are elevated. Histopathologic findings on initial liver biopsy specimens are of great importance in the management of patients with biliary atresia. Early in the course, the hepatic architecture is generally preserved with a variable degree of bile duct proliferation, canalicular and cellular bile stasis, and portal tract edema and fibrosis (see figure from question 625). The presence of bile plugs in portal triads is highly suggestive of large duct obstruction. Bile duct epithelium shows varying degrees of injury, including swelling, vacuolization, and even sloughing of cells into the lumen. Portal tracts may be infiltrated with inflammatory cells, and in approximately 25% of patients, there may be giant cell transformation of hepatocytes to a degree more commonly observed in neonatal hepatitis. Bile ductules occasionally may assume a ductal plate configuration, suggesting that the disease process has interfered with the ductular remodeling that occurs during prenatal development. Biliary cirrhosis may be present initially or evolve rapidly over the first months of life, whether or not bile flow is successfully restored.

626 **D** (S&F, ch68)
The most common locations for cholangiocarcinoma in patients with PSC are the bile duct and hilum, although it can occur anywhere in the biliary tree. Brush cytology of dominant strictures in the biliary tree is no more than 60% sensitive for the detection of cholangiocarcinoma. CA 19-9 is not sensitive or specific for the presence of cholangiocarcinoma. EUS with fine-needle aspiration may help in improving yield to obtain a cytologic diagnosis in selected cases.

627 **B** (S&F, ch65)
This patient may have *chronic cholecystitis*, a term that is less commonly used today. The most common histologic change observed in patients with biliary pain is mild fibrosis of the gallbladder wall with a chronic inflammatory cell infiltrate and an intact mucosa. However, recurrent episodes of biliary pain can be associated with a scarred, shrunken gallbladder and Rokitansky-Aschoff sinuses (intramural diverticula). An acute neutrophilic infiltrate could be expected with acute cholecystitis, which this patient does not have. Caseating granulomas are not characteristic of acute or chronic cholecystitis nor is eosinophilic infiltration of the gallbladder.

628 **D** (S&F, ch66)
In this question, it is unclear whether the patient's symptoms are related to gallstones or to the gastrointestinal dyspepsia and malabsorption induced by the fatty, greasy meal that she consumed. Patients of Native American heritage and those with a porcelain gallbladder are at elevated risk of gallbladder cancer, and cholecystectomy is recommended even in asymptomatic patients. Morbidly obese patients and those with heart-lung transplant are at higher risk of serious complications of gallstone disease. Renal transplant recipients with asymptomatic gallstones have a low risk of the development of complications related to gallstone disease and, therefore, should not be considered for prophylactic cholecystectomy.

629 **B** (S&F, ch70)
Placement of an uncovered SEMS is reasonable in patients with malignant biliary stricture given that it is usually resected at the time of surgery. If performed, care should be taken to allow an adequate segment of the common hepatic duct to be proximal to the SEMS to allow for the choledochojejunal anastomosis. Placement of an SEMS is cost-effective if a patient survives longer than three to six months. Covered SEMSs migrate more often than uncovered stents. Occlusion of an SEMS should be managed with a repeat ERCP for clearance of the original SEMS and possible placement of a second stent within the occluded one.

630 **A** (S&F, ch62)
Spontaneous perforation of the bile duct is rare but can occur during infancy. The perforation usually occurs at the junction of the cystic and common ducts. The cause is unknown, but in some cases, there is evidence of obstruction, secondary to stenosis or inspissated bile, at the distal end of the bile duct. Congenital weakness and injury due to infection have also been implicated in some cases.

631 **A** (S&F, ch67)
Acalculous cholecystitis typically occurs in patients hospitalized in the intensive care unit with severe illness resulting in hemodynamic compromise and lack of oral nutrition. Fasting results in concentration of bile acids within the gallbladder due to the absence of CCK-stimulated gallbladder contraction (chemical injury), and splanchnic vasoconstriction occurs because of hemodynamic compromise (ischemic injury). Classic symptoms of acute cholecystitis, such as abdominal pain, may be initially absent in as many as 75% of patients. Ultrasonography, CT, and hepatobiliary scintigraphy have all been used to establish this diagnosis. The presence of wall thickening of the gallbladder and pericholecystic fluid is an abnormal gallbladder finding.

632 **C** (S&F, ch66)
Oral dissolution should be considered for patients with uncomplicated gallstone disease. This includes patients with mild, infrequent biliary pain. Patients with severe or frequent biliary pain and patients with complications of gallstones, including cholecystitis, pancreatitis, and cholangitis, should not be treated with dissolution. These patients should be referred for surgery. Oral dissolution only works on cholesterol stones; the patient with sickle cell disease likely has pigmented stones related to hemolysis. Oral dissolution therapy has been effective in stones as large as 10 mm, with results being superior for stones smaller than 5 mm.

633 **D** (S&F, ch70)
Patients with indeterminate strictures may not have a definitive diagnosis before going to surgery, and the ultimate surgical plan may be determined intraoperatively. There is no role for corticosteroids or photodynamic therapy as a diagnostic or therapeutic modality. Choledochoscopy may be able to

better assess these strictures through direct imaging and targeted biopsies.

634 **B** (S&F, ch62)

635 **B** (S&F, ch65)
The patient's presenting symptoms, laboratory study results, and imaging are all consistent with an obstructing bile duct stone. Even though the stone itself was not seen on a transabdominal ultrasound scan and the patient's symptoms have improved, his liver function tests have worsened, suggesting persistent (incomplete) biliary obstruction. In this situation, ERCP is the most cost-effective diagnostic study because it is highly sensitive (95%) for diagnosing choledocholithiasis and can provide for therapy (sphincterotomy and stone extraction) at the same time. If the patient's laboratory test results had started to improve, suggesting possible stone passage, MRCP or EUS would be the preferred modality, although in this case, because of the patient's pacemaker, MRCP would not be an option.

636 **B** (S&F, ch66)
This patient has Bouveret syndrome, which is characterized by gastric outlet obstruction due to duodenal impaction of a large gallstone that has migrated through a cholecystoduodenal fistula. More commonly, patients with traditional gallstone ileus have intermittent obstruction as the stone passes through the intestinal tract and ultimately completely obstructs the ileum, where the small intestine is the narrowest. In this case, imaging would also reveal dilated loops of small bowel.

637 **C** (S&F, ch62)
Acute noncalculous, noninflammatory distention of the gallbladder may occur in infants and children. The gallbladder is not acutely inflamed, and cultures of the bile are usually sterile. The absence of gallbladder inflammation is what distinguishes acute hydrops from acute cholecystitis. Acute hydrops has been associated with Kawasaki's disease and Henoch-Schönlein purpura. Patients present with acute onset of crampy abdominal pain and, often, nausea and vomiting. The right upper quadrant is tender, and the gallbladder may be palpable. Ultrasonography reveals an enlarged, distended gallbladder without calculi or wall thickening. Gallbladder hydrops often responds to nonsurgical treatment; with supportive care and management of the current illness, the prognosis for return of normal gallbladder function is excellent.

638 **D** (S&F, ch69)
The risk of cholangiocarcinoma is elevated in those with Caroli disease, choledochal cysts, and PSC. Tobacco smoking is not a well-documented risk factor for cholangiocarcinoma.

639 **C** (S&F, ch68)
Recurrent cholangitis or pruritus that is refractory to medical or endoscopic management may be an indication for liver transplantation. Survival rates for patients undergoing liver transplantation for PSC are higher than for patients undergoing transplantation for hepatitis B and hepatitis C. Colectomy at the time of liver transplantation is not indicated for those patients with ulcerative colitis. Cholangioscopic evaluation is not a routine part of the pretransplantation evaluation.

640 **A** (S&F, ch70)
This patient is presenting with acute cholecystitis with obstruction of the cystic duct. Percutaneous drainage with a cholecystostomy is the next step in managing this patient. Sphincterotomy of the biliary sphincter will not alleviate obstruction of the cystic duct. Stenting of the cystic duct is occasionally possible but often difficult due to the spiral valves within the duct and is not a durable long-term solution for this high-risk surgical candidate. EUS-guided transgastric drainage of the gallbladder is not indicated and would put the patient at greater risk of complications than the percutaneous route.

641 **A** (S&F, ch63)
Although controversial, most evidence indicates that typical biliary-type pain and delayed gallbladder emptying in patients are predictive of relief of symptoms by cholecystectomy. Further prospective trials need to be done to define the role of CCK cholescintigraphy.

642 **D** (S&F, ch67)
The patient most likely has a gallbladder adenoma. Gallbladder polyps larger than 18 mm pose a significant risk of malignancy and should therefore be resected. Polyps 10 to 18 mm in size should be resected in patients unless they are high-risk surgical candidates, in which case, annual or biannual monitoring should be performed. Polyps smaller than 10 mm in diameter have a very low risk of malignancy, and surveillance is appropriate.

643 **B** (S&F, ch65)
Through the enterohepatic circulation, more than 95% of bile salt molecules secreted into bile are reabsorbed, mostly in the distal ileum via an active transport system, and returned to the liver. A small fraction (<5%) of bile salts is excreted in the feces; however, this loss is compensated by de novo bile salt synthesis in the liver. Interruption of the enterohepatic circulation (e.g., surgery, Crohn's ileitis, cholestyramine) results in up-regulation of bile salt synthesis in the liver, which could restore bile salt secretion rates to approximately 25% of their native values.

644 **C** (S&F, ch62)
The hallmark of Alagille syndrome is a paucity of interlobular bile ducts. Paucity may be defined as a significantly decreased ratio (<0.4) of the numbers of interlobular portal bile ducts to portal tracts. The histologic features of liver biopsy specimens from patients with Alagille syndrome presenting during the first months of life may overlap with those of neonatal hepatitis in that specimens in both cases may show evidence of ballooning of hepatocytes, variable cholestasis, portal inflammation, and giant cell transformation.

Often, the number of interlobular bile ducts is not decreased in the initial liver biopsy specimen. However, there may be evidence of bile duct injury consisting of cellular infiltration of portal triads contiguous to interlobular bile ducts, lymphocytic infiltration, pyknosis of biliary epithelium, and periductal fibrosis. Serial biopsies of an individual patient may show bile duct proliferation initially, followed by a paucity of bile ducts, with a paucity of interlobular bile ducts usually becoming apparent by three months after diagnosis. There may also be mild periportal fibrosis, but progression to cirrhosis is uncommon. The extrahepatic bile ducts are patent but usually narrowed or hypoplastic.

645 **A** (S&F, ch65)
Forty percent of this third-generation cephalosporin is secreted into bile in an unmetabolized form, reaching 100 to 200 times the concentration in plasma. Once the saturation level is exceeded, ceftriaxone complexes with calcium, resulting in the formation of biliary sludge. It is reported that 43% of children receiving high-dose ceftriaxone develop biliary sludge, and 19% of these become symptomatic. Biliary sludge spontaneously resolves after withdrawal of the drug.

646 **C** (S&F, ch67)
Cholesterolosis is an acquired histologic abnormality of the gallbladder epithelium characterized by excessive accumulation of cholesterol esters and triglyceride within epithelial macrophages. Cholesterolosis is more common in women before the age of 65; after this age, the sex differences are less pronounced. Cholesterolosis and cholesterol stones occur independently but can occur together. Cholesterolosis is present in 5% to 40% of autopsy specimens and is almost always an incidental finding. Symptoms are rare. No racial, ethnic, or geographic differences in prevalence have been described.

647 **D** (S&F, ch68)
Fatigue and abdominal pain are the most frequent symptoms in patients with PSC, whereas few have ascites or splenomegaly at diagnosis. Weight loss is uncommon, and although fat-soluble vitamin deficiency may occur, it is rarely life threatening.

648 **D** (S&F, ch63)
The modified Milwaukee classification system is used to divide patients into three categories based on diagnostic criteria. These categories are relevant to clinical practice in the utilization of diagnostic and therapeutic ERCP. The diagnostic criteria include biliary-type pain, serum liver enzyme levels more than 1.1 times the upper limit of normal on one occasion, and bile duct dilation to greater than 10 mm. The previous diagnostic criteria, called the original Milwaukee classification, included biliary dilation to greater than 12 mm, delayed drainage (>45 minutes) of bile into the duodenum at cholangiography, and serum liver enzymes elevated more than twice the upper limit of normal on at least two separate occasions. Studies have called into question the greater stringency of

the "old" criteria, and they are no longer used in clinical practice.

649 **B** (S&F, ch65)
At least five primary defects must be present simultaneously in gallbladder bile for cholesterol gallstone formation: genetic factors and *LITH* genes, hepatic hypersecretion, gallbladder hypomotility, rapid phase transitions, and intestinal factors. There is no clear evidence that taking calcium supplements or consuming a diet high in calcium plays a significant role in cholesterol gallstone formation.

650 **C** (S&F, ch68)
The diagnosis of PSC with a normal cholangiogram at ERCP may occur and as a result may be confused with primary biliary cirrhosis. Because primary biliary cirrhosis does not affect the extrahepatic biliary tree, the presence of disease in this location distinguishes PSC from primary biliary cirrhosis. IgG_2 is not related to PSC. PSC is possible without extrahepatic biliary disease. Gallbladder disease is seen in as many as 15% of patients with PSC.

651 **E** (S&F ch66)
This patient has a benign bile duct stricture from surgical clips placed on the bile duct. ERCP and endoscopic placement of a plastic bile duct stent would be an acceptable choice, but of the choices listed here, surgery is the best option. Surgical repair is highly effective and usually involves resection of the stricture and end-to-side Roux-en-Y choledochojejunostomy or hepaticojejunostomy.

652 **C** (S&F, ch62)
Paucity of bile ducts can be an isolated and unexplained finding in infants and children with idiopathic cholestasis or a feature of a heterogeneous group of disorders that include congenital infections with rubella and cytomegalovirus and genetic disorders such as α_1-antitrypsin deficiency and inborn errors of bile metabolism. It has also been observed in some cases of Williams syndrome and Noonan syndrome.

653 **C** (S&F, ch70)
Most bile duct injuries are related to the surgeon's not definitively confirming the anatomy of the cystic duct in relation to the bile duct or due to anatomic variations of the right biliary system. Bile duct injuries and right segmental injuries are the most common forms of iatrogenic injury in this setting. It is not recommended that patients routinely undergo preoperative MRCP or ERCP.

654 **A** (S&F, ch68)
More than 75% of patients with PSC have inflammatory bowel disease. The two diseases often do not progress together. Patients with Crohn's disease are not known to have a higher likelihood of severe PSC compared with those patients with ulcerative colitis and PSC. PSC is present in 2.4% to 4.0% of all patients with chronic ulcerative colitis and 1.4% to 3.4% of patients with Crohn's disease.

655 **B** (S&F, ch64)

Bile salts are absorbed in the distal ileum. When more than 100 cm of distal ileum is removed, bile salt malabsorption almost invariably occurs. Unabsorbed bile acids inhibit water absorption and induce water secretion in the colon, resulting in a mild, watery diarrhea. Bile acids cause water secretion by increasing chloride secretion in the perfused colon through an inositol 1,4,5-triphosphate and calcium-dependent mechanism. Dihydroxy bile acids induce net fluid secretion into the lumen at high concentrations seen in those with malabsorption of bile salts and block absorption of fluid and water at low concentrations.

656 **C** (S&F, ch63)

Using the modified Milwaukee classification, the patient meets the criteria for type I SOD in that she has biliary-type pain, AST elevation greater than two times normal on at least two occasions, and a bile duct dilated to more than 12 mm. Of patients with type I SOD, 86% have an elevated basal SOD pressure. Because at least 90% of such patients have a favorable clinical response to endoscopic sphincterotomy, no further diagnostic studies or therapeutic trials are necessary; this response rate is independent of the results of biliary manometry.

657 **B** (S&F, ch65)

Cholangitis due to purulent material under pressure in the biliary tree is the most rapidly fatal complication of gallstone disease. Infection can quickly spread to the bloodstream and cause septicemia. *Escherichia coli*, *Klebsiella*, *Pseudomonas*, *Enterococcus*, and *Proteus* species and anaerobic species such as *Bacteroides fragilis* and *Clostridium perfringens* are found in approximately 15% of appropriately cultured bile specimens. Anaerobes usually accompany aerobes, especially *E. coli*. Early diagnosis and prompt treatment with intravenous antibiotics and biliary decompression are essential.

658 **B** (S&F, ch62)

Nonobstructive saccular or fusiform dilation of the intrahepatic bile ducts is a rare congenital disorder. In the pure form, known as Caroli disease, dilation is classically segmental and saccular and associated with stone formation and recurrent bacterial cholangitis. A more common type, Caroli syndrome, is associated with a portal tract lesion typical of congenital hepatic fibrosis. Dilation of the extrahepatic bile ducts (choledochal cysts) also may be present. Renal disease occurs in both forms. Renal tubular ectasia occurs with the simple form, and both conditions can be associated with autosomal recessive polycystic renal disease or, rarely, autosomal dominant polycystic renal disease. There may be slight to moderate elevations of serum bilirubin, alkaline phosphatase, and aminotransferase levels. Liver function may be normal initially, but repeated episodes of infection and biliary obstruction within the cystic bile ducts may eventually lead to hepatic failure. Inability to concentrate urine is the most frequent abnormality of renal function; variable elevations of blood urea nitrogen and serum creatinine levels reflect the severity of the underlying kidney disease. Ultrasonography, MRI cholangiography, and CT are of great value in demonstrating intrahepatic cystic dilation. Renal cysts or hyperechogenicity of papillae may be detected. Cholangiography usually demonstrates a normal common duct with segmental, saccular dilations of the intrahepatic bile ducts. Rarely, the process may be limited to one lobe of the liver.

659 **A** (S&F, ch70)

Unilateral biliary drainage is sufficient for palliation of the obstructive jaundice from a hilar malignancy. SEMSs are not associated with higher complication rates but may require more expertise to achieve appropriate placement. Percutaneous drainage of hilar obstruction does not carry fewer complications compared with endoscopic stent placement. Drainage of an atrophied lobe is not necessary.

660 **C** (S&F, ch67)

Non-neoplastic polyps account for the majority of gallbladder polyps (95%). Of these, the most common type of gallbladder polyp is a cholesterol polyp. It is a benign variant of cholesterolosis resulting from infiltration of the lamina propria with lipid-laden foamy macrophages. The other types of polyps are much less common.

661 **A** (S&F, ch68)

This patient has an increased risk of colon cancer because of his history of pancolitis and PSC. The presence of PSC further increases his cancer risk above that of the colitis alone. He should undergo colonoscopic screening for colon cancer annually. Liver transplantation is not known to decrease the risk, and in fact, immunosuppression may indeed increase the overall cancer risk. Ursodeoxycholic acid may decrease the risk of colonic dysplasia, although the magnitude of this benefit and the impact on the incidence of malignancy are not well defined.

662 **C** (S&F, ch63)

Type I SOD patients experience pain accompanied by elevation of liver enzymes and biliary dilation, whereas type II SOD patients have pain and either elevated enzymes or biliary dilation, but not both. Patients with type III SOD have biliary-type pain without bile duct dilation or abnormal liver enzymes. Many experts advocate empirical sphincterotomy for patients with SOD types I and II due to the high risk of complications in patients undergoing biliary manometry. Because the response rate to sphincterotomy is less than 10% when the results of biliary manometry are normal (and 55% to 60% when the results are abnormal), biliary manometry is advocated before sphincterotomy for those with type III SOD.

663 **B** (S&F, ch64)

Bile acids are stored in the proximal small intestine where they are able to mix with food. After a meal, intestinal contractions propel the stored bile acids to the distal small intestine where they are actively reabsorbed.

664 **E** (S&F, ch62)

Bile plug syndrome results from thick, inspissated bile and mucus that causes biliary obstruction.

Healthy infants can be affected; however, it occurs more commonly in sick premature infants who cannot be fed and require prolonged parenteral nutrition or may occur in the setting of brisk hemolysis. Pathogenesis is thought to involve bile stasis, fasting, infection, and an increased bilirubin load. The clinical presentation can be similar to that of biliary atresia. Diagnosis is usually made by exploratory laparotomy or cholangiography. Treatment is with repeated bile duct irrigation and treatment of the underlying cause (e.g., initiating enteral feeding).

665 **A** (S&F, ch65)
The majority of gallstones are composed predominantly of cholesterol. The remaining stones are pigmented stones. This patient likely has black-pigmented gallstones, which are common in patients with chronic hemolytic disorders. These stones are composed predominantly of calcium bilirubinate, with substantial amounts of crystalline calcium carbonate and phosphate. In those with sickle cell disease, the risk of gallstones increases with age; stones are diagnosed in at least 14% of children younger than 10 years of age and 36% of those between ages 10 and 20 years.

666 **C** (S&F, ch66)
Ten-year follow-up data reveal 27%, 41%, and 54% cumulative recurrence rates at three, five, and 10 years, respectively. Recurrence is most often related to the presence of lithogenic bile composition and gallbladder dysmotility rather than patient variables such as sex, age, and weight. Factors predictive of higher rates of treatment failure include stones larger than 16 mm, multiple stones, and stones with CT density of greater than 84 Hounsfield units. Recurrent stones are usually small and multiple and cause recurrent biliary pain.

667 **D** (S&F, ch64)
Canalicular secretion is the rate-limiting step in the hepatic transport of bile acids.

668 **C** (S&F, ch69)
This patient has a distal bile duct cholangiocarcinoma in the presence of PSC, but no cirrhosis. Primary resection with pancreatoduodenectomy with curative intent is indicated. Transplantation evaluation for mild diffuse disease is not indicated at this time; moreover, in contrast to a hilar carcinoma, distal biliary cholangiocarcinoma does not require removal of the liver. Chemoradiation and/or photodynamic therapy may be used for those who are not surgical candidates, but cure requires surgery.

669 **D** (S&F, ch67)
This patient has a typical presentation of acalculous cholecystitis. In patients who are not at high risk, cholecystectomy provides definitive treatment. In patients with significant surgical risk factors, however, percutaneous cholecystostomy tube placement is a highly effective treatment. Ursodeoxycholic acid has no role in the treatment of acalculous cholecystitis. Endoscopic, transpapillary decompression of the gallbladder via selective cystic duct cannulation and stent placement is an alternative treatment in patients who are not candidates for cholecystectomy or percutaneous cholecystostomy. Early reports of endoscopic cholecystoduodenostomy and stent placement (much like draining a pseudocyst) have demonstrated significant risks (e.g., bile leak) and at present should still be considered experimental.

670 **C** (S&F, ch68)
This patient should have regular surveillance for early detection of cholangiocarcinoma. This typically consists of cross-sectional imaging and serum tumor markers. The presence of normal liver enzymes does not ensure that histologic progression is not occurring silently. Ursodeoxycholic acid should still be continued. Tacrolimus has not yet been shown to slow the histologic progression of PSC.

671 **B** (S&F, ch62)

672 **D** (S&F, ch65)
The figure from question 672 shows ERCP demonstrating a bile duct stone. The majority of gallstones are of the cholesterol variety. There is evidence that all these *LITH* genes play a role in the formation of cholesterol stone formation.

673 **C** (S&F, ch64)
The volume of bile secreted by the liver each day ranges from 500 to 600 mL. The predominant organic components are bile acids. Bile acids are almost completely reabsorbed by the terminal ileum and returned via the portal circulation to the liver.

674 **C** (S&F, ch68)
Small focal cholangiocarcinoma is not an absolute contraindication to transplantation, although patients should be referred to centers with protocols for liver transplantation for this indication. The one-year survival rate in these patients is approximately 65%. A living related donor is not preferred as a source for transplantation in patients with PSC. Endoscopic surveillance is not more than 60% sensitive in detecting cholangiocarcinoma in the setting of PSC.

675 **E** (S&F, ch70)
Congenital hepatic fibrosis is manifested as hepatic parenchyma fibrosis and evolution to synthetic dysfunction. Biliary strictures are not a common part of the spectrum of this disease. The other options are all causes of benign biliary obstruction.

676 **E** (S&F, ch65)
This patient has symptoms that could be related to biliary colic; however, an extensive workup including EUS has not revealed the presence of gallstones. In this situation, one must also consider nonbiliary causes of abdominal pain, including angina pectoris, gastroesophageal reflux disease, irritable bowel syndrome, peptic ulcer disease, pancreatitis, diverticulitis, and intestinal or colonic malignancy.

677 **A** (S&F, ch68)
Biliary epithelial cells have been shown to aberrantly express major histocompatibility complex

class II antigens. IgG-4 is present in as many as 53% of patients and perinuclear antineutrophilic cytoplasmic antibody is seen in as many as 88% of patients. Elevated serum IgG$_4$ is not associated with PSC.

678 **B** (S&F, ch65)
This patient has recurrent pyogenic cholangitis. The leading theory links biliary infection with the parasites *Clonorchis sinensis*, *Opisthorchis* sp., and *Ascaris lumbricoides*. These infections are endemic in Asia and can be cultured from biliary stones, bile, and stool. These patients may also lack an inhibitor of bacterial glucuronidase, an enzyme that deconjugates bilirubin and thereby promotes formation of brown-pigmented calcium bilirubinate stones.

679 **D** (S&F, ch62)
The sphincter ampullae is comprised of longitudinal muscle fibers that surround the circular fibers of the ampulla of Vater. When these fibers contract, the ampullary folds are approximated resulting in obstruction of pancreaticobiliary flow and prevention of reflux of duodenal content. The pancreatic duct and bile duct enter the duodenum together in 85% of individuals. The sphincter pancreaticus is absent in 30% of individuals but the sphincter choledochus is uniformly present. Biliary, not pancreatic, secretion is partly regulated by fasciculi longitudinales.

680 **C** (S&F, ch64)
Transporter gene mutations have been identified in a number of diseases affecting bile acid metabolism. These include primary bile acid malabsorption, intrahepatic cholestasis of pregnancy, progressive familial intrahepatic cholestasis, low phospholipid-associated cholelithiasis, and Dubin-Johnson syndrome. Primary biliary cirrhosis, however, is not associated with mutations in the bile acid transporter genes.

681 **A** (S&F, ch67)
Less than 50% of patients with acalculous biliary pain have a depressed gallbladder ejection fraction; however, of those who do, a majority will obtain some symptom relief after cholecystectomy. Some studies show that more than 80% of patients with acalculous biliary pain are female, with a mean age of 30. Some studies have found that as many as one half of patients with acalculous biliary pain actually have microscopic cholelithiasis in resected gallbladder specimens, suggesting an initial false-positive transabdominal ultrasound scan finding. A strong link between acalculous biliary pain and other functional bowel disorders suggests that visceral hypersensitivity may also contribute to biliary pain in patients with a normal gallbladder; acalculous biliary pain is listed as a functional gastrointestinal disorder by a multinational working committee of gastrointestinal investigators (Rome III classification).

682 **D** (S&F, ch70)
This patient has an unexplained etiology of recurrent pancreatitis. The diagnostic options include manometry to assess the biliary and pancreatic sphincter pressures. Hypertension of either sphincter may cause recurrent episodes of pancreatic duct obstruction. Cholangioscopy is not indicated because MRCP has excluded biliary obstruction. A CCK analog will not provide additional information in the setting of previous cholecystectomy. A transpapillary biliary stent is not indicated because it will not provide drainage of the pancreatic duct.

683 **B** (S&F, ch66)
Indications for cholecystectomy during pregnancy include complicated gallstone diseases, such as acute cholecystitis and pancreatitis, as well as the inability of the mother to maintain adequate oral intake as a result of biliary colic. Surgery poses the lowest risk to the fetus and mother during the second trimester.

684 **D** (S&F, ch68)
The patient should be counseled that, to date, no medical treatment has been shown clearly to alter the course of PSC. There is no indication for annual liver biopsy. Budesonide is not known to affect the natural history of PSC. Standard-dose ursodeoxycholic acid does not decrease death in patients with this disease and has a questionable impact on histologic progression. High-dose regimens are under study.

685 **D** (S&F, ch65)
MRCP is a sensitive and specific noninvasive study for choledocholithiasis with biliary obstruction. Although EUS has sensitivity and specificity rates of 98%, this is more invasive than MRCP (this is also true for ERCP, with 95% sensitivity and specificity rates). Transabdominal ultrasonography demonstrates bile duct stones only in approximately 50% of suspected cases. CT is not the preferred imaging modality for choledocholithiasis.

686 **E** (S&F, ch62)
PSC is an uncommon, chronic, progressive disease of the biliary tract characterized by inflammation and fibrosis of the intrahepatic and extrahepatic biliary ductal systems leading to biliary cirrhosis. In adults, carcinoma of the bile ducts also must be excluded; however, this complication has not been reported in children. PSC is associated with inflammatory bowel disease (most often, ulcerative colitis) in 70% of adults and 50% to 80% of children with the disorder. A male preponderance has been reported in some, but not all, large series of children with PSC. Inflammatory bowel disease–associated PSC most often occurs with ulcerative colitis, although cases have been reported in patients with Crohn's disease. The bowel symptoms can precede, occur simultaneously with, or appear years after the diagnosis of PSC. As in adults, treatment of the bowel disease in infants, including colectomy, does not influence the progression of PSC. The prognosis of PSC in children is guarded. The clinical course of the disorder is variable but usually progressive. Analysis of survival factors at presentation indicates that older age, splenomegaly, and prolonged prothrombin time predict a poor outcome. The occurrence of jaundice after the neonatal period with a persistent serum bilirubin level of more than five times the

upper limit of normal was also associated with a poor outcome. Hepatocellular carcinoma also may occur, but cholangiocarcinoma, an important complication of adult PSC, has not been reported in children.

687 **B** (S&F, ch66)
This patient has asymptomatic cholelithiasis. Decision analyses suggest that the risks of cholecystectomy approximate the potential benefit in preventing future serious sequelae of the gallstones. Although this patient is diabetic, initial perceptions that individuals with diabetes are more prone to the development of complications from asymptomatic stones are unwarranted; especially when confounding variables such as hyperlipidemia, obesity, and cardiovascular disease are taken into account. When symptoms related to gallstones do develop in diabetic patients, however, early intervention is indicated because such patients are at increased risk of the development of complications such as gangrenous cholecystitis.

688 **B** (S&F, ch70)
Patients with hepaticojejunostomies after liver transplantation usually have an anatomic composition that makes retrograde cholangiography challenging. Although overtube-assisted endoscopy has revolutionized the ability to perform ERCP in those with altered anatomy, percutaneous cholangiography is a reasonable first-line approach. Choledochocholedochal (duct-to-duct) anastomoses are accessible via the intact ampulla and may be cannulated endoscopically. Post-transplantation anastomotic strictures are successfully managed more than 70% of the time by ERCP, and thus surgery is not usually required. Strictures resulting from stenosis and occlusion of the hepatic artery and smaller peribiliary arteries are a well-documented complication of liver transplantation. Spontaneous rupture is not within the spectrum of complications of these strictures.

689 **B** (S&F, ch69)
Liver transplantation is an option for suitable candidates with localized hilar disease and has led to a five-year survival rate of 76%. Cholangioscopy is not used to define the extent of disease and is most useful to determine the etiology of an indeterminate stricture. Positron emission tomography is inaccurate for local nodal metastasis and is not indicated to determine the resectability of the primary tumor. EUS is not indicated for staging hilar cholangiocarcinoma.

690 **E** (S&F, ch64)
Bile plays a central role in lipid digestion and absorption and therefore cholesterol homeostasis. Additionally, a host of additional compounds and chemicals are secreted by bile, including lipid-soluble xenobiotics, drug metabolites, and heavy metals. Short-chain fatty acid enterohepatic circulation occurs via direct uptake mechanisms that do not require bile acids.

691 **D** (S&F, ch62)
The infantile form of choledochal cyst disease must be distinguished from other forms of hepatobiliary disease of the neonate, particularly biliary atresia. Sequelae of a choledochal cyst often appear during the first months of life, and as many as 80% of patients have cholestatic jaundice and acholic stools. Vomiting, irritability, and failure to thrive may occur. Examination reveals hepatomegaly, and in approximately one half of patients, there is a palpable abdominal mass. In a series of 72 patients in whom a cyst was diagnosed postnatally, jaundice was the most common symptom followed by abdominal pain. Spontaneous perforation of a choledochal cyst may occur, particularly when bile flow is obstructed. Progressive hepatic injury can occur during the first months of life as a result of biliary obstruction. The diagnosis of a choledochal cyst is best established by ultrasonography (see figure from question 691, in which the arrow points to a type I choledochal cyst off the bile duct of an infant).

692 **C** (S&F, ch64)
In patients with inherited disorders of bile acid conjugation, fat-soluble vitamin deficiency and steatorrhea develop. One would not expect vitamin B_{12} deficiency, fluid overload, or ascites.

693 **D** (S&F, ch66)
The patient is presenting with acute cholecystitis that is severe, and she should receive broad-spectrum antibiotics. Dual therapy with a third-generation cephalosporin and metronidazole would also be acceptable. If the patient had presented with only mild signs and symptoms, intravenous cefotoxin would have been sufficient. Intravenous antibiotics are indicated because bile or gallbladder wall cultures are positive for bacteria in more than 40% of cases. This patient should undergo cholecystectomy, preferably early in her hospital course.

694 **B** (S&F, ch70)
This patient has type I SOD, and empirical sphincterotomy is appropriate in this situation. Performing biliary manometry is not necessary given the high likelihood of response from biliary sphincterotomy and would subject the patient to the associated high risk of pancreatitis. A workup for chronic liver disease is not yet indicated.

695 **A** (S&F, ch69)
EUS is the most sensitive means of determining the local extent of tumor and regional adenopathy. After EUS, a surgical consultation may be obtained. Should the patient be found to be a surgical candidate, she should proceed directly to surgery without neoadjuvant therapy. Photodynamic therapy is not standard treatment for ampullary malignancy.

696 **A** (S&F, ch68)
PSC is associated with nonhepatic autoimmune phenomena including celiac sprue, Sjögren syndrome, Peyronie disease, and rheumatoid arthritis. An increased prevalence of PSC is seen in ulcerative colitis as well as in Crohn's disease. Screening for proteinuria is not indicated in patients with PSC. Smoking may confer a decreased risk of PSC.

697 **B** (S&F, ch66)
Decision analyses and randomized trials have shown that combined laparoscopic cholecystectomy with bile duct exploration via either a transcystic or transcholedochal approach offers less morbidity, less mortality, shorter hospital stay, quicker return to health, and fewer procedures compared with a preoperative endoscopic retrieval followed by laparoscopic cholecystectomy, and when performed by experienced surgeons, the success rates range from 83% to 97%. Because the technique is technically demanding and its success often depends on the experience of the surgeon, however, endoscopic stone retrieval via endoscopic retrograde cholangiography is a widely practiced and acceptable strategy for the patient with known choledocholithiasis. A percutaneous approach carries greater morbidity and is also inconvenient for the patient who would require that a temporary drain remain in the postoperative period.

698 **B** (S&F, ch70)
EUS and ERCP have a similar sensitivity for detecting choledocholithiasis, which is greater than 90%. The sensitivity of transabdominal ultrasonography in detecting stones is not greater than 68% and in many studies is less than 50%. MRI/MRCP has a sensitivity of between 81% and 100%.

699 **C** (S&F, ch65)
The U.S. National Cooperative Gallstone Study found that, in persons who have an episode of uncomplicated biliary pain in the year before entering the study, the rate of recurrent biliary pain is 38% per year. Other investigators have reported a rate of recurrent biliary pain as high as 50% per year in persons with symptomatic gallstones. Biliary complications also are more likely to develop in persons with symptomatic gallstones.

700 **A** (S&F, ch66)
The most likely cause of pancreatitis in this patient is gallstones, which are seen in the image of the patient's ultrasound scan. The other common cause of pancreatitis in developed countries is alcohol, which this patient does not consume. Cholecystectomy can be safely performed during the initial hospitalization after the acute episode of pancreatitis begins to resolve. When surgery is delayed, as many as one half of patients with have further episodes of pancreatitis or complications of gallstone disease.

701 **A** (S&F, ch68)
Infection with *C. sinensis*, *Opisthorchis* species, and *A. lumbricoides* is endemic to the same geographic region where PRC is prevalent. The majority of these patients present with intrahepatic biliary stones and repeated bouts of infectious cholangitis. The risk of cholangiocarcinoma is increased in those with RPC, but the risk of duodenal carcinoma is not. There is no association with urinary tract infection.

702 **B** (S&F, ch67)
This patient most likely has adenomyomatosis, incidentally discovered on an ultrasound scan performed for a different reason. Carefully performed studies in which radiologic and ultrasonographic findings of adenomyomatosis were correlated with pathologic findings have shown that diffuse or segmental thickening of the gallbladder wall in association with intramural diverticula (seen as round anechoic foci) accurately predicts adenomyomatosis. If these intramural diverticula (dilated Rokitansky-Aschoff sinuses) are filled with sludge or small calculi, the lesions may appear echogenic with acoustic shadowing, which may be mistaken for true cholelithiasis.

703 **B** (S&F, ch65)
The rate at which biliary pain develops in persons with asymptomatic gallstones is approximately 2% per year for the first five years; it then decreases over time.

704 **B** (S&F, ch64)

705 **B** (S&F, ch69)

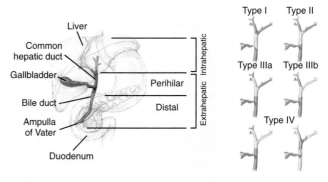

Figure for answer **705**

706 **A** (S&F, ch70)
Biliary access can be achieved either through the right or left hepatic lobe, depending on the individual's anatomy and disease process and the expertise of the interventional radiologist. PTC has no role in SOD. The PTC catheter has a life span of several weeks before it becomes dysfunctional and usually has to be replaced. When hemobilia occurs secondary to percutaneous biliary access, it is rarely fatal.

707 **B** (S&F, ch69)
Photodynamic therapy has been demonstrated in randomized trials to improve survival and quality of life in patients with cholangiocarcinoma. Endoscopic management is achieved by unilateral biliary decompression of either the right or left hepatic duct. Transcutaneous drainage is not more durable than SEMS for hilar malignancy.

708 **D** (S&F, ch70)
This patient had an impacted stone at the ampulla with probable low-grade and early cholangitis. The risk of pancreatitis is close to 5% to 10%, not 50%. There is no evidence of an anatomic variant. She will require elective cholecystectomy; no stent is needed, because the obstruction has been eliminated.

709 **C** (S&F, ch64)

Free bile acids in the colon both inhibit water absorption and induce water secretion, resulting in watery diarrhea. Symptomatic relief from diarrhea induced by bile acid malabsorption can be achieved by administration of a bile acid sequestrant, thereby reversing these effects.

710 **B** (S&F, ch70)

The serial placement of a single stent is usually insufficient to manage a benign biliary stricture. Multiple stents lead to resolution in 50% to 80% of patients. Although covered SEMSs have been used for benign stricture, uncovered stents should not be used. Although biliary strictures secondary to chronic pancreatitis may require surgical biliary bypass, endoscopic therapy has been successful and should be considered for selected individuals, particularly those with concomitant cirrhosis who are at increased risk of surgery.

711 **B** (S&F, ch65)

The CT scan shows gallbladder cancer. The relationship between gallbladder cancer and gallstones is well established. At least 80% to 90% of patients with this malignancy have gallstones. Gallbladder cancer is three to four times more common in women and occurs primarily in the elderly. Although as many as 30% of patients with gallbladder cancer present with jaundice, abdominal pain is the most common symptom and occurs in more than 80% of patients with gallbladder cancer.

712 **B** (S&F, ch63)

Numerous medications have been studied with respect to their effect on SOD because there are implications for the patient undergoing SOD manometry. Narcotics, such as morphine, stimulate the sphincter of Oddi and increase the basal pressure. Based on this observation, some experts advocate using morphine provocation tests to diagnose SOD. The exception is meperidine, which does not affect sphincter of Oddi pressure when used at a moderate dose (1 mg/kg). Calcium channel blockers such as verapamil relax the sphincter of Oddi. Diazepam does not affect sphincter of Oddi pressure, but midazolam may lower basal pressure in hypertensive sphincters and should be avoided when performing biliary manometry because it may confound results.

713 **B** (S&F, ch70)

The presence of ascites predisposes to complications with percutaneous biliary access. The presence of intra-abdominal fluid results in separation of the gallbladder or bile ducts from the site of puncture, thereby preventing adequate track formation. Maturation of T-tube tracks requires six weeks, and thus any manipulation of the tube should be postponed until a mature track has formed. Diagnosis and treatment of bile duct stones should be performed by ERCP as the initial procedure of choice. Endoscopic techniques such as papillotomy, dilation, and mechanical or laser lithotripsy may be used effectively for stone removal. Malignant biliary obstruction may be effectively palliated by endoscopic or percutaneous means. For the patient who has established percutaneous biliary access, a permanent stent may be placed radiologically.

714 **C** (S&F, ch65)

Given the rapid onset of the patient's jaundice and pain, he most likely has Mirrizi syndrome, a rare complication in which a stone impacted in the neck of the gallbladder or cystic duct extrinsically compresses the common hepatic duct with resulting proximal biliary obstruction. Occasionally, the stone can cause a fistula between the gallbladder or cystic duct and common hepatic duct. There are no other aspects of the patient's history, presentation, or imaging that suggest a gallbladder carcinoma or pancreatic malignancy. Hepatic artery thrombosis in this patient is rare without antecedent cause.

715 **A** (S&F, ch62)

Ultrasonography can be used to assess the size and echogenicity of the liver. Even in neonates, high-frequency, real-time ultrasonography can usually outline the gallbladder so that its size and contours can be estimated. Ultrasonography may also reveal stones and sludge in the bile ducts and gallbladder and cystic or obstructive dilation of the biliary system. Extrahepatic anomalies also may be identified. The outline of a triangle 3 mm or greater in thickness of a cone-shaped fibrotic mass cranial to the portal vein is diagnostic of biliary atresia. The "ghost" triad of gallbladder length less than 1.9 cm, lack of a smooth (complete echogenic) mucosal lining, and an indistinct wall and irregular or lobular contour of the gallbladder on ultrasonography has also been proposed as diagnostic for biliary atresia.

716 **B** (S&F, ch66)

Strictures that develop after laparoscopic cholecystectomy tend to occur in the common hepatic duct. Symptoms that present several months after surgery are often the result of thermal injury to the bile duct, as may occur when cautery is used to control hemorrhage.

717 **A** (S&F, ch70)

EUS provides detailed pancreatic imaging due to its proximity within the gastroduodenal lumen and the high-resolution imaging. The sensitivity of EUS for bile duct stones is greater than 90%, although it is not a modality for detecting SOD. EUS is not very good for detecting lesions in the right lobe of the liver given the distance from the right lobe, so it is poorly sensitive in that regard.

718 **A** (S&F, ch68)

Ampullary papillitis and SOD have been described in patients with RPC. Ova and parasites are typically not found within the stones of patients with RPC. Cholangiocarcinoma develops in approximately 3% of patients with RPC. RPC is not associated with IgA deficiency.

719 **B** (S&F, ch67)

Adenomyomatosis is characterized by excessive proliferation of surface epithelium with invaginations into a thickened muscularis. Despite its name, this condition is not associated with adenomas and is not thought to be a premalignant condition. As many as one half of resected gallbladders with adenomyomatosis have concomitant gallstones; in these cases, biliary colic is thought to be due to the gallstones rather than to the adenomyomatosis. In simple, uncomplicated cases, this condition does not warrant cholecystectomy.

720 **C** (S&F, ch70)
This patient has a bile leak after cholecystectomy, and the most likely cause is a cystic stump leak or a duct of Luschka leak. It is usually not necessary to perform surgery, and ERCP with biliary stent placement is successful more than 80% of the time. The fluid collection may need to be drained, but it is not unreasonable to have the stent placed before draining the fluid collection.

721 **D** (S&F, ch69)
Local resection of ampullary carcinoma, either by ampullectomy or transduodenal resection, is associated with an inferior survival outcome compared with pancreaticoduodenectomy. Pancreatitis is not a common presentation in these patients, who typically present with jaundice. Endoscopic biopsies are usually sufficient to obtain a histologic diagnosis.

722 **D** (S&F, ch65)
This patient has emphysematous cholecystitis, as evidenced by air in the gallbladder wall, which is caused by infection of the gallbladder wall with gas-forming organisms. This is a rare complication of acute cholecystitis, occurring in less than 1% of cases. The risk of gallbladder perforation is high, and broad-spectrum antibiotics should therefore be initiated immediately, with plans for early cholecystectomy. It more often occurs in diabetic persons or older men who do not have gallstones in whom atherosclerosis of the cystic artery with resulting ischemia may be the initiating event.

723 **B** (S&F, ch69)
A T1a gallbladder cancer is confined to the duodenal wall, invading only the lamina propria. The five-year survival rate of patients with T1a gallbladder cancer is between 85% and 100%. Adjuvant chemotherapy is not recommended. Re-exploration for lymph node metastases is usually not necessary to complete surgical staging. A pancreaticoduodenectomy is not indicated.

724 **A** (S&F, ch70)
Mechanical lithotripsy is usually highly effective for achieving stone removal with success rates of 80% to 90% in most series. The use of a balloon or basket is a personal preference of the operator, and a basket is no more traumatic when used appropriately. Sphincteroplasty of the sphincter of Oddi carries a higher risk of pancreatitis than sphincterotomy. Extracorporeal shock wave lithotripsy can be performed safely for some patients with large bile duct stones.

725 **A** (S&F, ch67)
In the evaluation of patients with suspected acute acalculous cholecystitis, ultrasonography offers the distinct advantages of being widely available and easily transportable to the bedside. In the image presented with this question, there is thickening of the gallbladder wall to 17 mm (denoted by asterisks) without the presence of stones, characteristic of acute acalculous cholecystitis. Other characteristic features during ultrasonography are a sonographic Murphy's sign and pericholecystic fluid.

CHAPTER
8

Liver

QUESTIONS

726 A 36-year-old woman has recurrent bouts of severe abdominal pain that have defied diagnosis. No abnormalities have been discovered by radiologic or endoscopic procedures. Serum and fecal porphyrin tests are ordered based on this clinical history. What is the most likely diagnosis?
A. Erythropoietic protoporphyria
B. Hepatoerythropoietic porphyria
C. Porphyria cutanea tarda (PCT)
D. Variegate coproporphyria

727 A 38-year-old man with recent recovery from a bout of alcoholic hepatitis is seen in follow-up. He has a body mass index of 33, smokes a pack of cigarettes per day, and frequently smokes marijuana. In addition to alcohol abstinence, which is the lifestyle modification that is most likely to improve his outcome?
A. Cigarette smoking cessation
B. Marijuana smoking cessation
C. Nutritional protein supplementation
D. Weight loss

728 A 69-year-old man with a history of mitral valve replacement undergoes liver function testing, and the results indicate a combination of cholestatic and hepatocellular disease. Ultrasonography shows no abnormality. Liver biopsy reveals steatosis, portal acute and chronic inflammatory infiltrates, and central hyaline sclerosis. Which drug is most likely to have caused this patient's condition?
A. Amiodarone
B. Androgenic steroids
C. Methotrexate
D. Phenytoin
E. Pioglitazone

729 A 33-year-old woman presents for evaluation of chronic hepatitis C virus (HCV) infection discov-

ered during a life insurance physical examination. Her risk factor for HCV infection was a blood transfusion after a motor vehicle accident at the age of nine years. Her husband of seven years tests negative for anti-HCV antibody. The couple wishes to conceive a child. Which of the following recommendations is most appropriate?
A. Avoid breast-feeding the baby.
B. Plan delivery of the baby by cesarean section.
C. Administer HCV immunoglobulin to the infant at the time of delivery.
D. Test the infant for HCV after the age of 18 months.
E. Use latex condoms.

730 Which of the following statements regarding the hepatic arteries is true?
A. Arterial ligation is usually well tolerated in persons with normal liver function.
B. The common hepatic artery usually arises from the superior mesenteric artery.
C. The cystic arteries usually arise from the celiac artery.
D. The hepatic artery supplies 70% of the blood flow to the hepatic parenchyma.

731 A 60-year-old man with a history of alcohol-induced cirrhosis presents three months after liver transplantation with jaundice and an alkaline phosphatase level that is three times the upper limit of normal, accompanied by a threefold elevation of the gamma glutamyl transpeptidase (GGTP). A Doppler ultrasound scan shows normal arterial flow, no masses, and no bile duct dilation. A liver biopsy specimen shows bile duct proliferation and no rejection. What test should be performed next?
A. Abdominal computed tomography (CT) with intravenous contrast
B. Bone scan

C. Endoscopic retrograde cholangiopancreatography (ERCP)
D. Hepatic arteriogram

732 Which of the following treatments for nonalcoholic fatty liver disease (NAFLD) is the most appropriate?
A. Antioxidant drug therapy
B. Bariatric surgery for morbid obesity
C. Iron reduction therapy
D. Treatment of the underlying disorder

733 A 37-year-old woman presents with blisters and scarring on the backs of both hands. PCT is diagnosed. Which of the following is most appropriate for management of this condition?
A. Chloroquine
B. Fasting during an outbreak
C. Hematin infusion
D. Phlebotomy
E. Ultraviolet light therapy

734 A 23-year-old woman without known liver disease presents with increasing abdominal girth and right upper quadrant abdominal pain. A 10-cm mass is found in the right lobe of the liver. What is histologic evaluation of the mass likely to show?
A. Hepatocellular carcinoma, fibrolamellar histology
B. Hepatocellular carcinoma, standard histology
C. Lymphoma
D. Metastatic adenocarcinoma

735 A 43-year-old woman has the following laboratory test results: serum bilirubin, total 4.6 mg/dL and direct 0.3 mg/dL; serum alkaline phosphatase, 108 U/L; serum aminotransaminase, aspartate aminotransferase (AST) 18 U/L and alanine aminotransferase (ALT) 22 U/L. What is the most likely diagnosis?
A. Chronic hepatitis C virus infection
B. Dubin-Johnson syndrome
C. Hemolytic anemia
D. Primary biliary cirrhosis
E. Primary sclerosing cholangitis

736 Which of the following changes occurs in the sinusoids with the development of cirrhosis?
A. The passage of macromolecules across the sinusoidal walls is increased.
B. Subendothelial material becomes scanty.
C. The endothelial fenestrations increase in size and number.
D. Disse spaces become widened with collagen.

737 After a three-day fast, which of the following is the primary source of glucose supplied to the brain?
A. Beta oxidation of fatty acids
B. Hepatic gluconeogenesis
C. Hepatic glycogen
D. Muscle glycogen

738 A 45-year-old homosexual man with a new diagnosis of acute hepatitis A virus (HAV) infection asks whether any precautions should be taken to prevent transmission of HAV to his sexual partner. Which of the following strategies would be best for his partner?
A. First dose of HAV vaccine alone
B. HAV serum immunoglobulin and first dose of HAV vaccine
C. HAV serum immunoglobulin alone
D. No prophylaxis necessary

739 A 50-year-old man with decompensated cirrhosis secondary to hepatitis B virus (HBV) is being evaluated for liver transplantation. Pretransplantation testing reveals that the patient is infected with GB virus type C (GBV-C) (hepatitis G virus). GBV-C virus poses a risk of which of the following complications for this patient?
A. Fulminant hepatic failure
B. Increased risk of HBV flare post-transplantation
C. Increased post-transplantation mortality
D. New onset of pancytopenia
E. No clinically significant complications

740 A 41-year-old woman chronically infected with HCV, genotype 1a, 580,000 IU/mL, whose liver biopsy specimen showed stage 2, grade 1 disease has been receiving 180 μg peginterferon alfa-2b subcutaneously per week and 600 mg ribavirin orally twice daily. After 12 weeks of therapy she has had no adverse effects of therapy, her absolute neutrophil count is 800/mL, her hemoglobin level is 10.8 g/dL, her platelet count is 127,000/mL, and her HCV RNA level is 25,000 IU/mL. Which of the following is the most appropriate next step in this patient's care?
A. Add 40,000 IU erythropoietin per week to her medication regimen.
B. Continue current therapy for 12 weeks and then recheck HCV RNA level.
C. Decrease ribavirin to 400 mg twice daily.
D. Discontinue therapy.
E. Increase peginterferon to 180 μg/week.

741 A 17-year-old otherwise healthy girl notes that her urine has become darker than usual and she is having a difficult time concentrating in school. Routine blood work is found to be significant for a hemoglobin level of 8 g/dL. Liver test results are significant for a total bilirubin of 9 mg/dL, alkaline phosphatase of 90 U/L, AST of 700 U/L, and ALT of 890 U/L. Hepatitis A/B/C serology results are negative. Which is the most likely diagnosis?
A. Alcoholic hepatitis
B. Ischemic hepatitis
C. Wilson disease
D. *Amanita phalloides* poisoning
E. Autoimmune hepatitis (AIH)

742 A 55-year-old man presents with new-onset ascites. The ascitic fluid has a protein level of 2.8 g/dL and an albumin level of 2.1 g/dL. A simultaneously obtained serum sample has an albumin level of 3.4 g/dL. Which of the following is the most likely cause of ascites in this case?
A. Cirrhosis
B. Cardiac disease
C. Nephrotic syndrome
D. Pancreatic disease
E. Peritoneal carcinomatosis

743 Bacillary angiomatosis is most commonly associated with which systemic illness?
A. Cirrhosis
B. Colon cancer
C. Acquired immunodeficiency syndrome
D. Hemochromatosis
E. Sarcoidosis

744 A 54-year-old man with HCV-related cirrhosis has just been listed for orthotopic liver transplantation at his local tertiary care hospital. His other viral serology findings are as follows: hepatitis B surface antigen (HBsAg) negative, HBV surface antibody (HBsAb) positive, HBV core antibody (HBcAb) IgG negative, and anti-HAV IgG negative. In addition to routine screening for hepatocellular carcinoma, what additional preventive care measure should be offered to the patient?
A. HAV and HBV vaccination
B. HAV immunoglobulin
C. HAV vaccination only
D. HBV immunoglobulin
E. HBV vaccination only

745 After experiencing a sporadic epidemic of acute hepatitis E virus (HEV), a town in Nepal wants to take measures to prevent another outbreak. Which of the following strategies would be most effective?
A. Boil water for personal use.
B. Discontinue use of multiuse syringes.
C. Discontinue use of well water.
D. HEV immunoglobulin administration to patient contacts
E. Increased use of condoms

746 A 55-year-old man who is three months status post-orthotopic liver transplantation for alcohol-related cirrhosis presents to the emergency department with new-onset jaundice. He has a moderate aminotransferase elevation and leukopenia on laboratory studies. An ultrasound scan reveals no biliary obstruction. A liver biopsy is ordered to help make a diagnosis. Based on the histologic appearance of his biopsy specimen (see figure), what is the most likely diagnosis?

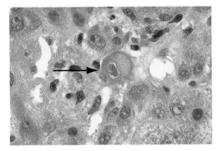

Figure for question **746**

A. Acute rejection
B. Acute alcoholic hepatitis
C. Cytomegalovirus (CMV) infection

D. Drug-induced liver injury
E. Herpes simplex virus (HSV) infection

747 A 55-year-old woman with cirrhosis and a history of hepatic encephalopathy is admitted to the hospital for the third time in one month with tense ascites. At each previous admission, she underwent therapeutic paracentesis with removal of 2 to 3 L of fluid. She has been following a diet restricted to 2 g of sodium per day and taking 160 mg furosemide and 400 mg spironolactone daily for diuresis. Her urine sodium concentration is low, confirming her compliance with a low-sodium diet. Serum sodium and potassium levels are 125 mEq/L and 4.2 mEq/L, respectively. Which of the following is the most appropriate initial approach to managing this patient's ascites?
A. Administer intravenous furosemide.
B. Remove all ascitic fluid possible and add amiloride to her medication regimen.
C. Remove all ascitic fluid possible and start intravenous albumin replacement.
D. Remove as much as 5 L of ascitic fluid and increase the doses of both diuretics.
E. Place a transjugular intrahepatic portosystemic shunt (TIPS).

748 A 48-year-old man who is 18 months status posthotopic liver transplantation for HCV cirrhosis is found to have elevated aminotransferase enzymes. He was treated successfully for post-transplantation recurrent HCV with peginterferon alfa-2a and ribavirin and has no detectable HCV in his serum. Test results for CMV antigenemia are negative, and he is immune to HBV. A liver biopsy specimen shows no evidence of acute rejection, but does show centrilobular necrosis. What is the most likely diagnosis?
A. CMV infection
B. De novo autoimmune hepatitis
C. GBV-C infection
D. HSV infection
E. Recurrent HCV

749 A 60-year-old woman with a 15-year history of primary biliary cirrhosis (PBC) maintained on 15 mg/kg ursodeoxycholic acid (UDCA) daily presents to the emergency department with hematemesis. An urgent upper endoscopy reveals bleeding from large esophageal varices. After endoscopic band ligation and initiation of an intravenous octreotide infusion, the patient becomes more stable and is discharged home five days later on propranolol. The appropriate next step in the management of her PBC should be which of the following?
A. Cholestyramine
B. Glucocorticoids
C. Liver biopsy
D. Liver transplantation evaluation
E. Methotrexate

750 Which of the following criteria are used in predicting the need for liver transplantation in cases of acute liver failure secondary to acetaminophen toxicity?

A. Platelet count, lactate level, hemoglobin level, creatinine level, presence of encephalopathy
B. Platelet count, lactate level, international normalized ratio (INR), creatinine level, presence of encephalopathy
C. pH, lactate level, INR, bilirubin level, albumin level
D. pH, lactate level, INR, creatinine level, presence of encephalopathy
E. pH, lactate level, INR, creatinine level, transaminase levels

751 A 41-year-old woman who is undergoing an ultrasound scan for infertility evaluation is noted to have a 3-cm hyperechoic mass in the left lobe of her liver. She is otherwise well and has no risk factors for or physical examination findings consistent with chronic liver disease. Liver function test results and serum alpha fetoprotein levels are normal. Which is the most appropriate next step in the care of this patient?
A. Hepatic artery embolization
B. Contrast-enhanced magnetic resonance imaging (MRI)
C. No further treatment or testing
D. Radiography-guided biopsy of the mass
E. Surgical resection of the mass

752 Drug-mediated hepatotoxicity that results in formation of intracellular collagen is likely related to activation of which hepatic cell type?
A. Endothelial cells
B. Hepatocytes
C. Kupffer cells
D. Stellate cells

753 A drug in phase II trials caused elevations of ALT to more than eight times the upper limit of normal in 2 of 2500 subjects who received the drug. According to "Hy's rule," this finding during the trial indicates that during the marketing phase, one case of acute liver failure would be expected per every
A. 2500 persons receiving the drug
B. 12,500 persons receiving the drug
C. 50,000 persons receiving the drug
D. 100,000 persons receiving the drug
E. 1,000,000 persons receiving the drug

754 A patient inquires whether he is at risk of deleterious effects on his liver from alcohol. Which of these cofactors puts him at higher risk of such effects?
A. Advanced age
B. Chronic HCV infection
C. Diabetes mellitus and insulin sensitivity
D. Obesity and smoking

755 A 25-year-old woman presents with fever and right upper quadrant abdominal pain. She states that recently she became sexually active with a new partner. You perform a pelvic examination and note a very tender cervix with thick discharge. What is the most likely diagnosis?
A. Hepatic abscess
B. Fitz-Hugh-Curtis disease

C. Cholecystitis
D. Acute viral hepatitis
E. Acute alcoholic hepatitis

756 A cardiologist expresses concern about increased risk of cardiovascular disease in your patient with PBC who has been found to have an elevated low-density lipoprotein (LDL) level. Which of the following is the most appropriate recommendation to address the abnormal LDL level?
A. Prescribe an exercise regimen.
B. Prescribe a low-fat diet.
C. Prescribe a niacin supplement.
D. Order a stress test.
E. No intervention is necessary.

757 A 52-year-old man with chronic back pain is prescribed acetaminophen with oxycodone for pain control. He also has been taking his wife's pain medicine for breakthrough pain. His typical alcohol intake is six beers daily with dinner. He presents to the emergency department of a community hospital with new-onset jaundice, nausea, and renal failure. On examination, he is noted to be oriented but has asterixis. Treatment with *N*-acetylcysteine is started. What is the next step in treating this patient?
A. Admit him to a medical-surgical unit and observe.
B. Begin antibiotic therapy.
C. Discharge him home with close follow-up.
D. Perform a liver biopsy.
E. Refer him to a transplantation center.

758 HCV infection recurs after liver transplantation in all patients who have HCV infection before transplantation. Graft failure due to HCV infection may occur after transplantation. Among others, one predictor of recurrence includes which of the following?
A. The age of the recipient
B. Older deceased donor
C. A low pretransplantation viral load
D. The duration of the operative procedure

759 A 36-year-old woman presents to the emergency department with brisk gastrointestinal hemorrhage. After volume resuscitation and achievement of hemodynamic stability, she undergoes esophagogastroduodenoscopy (EGD). Bleeding esophageal varices are noted; hemostasis is achieved using band ligation. Which of the following is the best way to estimate this patient's portal venous pressure?
A. Measure the portal pressure directly.
B. Measure the variceal pressure endoscopically.
C. Determine the hepatic vein pressure gradient (HVPG).
D. Measure the splenic pulp pressure.

760 A 20-year-old intravenous drug user who is known to be infected with human immunodeficiency virus (HIV) is admitted to the medical intensive care unit with jaundice, asterixis, confusion, and markedly elevated transaminase levels. His sister reports that his primary care physician recently started him on acyclovir for a "cold sore." Based on the histologic appearance of a liver biopsy specimen (see figure), what is the most likely diagnosis?

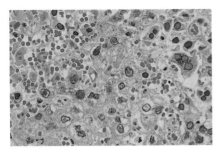

Figure for question 760

A. Acyclovir toxicity
B. HSV infection
C. HBV infection
D. HAV infection
E. Epstein-Barr virus infection

761 A 47-year-old woman presents with severe alcoholic hepatitis. In which of the following circumstances is pentoxifylline more appropriate than glucocorticoids?
A. Ascites and spontaneous bacterial peritonitis
B. Mild jaundice and encephalopathy with active infection
C. Severe jaundice, coagulopathy, and encephalopathy
D. Severe jaundice, encephalopathy, and hepatorenal syndrome (HRS)

762 A 65-year-old woman with a history of PBC (MELD [Model for End-Stage Liver Disease] score of 12) presents with upper gastrointestinal hemorrhage. After she has been resuscitated, she undergoes EGD, which reveals bleeding esophageal varices. Hemostasis is achieved using band ligation, but rebleeding occurs six hours later. On repeat EGD, the bands placed previously are in place, but there is brisk bleeding. More bands are applied, and they control bleeding briefly, but rebleeding occurs again later that day. Which of the following is the most appropriate therapy for this patient at this time?
A. Distal splenorenal shunt
B. Endoscopic sclerotherapy
C. Repeat band ligation
D. Sengstaken-Blakemore tube placement
E. TIPS insertion

763 A patient with Wilson's disease has been taking penicillamine for a number of years. He presents to his physician with the development of a painful vesicular rash along his chest, back, and arms. Which of the following is the correct treatment for this patient?
A. Initiate valganciclovir for zoster infection.
B. Discontinue penicillamine, and start the patient on trientene.
C. Continue penicillamine, and have the patient take an antihistamine.

D. Have the patient stop penicillamine until the rash subsides, and then have the patient resume the medication.
E. Have the patient stop the medication, and monitor the urinary copper levels.

764 A 54-year-old man with a history of end-stage liver disease secondary to hereditary hemochromatosis deficiency presents with upper gastrointestinal hemorrhage. Volume resuscitation and intravenous octreotide are started. On upper endoscopy, active bleeding in the esophagus impedes visibility. This condition should be managed by which of the following?
A. Band ligation of the esophagus every 2 cm in a spiral pattern
B. Circumferential band ligation of the lower esophagus
C. Endoscopic sclerotherapy
D. Withdrawal of the endoscope and esophageal balloon tamponade
E. Withdrawal of the endoscope and immediate placement of a TIPS

765 A 42-year-old woman with cirrhosis secondary to HBV infection is hospitalized with a 3-day history of abdominal pain and fever. Her prehospitalization medication regimen included spironolactone, furosemide, and nadolol. Her temperature is 103.1°F; her blood pressure is 100/65 mm Hg; she has moderate ascites; she has no signs of hepatic encephalopathy. Laboratory test results show a white blood cell count of 6000/μL, platelet count of 85,000/μL, albumin of 2.6 g/dL, total bilirubin of 2.2 mg/dL, and INR of 2.5. Spontaneous bacterial peritonitis (SBP) is suspected. What is the most appropriate next step in the management of this patient's condition?
A. Treat SBP empirically and perform paracentesis when the INR falls to below 1.5.
B. Administer fresh-frozen plasma and then perform paracentesis.
C. Perform paracentesis now.
D. Administer vitamin K subcutaneously and then perform paracentesis.

766 A 55-year-old woman recently moved to the United States from the Far East. She presents to her primary care doctor for symptoms of abdominal bloating, lower extremity edema, and jaundice. She describes having an illness six months before moving to the United States consisting of fever, cough, and arthralgias. She was told she had an upper respiratory infection and was treated symptomatically. On examination, she has scleral icterus tense ascites and lower extremity edema. A CT scan confirms large ascites with splenomegaly. Blood work reveals thrombocytopenia and eosinophilia. Hepatitis viral serologies are negative. The serum IgE level is elevated, and she has leukocytosis. She is HIV negative. What is the most likely diagnosis?
A. Ascariasis
B. Sarcoidosis
C. *Bartonella henselae*
D. Schistosomiasis
E. Malignant ascites

767 Which of the following is positively associated with a sustained virologic response as a result of treatment of HCV infection?
A. African-American ethnicity
B. Co-infection with HIV
C. Biopsy-proven bridging fibrosis or cirrhosis
D. HCV genotype 2
E. Presence of steatosis on biopsy

768 A 35-year-old man presents to the emergency department with the development of abdominal pain and distention over the past week. On examination, he is found to have tender hepatomegaly and ascites but no asterixis. He does not take any medications. His blood work is significant for hemolysis. Urinalysis shows hemoglobinuria. Which of the following is the most likely diagnosis?
A. Acetaminophen-induced liver failure
B. Acute HBV infection
C. α_1-Antitrypsin deficiency
D. Budd-Chiari syndrome
E. Hemochromatosis

769 A 50-year-old man is brought to the emergency department by fire rescue after collapsing at work. He was successfully resuscitated in the ambulance after ventricular fibrillation. An echocardiogram is obtained, and he is noted to have a significant cardiomyopathy. During his hospitalization, he is also diagnosed with diabetes and thrombocytopenia. On review of symptoms, he describes fatigue, loss of libido, and worsening arthritic symptoms. He denies alcohol use. An ultrasound scan of the liver reveals an irregular contour suggestive of cirrhosis. What is the most likely cause of this patient's cirrhosis?
A. Alcohol
B. AIH
C. Hemochromatosis
D. HCV infection
E. Nonalcoholic fatty liver disease

770 A patient with newly diagnosed lung cancer is referred to your office for an elevated ferritin of 580 ng/mL. Transferrin saturation is 45% and testing for the HFE genotype identifies him as homozygous for H63D. His liver test results are normal, he has no risk factors for viral hepatitis, and he does not drink alcohol. Which is the most appropriate management of this patient's condition?
A. Weekly phlebotomy
B. Liver biopsy
C. Iron chelation
D. MRI to screen for hepatocellular carcinoma
E. No further management

771 Which structure is involved in the transport to hepatocyte cytoplasm of messenger RNAs synthesized in hepatocyte nuclei?
A. Endoplasmic reticulum
B. Golgi complex
C. Lysosome
D. Nuclear pore complex
E. Peroxisome

772 A 58-year-old patient with advanced cirrhosis who is on the liver transplantation list is admitted with

hepatic encephalopathy for the third time in a month. His wife reports that he has been compliant with lactulose since his last discharge and has four to five loose bowel movements daily. He had a TIPS placed six weeks ago for refractory ascites. A complete evaluation does not reveal a precipitating factor for his encephalopathy. What is the most appropriate management option?
A. Decrease the dietary protein intake to 1 g/kg/day.
B. Remove the TIPS.
C. Increase lactulose to 1 tablespoon every two hours.
D. Rifaximin 400 mg orally three times daily

773 A 70-year-old woman is brought to the emergency department because of several days of profuse watery diarrhea and vomiting. Her admitting vital signs are significant for a blood pressure of 68/40 mm Hg and a heart rate of 120 beats per minute. Her admission blood work reveals an AST of 3750 U/L and an ALT of 4260 U/L. The bilirubin is 3.1 mg/dL and the INR is 1.9. The following day after administration of intravenous fluids, her AST and ALT are rapidly decreasing and her INR is 1.4. Which is the most likely diagnosis?
A. Acute HCV infection
B. Fulminant liver failure
C. Ischemic hepatitis
D. Acute alcoholic hepatitis
E. Choledocholithiasis

774 Spontaneous HBV e antigen (HBeAg) seroconversion is seen in approximately what percentage of patients chronically infected with HBV annually?
A. 10%
B. 25%
C. 50%
D. 75%

775 Classic histologic findings of alcoholic hepatitis include which of the following?
A. Hepatocellular necrosis, bridging fibrosis, steatosis
B. Hepatocyte ballooning, Mallory hyaline bodies, neutrophilic infiltrate
C. Regenerative nodule formation with Mallory hyaline bodies
D. Steatosis with chronic inflammatory infiltrate

776 Fibrogenesis involves which type of liver cells?
A. Kupffer cells
B. Cholangiocytes
C. Ito cells
D. Sinusoidal cells

777 A 36-year-old man is noted to have jaundice two days after uncomplicated appendectomy. The surgery and postoperative course were uneventful, without documented episodes of hemodynamic instability, and his surgical incision has no signs of infection. He is found to have an elevated indirect bilirubin level with a serum ALT level 1.5 times the upper limit of normal. The results of a complete blood count with differential are normal. Which of the following is the most likely diagnosis?

A. Analgesic agent–induced hepatotoxicity
B. Anesthetic agent–induced hepatotoxicity
C. Hemolytic anemia
D. Ischemic hepatitis
E. Postoperative cholestasis

778 A 25-year-old Chinese woman presents for a routine evaluation. The results of a test for HBsAg are positive despite normal results of liver function tests. How did this patient most likely acquire chronic HBV infection?
A. Horizontal transmission
B. Parenteral transmission
C. Sexual transmission
D. Vertical transmission

779 A 43-year-old woman with a diagnosis of cutaneous porphyria is referred by a dermatologist. Further testing reveals a severe Coombs-negative hemolytic anemia. Which is the most likely diagnosis?
A. Congenital erythropoietic porphyria
B. Erythropoietic protoporphyria
C. Hepatoerythropoietic porphyria
D. PCT

780 A 12-year-old boy is seen in consultation for growth retardation, episodic irritability, lethargy, and refusal to eat animal protein such as milk, eggs, and meat. Which of the following abnormalities is most characteristic of ornithine transcarbamylase deficiency?
A. Elevated plasma ammonia
B. Elevated plasma citrulline
C. Metabolic acidosis
D. Serum aminotransaminase levels of less than 1000 U/L

781 A 57-year-old recent immigrant from Egypt has acute hepatitis with IgM antibody against HEV. How did he most likely become infected?
A. Blood transfusion
B. Consumption of contaminated drinking water
C. Consumption of raw pork
D. Exposure to an infected relative
E. Vertical transmission

782 A 35-year-old woman presents to her primary care physician with malaise and jaundice. Laboratory studies are notable for an AST of 1300 U/L and ALT of 1100 U/L. The bilirubin is elevated at 3.5 mg/dL. She is completely oriented but her INR is elevated to 1.9. Her creatinine is also elevated at 2.5 mg/dL, and although blood is reported in the urine, no red blood cells are seen. She denies any use of intravenous drugs but was at a party two nights before. What is the most likely exposure leading to these abnormalities?
A. Alcohol
B. HCV
C. Marijuana
D. Cocaine
E. HAV

783 A 52-year-old man is brought to the emergency department with fever and sharp, diffuse abdominal pain. His temperature is 102.2°F, pulse is 90 beats per minute, and blood pressure is 110/78 mm Hg.

His abdomen is distended with ascites and diffusely tender without rebound or guarding. Diagnostic paracentesis is performed. Which of the following results for total protein, glucose, and lactate dehydrogenase (LDH) is consistent with a diagnosis of secondary bacterial peritonitis?
A. Total protein 0.6 g/dL, glucose 120 mg/dL, LDH 300 U/L
B. Total protein 0.6 g/dL, glucose 20 mg/dL, LDH 100 U/L
C. Total protein 1.0 g/dL, glucose 100 mg/dL, LDH 150 U/L
D. Total protein 2.0 g/dL, glucose 100 mg/dL, LDH 150 U/L
E. Total protein 2.0 g/dL, glucose 20 mg/dL, LDH 300 U/L

784 Of these patients with acute alcoholic hepatitis, which would be most appropriately treated with glucocorticoids to reduce short-term mortality?
A. A 40-year-old man with jaundice, encephalopathy, severe coagulopathy, and renal failure
B. A 40-year-old woman with jaundice and encephalopathy but with no evidence of infection, renal failure, or gastrointestinal bleeding
C. A 60-year-old man with mild jaundice but with no coagulopathy, infection, renal failure, or encephalopathy
D. None; glucocorticoids have not been shown to reduce short-term mortality in patients with alcoholic hepatitis.

785 A 42-year-old woman presents with a three-week history of progressive fatigue, right upper quadrant discomfort, nausea, and jaundice. Her serum ALT level is 10 times the upper limit of normal. The presence of which of the following in a blood sample is most indicative of acute HBV infection?
A. Anti-HBc IgG
B. Anti-HBc IgM
C. Anti-HBs
D. HBsAg

786 A 58-year-old woman with chronic HCV infection was treated with 24 weeks of peginterferon/ribavirin, but had no virologic response. Because of the presence of hepatic fibrosis, she is being considered for further therapy. Which is the most accurate estimate of sustained virologic response in her situation?
A. Less than 5%
B. 10%
C. 35%
D. 50%
E. 85%

787 A 67-year-old man with HCV-induced cirrhosis is noted on screening EGD to have large esophageal varices with no signs of recent hemorrhage. He has no clinical signs or symptoms of blood loss. Which of the following is the most appropriate course of action for this patient?
A. Administer octreotide intravenously.
B. Begin nonselective beta blocker therapy.
C. Begin oral nitrate therapy.

D. Perform band ligation of the esophageal varices.
E. Perform sclerotherapy of varices.

788 A 56-year-old man has been noted to have a fatty liver on ultrasonography. A liver biopsy is suggested to establish the prognosis, but the patient would rather pursue a noninvasive evaluation. Which option is most accurate for predicting fibrosis in NAFLD?
A. FibroTest
B. Ultrasonography
C. MRI with gadolinium
D. Liver-spleen scan
E. Fasting triglycerides

789 An 83-year-old man presents to the emergency department with abdominal pain and hypotension. An 8-cm vascular mass, actively bleeding, is seen in the right lobe of the liver on angiography. Exploratory laparotomy is performed to control the bleeding, and a biopsy of the mass is performed. The results of histologic evaluation of the biopsy specimen are consistent with angiosarcoma. Which occupational exposure is likely to have contributed to the development of this patient's cancer?
A. Asbestos
B. Pesticides
C. Petroleum
D. Plastics

790 A 54-year-old homeless man with a long history of tobacco and intravenous drug abuse is evaluated for new-onset ascites. He has not seen a physician for 25 years and is taking no medications. Physical examination is notable for bitemporal atrophy, muscle wasting in the upper extremities, moderate ascites, and ankle edema. Ascites fluid analysis shows a leukocyte count of 1000/μL (35% polymorphonuclear leukocytes, 65% lymphocytes) and a serum-ascites albumin gradient (SAAG) of 1.0 g/dL. Gram staining shows no bacteria, and culture results are pending. What is the most likely diagnosis?
A. Cardiac ascites
B. Cirrhosis
C. Peritoneal carcinomatosis
D. Spontaneous bacterial peritonitis
E. Tuberculous peritonitis

791 A 73-year-old man presents with a six-week history of fatigue and dull right upper quadrant discomfort followed by a four-week history of jaundice. He has had frequent bouts of prostatitis, which have been treated with antibiotics. He has an elevated direct bilirubin level, minimally elevated alkaline phosphatase level, aminotransferase levels 10 times the upper limit of normal, and normal albumin. His antinuclear antibody titer is 1:40. Which of the following is the most likely cause of his drug-induced hepatic injury?
A. Amoxicillin
B. Cephalexin
C. Ciprofloxacin
D. Nitrofurantoin
E. Trimethoprim/sulfamethoxazole

792 A 19-year-old female college student presents to the emergency department after her roommate noticed

that she had developed jaundice. Initial blood work shows total bilirubin of 12.4 mg/dL, direct bilirubin of 7.2 mg/dL, AST of 1200 U/L, and ALT of 1374 U/L. Which is the most likely cause of her liver injury?
A. Depo-Provera
B. Multivitamin
C. Levothyroxine
D. "Weight loss" supplement
E. Nicotine patch

793 A 50-year-old woman presents with persistently elevated serum aminotransaminase levels and a body mass index of 40 kg/m². Serologic test results are negative for autoimmune, infectious, and metabolic diseases. Ultrasonography demonstrates a fatty liver, and evaluation of a biopsy specimen shows steatosis, lobular inflammation, and fibrosis. Which feature of this patient's presentation is most predictive of progression to advanced liver disease?
A. Elevated serum transaminase levels
B. Her sex and age
C. Inflammation and fibrosis on biopsy specimen
D. High body mass index (obesity)
E. Steatosis on biopsy specimen

794 Which of the following is most infectious?
A. HBV
B. HCV
C. HIV

795 A 33-year-old man taking isoniazid prophylactically is noted to have increased serum levels of aminotransaminases and bilirubin. Which of the following courses of action will be most effective?
A. Start cholestyramine.
B. Discontinue isoniazid.
C. Start glucocorticoids.
D. Start N-acetylcysteine.
E. Start UDCA.

796 Which hepatic structure allows a difference in concentration of solutes between the cytoplasm and bile canaliculus?
A. Anchoring junction
B. Gap junction
C. Lipid rafts
D. Tight junction

797 A 66-year-old woman presents with jaundice. She was recently started on a new medication, but cannot recall the name. Which of the following agents is the most likely to cause hepatotoxicity?
A. Amoxicillin/clavulanic acid
B. Ibuprofen
C. Isoniazid
D. Tamoxifen
E. Trimethoprim/sulfamethoxazole

798 A 56-year-old woman presents for management of chronic HCV after being refused as a blood donor. Her risk factor for HCV infection is a brief period of intravenous drug use while in her teens. She has no symptoms, the results of her physical examination are unremarkable, her serum ALT level was slightly elevated on two occasions, and she is found to have an HCV RNA (genotype 1a) level

of 430,000 IU/mL. Which of the following is most helpful in determining her prognosis?
A. ALT level
B. Duration of HCV infection
C. HCV genotype
D. HCV viral load
E. Results of a liver biopsy

799 A 17-year-old girl has abnormal serum aminotransaminase levels. Serologic evaluation and liver biopsy are undertaken. The liver biopsy specimen (see figure) shows the presence of periodic acid-Schiff (PAS)–positive, diastase-resistant periportal globules. Which protease inhibitor (Pi) genotype (allelic representation) is the serologic evaluation likely to show?

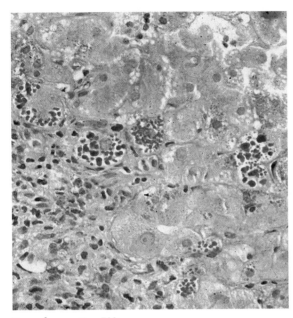

Figure for question **799**

A. PiMM
B. PiMZ
C. PiSS
D. PiSZ
E. PiZZ

800 Immediately after orthotopic liver transplantation, which constellation of findings most strongly indicates poor graft function?
A. Electrolyte imbalance and renal failure
B. Liver enzyme levels 10 times the upper limit of normal on the first postoperative day
C. Nonanion gap acidosis
D. Persistent coagulopathy and impaired cognition

801 A 52-year-old man is referred for evaluation of persistently elevated serum levels of liver enzymes. His medical history is notable for chronic atrial fibrillation, hypertension, and diabetes mellitus. His medication regimen includes nifedipine, warfarin, and metformin. He has had no exposure to hepatotropic viruses, nor does he drink alcohol. His laboratory test results are as follows: serum

bilirubin, total 0.6 mg/dL and direct 0.1 mg/dL; alkaline phosphatase 78 U/L; GGTP 250 U/L; serum aminotransaminases AST 23 U/L; ALT 16 U/L. Which of the following is the most appropriate next step in management for this patient?
A. Abdominal ultrasound scan
B. ERCP
C. Liver biopsy
D. No further testing
E. Serum 5´-nucleotidase level

802 A 25-year-old woman presents reporting fatigue, sore throat, and intermittent fever. Lymphadenopathy is present on physical examination, and her laboratory studies reveal abnormal serum aminotransaminase levels. Which of the following is the most likely cause of her signs and symptoms?
A. HSV infection
B. Group A *Streptococcus* infection
C. HAV infection
D. Epstein-Barr virus infection
E. Transfusion-transmitted virus infection

803 A 35-year-old Chinese woman who has been HBsAg positive and anti-HBe positive is pregnant. Which is the most accurate estimate of transmitting HBV to her newborn infant?
A. 90%
B. 80%
C. 20%
D. 5%

804 Where is the site of fatty acid synthesis within the liver?
A. Cytosol
B. Membrane-bound proteins
C. Mitochondria
D. Nucleus

805 A 45-year-old woman with newly diagnosed PBC seeks your opinion on what medical therapy is available to treat her condition. You inform her that the only medical therapy approved by the U.S. Food and Drug Administration for PBC is
A. Diphenhydramine
B. Ursodeoxycholic acid
C. Prednisone
D. Rifampin
E. Cholestyramine

806 A 62-year-old man presents to the emergency department with nausea, vomiting, lethargy, and jaundice. In reviewing his medical history, he states that he recently returned from visiting his family in Oregon. While there, he and his brother went mushroom picking and ate what they found. He is not concerned because he cooked the mushrooms completely. His blood work reveals an AST level of 3500 and an ALT level of 6100. His bilirubin is 12.5, his INR is 2.1, and his creatinine is 1.8. You initiate the following therapy for *Amanita phalloides* poisoning as you begin the liver transplant evaluation:
A. Hemodialysis
B. Penicillamine
C. Penicillin
D. Plasmapheresis
E. Steroids

807 A 57-year-old man with Child-Pugh class B cirrhosis due to chronic HCV infection is found to have a 3-cm hepatocellular carcinoma in the right lobe on MRI. There is an enhancing thrombus in the right portal vein. Which of the following is the most appropriate approach to treatment of this patient?
A. Chemoembolization followed by transplantation
B. Liver transplantation
C. Radiofrequency ablation or ethanol injection
D. Surgical resection

808 A 42-year-old woman is incidentally noted to have a 4-cm cyst in the right lobe of the liver. She denies abdominal pain, fever, or recent travel. The cyst has no internal echoes on ultrasonography. Which is the most appropriate management?
A. Aspiration
B. Cyst cavity sclerosis
C. Laparoscopic fenestration
D. Observation only
E. Percutaneous drain

809 A 52-year-old woman with a known history of chronic HCV infection has active upper gastrointestinal hemorrhage, scleral icterus, gynecomastia, spider angiomata, and splenomegaly. Which of the following medications should be prescribed first?
A. Nitroglycerin
B. Octreotide
C. Propranolol
D. Terlipressin
E. Losartan

810 Women have greater susceptibility than men to the injurious effects of alcohol on the liver. Risk factors that predispose to this heightened susceptibility in women include which of the following?
A. Increased endotoxemia and lipid peroxidation
B. Lower body mass index
C. Less gastric mucosal secretion of alcohol dehydrogenase
D. Slower alcohol metabolism

811 A 67-year-old man presents to the hospital with variceal hemorrhage. In deciding how to control the hemorrhage, the endoscopist should be aware of which of the following possible complications of sclerotherapy that is not seen with band ligation?
A. Elevation of hepatic venous pressure gradient
B. Esophageal perforation
C. Esophageal stricture
D. Esophageal ulceration

812 A 38-year-old man is newly diagnosed with decompensated AIH manifested by onset of ascites and encephalopathy. He is started on diuretic therapy and lactulose. What is the next best step in managing this patient's condition?
A. Azathioprine
B. Tacrolimus
C. Steroids only
D. Steroids and transplantation evaluation
E. Transplantation evaluation only

813 A 16-year-old high school student is brought to the emergency department by his mother because over the past two or three days he has become lethargic and confused. His family has noticed that over the past few months, he has become withdrawn and irritable and started to have problems with homework. Laboratory test results show that his hemoglobin level is 10.6 g/dL, total bilirubin is 26.4 mg/dL, direct bilirubin is 7.9 mg/dL, AST is 934 U/L, ALT is 788 U/L, alkaline phosphatase is 104 U/L, and INR is 1.7. Which of the following is the most appropriate course of treatment for this patient?
A. Administer intravenous *N*-acetylcysteine.
B. Initiate a transplantation evaluation.
C. Initiate penicillamine therapy.
D. Infuse α_1-antitrypsin.
E. Begin therapeutic phlebotomy.

814 A 75-year-old woman with congestive heart failure and respiratory failure experiences cardiopulmonary arrest but is successfully resuscitated within three minutes. The next morning, she has markedly elevated liver function enzymes (AST is 12,000 U/L and ALT is 9000 U/L). Her INR is also elevated at 2.4. The most appropriate treatment for this patient would be which of the following?
A. Anticoagulation therapy
B. Administration of HBV immunoglobulin and initiation of lamivudine therapy
C. Administration of *N*-acetylcysteine
D. A course of prednisone
E. Provision of supportive care and treatment of her underlying conditions

815 A 65-year-old woman has had pruritus, fever, and weight loss for three weeks. She does not have icterus, but there are bilateral temporal wasting and a palpable, smooth liver edge. Her bilirubin and aminotransaminase levels are normal, but her alkaline phosphatase level is four times the upper limit of normal and her GGTP level is elevated. Ultrasonography shows an echogenic liver without ductal dilation. On the basis of these findings, which of the following is the most likely diagnosis?
A. Extrahepatic biliary obstruction
B. Granulomatous hepatitis
C. Nonalcoholic fatty liver disease
D. Paget's disease of bone
E. Renal cell carcinoma

816 A 43-year-old woman known to have advanced PBC presents to the emergency department after a minor motor vehicle accident that she believes was caused by worsening night vision. She also reports easy bruising on her skin, which is evident on examination. She has no asterixis and is alert and oriented to person, place, and time. After being cleared by the emergency department physicians of any serious injury, you should recommend which of the following nutritional therapies?
A. Fat-soluble vitamin supplementation
B. Vitamin B_{12} supplementation
C. Vitamin C supplementation
D. Thiamine supplementation
E. Calcium supplementation

817 Since 1995, the incidence of HAV infection has decreased by 90% in the United States. Among which of the following subgroups was the rate of decrease the greatest?

A. Children 5 to 14 years old
B. Adults 20 to 44 years old
C. Adults 45 to 65 years old
D. Homosexual men of any age
E. Intravenous drug users of any age

818 A 48-year-old man with HCV- and alcohol-related cirrhosis is hospitalized with a two-day history of fever and abdominal discomfort. His temperature is 102.2°F, he has abdominal distention with shifting dullness, and a small, reducible umbilical hernia is noted. Laboratory test results reveal a sodium level of 130 mEq/L, albumin of 2.5 g/dL, and ALT of 75 U/L. Ascitic fluid has an albumin level of 1 g/dL and a polymorphonuclear leukocyte count of 500/μL. Which of the following is the most appropriate next step in managing this patient?
A. Administration of ampicillin plus an aminoglycoside
B. Large-volume paracentesis
C. Surgery to correct the umbilical hernia
D. Administration of a third-generation cephalosporin
E. Placement of a TIPS

819 A 30-year-old woman has a new diagnosis of AIH confirmed by liver biopsy. The first choice for single-drug therapy for this patient would be which of the following?
A. Prednisone
B. Azathioprine
C. Cyclosporine
D. Tacrolimus
E. UDCA

820 A 52-year-old African-American woman with cryptogenic cirrhosis notes progressive exertional dyspnea, despite being fully compliant with a salt-restricted diet and a high-dose diuretic medication regimen. Pulse oximetry shows an oxygen saturation of 92% while sitting and 88% when standing. The results of her cardiac and pulmonary system examinations are normal, she has minimal ascites and trace ankle edema, and her weight has been stable over the past several months. Which of the following is the most likely diagnosis in this case?
A. Hepatopulmonary syndrome (HPS)
B. Portopulmonary hypertension
C. Sarcoidosis
D. Hepatic hydrothorax

821 A 44-year-old man with HCV cirrhosis presents with increasing abdominal girth, ankle edema, and a 20-lb weight gain over the past four months. On physical examination, he has scleral icterus and moderate ascites. Laboratory test findings include the following: sodium 132 mEq/L, potassium 3.8 mEq/L, creatinine 1.1 mg/dL, albumin 3.0 g/dL, and total bilirubin 2.7 mg/dL. Ascitic fluid analysis showed an albumin level of 1.2 g/dL and neutrophil count of 180/μL. In addition to a salt-restricted diet, which of the following is recommended to manage his ascites?
A. Diuretic therapy with a loop diuretic
B. Diuretic therapy with a loop diuretic and spironolactone
C. Fluid restriction

D. Serial large-volume paracentesis
E. TIPS placement

822 A 50-year-old Asian man presents with cirrhosis due to HBV complicated by ascites that has been controlled with diuretics and a 2.5-cm hepatocellular carcinoma. His alanine aminotransferase level is three times the upper limit of normal. The result of a test for HBsAg is positive, the HBeAg test result is negative, and the HBV DNA level is 5 million copies/mL. It is decided that the patient would benefit from liver transplantation. Which therapy would be most likely to minimize the risk of recurrence of HBV after liver transplantation?
A. Nucleoside/nucleotide analog, administered orally
B. Chemoembolization of the tumor
C. Immediate listing for liver transplantation
D. Peginterferon combined with oral lamivudine

823 A 39-year-old woman has had elevated serum aminotransferase levels for more than a year. Her medical history is notable for type 2 diabetes mellitus and hypertriglyceridemia. Serum test results for possible liver pathogens are negative. Ultrasonography reveals increased hepatic echogenicity. What is the most likely finding on histologic evaluation of a biopsy specimen?
A. Interface hepatitis with lymphocytoplasmic infiltrate
B. Nonsuppurative destructive cholangitis
C. PAS-positive diastase-resistant periportal globules
D. Perisinusoidal fibrosis and Mallory hyaline bodies
E. Portal lymphoid aggregates with germinal centers

824 A 35-year-old liver transplant recipient with HCV infection who is in her third postoperative year presents with hypertension and renal insufficiency. What is the most likely cause?
A. Calcineurin inhibitor–induced nephrotoxicity
B. Immunosuppression-related renal cell cancer
C. New-onset diabetes mellitus
D. Recurrent HCV infection complicated by membranoproliferative renal disease

825 A 39-year-old patient with cirrhosis and ascites has been gaining an average of 500 g of weight every day despite taking 40 mg furosemide and 100 mg spironolactone daily. Her serum sodium level is 128 mEq/L, potassium is 3.8 mEq/L, and creatinine is 1.5 mg/dL. She is excreting 120 mEq of sodium in the urine daily. What is the most appropriate management?
A. Increase furosemide to 80 mg/day
B. Increase spironolactone to 200 mg/day
C. Increase furosemide to 80 mg/day and spironolactone to 200 mg/day
D. Keep sodium restriction to 88 mEq/day
E. Add metolazone 2.5 mg/day

826 A 55-year-old man presents to your clinic concerned that he has hereditary hemochromatosis. He explains to you that his cousin was just diagnosed with this disease at age 50 and has been found to have cirrhosis. The patient has noticed that he has been having a more difficult time achieving an erection and describes a loss in libido. His serum iron and ferritin levels are within normal limits. Which is the most appropriate next step in management?

A. Phlebotomy therapy
B. Genetic testing for hereditary hemochromatosis
C. Liver biopsy
D. Reassure the patient.
E. Screening for liver cancer

827 Cholestasis and hepatocellular inflammation develop in a 55-year-old man after treatment with an aminopenicillin. Which of the following techniques is most specific for a diagnosis of drug-induced hepatotoxicity?

A. Drug rechallenge
B. In vitro testing
C. Liver biopsy
D. Peripheral eosinophil count
E. Skin biopsy

828 In which of the following patients with elevated liver enzymes would a diagnosis of NAFLD be most likely, excluding other causes?

A. A 40-year-old female patient with insulin resistance
B. A 55-year-old male patient with hypertension
C. A 65-year-old male patient who consumes 15 g of alcohol per day
D. A 70-year-old female patient with a body mass index of 28

829 A 63-year-old man with alcohol-related cirrhosis is noted on CT to have a patent periumbilical vein. Considering the mechanisms involved in portal hypertension, which of the following is likely to be present?

A. Decreased cardiac output
B. Increased mean arterial pressure
C. Peripheral vasoconstriction
D. Splanchnic vasodilation

830 A 26-year-old woman in her third trimester of pregnancy returns from a six-week medical school rotation in India. She seeks medical attention after developing flu-like symptoms followed by dark urine, jaundice, and clay-colored stools. A right upper quadrant ultrasound scan shows a normal biliary tree. She denies a history of intravenous drug use and has not been sexually active for the past two months. She has IgG antibodies to HAV and was vaccinated for HBV before starting medical school. Which of the following is the most likely diagnosis in this case?

A. Acute HAV infection
B. Acute HBV infection
C. Acute HCV infection
D. Acute hepatitis D virus infection
E. Acute HEV infection

831 A 28-year-old female health care worker presents after an accidental self-puncture with an 18-gauge hollow-bore needle that had been used to withdraw blood from an HCV-infected patient. At the time of presentation, she tests negative for anti-HCV antibodies, HCV RNA is detectable at a level of 5690 IU/mL, and serum transaminase levels are normal.

Which of the following is the most appropriate management of this case?

A. Administer HCV immunoglobulin, 1.5 mL intramuscularly.
B. Start peginterferon therapy at 180 μg/week for 24 weeks.
C. No further evaluation is necessary.
D. Start peginterferon, 180 μg/week, and ribavirin, 600 mg orally twice daily, for 48 weeks.
E. Recheck for viremia at three months.

832 A 45-year-old woman with cirrhosis due to AIH presents with encephalopathy and ascites. The ascites persists despite dietary salt restriction and a diuretic regimen. She has no comorbid illnesses and lives with her extended family. What intervention will have the greatest impact on the patient's survival?

A. Prescribe high-dose diuretic therapy and nonabsorbable antibiotic therapy.
B. Evaluate for liver transplantation.
C. Insert a splenorenal shunt.
D. Place a TIPS.

833 Which of the following is synthesized primarily outside the liver?

A. Apolipoproteins
B. Fatty acids
C. 3-Hydroxy-3-methylglutaryl–coenzyme A (CoA) reductase
D. Lipoprotein lipase

834 A 2-year-old infant is admitted to the hospital with severe drug-induced hepatotoxicity. Which of the following agents is most likely to be implicated?

A. Diclofenac
B. Isoniazid
C. Nitrofurantoin
D. Phenytoin
E. Valproic acid

835 A 20-year-old man from Afghanistan presents with increasing abdominal girth and painful hepatomegaly. The hepatic venous system appears to be patent, but a liver biopsy specimen shows evidence of hepatic veno-occlusive disease (VOD). Which of the following herbal therapies has most likely caused liver disease in this case?

A. Chaparral (*Larrea tridentata*)
B. Comfrey (*Symphytum officinale*)
C. Germander (*Teucrium chamaedrys*)
D. Kava kava (*Piper methysticum*)
E. Pennyroyal (*Hedeoma pulegoides*)

836 A 37-year-old woman with splenic vein thrombosis presents with brisk hematemesis. The patient is hemodynamically stable. She is given transfusion products, started on octreotide and antibiotics, and then is sent for endoscopy. At endoscopy, a large pool of blood is seen in the fundus, and inferior to this pool are bleeding gastric varices, estimated at 15 mm in size. Which of the following is the most appropriate next step in managing this patient's condition?

A. Balloon tamponade
B. Endoscopic band ligation
C. Endoscopic sclerotherapy

D. Epinephrine injection
E. TIPS placement

837 A patient has abnormal aminotransaminase levels and suspected NAFLD based on negative results of serum tests for liver pathogens or other infectious agents and imaging studies to evaluate for other liver diseases. What is the best rationale for performing a percutaneous liver biopsy in this patient?
A. To exclude occult iron overload disorders
B. To counsel the patient on the possible risk of future complications
C. To establish the diagnosis
D. To identify the most appropriate pharmacotherapeutic approach

838 A 38-year-old woman who has been taking oral contraceptives for 12 years undergoes an abdominal ultrasound scan because of a bout of right upper quadrant pain, and a mass is seen. She is otherwise well. Her only medication is oral contraceptives. MRI shows a brightly enhancing 6-cm mass in the periphery of the right lobe of the liver. The mass has a "spoke-wheel" appearance but no central scar. Which of the following is most appropriate for managing this patient's condition?
A. Arterial embolization
B. Exploratory laparoscopy
C. Radiologic percutaneous biopsy
D. Repeat MRI in six months
E. Surgical resection

839 A 50-year-old woman presents with fatigue and persistently abnormal aminotransaminase levels. The results of a right upper quadrant ultrasound scan are normal. She has no abdominal pain, weight loss, or diarrhea. Blood test results for evidence of viral hepatitis are negative. She was recently diagnosed with Graves disease. Her laboratory test results show an antinuclear antibody (ANA) titer of 1:320, a ferritin level of 200 ng/mL, an α_1-antitrypsin MM phenotype, a normal ceruloplasmin level, and negative antimitochondrial antibody. Which of the following serologic tests would support the likely diagnosis?
A. Anti-Ro, Anti-La
B. Elevated IgM fraction on serum protein electrophoresis
C. Anti–smooth muscle antibody
D. HFE genotype
E. Liver/kidney microsome type 1 antibody

840 A 55-year-old man with a history of alcohol-induced cirrhosis has abstained from alcohol use for three years. He has been vaccinated against HAV and HBV and has twice-yearly alpha fetoprotein determinations and regular cross-sectional images of the liver. Which of the following is most important in determining his prognosis?
A. Hepatic venous pressure gradient
B. Liver size on CT or MRI
C. Serum albumin level
D. Size of esophageal varices

841 A 48-year-old man is noted to be coinfected with HCV and HIV. Compared with HCV monoinfected patients, which of the following is correct?

A. Antiviral therapy can be given regardless of the CD4$^+$ count.
B. Coinfected patients are more likely to spontaneously clear HCV.
C. Coinfected patients have slower rates of hepatic fibrosis.
D. Rates of interferon-induced sustained virologic response are higher.
E. Ribavirin should not be used with didanosine.

842 A 50-year-old Asian woman notes the gradual appearance of ascites and leg edema. The urine has 4+ proteinuria, and the serum albumin is 2.8 g/L. She has been HBsAg positive with a slightly elevated ALT level in the past. Her mother died of hepatocellular carcinoma and her siblings are all HBsAg positive, with one of them having decompensated cirrhosis. Her kidney biopsy specimen shows membranous glomerulonephritis. The HBV DNA is 1000 IU/mL. Which of the following is the best management for this patient?
A. Treatment with diuretics
B. High-protein diet
C. Nucleoside analog treatment

843 A patient with cirrhotic ascites is admitted for SBP. He has significant coagulopathy and pancytopenia and is jaundiced. In addition to intravenous antibiotics, which other therapy is indicated for the management of SBP?
A. Correction of coagulopathy with vitamin K
B. Intravenous octreotide
C. Blood transfusion
D. Correction of coagulopathy with fresh-frozen plasma
E. Intravenous albumin

844 A 22-year-old man with a history of cystic fibrosis (CF) is referred for evaluation of constant, achy right upper quadrant discomfort. Ultrasonography shows notable nodularity of the liver and evidence of portal hypertension. Histologic examination of a needle biopsy specimen is likely to show which of the following?
A. Inflammatory changes and bile duct proliferation
B. PAS-positive, diastase-resistant periportal globules
C. Steatosis, hepatocyte ballooning, and Mallory hyaline bodies
D. Widespread staining with Prussian blue

845 A 23-year-old man is brought to the emergency department with rhabdomyolysis, hypotension, hyperpyrexia, disseminated intravascular coagulation, and renal failure. Serum aminotransaminase levels are in excess of 1000 U/L. Ingestion of which substance is most likely responsible for this patient's condition?
A. Cocaine
B. Ecstasy (3,4-methylenedioxymethamphetamine)
C. Heroin
D. Methamphetamine
E. Phencyclidine ("angel dust")

846 A 24-year-old man is admitted to the intensive care unit after intentional acetaminophen overdose. He is intubated, unresponsive, and mildly hypotensive and has no signs of chronic liver disease. His transaminase levels are in excess of 3000 U/L, INR is 4.5, and creatinine is 3.7 mg/dL. What will be the most likely cause of death?

A. Cerebral herniation
B. Coagulopathy with bleeding
C. Hemodynamic collapse
D. Liver synthetic failure
E. Renal failure

847 A 22-year-old man develops acute hepatitis, ultimately found to be due to acute HBV infection. The infection is self-limited, with full recovery after a period of jaundice. Which is the most accurate estimate of this man's risk of chronic HBV infection?

A. 5%
B. 15%
C. 50%
D. 75%
E. 90%

848 A 72-year-old Asian man with chronic *Clonorchis sinensis* infection has had multiple admissions to the hospital with fever, right upper quadrant pain, tender hepatomegaly, and eosinophilia. At this admission, he presented with weight loss and a palpable abdominal mass. Imaging reveals an enhancing intrahepatic mass. Which of the following is the most likely diagnosis?

A. Angiosarcoma
B. Cholangiocarcinoma
C. Hemangiosarcoma
D. Hepatocellular carcinoma
E. Metastatic gastric adenocarcinoma

849 A 55-year-old man with a history of HCV-related cirrhosis undergoes orthotopic liver transplantation. The surgery is uneventful; the patient is extubated on day 2 and is discharged from the hospital on day 8. Two months later, jaundice associated with an elevated alkaline phosphatase level and slightly increased serum aminotransminase levels develops. Ultrasonography shows that hepatic vessels are patent, and a cholangiogram reveals a normal biliary anastomosis. Liver biopsy reveals profound cholestasis, minimal chronic portal inflammatory infiltrates, and extensive portal-portal fibrous bridging. Which of the following is the most accurate prediction of this patient's clinical course?

A. The development of cholestasis, biochemical and histologic, may signal the rapid development of graft failure.
B. Resolution of recurrent disease with therapy
C. Resolution of laboratory test abnormalities over six months
D. Retransplantation within one year

850 A 35-year-old man with a two-year history of abnormal results of serum tests of liver function is found to have steatohepatitis, and evaluation of a liver biopsy specimen shows fibrosis. He attempts to lose weight, but is unsuccessful; elevations persist on liver tests. Citing a newsletter that he receives, the patient requests a prescription for pioglitazone for his condition. Which of the following is a likely effect of pioglitazone?

A. Reduction in fibrosis
B. Reduction in transaminases
C. Sustained effect with drug discontinuation
D. Weight loss

851 A 63-year-old woman with a 30-year history of chronic HCV infection presents with leg swelling and purpura consisting of round, 1- to 3-mm palpable lesions that coalesce to form plaques in some areas. Testing is most important for which of the following?

A. Anti–glomerular basement membrane antibody
B. Antineutrophil cytoplasmic antibody
C. ANA
D. Rheumatoid factor
E. Serum cryoglobulin

852 A 47-year-old man has had fever and right upper quadrant discomfort for the past six to eight weeks. His history is significant for a recent episode of diverticulitis. He states that he was treated with antibiotics for this infection; however, he stopped taking the antibiotics after several days when his symptoms of diverticulitis improved. You perform a CT scan and identify a 7-cm liver abscess. Which of the following should you recommend?

A. Resection of abscess and antimicrobial therapy
B. Percutaneous drainage and antimicrobial therapy
C. Antimicrobial therapy alone
D. Initiation of metronidazole
E. Test stool for ova and parasites

853 A six-week-old infant presents with lethargy and seizures. Physical examination is notable for a protruding abdomen, hepatomegaly, and muscular hypotonia. Laboratory evaluation is notable for metabolic acidosis. Which of the following tests is the best to establish the diagnosis of glycogen storage disease type I?

A. Abdominal CT with contrast
B. Fasting serum glucose measurement
C. Glucagon response test
D. Liver biopsy

854 A patient who raises livestock for a living presents to your office after a CT scan obtained in the emergency department for abdominal pain reveals a calcified sharply circumscribed cyst containing two "daughter" cysts. Which of the following is the most likely diagnosis?

A. Schistosomiasis
B. *Entamoeba histolytica*
C. *Strongyloides*
D. *Echinococcus* sp.
E. Metastatic colon cancer

855 A 67-year-old woman recently emigrated from India. She is brought to the emergency department for abdominal distention, weight gain, and jaundice. She does not take any medications on a regular basis and explains that she drinks medicinal hot tea almost daily. She undergoes a liver biopsy, and histologic evaluation of the biopsy specimen shows sinusoidal dilation and severe hepatic congestion. Inflammation is notably absent. Which of the following is the most likely diagnosis?

A. Budd-Chiari syndrome
B. Congestive heart failure
C. Drug toxicity
D. Graft-versus-host disease
E. VOD

856 A 28-year-old Hispanic man presents with a two-week history of abdominal pain, fever, malaise, and myalgias. He is found to have a fluid-filled abscess in his liver. The radiologist who aspirated the fluid for diagnostic purposes describes the aspirate as reddish brown and pasty. Trophozoites are identified on microscopic examination. Which of the following is the best treatment for this liver abscess?
A. Third-generation cephalosporin
B. Resection
C. Metronidazole
D. Praziquantal
E. Albendazole

857 A 30-year-old woman was recently diagnosed with autoimmune hepatitis by positive ANA with a titer of 1:320 and a characteristic liver biopsy specimen. The medical student on rotation with you asks how to describe the characteristic histologic findings of AIH on biopsy. Which of the following should be your response?
A. Florid bile duct lesion, granulomas, ductopenia
B. Ground-glass appearance of hepatocytes
C. Interface hepatitis, lymphoplasmacytic infiltration, rosette formation
D. Microvesicular fat and Mallory hyaline bodies
E. Piecemeal necrosis, lymphocytic infiltration

858 A liver biopsy specimen obtained from a patient with newly diagnosed PBC would most likely show which of the following?
A. Ground-glass appearance of hepatocytes
B. Ductopenia and florid bile duct lesion
C. Microvesicular fat and hyaline bodies
D. Obliterative fibrosis cholangitis
E. "Owl's-eye" inclusions

859 Autoimmune thyroiditis, Graves disease, and ulcerative colitis are the most common extrahepatic immune-mediated diseases associated with which of the following conditions?
A. PBC
B. Celiac disease
C. Type 1 AIH
D. Type 2 AIH
E. HCV

860 A 62-year-old woman with alcoholic cirrhosis has become progressively lethargic over the past few days. On physical examination, she is somnolent but oriented and able to follow commands and has asterixis and sluggish reflexes. Which of the following statements regarding ammonia (NH3) measurements and hepatic encephalopathy (HE) is true?
A. The blood level of NH3 is more accurately measured in a sample of arterial blood than in a sample of venous blood.
B. A normal serum NH3 level excludes the diagnosis of HE.
C. Serial measurements of NH3 levels are indicated to assess response to treatment.

D. The serum NH3 level correlates poorly with the severity of HE.

861 A 25-year-old intravenous drug user presents to the emergency department with jaundice, fever, hypotension, elevated transaminase levels, and an elevated INR. Determining the level of which of the following factors may help to distinguish sepsis from acute liver failure?
A. Factor II
B. Factor V
C. Factor VII
D. Factor VIII
E. Factor IX

862 A 75-year-old man is brought to the emergency department after being found unconscious at home. He is nonresponsive, hypothermic, and hypotensive. Initial laboratory studies reveal abnormal liver chemistries: serum bilirubin, total 1.4 mg/dL and direct 0.3 mg/dL; serum alkaline phosphatase 84 U/L; serum aminotransaminases, AST 1570 U/L and ALT 128 U/L. Which of the following is the most likely diagnosis?
A. Acetaminophen overdose
B. Acute alcoholic hepatitis
C. Ischemic hepatitis
D. Mesenteric vasculitis
E. Rhabdomyolysis

863 A 25-year-old man in whom acute HAV infection was diagnosed approximately one month ago reports continued jaundice, fatigue, and dark urine. He denies having fever or abdominal pain. His laboratory test results are positive for HAV IgM, negative for HBsAg, and negative for HCV antibody. A right upper quadrant ultrasound scan shows a nondilated biliary tree and no gallstones. What is the best course of action for treatment at this time?
A. Liver biopsy
B. Continue symptomatic care.
C. MRCP of the abdomen and pelvis
D. ERCP

864 A 55-year-old woman from South America who works as a fruit vendor in her country is visiting family. During her visit, it is noted that jaundice has developed. She is brought to the emergency department for evaluation. A chest x-ray shows an infiltrate, and laboratory test results reveal eosinophilia, a total bilirubin of 4.2 mg/dL, direct bilirubin of 2.8 mg/dL, and alkaline phosphatase of 541 U/L. MRI with magnetic resonance cholangiopancreatography is performed, and bile duct dilation is noted. She is scheduled for a therapeutic ERCP. What is the most likely cause of this patient's biliary obstruction?
A. Ascariasis
B. Cholangiocarcinoma
C. Choledocholithiasis
D. Metastatic colon cancer
E. Sarcoidosis

865 A 30-year-old woman is diagnosed with acute HEV infection. Urine human chorionic gonadotropin testing is negative. This condition is most likely to progress to which of the following?

A. Fulminant hepatic failure
B. Chronic hepatitis
C. Resolution
D. Cirrhosis
E. Hepatocellular cancer

866 A 63-year-old man from China presents with right upper quadrant abdominal pain and jaundice. CT of the abdomen reveals a 6-cm enhancing mass in the left hepatic lobe. His serum alpha fetoprotein level is 598 ng/mL. What is the likelihood of hepatocellular carcinoma?
A. 10%
B. 50%
C. 75%
D. 100%

867 Which of the following is the best initial approach to treat systemic hypertension in the absence of volume overload after liver transplantation?
A. Angiotensin-converting enzyme inhibitor
B. Furosemide
C. Nifedipine
D. Reduction in doses of immunosuppressant medications

868 Which of the following regarding the surface anatomy of the liver is true?
A. At the porta hepatis, the portal vein is anterior to the hepatic artery.
B. The caudate lobe of the liver is posterior to the transverse fissure.
C. The falciform ligament contains the obliterated umbilical artery.
D. All surfaces of the liver lie within the peritoneum.

869 A 45-year-old man with alcoholic cirrhosis is hospitalized with refractory ascites, oliguria, and failure to thrive. On physical examination, he looks chronically ill and has noticeable ascites, but no fever, jaundice, peripheral edema, or encephalopathy. His blood urea nitrogen (BUN) and creatinine levels have increased over the past six weeks from 18 mg/dL and 1.5 mg/dL to 20 mg/dL and 1.8 mg/dL, respectively. The results of routine blood and urine cultures are negative; a sample of ascitic fluid shows 120 neutrophils. A sample of nasogastric lavage fluid is negative for blood. What is the best next step in managing this patient?
A. Start antibiotic therapy for SBP.
B. Perform EGD.
C. Increase the dose of his current diuretic medication.
D. Administer intravenous fluids for intravascular volume expansion.
E. Insert a transvenous intrahepatic portosystemic shunt.

870 Infections with transfusion-transmitted virus and SEN virus are similar because both viruses
A. Can adversely affect treatment for chronic HCV infection
B. Are associated with increased mortality
C. Can progress to chronic infection and cirrhosis
D. Can be acquired through parenteral and fecal-oral transmission

E. Are predominantly acquired through sexual transmission

871 You are asked to evaluate a 76-year-old man in the hospital for abnormal liver tests and an ultrasound scan that shows hepatomegaly and trace ascites with patent vessels. In reviewing the medical records, you learn that the patient has a history of coronary artery disease and was admitted with dyspnea and lower extremity edema. The liver tests show total bilirubin of 2.5 mg/dL, direct bilirubin of 1.5 mg/dL, alkaline phosphatase of 185 U/L, and normal transaminase levels. Paracentesis yields fluid with 145 white blood cells per milliliter, an SAAG of 2.2, and a normal total protein level. Which of the following is the most likely diagnosis?
A. Alcoholic cirrhosis
B. Choledocholithiasis
C. Congestive hepatopathy
D. Budd-Chiari syndrome
E. PBC

872 A 54-year-old woman with HCV cirrhosis and ascites has been compliant with a sodium-restricted (2 g/day) diet and her diuretic regimen of 200 mg spironolactone daily and 80 mg furosemide daily. She has gained 8 lb over six weeks. A blood sample obtained at the time of evaluation shows a sodium level of 128 mEq/dL, potassium of 3.9 mEq/dL, and creatinine of 0.7 mg/dL, and a urine sample shows a sodium/potassium ratio of 0.8. What should be done to address this patient's weight gain?
A. Admit the patient for intravenous administration of furosemide.
B. Further restrict sodium intake to 500 mg/day.
C. Educate the patient about how to follow a low-sodium diet.
D. Increase her dose of spironolactone.
E. Increase her doses of spironolactone and furosemide.

873 A 28-year-old man presents with asymptomatic elevation of serum aminotransaminase levels. Serologic evaluation reveals the presence of anti-HCV antibodies. From an epidemiologic perspective, which is the most likely source of viral transmission?
A. Blood transfusion
B. Intravenous drug use
C. Occupational needle-stick injury
D. Perinatal transmission
E. Sex with an HCV-infected partner

874 A 56-year-old man presents with alcohol-related cirrhosis. Which of the following is thought to be the principal mechanism of liver fibrosis in this patient?
A. Alcohol-mediated free radical injury
B. Chronic intrahepatic cholestasis
C. Increase in matrix degradation
D. Increase in stellate cell activation

875 A 41-year-old woman who is diagnosed with breast cancer needs chemotherapy. She has been known to be an HBsAg-positive carrier for years but with normal liver function. What advice would you provide the oncologist?

A. Prophylactic treatment with a nucleoside analog

B. Treatment with a nucleoside analog if the HBV DNA is greater than 105 copies/mL

C. Treatment with a nucleoside analog if ALT flares during chemotherapy

D. Prophylactic treatment with HBV immunoglobulin

876 A 54-year-old man with a history of end-stage liver disease secondary to hereditary hemochromatosis deficiency presents with upper gastrointestinal hemorrhage. Volume resuscitation and intravenous octreotide are started. On upper endoscopy, active bleeding in the esophagus impedes visibility. This condition should be managed by which of the following?

A. Band ligation of the esophagus every 2 cm in a spiral pattern

B. Circumferential band ligation of the lower esophagus

C. Endoscopic sclerotherapy

D. Withdrawal of the endoscope and esophageal balloon tamponade

E. Withdrawal of the endoscope and immediate placement of a TIPS

877 A 43-year-old depressed woman is brought to the emergency department with nausea, vomiting, diarrhea, and jaundice. Laboratory tests reveal indirect hyperbilirubinemia, hemolysis, elevated serum transaminase rhabdomyolysis, and evidence of renal failure. This patient's condition is most likely due to which of the following?

A. Acetaminophen

B. *Amanita phalloides*

C. Carbon tetrachloride

D. Copper

878 A 38-year-old woman presents for further evaluation of vague right upper quadrant pain, pruritus, and abnormal liver test results. Her primary care physician has already ordered a right upper quadrant ultrasound scan, which showed cholelithiasis without gallbladder wall thickening, pericholecystic fluid, or ductal dilation, and a quantitative hepatobiliary iminodiacetic acid scan, which showed a normal gallbladder ejection fraction. Her laboratory test results reveal the following: an albumin level of 4.0 g/dL, bilirubin 1.2 mg/dL, alkaline phosphatase 350 U/L, AST 65 U/L, ALT 72 U/L, antimitochondrial antibody 1:1280, ANA 1:20, HCV antibody negative, antibody to anti-HBc negative, HBsAg negative, and anti-HBs positive. What is this patient's most likely diagnosis?

A. AIH

B. Symptomatic cholelithiasis

C. HBV infection

D. HCV infection

E. PBC

879 A 45-year-old man is referred for evaluation of abnormal liver test results. He has a medical history of dyslipidemia and hypertension. Physical examination reveals central obesity and a smooth, palpable liver edge. His serum aminotransaminase levels are twice the upper limit of normal with maintained hepatic synthetic function. Which of the following studies is best able to differentiate between steatosis and steatohepatitis?

A. CT

B. Liver biopsy

C. MRI

D. Positron emission tomography

E. Ultrasonography

880 The most common cause of acute liver failure worldwide is which of the following?

A. Acetaminophen

B. AIH

C. Budd-Chiari syndrome

D. HAV infection

E. HBV infection

881 A 33-year-old woman attends a holiday party on a cruise ship. She has some alcoholic drinks and eats freely from the buffet table. Two weeks later, she presents with diarrhea, fever, myalgias, and periorbital edema. A complete blood count shows leukocytosis and eosinophilia. A muscle biopsy is diagnostic, and she is treated promptly with albendazole. What was the food that was most likely the source of the pathogen causing her infection?

A. Canned fruit

B. Cream pie

C. Pork

D. Potato salad

E. Refried rice

882 A 24-year-old woman is found to be jaundiced. She is otherwise healthy. Physical examination shows only scleral icterus. Laboratory studies are most notable for a total bilirubin of 5.6 mg/dL, alkaline phosphatase of 190 U/L, and normal serum aminotransferases. Which drug is the most likely cause of her cholestasis?

A. Aminopenicillin

B. Phenytoin

C. Nitrofurantoin

D. Oral contraceptive

ANSWERS

726 **D** (S&F, ch76)

Porphyrias are commonly classified according to clinical features into two main groups: acute porphyrias, which are characterized by dramatic and potentially life-threatening neurologic symptoms, and cutaneous porphyrias, which typically cause few or no neurologic symptoms but instead give rise to a variety of severe skin lesions (see table at the end of chapter). Variegate coproporphyria is the only example given of an acute porphyria; the other conditions listed are cutaneous porphyrias. The signs and symptoms of the acute neurovisceral attacks that occur in the four acute porphyrias vary considerably. Abdominal pain is present in more than 90% of patients, followed by tachycardia and dark urine in approximately 80% of patients. The other acute porphyrias are alanine dehydratase deficiency, acute intermittent porphyria, and hereditary coproporphyria.

727 **D** (S&F, ch84)

The risk of liver disease is two to three times higher in drinkers who are obese than in drinkers who have a normal body mass. Although an increased risk of fatty liver is not surprising in obese persons, obesity also seems to be an independent risk factor for both alcoholic hepatitis and cirrhosis. Cigarette smoking also has been shown to accelerate the progression of fibrosis in patients with alcoholic liver disease as well as accelerate disease progression in patients with HCV infection who drink heavily.

728 **A** (S&F, ch86)

Amiodarone is an iodinated benzofuran derivative used for therapy-resistant ventricular tachyarrhythmias. Adverse effects lead to discontinuation of therapy in 25% of patients. These adverse effects include pulmonary infiltrates, worsening cardiac failure, hypothyroidism, peripheral neuropathy, nephrotoxicity, and corneal deposits, but liver disease is one of the most serious. The spectrum of abnormalities includes abnormal liver biochemical test levels in 15% to 80% of patients and clinically significant liver disease, including rare cases of acute liver failure, in 0.6%. Liver disease also has been reported in patients who receive an intravenous loading dose of amiodarone; the toxic ingredient is likely to be the vehicle (polysorbate 80) rather than amiodarone because oral amiodarone has been used subsequently in these cases without a problem. The most typical hepatic lesion is steatohepatitis; cirrhosis develops in 15% to 50% of patients with hepatoxicity.

729 **D** (S&F, ch79)

Monogamous sexual partners who do not engage in high-risk sexual activity have a negligible risk of transmission. In view of the low rate of vertical transmission, pregnancy and breast-feeding are not contraindicated in HCV-infected women. Data regarding the risk associated with vaginal delivery as opposed to cesarean delivery are uncontrolled, but evidence of a higher risk of HCV transmission with vaginal delivery is unconvincing. This issue remains controversial, and some authorities recommend elective cesarean section before membrane rupture. Because HCV antibodies can be acquired passively by the infant, molecular testing is required if the diagnosis of HCV infection is suspected. Infants of infected mothers should not undergo serologic testing for HCV antibodies before the age of 18 months because maternal antibodies may persist in the infant's serum and lead to diagnostic confusion.

730 **A** (S&F, ch71)

The portal vein supplies 70% of the blood flow to the hepatic parenchyma. The common hepatic artery arises from the celiac artery. The cystic arteries usually arise from the right hepatic artery. Arterial ligation is usually well tolerated by persons with normal liver function.

731 **C** (S&F, ch95)

This patient's alkaline phosphatase level indicates bile duct obstruction or injury. The ultrasound scan results do not suggest large bile duct obstruction; however, the histologic findings strongly suggest obstruction, so the lack of obstruction must be confirmed by ERCP. Another reason to perform ERCP is that it would identify anastomotic strictures that may be present in the patient as a consequence of surgery. A CT scan is not likely to alter the need for ERCP. The elevation of the GGTP level makes an extrahepatic source for alkaline phosphatase, such as bone, unlikely; thus, a bone scan is not indicated. Finally, because the Doppler ultrasound scan results are normal, a hepatic arteriogram is not indicated at this time.

732 **D** (S&F, ch85)

The optimal therapy for NAFLD has not been established. To date, no large, randomized treatment trials demonstrating resolution of steatosis, inflammation, and fibrosis have been conducted in patients with NAFLD. Small numbers, varying inclusion criteria, and varying endpoints have limited the clinical impact of published studies. Historically, the treatment of NAFLD has consisted of weight loss, removal of offending drugs and toxins, and control of associated metabolic disorders, including diabetes mellitus and hyperlipidemia. Several case reports and small studies of diet and exercise have shown improvements in biochemical, ultrasonographic, and, in some cases, histologic abnormalities in children and adults with NAFLD.

733 **D** (S&F, ch76)

PCT, the most common of the porphyrias, typically involves a 50% reduction in activity of the enzyme uroporphyrinogen decarboxylase. PCT is strongly associated with high alcohol intake, estrogen therapy, and systemic illnesses, including systemic lupus erythematosus, diabetes mellitus, chronic renal failure, and acquired immunodeficiency syndrome. For unclear reasons, concomitant HCV infection is strongly associated with expression of PCT. Treatment of PCT initially consists of removal of any offending agent. Historically, treatment has included phlebotomy to decrease iron overload and hepatic siderosis. This approach may provide relief of cutaneous symptoms in four to six months. Chloroquine complexes with uroporphyrin and facilitates its excretion, but caution must be used during chloroquine therapy because the drug is potentially hepatotoxic. Chloroquine therapy has been variably effective in patients with PCT who are homozygous for mutations in the hemochromatosis *HFE* gene; for them, phlebotomy should be first-line therapy.

734 **A** (S&F, ch94)

The fibrolamellar variant of hepatocellular carcinoma typically occurs in young patients, has an approximately equal sex distribution, does not secrete alpha fetoprotein, is not caused by chronic

HBV or HCV, and almost always arises in a noncirrhotic liver. Fibrolamellar hepatocellular carcinoma is more often amenable to surgical treatment and therefore generally carries a better prognosis than that for conventional hepatocellular carcinoma. It does not, however, respond to chemotherapy any better than do other forms of hepatocellular carcinoma. Chronic ulcerative colitis is a risk factor for primary sclerosing cholangitis, which is, in turn, a risk factor for cholangiocarcinoma. In the Far East, the most common risk factors for cholangiocarcinoma are chronic biliary infections, especially infections with *C. sinensis*.

735 **C** (S&F, ch73)
The first step in the evaluation of a patient with an isolated elevation of the serum bilirubin level is to fractionate the bilirubin to determine whether it is conjugated or unconjugated bilirubin (see figure). If less than 15% of the total is conjugated, one can be assured that virtually all the serum bilirubin is unconjugated. An overproduction of bilirubin as a result of excessive breakdown of hemoglobin can occur with any of a number of inherited or acquired disorders, including hemolytic anemia (see table at end of chapter). The patient's medication history should be reviewed for drugs that can cause impaired hepatocellular uptake of bilirubin. If no cause is identified, a genetic enzyme deficiency that results in impaired conjugation of bilirubin, the most common of which is Gilbert's syndrome, is likely. The remaining choices are causes of conjugated bilirubin elevations.

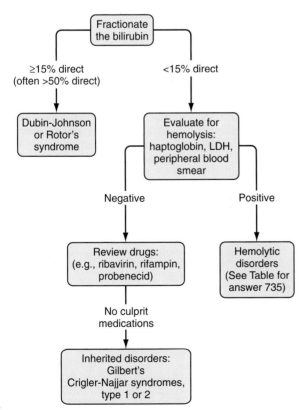

Figure for answer **735**

736 **D** (S&F, ch71)
During the development of cirrhosis, the sinusoids acquire some features of systemic capillaries; the Disse space becomes widened with collagen, basement membrane material is deposited, and endothelial fenestrations become smaller and less numerous, all leading to decreased transport across sinusoidal walls.

737 **B** (S&F, ch72)
Glycogen stored in the liver is the main source of rapidly available glucose for the glucose-dependent tissues, such as red blood cells, retina, renal medulla, and brain. Hepatic glycogen stores contain as much as a two-day supply of glucose before gluconeogenesis occurs, mainly from lactate, a three-carbon end-product of anaerobic glucose metabolism. Hepatic gluconeogenesis produces as much as 240 mg of glucose a day, which is approximately twice the metabolic need of the red blood cells, retina, and brain. During fasting, a decrease in plasma insulin levels removes the inhibition of the gluconeogenic enzymes PEPCK and fruc-1,6-P2ase. Simultaneously, an increase in glucagon and β-adrenergic agonists increases intracellular cyclic adenosine monophosphate levels, leading to inhibition of 6-PK-2 kinase activity and stimulation of fruc-2,6-Pase, thereby reducing fruc-2,6-P2 concentration and activation of fruc-1,62Pase, with a net increase in gluconeogenesis. After a prolonged fast, gluconeogenesis is further stimulated by an increase in the supply of substrate and alterations in the concentration of various enzymes.

738 **B** (S&F, ch77)
Administration of serum immunoglobulin and the first dose of HAV vaccine, along with good hygiene practices are the mainstays of preventing HAV infection. In June 2007, the HAV vaccine was approved for use in postexposure prophylaxis of immunocompetent persons, ages 12 months to 40 years, without chronic liver disease. When immunoglobulin is used for postexposure prophylaxis, it should be given within two weeks of exposure at a recommended dose of 0.02 mL/kg by intramuscular injection. Although considered safe, immunoglobulin can cause fever, myalgias, and pain at the injection site. Postexposure prophylaxis with immunoglobulin can be accompanied safely with initiation of active immunization with the vaccine, and this course is recommended rather than immunoglobulin alone.

739 **E** (S&F, ch81)
GBV-C is a positive-strand RNA virus, is found worldwide, and is present in approximately 20% of HCV-infected persons. GBV-C infection does not seem to cause liver disease or any other disorder. In addition, it does not seem to modulate the course or response to treatment of chronic HCV or HBV infection. GBV-C infection also does not affect the outcome of liver transplantation. Although liver transplant recipients have high rates of GBV-C infection, the outcome of transplantation is unaffected by current or past GBV-C infection.

740 **D** (S&F, ch79)

A serum HCV RNA level should be obtained at baseline in all patients. Assessment of the decrease in the HCV RNA level during treatment predicts the likelihood of a sustained viral response (SVR), can be used to determine the duration of therapy, and is essential for determining treatment failure in genotype 1–infected patients. Therefore, quantitative HCV RNA levels should be drawn at baseline and at weeks 4 and 12. If HCV RNA is still detectable in serum at week 12, a level should also be drawn at week 24. If the HCV RNA level has not been lowered by at least 2 logs (99%) after 12 weeks of treatment or is still detectable at week 24, treatment should be stopped. Use of the serum HCV RNA level at week 12 to indicate an early virologic response does not apply to patients with genotype 2 or 3 infection.

741 **C** (S&F, ch75)

This patient has Wilson's disease. Wilson's disease is most commonly diagnosed in children and young adults and should be suspected in this age group. This disorder results from a defect in the *ATP7A* gene and results in copper retention in the liver resulting in hepatocyte injury. Patients can present in various ways, from asymptomatic abnormalities in blood work to fulminant hepatic failure. Patients presenting with severe acute Wilson's disease are often noted to have hemolysis with an elevated hyperbilirubinemia and anemia resulting in jaundice. AST and ALT levels are often quite elevated compared with the alkaline phosphatase, which is either normal or below normal in acute settings. Patients presenting in this manner need to be diagnosed expeditiously and transferred to a liver transplantation facility as copper chelators are not beneficial in this setting.

742 **B** (S&F, ch91)

Appropriate treatment of ascites depends on the cause of fluid retention. Accurate determination of the etiology of ascites is crucial. The SAAG is helpful diagnostically and for therapeutic decision making. Patients with a low SAAG usually do not have portal hypertension and do not respond to salt restriction and diuretics (except for those with nephrotic syndrome). Conversely, patients with a high SAAG have portal hypertension and are usually responsive to these measures. Among the choices listed, only cardiac ascites is associated with an SAAG of more than 1.1 g/dL and a protein level greater than 2.5 g/dL.

743 **C** (S&F, ch82)

Bacillary angiomatosis is a gram-negative bacillus that primarily infects patients with acquired immunodeficiency syndrome. This disease manifests in most patients by the development of multiple blood-red papular skin lesions. However, systemic illness can also be seen and can lead to sepsis with multiorgan system failure. In the liver, this disease can manifest as peliosis hepatitis. The bacteria can be identified by polymerase chain reaction (PCR) and the treatment is with erythromycin or doxycycline.

744 **C** (S&F, ch77)

Persons with chronic liver disease are at increased risk of HAV-related morbidity and mortality if they acquire the infection. Therefore, preexposure prophylaxis with the HAV vaccine has been recommended for patients with chronic liver disease who are susceptible to HAV. This recommendation should be extended to patients awaiting liver transplantation as well as those who have already undergone liver transplantation, although the immunogenicity of the HAV vaccine is reduced in such persons. This patient already has immunity to HBV, as evidenced by HBsAb positivity, so he does not require immunization or immunoglobulin against HBV. HAV immunoglobulin is not indicated in the absence of an exposure to HAV.

745 **A** (S&F, ch80)

In the epidemic setting, measures to improve the quality of water, including boiling water for personal use, have been shown to decrease the number of new cases. The occurrence of large epidemics of HEV among adults in endemic areas suggests either that anti-HEV is not fully protective or that antibody levels in serum decline with time, gradually reaching a nonprotective level. In the few studies that have evaluated the role of immunoglobulin manufactured in endemic areas for pre- or postexposure prophylaxis, no significant reduction in disease rates with use of this agent was found. A vaccine for HE is not currently available, although one is undergoing phase II testing at the current time. The experimental vaccine showed 95.5% protective efficacy against HEV among those receiving three doses over six months and may prove to be an important intervention in the future.

746 **C** (S&F, ch81)

The biopsy (see figure for question 746) shows an enlarged hepatocyte with a large nucleus that contains an "owl's-eye" inclusion and is characteristic of CMV infection. Multinucleated giant cells with mononuclear portal and parenchymal inflammatory infiltrates and cholestasis are commonly seen on liver biopsy specimens from patients with CMV hepatitis. Large nuclear "owl's-eye" inclusions may be seen in hepatocytes or biliary epithelial cells. CMV hepatitis can be difficult to distinguish from graft rejection in liver transplant recipients. Because CMV viremia precedes organ involvement, testing for CMV antigenemia or CMV PCR testing of blood are useful screening tools in immunocompromised patients.

747 **C** (S&F, ch91)

Therapeutic paracentesis is the accepted first-line therapy for patients with tense ascites. Because this patient has recurrent ascites despite maximal doses of diuretics, removal of all ascitic fluid possible is indicated. In addition, albumin replacement with large-volume paracentesis has been shown to decrease mortality and renal failure. TIPS placement is a second-line choice because it is associated with an increased risk of hepatic encephalopathy.

748 **B** (S&F, ch88)

De novo AIH is a clinical syndrome that affects both children and adults who undergo transplantation for nonautoimmune liver disease. Patients with de novo AIH in whom glucocorticoid therapy fails experience worsening hepatic fibrosis with possible graft loss, and those who do not receive glucocorticoids progress to cirrhosis, require retransplantation, or die of liver failure. De novo AIH in some adults has been associated with severe centrilobular necrosis, and adult patients have been reported to express an atypical anti–liver-kidney cytosolic antibody of uncertain pathogenic significance. AIH should be included in the differential diagnosis of allograft dysfunction in all transplant recipients.

749 **D** (S&F, ch89)

The best therapeutic alternative for patients with end-stage PBC is liver transplantation. Evaluation for liver transplantation should be prompted by complications related to portal hypertension, including bleeding from gastroesophageal varices, diuretic-resistant ascites, HRS, and hepatic encephalopathy. In patients with PBC, the development of complications associated with chronic cholestasis, such as a poor quality of life secondary to disabling fatigue, intractable pruritus, and severe muscle wasting, as well as persistent increases in the serum bilirubin level in the absence of hepatic malignancy, should also prompt clinicians to consider referral for liver transplantation, even in patients without cirrhosis on a liver biopsy specimen. A liver biopsy is unlikely to change management at this time. Cholestyramine may help with pruritus in PBC but has no adjuvant role to UDCA. Methotrexate or glucocorticoid is not recommended as monotherapy or as an adjuvant to UDCA in PBC.

750 **D** (S&F, ch93)

Investigators at King's College in London performed a multivariate analysis of clinical and biochemical variables and their relationship to mortality in 588 patients with acute liver failure. In this analysis, a major distinction was made between acetaminophen toxicity and other causes of acute liver failure. For liver failure due to acetaminophen toxicity, the King's College criteria for liver transplantation were as follows: (1) pH less than 7.3 or arterial lactate greater than 3.5 mmol/L at four hours or arterial lactate greater than 3.0 mmol/L at 12 hours or (2) INR greater than 6.5 (prothrombin time >100 seconds), (3) serum creatinine greater than 3.4 mg/dL, and (4) stage 3 or 4 encephalopathy.

751 **B** (S&F, ch94)

This incidentally discovered mass is likely to be a cavernous hemangioma, the most common benign tumor of the liver. Although the ultrasonographic appearance of this tumor is variable, the lesion is usually echogenic. Contrast-enhanced CT or MRI is diagnostic. Biopsy is unnecessary, and, in fact, some reports on series of patients with this tumor have suggested that biopsy in these cases is associated with an increased risk of bleeding. Hemangioma rarely requires resection, which is usually only performed when a patient has severe symptoms or hemorrhage.

752 **D** (S&F, ch72)

Hepatic stellate cells (formerly referred to as fat-storing or Ito cells) are the principal liver cell type involved in matrix deposition and hepatic fibrosis. Stellate cells are activated in methotrexate-induced hepatic fibrosis, and the possibility that vitamin A, drugs, or drug metabolites can transform stellate cells into collagen-synthesizing myofibroblasts is of considerable interest.

753 **B** (S&F, ch86)

A relationship may exist between the frequency and severity of serum ALT elevations that indicate liver injury and the risk of severe hepatotoxicity. This relationship was proposed in the 1970s by the late Hyman Zimmerman. According to "Hy's rule," elevations of serum ALT levels to eightfold or more above the upper limit of normal or associated increases in the serum bilirubin concentration indicate a potential for the drug to cause acute liver failure at a rate of approximately 10% of the number of cases of jaundice. Therefore, if two cases of jaundice associated with drug-induced liver injury are observed in a total phase III clinical trial experience of 2500 patients, approximately one case of acute liver failure would be expected for every 12,500 subjects prescribed the drug during the marketing phase.

754 **B** (S&F, ch84)

The cofactor that influences progression of alcoholic liver disease most profoundly is HCV infection. Between one fourth and one third of patients with alcoholic liver disease have serologic or virologic evidence (or both) of HCV infection. The prevalence of HCV infection is highest in patients who have used injection drugs; however, the risk is high even among those who deny drug use. Histologic features of focal lymphoid aggregates, portal inflammation, and periportal or bridging fibrosis are common in liver biopsy specimens from alcoholics with HCV infection. Of greater importance, liver disease is more severe, advanced disease develops at a younger age, and survival is shorter in patients with both alcoholic liver disease and HCV infection than in patients with alcoholic liver disease and no evidence of HCV infection. In one of the more striking examples of the interaction between alcohol abuse and hepatitis C, Corrao and colleagues found that the relative risk of cirrhosis was 10-fold higher among heavy drinkers with chronic HCV than among those who had no evidence of HCV infection. In addition, there seems to be synergism between alcohol and HCV in the development of hepatocellular carcinoma.

755 **B** (S&F, ch82)

This patient has classic symptoms of pelvic inflammatory disease, especially with the history of a new sexual partner and the very tender cervical examination. The additional symptom of right upper quadrant pain is most likely secondary to pelvic inflammatory disease with perihepatic involvement. Often one can appreciate a hepatic rub on examination. Most often the liver tests are normal, and the diagnosis, if in question, can be confirmed with laparoscopic visualization. Most common pathologic organisms involved in this disease are gonorrhea and *Chlamydia*. She should be treated for both bacteria with a combination of ceftriaxone and azithromycin or doxycycline.

756 **E** (S&F, ch89)

Lipid abnormalities are found in as many as 85% of patients with PBC. High-density lipoprotein cholesterol levels are usually most prominently elevated in the early stages of PBC. As the disease progresses, high-density lipoprotein cholesterol levels decrease and LDL cholesterol levels increase. However, the risk of atherosclerosis in these patients with PBC and hyperlipidemia does not seem to be increased. Therapy with UDCA has been shown to lower the LDL cholesterol levels in patients with PBC and has been useful in some patients with xanthelasmas. Simvastatin may also decrease LDL levels in patients with PBC and is still undergoing investigation.

757 **E** (S&F, ch93)

Acute liver failure is defined as the rapid development of hepatocellular dysfunction (i.e., coagulopathy) and mental status changes (i.e., encephalopathy). The reported incidence of acute liver failure due to acetaminophen overdose has been increasing recently. In many of these "therapeutic misadventures," patients ingested over-the-counter products containing acetaminophen along with prescription narcotic-acetaminophen congeners. Long-term heavy ethanol consumption may lower the threshold for acetaminophen toxicity in some patients via induction of cytochrome P-450 enzyme activity. Only liver transplantation has been effective in treating patients with irreversible liver failure. Unfortunately, many patients with irreversible acute liver failure do not undergo transplantation because of late referral, contraindications, or lack of donor livers. Therefore, patients in acute liver failure should be evaluated for liver transplantation as soon as possible and, if no contraindications are identified, placed on a liver transplantation waiting list.

758 **A** (S&F, ch95)

Various factors have been implicated as predictors of recurrent HCV infection after liver transplantation. These include higher serum viral levels before and immediately after liver transplantation, older deceased donor age, and episodes of acute rejection.

759 **C** (S&F, ch90)

Measurement of the HVPG has been proposed for the following indications: (1) to monitor portal pressure in patients taking drugs used to prevent variceal bleeding, (2) as a prognostic marker, (3) as an endpoint in trials using pharmacologic agents for the treatment of portal hypertension, (4) to assess the risk of hepatic resection in patients with cirrhosis, and (5) to delineate the cause of portal hypertension (that is, presinusoidal, sinusoidal, or postsinusoidal) (see table at end of chapter), usually in combination with venography, right-sided heart pressure measurements, and transjugular liver biopsy. Although the indication for HVPG measurement with the most potential for widespread use is monitoring the efficacy of therapies to reduce portal pressure, HVPG monitoring is not done routinely in clinical practice because no controlled trials have yet demonstrated its usefulness. Splenic pulp pressure is an indirect method of measuring portal pressure and involves puncture of the splenic pulp with a needle catheter. Because of potential risks of splenic puncture, however, the procedure is now rarely used. Direct portal pressure measurements are performed when HVPG cannot be measured, as in patients with Budd-Chiari syndrome with occluded hepatic veins in whom a surgical portosystemic shunt is being contemplated or in patients with intrahepatic, presinusoidal causes of portal hypertension such as idiopathic portal hypertension (in which case HVPG may be normal). Variceal pressure can be measured by inserting into the varices a needle connected to a fluid-filled catheter that is in turn connected to a pressure transducer; use of this method is not justified unless variceal pressure measurement can be followed by variceal injection sclerotherapy. Because variceal sclerotherapy has fallen out of favor, measuring variceal pressure by variceal puncture is seldom performed except in research protocols.

760 **B** (S&F, ch81)

HSV hepatitis is seen in neonates, pregnant women, and immunocompromised patients and can be aggressive and possibly life-threatening. Mucocutaneous lesions are present in only one half of the cases; therefore, a high index of clinical suspicion is important in making a timely diagnosis. Hepatitis is more common with acute infection than with reactivation. The individual with HSV hepatitis typically presents with fever, leukopenia, and markedly elevated aminotransaminase levels. Disseminated intravascular coagulation and jaundice may also be seen. Liver biopsy is essential for diagnosis, especially during pregnancy. Focal or extensive hemorrhagic or coagulative necrosis is seen with few inflammatory infiltrates. Intranuclear inclusions (Cowdry type A inclusions) may be identified in hepatocytes at the margins of the necrosis. In addition, some multinucleated periportal hepatocytes show a ground-glass appearance suggestive of viral inclusions. Electron microscopy, immunohistochemical staining, and PCR amplification techniques can be used to confirm the diagnosis.

761 **D** (S&F, ch84)

Akriviadis and colleagues performed a prospective, randomized, double-blind clinical trial of pentoxifylline in patients with severe alcoholic hepatitis (discriminant function >32). Forty-nine patients received 400 mg pentoxifylline orally three times daily and 52 received placebo (vitamin B_{12}) for four weeks. Only 12 patients (24.5%) who received pentoxifylline died compared with 24 (46%) who received placebo (see figure). Pentoxifylline therapy was associated with a significant decrease in the frequency of HRS as a cause of death and was well tolerated with no major side effects. On the basis of this single trial, pentoxifylline seems to be a viable alternative to glucocorticoids, particularly in patients with clinically important renal dysfunction.

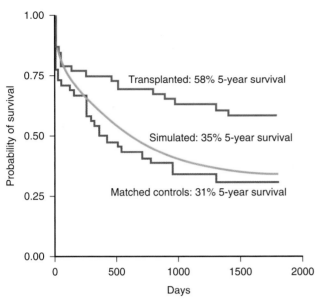

Figure for answer **761**

---

762 **E** (S&F, ch90)
The most common indication for placement of a TIPS is refractory variceal bleeding. A TIPS has been used to control acute variceal bleeding and to prevent variceal rebleeding when pharmacologic and endoscopic therapies have failed, especially in patients with Child class B or C cirrhosis in whom bleeding is more likely to be refractory to therapy than in patients with Child class A cirrhosis. Refractory ascites and prevention of variceal rebleeding are the only indications for TIPS placement that have been subjected to controlled trials. When bleeding from varices cannot be controlled after two sessions of endoscopic therapy within a 24-hour period, TIPS placement is the usual salvage treatment. A TIPS also is used to treat bleeding from isolated gastric fundal varices, for both control of bleeding and prevention of rebleeding. A surgical portosystemic shunt may be preferred over a TIPS in patients with preserved synthetic liver function (Child class A) in centers that have the surgical expertise.

763 **B** (S&F, ch75)
Adverse reactions from penicillamine are not common and include nephrotic range proteinuria, leukopenia, thrombocytopenia, aplastic anemia, myasthenia symptoms, Goodpasture syndrome, arthralgias, and gastrointestinal upset. Side effects involving the skin include various types of rashes, pemphigus, and elastosis perforans serpiginosa. Severe side effects from this therapy are seen to develop in as many as 30% of patients with Wilson's disease. This patient has pemphigus from penicillamine therapy. The medication should be discontinued, and the patient should not be rechallenged with this same treatment. Instead he should

be changed to the equally effective chelator trientene, which tends to have fewer side effects than penicillamine.

764 **B** (S&F, ch90)
Ligation initially should be at the bleeding site or immediately below the bleeding site. Other large varices should also be banded in the same session. If active bleeding is not noted, then ligation is performed beginning at the gastroesophageal junction and proceeding proximally at a distance of every 2 cm in a spiral fashion. If bleeding obscures the varices, then multiple bands are placed at the gastroesophageal junction circumferentially until bleeding can be controlled, but the long-term risks of esophageal stricture increase in such patients. Bleeding can be controlled in as many as 90% of patients by a combination of pharmacologic and endoscopic methods.

765 **C** (S&F, ch91)
Early detection of SBP, before symptoms of infection occur, may reduce mortality. Therefore, ascitic fluid should be sampled in all patients with ascites who are admitted to the hospital, especially if infection is suspected. Few contraindications to paracentesis have been recognized. Coagulopathy is a potential contraindication; however, most patients with cirrhotic ascites have coagulopathy, and if mild to moderate coagulopathy were viewed as a contraindication to paracentesis, few patients with cirrhosis would undergo this procedure. Coagulopathy should preclude paracentesis only when clinically evident fibrinolysis or disseminated intravascular coagulation is present. These conditions occur in fewer than 1 per 1000 paracenteses. No data are available to support cutoff values for coagulation parameters beyond which paracentesis should be avoided. Global coagulation is usually normal in the setting of cirrhosis despite abnormal tests of coagulation because there is a balanced deficiency of procoagulants and anticoagulants. Even after multiple paracenteses, bloody ascites usually does not develop in patients with severe prolongation of the prothrombin time. Patients with cirrhosis and without clinically obvious coagulopathy simply do not bleed excessively from needlesticks unless a blood vessel is entered. Giving fresh-frozen plasma or vitamin K routinely before paracentesis in patients with cirrhosis and coagulopathy is not supported by data.

766 **D** (S&F, ch82)
This patient has schistosomiasis infection. This trematode is more commonly found in endemic areas such as Africa and the Far East. Humans are infected initially when cercariae found in fresh water bore through the skin, usually the feet. Initially patients will have an acute systemic response manifested by fever and cough as the cercariae reach the pulmonary vessels and then are coughed up and ingested, ultimately reaching the portal circulation. They then lodge in multiple organs, including the liver, where they mate and begin to lay large numbers of eggs. These eggs lead to periportal fibrosis through a rigorous tumor necrosis factor-α response and sinusoidal obstruction. This ultimately leads to portal hypertension. Diagnosis

is made by identification of ova in stool or enzyme-linked immunosorbent assay. However, enzyme-linked immunosorbent assay cannot differentiate between new or old infection. Treatment with praziquantel is usually effective.

767 **D** (S&F, ch79)
Pretreatment factors associated with a greater chance of an SVR include infection with non–genotype 1 HCV, a low baseline serum HCV RNA level, the absence of bridging fibrosis or cirrhosis on a liver biopsy specimen, age younger than 40 years, the absence of obesity, the lack of hepatic steatosis or insulin resistance, the absence of HIV infection, and white race (see figure). Although the likelihood of an SVR is marginally lower in patients without these favorable factors, patients should not be discouraged and treatment should not be withheld because of the presence of any or all of these factors. Of known pretreatment variables, the most powerful predictor of a response to treatment is the viral genotype.

768 **D** (S&F, ch83)
Budd-Chiari syndrome is characterized by hepatic venous outflow obstruction. Classic Budd-Chiari syndrome is due to thrombosis of one or more hepatic veins at their opening into the inferior vena cava, which results in hepatomegaly, pain, ascites, and impaired hepatic function. Any hypercoagulable state can predispose a patient to the development of Budd-Chiari. This patient has paroxysmal nocturnal hemoglobinuria. Oral contraceptives in women can also be a predisposing factor. Other risk factors include malignancies, pregnancy, and inherited hypercoagulable states, among others.

769 **C** (S&F, ch74)
Most patients with symptomatic hemochromatosis are between 40 and 50 years of age at the time of diagnosis. Although the defective gene is equally distributed between men and women, men have predominated in most clinical series. When patients present with symptoms, the most common symptoms are weakness, lethargy, arthralgias, abdominal pain, loss of libido, and impotence. Physical findings include hepatomegaly, splenomegaly, ascites, edema, and jaundice. Diabetes is typically not seen in the absence of cirrhosis. The bronze or slate-gray skin pigmentation of hereditary hemochromatosis is often a subtle finding. Cardiomyopathy, atrial and ventricular dysrhythmias, and congestive heart failure can occur. Although alcoholism can lead to cardiomyopathy, this patient had many clinical signs of hereditary hemochromatosis that make this diagnosis more likely. Furthermore, the patient does not have a significant alcohol use history.

770 **A** (S&F, ch74)
Those in whom hereditary hemochromatosis is diagnosed most frequently have the genotype C282Y/C282Y or C282Y/H63D. This patient does not have hereditary hemochromatosis but rather has secondary mild iron overload along with an elevated ferritin level in response to his new diagnosis of lung cancer. This patient does not need to undergo either phlebotomy or chelation therapy. Because he does not have a liver disease, he does not need an MRI to screen for hepatocellular cancer. He requires only treatment of his underlying lung malignancy.

771 **D** (S&F, ch71)
Pores of the nuclear envelope are associated with a large number of proteins that are organized in an octagonal array. The nuclear pore complex is a large macromolecule assembly that protrudes into both the cytoplasm and the nucleoplasm. Bidirectional nucleocytoplasmic transport occurs through the central aqueous channel in the nuclear pore complex.

772 **D** (S&F, ch92)
Protein restriction will lead to negative nitrogen balance and malnutrition and is not advised. The lactulose dose should be titrated to three daily bowel movements. If HE develops after placement of a TIPS, the diameter of the shunt can be reduced by interventional techniques. Rifaximin has been studied and approved by the U.S. Food and Drug Administration for the treatment of chronic HE on the basis of the results of a multicentered, randomized, controlled trial in which the overall clinical efficacy and rate of side effects were similar in patients treated with lactitol and those treated with rifaximin. The usual dose is 400 mg orally three times daily. Two systematic reviews of

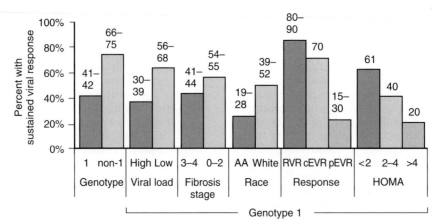

Figure for answer **767**

randomized, controlled trials that compared rifaximin with other therapies (nonabsorbable disaccharides and other antibiotics) for the treatment of acute or chronic HE have confirmed that the efficacy and side effect profiles are comparable. Other antibiotics, including metronidazole and vancomycin, have been reported to be effective in small trials and case series, but the data to support their use are insufficient.

773 C (S&F, ch83)

This elderly woman has ischemic hepatitis secondary to profound dehydration and hypotension. Ischemic hepatitis commonly causes a significant elevation of the transaminases as well as a mild elevation of the bilirubin and the INR. Although viral hepatitis can cause a similar biochemical profile, this patient's clinical presentation along with the rapid improvement with correction of the underlying precipitating factor is most consistent with the diagnosis of ischemic hepatitis. Characteristically, serum aminotransferase levels peak one to three days after the hemodynamic insult and return to normal within 7 to 10 days.

774 A (S&F, ch78)

Spontaneous HBeAg seroconversion is seen annually in only approximately 10% of patients with chronic HBV infection. Early changes in serum markers in patients with HBV infection that progresses to chronicity are similar to those in patients with acute HBV infection that resolves. However, with chronic infection, HBsAg, HBeAg, and HBV DNA remain positive for six months or longer. After the acute phase of infection, serum ALT levels fall but often remain persistently abnormal (between 50 and 200 U/L). Anti-HBc IgM titers typically falls to undetectable levels after six months but may become detectable again during reactivation of infection. Detectable levels of anti-HBc IgG persist indefinitely. HBV DNA is detectable by hybridization assays during the acute and chronic phases of disease. With time, there may be a spontaneous decrease in levels of HBV DNA and HBeAg, frequently in association with a flare of serum ALT levels and seroconversion to anti-HBeAg positivity. Spontaneous loss of reactivity to HBsAg is rare. Anti-HBsAg may be detected simultaneously with HBsAg in serum in less than 10% of cases. In some cases of chronic infection, active viral replication (HBV DNA positivity) occurs in the absence of HBeAg.

775 B (S&F, ch84)

The clinical diagnosis of alcoholic liver disease is quite sensitive and specific; therefore, liver biopsy is rarely needed to establish the diagnosis. A liver biopsy is essential for determining precisely the severity of hepatic injury, however, and for clarifying the diagnosis in atypical cases. Centrilobular and perivenular fatty infiltration in the liver is seen in most persons who drink more than 60 g of alcohol daily. Classic histologic features of alcoholic hepatitis include ballooning degeneration of hepatocytes, alcoholic hyaline (Mallory bodies) within damaged hepatocytes, and a surrounding infiltrate composed of polymorphonuclear leukocytes. Most patients have moderate to severe fatty infiltration. Varying degrees of fibrosis may be present, and many patients exhibit an unusual perisinusoidal distribution of fibrosis, at times with partial or complete obliteration of the terminal hepatic venules (sclerosing hyaline necrosis). Cirrhosis can be identified by the presence of nodules of hepatic tissue that are completely surrounded by fibrous tissue.

776 C (S&F, ch71)

Hepatic stellate cells, also known as Ito cells, are perisinusoidal cells that are sites of fat metabolism and vitamin A storage. When hepatic stellate cells are activated, they transform into myofibroblasts that express desmin and smooth muscle actin.

777 E (S&F, ch73)

Between 25% and 75% of patients undergoing surgery experience postoperative hepatic dysfunction, ranging from mild elevations in serum levels of liver enzymes to hepatic failure. Drugs that may cause hepatoxicity in this setting include antibiotics (e.g., erythromycin, amoxicillin-clavulanate, and sulfamethoxazole-trimethoprim) and the halogenated anesthetics; most produce injury by causing a hypersensitivity reaction that becomes evident within one to two weeks of administration. Postoperative cholestasis is characterized by a short-latency elevation in the level of indirect bilirubin, lack of rash or eosinophilia, and ensured recovery.

778 D (S&F, ch78)

Transmission of infection from an HBV carrier mother to her neonate accounts for the majority of new infections in the world today. Sixty percent to 90% of HBsAg-positive mothers who are HBeAg-positive transmit the disease to their offspring, whereas mothers who are positive for anti-HBe do so less frequently (15% to 20%). Other less common sources of infection are household contact with an HBV carrier, hemodialysis, exposure to infected health care workers, tattooing, body piercing, artificial insemination, and receipt of blood products or organs. Since routine screening of the blood supply was implemented in the early 1970s, transfusion-associated HBV has become rare in the United States. HBV can be transmitted by blood that tests negative for HBsAg but positive for anti-HBc because of low levels of circulating HBV DNA in such blood. HBsAg-negative blood that is positive for anti-HBc is excluded from the donor pool in the United States and many countries around the world. In up to 30% of persons who are seropositive for anti-HBcA alone, HBV DNA is detectable in serum by PCR testing.

779 A (S&F, ch76)

Congenital erythropoietic porphyria is a rare form of porphyria with autosomal recessive transmission that is caused by deficiency of uroporphyrinogen III cosynthase, which mainly affects erythropoietic tissue. Affected patients typically present in the first year of life with blisters and disfiguring skin lesions in exposed areas. Infants may present with pink urine and photosensitivity. As patients age, erythrodontia, a pathognomonic red or brownish discoloration of the teeth, is commonly seen.

Congenital erythropoietic porphyria can be distinguished clinically from hepatoerythropoietic porphyria by the presence in some cases of a Coombs-negative hemolytic anemia, which can be quite severe. Splenomegaly is common.

780   **A** (S&F, ch76)

If a urea cycle defect is considered, the following laboratory measurements should be obtained: serum ammonia, arterial blood gases, urine organic acids, serum amino acids, and urinary orotic acid (see table at end of chapter for review of expected laboratory results). Plasma ammonia levels are generally dramatically elevated in patients with urea cycle defects, sometimes to more than 2000 μmol/L (3400 μg/dL), with normal being 50 μmol/L (85 μg/dL) or less. This patient's blood gas values reflect respiratory alkalosis, which is secondary to hyperventilation triggered by the effects of ammonia on the central nervous system. Serum levels of liver enzymes are usually normal or minimally elevated in such cases. Citrulline levels are barely detectable in patients with ornithine transcarbamoylase or carbamoyl phosphate synthetase deficiencies but are markedly elevated in those with argininosuccinate synthetase and argininosuccinate lyase deficiencies.

781   **B** (S&F, ch80)

HEV transmission is predominantly via the fecal-oral route. Most reported outbreaks have been related to consumption of fecally contaminated drinking water. Recurrent epidemics are probably related to continuous fecal contamination of water. Person-to-person transmission is distinctly uncommon during epidemics, and secondary attack rates among household contacts are only 0.7% to 2.2%.

Although transmission by ingestion of undercooked meat or by receiving a blood transfusion has been reported, the frequency of infection by these mechanisms is low. Vertical transmission is well documented, but it would be unlikely for a 57-year-old man to develop acute HEV in this manner. The presence in serum of IgM antibody to HEV indicates acute infection, whereas detection of anti-HEV IgG may indicate the convalescent phase or past infection. IgM antibody to HEV appears in the early phase of clinical illness, lasts four to five months, and can be detected in 80% to 100% of cases during outbreaks of acute HEV.

782   **D** (S&F, ch87)

The most likely cause of her acute liver injury is cocaine use. Associated features include rhabdomyolysis, hypotension, hyperpyrexia, disseminated intravascular coagulation, and renal failure. Hepatic injury probably is the result of toxic metabolites (e.g., norcocaine nitroxide) formed by CYP2E1 and CYP2A. For this reason, enhanced hepatotoxicity can be seen in patients consuming large amounts of alcohol. Although acute viral hepatitis can lead to elevated transaminases, the time frame from the exposure to the development of disease manifestation is too short for this to be a likely consideration. Acute alcohol injury would not result in such a profound elevation of the transaminases.

783   **E** (S&F, ch91)

The diagnosis of secondary bacterial peritonitis requires the presence of at least two of the following three criteria: total protein more than 1 g/dL, glucose more than 50 mg/dL, and LDH more than the upper limit of normal for serum (see figure).

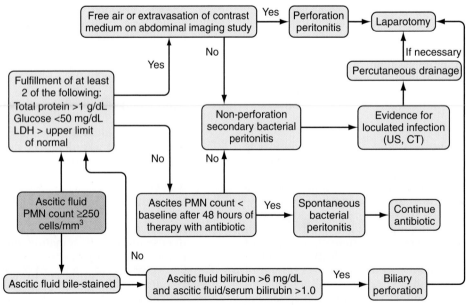

Figure for answer **783**

784 **B** (S&F, ch84)

In a meta-analysis performed by Imperiale and McCullough, only when patients who had gastrointestinal hemorrhage were excluded from consideration did treatment improve the chances for survival. Glucocorticoids did not increase the risk of gastrointestinal hemorrhage, but bleeding was independently associated with such a high mortality risk that it overrode the beneficial effect of glucocorticoids. Poor renal function at the time of randomization to glucocorticoid therapy can also limit the benefit of this treatment. Patients with alcoholic hepatitis who had serum creatinine levels greater than 2.5 mg/dL were at high risk of progression to renal failure, and the short-term mortality in this group was 75%, with or without glucocorticoid therapy. When evaluating patients for glucocorticoid therapy, certain confounding illnesses should be considered contraindications to therapy; these illnesses include active infection, pancreatitis, and possibly insulin-dependent diabetes mellitus.

785 **B** (S&F, ch78)

The incubation period (time from acute exposure to clinical symptoms) of HBV infection ranges from 60 to 180 days. The clinical presentation varies, from asymptomatic infection to cholestatic hepatitis with jaundice and, rarely, liver failure. In patients with acute infection, HBsAg and markers of active viral replication (HBeAg and HBV DNA) become detectable approximately six weeks after inoculation, before the onset of clinical symptoms or biochemical abnormalities. Biochemical abnormalities usually coincide with the prodromal phase of the acute illness and may persist for several months. With the onset of symptoms, anti-HBc IgM becomes detectable. Detectable levels of anti-HBc IgM may persist for many months, and detectable levels of anti-HBc IgG may persist for many years, if not a lifetime. Anti-HBs is the last serologic marker to become detectable, and its appearance (as HBsAg titers fall) indicates that the infection is resolving. Much has been made of the serologic window when neither HBsAg nor anti-HBs is detectable and anti-HBc IgM is the only marker of acute infection. However, with the ability of currently available serologic assays to detect low levels of marker proteins, this window occurs rarely.

786 **B** (S&F, ch79)

The decision to re-treat a patient who failed to respond to a previous course of antiviral therapy should take into consideration the previous regimen used, the appropriateness of the doses given throughout the course, the patient's ability to tolerate therapy, and the response to treatment, especially whether and when HCV RNA became undetectable. Retreatment SVR rates in previous nonresponders range from approximately 10% to as high as 15% with longer treatment durations. Maintenance therapy has not been shown to be of benefit.

787 **B** (S&F, ch90)

All patients with large varices (diameter >5 mm) should be considered for prophylactic therapy (primary prophylaxis) to prevent variceal bleeding. The presence of additional endoscopic signs such as red wales does not influence the decision regarding prophylactic therapy. Twelve trials addressed the use of a nonselective beta blocker for primary prophylaxis of variceal bleeding and demonstrated a decrease in the risk of variceal bleeding from 25% in patients in the control group to 15% in patients taking a beta blocker. The absolute risk reduction is thus approximately 10%, and the number needed to treat to prevent one variceal bleed is approximately 10 patients. Prophylactic sclerotherapy for the prevention of variceal bleeding has been studied extensively but cannot be recommended.

788 **E** (S&F, ch85)

Percutaneous liver biopsy remains the gold standard for the diagnosis of NAFLD. However, liver biopsy is costly, invasive, and associated with a small risk of complications. Sampling variability is common, and the large number of individuals with NAFLD far outstrips the manpower available to perform liver biopsies. Significant progress has been made in developing simple, noninvasive, and quantitative tests to estimate the degree of hepatic fibrosis in a number of liver diseases, including NAFLD. The FibroTest (called FibroSURE in the United States) is the best studied of these tests.

789 **D** (S&F, ch94)

Despite its rarity, hepatic angiosarcoma is of special interest because specific risk factors have been identified, although no cause is discerned in the majority of tumors. Hepatic angiosarcoma in workers exposed to vinyl chloride monomer was first reported in 1974. The monomer is converted by enzymes of the endoplasmic reticulum to reactive metabolites that form DNA adducts and G-to-A transitions in the *ras* and *TP53* genes. Angiosarcomas have occurred after exposures of 11 to 37 years (or after shorter periods with a heavy initial exposure). The mean age of patients at diagnosis is 48 years. In addition to angiosarcoma, persons exposed to vinyl chloride monomer may be at increased risk of hepatocellular carcinoma and soft-tissue sarcoma.

790 **E** (S&F, ch91)

Calculating the SAAG involves measuring the albumin concentration of serum and ascitic fluid specimens and simply subtracting the ascitic fluid value from the serum value. Unless a laboratory error has been made, the serum albumin concentration is always the larger value. The SAAG is calculated by subtraction and is not a ratio. If the SAAG is 1.1 g/dL (11 g/L) or greater, the patient can be considered to have portal hypertension with an accuracy of approximately 97%. The presence of a high SAAG does not confirm a diagnosis of cirrhosis; it simply indicates the presence of portal hypertension. Although peritoneal carcinomatosis is the most common cause of a low SAAG, other causes exist (see table at end of chapter). This patient has a SAAG of less than 1.1 g/dL, which is not consistent with answers **A**, **B**, or **D**. Also the predominance of mononuclear cells in the differential count provides a clue to the diagnosis of tuberculous peritonitis or peritoneal carcinomatosis. There is nothing in the history or physical examination to suggest malignancy.

791 **D** (S&F, ch86)

Nitrofurantoin, a synthetic furan-based compound, is a urinary antiseptic agent that continues to lead to cases of hepatic injury. The frequency of nitrofurantoin hepatic injury ranges from 0.3 to 3 cases per 100,000 exposed persons. The risk increases with age, particularly after the age of 64. Two thirds of acute cases occur in women, and the female-to-male ratio is 8:1 for chronic hepatitis. The range of liver diseases associated with nitrofurantoin includes acute hepatitis, occasionally with features of cholestasis, hepatic granulomas, chronic hepatitis with autoimmune phenomena, acute liver failure, and cirrhosis. Causality has been proved by rechallenge and no relationship to dose has been observed; cases even have been described after ingestion of milk from a nitrofurantoin-treated cow.

792 **D** (S&F, ch87)

Certain weight loss supplements have been identified to cause hepatotoxicity and should be considered the most likely cause of this young woman's liver abnormalities. Specifically, Chaso and Onshido are Chinese herbal dietary weight loss supplements that were reported to cause severe liver injury, with a mean serum ALT level of 1978 U/L (range, 283 to 4074 U/L), in 12 patients. Fulminant hepatic failure developed in two persons, one of whom died and one of whom survived after receiving a liver transplant. The suspected hepatotoxic ingredient was *N*-nitroso-fenfluramine, a derivative of the appetite suppressant fenfluramine, which was withdrawn from the U.S. market in 1997. Another dietary supplement used for weight loss, Lipokinetix (composed of norephedrine, sodium usniate (usnic acid), diiodothyronine, yohimbine, and caffeine) has been associated with acute hepatitis, including fulminant hepatic failure requiring liver transplantation.

793 **C** (S&F, ch85)

Liver biopsy is the standard means of diagnosis and the only test that can reliably differentiate simple steatosis from advanced NAFLD (nonalcoholic steatohepatitis), although noninvasive methods for assessing fibrosis are in development.

794 **A** (S&F, ch78)

HBV is transmitted efficiently by percutaneous and mucous membrane exposure to infectious body fluids. The virus is 100 times as infectious as HIV and 10 times as infectious as HCV. HBeAg seropositivity indicates a higher risk of transmission from mother to child, after needlestick exposure, and in the setting of household contact. HBV DNA has been detected by sensitive techniques such as PCR testing in most body fluids, except for stool that has not been contaminated with blood.

795 **B** (S&F, ch86)

Cases with a fatal outcome have been associated with a longer duration of treatment with isoniazid or continued ingestion of isoniazid after the onset of symptoms. Therefore, most deaths from isoniazid hepatitis could be prevented if patients report symptoms early in the course and isoniazid is discontinued. In the United States, isoniazid hepatotoxicity is second only to acetaminophen as an indication for liver transplantation. Children are less susceptible than adults, but serious hepatotoxicity can occur in children; over a 10-year period (1987-1997), eight children required liver transplantation for isoniazid hepatotoxicity in the United States (0.2% of pediatric liver transplantations).

796 **D** (S&F, ch71)

Tight junction complexes between neighboring hepatocytes separate the sinusoidal space from the bile canaliculi. Disruption of tight junctions can permit regurgitation of biliary solutes into the bloodstream. The liver's unique sinusoidal structure is well suited for the bidirectional transfer of a variety of solutes, including macromolecules, across the sinusoidal membrane. The low pressure allows blood to percolate slowly through the sinusoids and hepatic acinus. Fenestrae within the sinusoidal endothelium and the absence of a basement membrane permit direct contact of the portal blood with the hepatic sinusoidal surface in the subsinusoidal vascular space, referred to as the Disse space. Microvilli on the hepatic sinusoidal plasma membrane further facilitate interchange of nutrients between sinusoidal blood and hepatocytes.

797 **C** (S&F, ch86)

Isoniazid-induced liver injury has been characterized since the 1970s, but deaths still occur. Hepatitis develops in approximately 21 per 1000 persons exposed to isoniazid; 5% to 10% of cases are fatal. The risk and severity of isoniazid hepatitis increase with age; the risk is 0.3% in the third decade of life and increases to 2% or higher after age 50. Overall frequency rates are the same in men and women, but 70% of fatal cases are in women; black and Hispanic women may be at particular risk. The risk of toxicity is not related to the dose or blood level of isoniazid. The role of genetic factors has been controversial. Associations have been described with specific genes that code for enzymes involved in aspects of drug metabolism or detoxification (CYP2E1, *N*-acetyltransferase, glutathione-*S*-transferase), but data are conflicting. Long-term excessive alcohol intake increases the frequency and severity of isoniazid hepatotoxicity, as may rifampin and pyrazinamide.

798 **E** (S&F, ch79)

The risk of progressive hepatic injury from HCV infection varies considerably, with some patients showing little or no progression after decades of infection and others progressing rapidly to cirrhosis. Therefore, an assessment of the degree of liver injury is usually advisable. This assessment is usually done by percutaneous liver biopsy (see table at end of chapter), but indirect and noninvasive methods to assess liver injury and fibrosis are under study and becoming commercially available. Although noninvasive testing has dramatically improved, all currently available tests have limitations. First, these tests generally have not been applied to the evaluation of other potentially contributing disease processes, such as nonalcoholic steatohepatitis. Second, the degree of hepatic inflammation is not assessed by these tests. Third, the utility of these tests has not been evaluated in select populations such as dialysis patients, HIV-positive persons, liver transplant recipients, and persons with active autoimmune conditions. Fourth, although cirrhosis is accurately predicted by several noninvasive tests, the finer discrimination of fibrosis score is not as reliable as that with examination of liver biopsy specimens. Despite the limitations, in patients with a relative contraindication to liver biopsy (such as hemophilia or anticoagulation therapy in patients who are at high risk of the development of thrombotic events if treatment is interrupted) or in patients who refuse a liver biopsy, noninvasive testing can be helpful in disease management and assessing prognosis. Measurement of serum HCV RNA levels (viral load) may be useful in assessing the effectiveness of antiviral therapy and in evaluating the likelihood of a treatment response, but not in estimating the overall prognosis.

799 **E** (S&F, ch76)
Although liver disease is often (but not always) mild during infancy and childhood, patients with α_1-AT deficiency have an increased risk of the development of cirrhosis during adulthood; 42% of all PiZZ patients have histologic evidence of cirrhosis at autopsy. Moreover, homozygous α_1-AT deficiency increases the risk of the development of hepatocellular carcinoma, especially in men older than 50 years. The diagnosis of α_1-AT deficiency should be considered in any patient presenting with noninfectious chronic hepatitis, hepatosplenomegaly, cirrhosis, portal hypertension, or hepatocellular carcinoma. Histopathologic features of α_1-AT deficiency change as the affected patient ages. In infancy, liver biopsy specimens may show bile duct paucity, intracellular cholestasis with or without giant cell transformation, mild inflammatory changes, or steatosis, with few of the characteristic PAS-positive, diastase-resistant globules. These inclusions, which are due to polymerized α_1-ATZ protein, are most prominent in periportal hepatocytes but may also be seen in Kupffer cells. Immunohistochemistry with monoclonal antibody to α_1-ATZ can also be performed to verify the diagnosis. As the patient ages, these changes may resolve completely or progress to chronic hepatitis or cirrhosis.

800 **D** (S&F, ch95)
The period immediately after liver transplantation is characterized by acid/base abnormalities, fluid shifts, and striking elevations in liver enzyme levels. The most important indicators of graft function are clinical and include the patient's mental status and coagulation parameters; in those with a T tube, the amount and character of bile production is also used to judge graft function.

801 **D** (S&F, ch73)
GGTP is found in the cell membranes of a wide distribution of tissues including the liver (both hepatocytes and cholangiocytes), kidney, pancreas, spleen, heart, brain, and seminal vesicles. It is present in the serum of healthy persons. Serum levels are not different between men and women and do not increase in pregnancy. Although an elevated serum GGTP level has high sensitivity for hepatobiliary disease, its lack of specificity limits its clinical utility. The primary use of serum GGTP levels is to identify the source of an isolated elevation in the serum alkaline phosphatase level; the GGTP level is not elevated in bone disease (see figure). The GGTP level is elevated in patients taking phenytoin, barbiturates, and some drugs used in highly active antiretroviral therapy, including non-nucleoside reverse transcriptase inhibitors and the protease inhibitor abacavir.

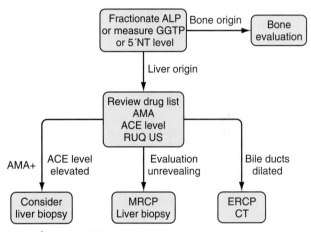

Figure for answer **801**

802 **D** (S&F, ch81)
Epstein-Barr virus infection is common and has a wide range of clinical presentations. Most affected infants or children are asymptomatic or have mild, nonspecific symptoms, whereas adolescents and adults typically present with the triad of pharyngitis, fever, and lymphadenopathy. Although usually subclinical, liver abnormalities are nearly universal in patients with Epstein-Barr virus mononucleosis and range from mild, self-limited elevations in serum aminotransaminase levels to, rarely, fulminant and even fatal hepatitis.

803 **C** (S&F, ch78)
In Asia, the most common mode of HBV transmission is perinatal infection during birth from the HBV carrier mother to the newborn. If the mother is HBsAg positive and HBeAg positive, the transmission rate is 60% to 90%, whereas if she is HBeAg negative and anti-HBe positive, the transmission rate is much lower (15% to 20%).

804 **A** (S&F, ch72)
Fatty acid synthesis occurs in the cytosol and is regulated closely by the availability of acetyl-CoA, which forms the basic subunit of the developing fatty acid carbon chain. Acetyl-CoA is synthesized predominantly in mitochondria and is derived mainly from carbohydrate metabolism, with a small

fraction coming from amino acids. Acetyl-CoA is condensed with oxaloacetate to form citrate, which is exported from the mitochondria and is then cleaved by the cytosolic adenotriphosphate citrate lyase to produce oxaloacetate and acetyl-CoA. Conversion of acetyl-CoA to malonyl-CoA by the action of acetyl-CoA carboxylase is the first step in fatty acid synthesis. Acetyl-CoA carboxylase is the key enzyme in regulating fatty acid synthesis because it provides the necessary building blocks for elongation of the fatty acid carbon chain.

805 **B** (S&F, ch89)

UDCA is the only medication approved by the U.S. Food and Drug Administration for the treatment of PBC. Several mechanisms for the protective actions of UDCA have been proposed, including inhibiting the absorption of toxic, hydrophobic, endogenous bile salts; stabilizing hepatocyte membranes against toxic bile salts; replacing endogenous bile acids, some of which may be hepatotoxic, with the non-hepatotoxic UDCA; and reduction in expression of major histocompatibility complex class I and II antigens. Treatment with UDCA leads to rapid improvement in liver test results and to improvement in the histologic severity of interface hepatitis, inflammation, cholestasis, bile duct paucity, and bile duct proliferation. UDCA also significantly decreases the risk of developing gastroesophageal varices and delays progression to cirrhosis. Diphenhydramine, cholestyramine, and rifampin all treat pruritus associated with PBC, but are not approved for treatment of PBC itself. Glucocorticoids may improve short-term liver test results and some histologic findings in patients with PBC, but side effects, particularly bone mass reduction, preclude their long-term use in PBC.

806 **C** (S&F, ch87)

This patient has acute poisoning from *Amanita phalloides*. Fatality can result from the ingestion of just one mushroom. Unfortunately, the toxins are not inactivated by cooking. Usually, within six to 20 hours of ingestion, the phalloidin toxin leads to typical gastrointestinal illness consisting of severe abdominal pain, diarrhea, and nausea. Hepatotoxicity results from the amatoxin, which inhibits protein synthesis, leading to cellular necrosis. Liver biopsy specimens often show necrosis with steatosis limited to zone 3 of the lobule. Many cases of poisoning result in liver failure and require transplantation. However, use of penicillin along with *N*-acetylcysteine should be implemented.

807 **C** (S&F, ch94)

Hepatocellular carcinoma with extension to the portal vein is not considered an indication for liver transplantation given the very high risk of recurrence. Chemoembolization is relatively contraindicated due to portal vein thrombosis. Surgical resection is reserved for hepatocellular carcinoma in patients without cirrhosis. Local ablative therapies would be most appropriate in this case. Sorafenib, an inhibitor of Raf kinase and the receptor tyrosine kinase activity of vascular endothelial growth factor receptors and platelet-derived growth factor receptor is the first of these new agents to

be shown to modestly improve survival compared with supportive care. It should be considered for patients with intact hepatic function (Child A) and portal vein thrombosis, extrahepatic disease, or failure of other therapies.

808 **D** (S&F, ch94)

Simple hepatic cysts are thought to be congenital in origin and have an incidence of approximately 2.5% of the population. The cysts usually are asymptomatic and discovered incidentally during upper abdominal imaging. They occur more often in women than in men, and their prevalence increases with age. Asymptomatic solitary hepatic cysts should be left alone. If intervention is required, percutaneous aspiration and sclerosis with alcohol or doxycycline will usually ablate the cyst, but recurrence is frequent. An alternative approach is laparoscopic (or, rarely, open surgical) fenestration, which is seldom followed by recurrence, but has a higher morbidity rate.

809 **B** (S&F, ch90)

Available evidence is insufficient to prove the superiority of somatostatin and its analogs to placebo in the control of acute variceal bleeding. Some randomized, controlled trials, however, support the view that somatostatin or octreotide may be equivalent in efficacy to sclerotherapy or terlipressin for controlling acute variceal bleeding. Also, early administration of vapreotide may be associated with improved control of bleeding but without a significant reduction in the mortality rate. In clinical practice, treatment with somatostatin or octreotide is combined with endoscopic management of variceal bleeding. Nonselective beta blocker drugs such as propranolol and nadolol are recommended as prophylaxis against a first variceal bleed in selected patients with portal hypertension. Nitrates are no longer recommended, either alone or in combination with beta blockers, for primary prophylaxis. For secondary prophylaxis, isosorbide mononitrate may be added to beta blocker therapy if the beta blocker drugs have not resulted in an appropriate decrease in the HVPG. Terlipressin, although not currently available in the United States, would be preferable to vasopressin due to its better safety profile and studies showing longer survival of patients with variceal bleeding treated with terlipressin. Losartan has not been shown in randomized, controlled trials to promote a clinically significant reduction in portal pressure.

810 **A** (S&F, ch84)

Female sex is now a well-accepted risk factor for the development and rapid progression of alcoholic liver disease. Although rates of metabolism and elimination of alcohol have been reported to be more rapid in women than in men, when adjusted for liver volume, elimination rates are similar between sexes. Studies in rats or mice fed alcohol long term have demonstrated that females are more susceptible than males to liver injury. Risk factors for the development of liver disease in women seem to include increased endotoxemia, lipid peroxidation, activation of the critical transcription factor nuclear factor κB, and chemokine (e.g., monocyte chemotactic protein-1) messenger RNA levels. These risk factors are critical for determining "safe" levels of alcohol consumption in women. Many authorities consider any amount of alcohol more than 20 g daily to be a risk factor for the development of liver disease in women; differences between men and women in levels of alcohol dehydrogenase in gastric mucosa are not thought to play a major role in the greater susceptibility of women to alcoholic liver injury.

811   **A** (S&F, ch90)

Endoscopic variceal ligation is associated with fewer complications than sclerotherapy and requires fewer sessions for variceal obliteration. Specifically, esophageal variceal ligation during an acute bleed is not associated with the sustained increase in the HVPG seen with sclerotherapy. Complications of endoscopic sclerotherapy may arise during or after the procedure. During injection, the patient may experience some degree of retrosternal discomfort, which may persist postoperatively. More serious complications include sclerosant-induced esophageal ulcer-related bleeding, strictures, and perforation. The risk of ulcers caused by sclerotherapy may be reduced by the use of sucralfate or a proton pump inhibitor after sclerotherapy. Compared with sclerotherapy, endoscopic band ligation of varices is less often associated with local complications such as esophageal ulcers, strictures, and dysmotility. However, ulcers that occur as a complication of banding can be large and potentially serious when gastric fundal varices have been banded. Now that overtubes are not used, the mechanical complications of mucosal tear or even esophageal perforation are uncommon.

812   **D** (S&F, ch88)

The presence of ascites or hepatic encephalopathy in patients with established AIH is indicative of a poor prognosis, but there is a chance that AIH may resolve completely with glucocorticoid therapy. In addition, liver transplantation is effective in the treatment of decompensated AIH. Decompensated patients with multilobular necrosis on histologic examination who have at least one laboratory parameter that fails to normalize or hyperbilirubinemia that does not improve after two weeks of treatment are at high risk of early mortality unless they undergo liver transplantation. Thus, the recommendation in this case is for glucocorticoid therapy and evaluation for liver transplantation.

813   **B** (S&F, ch75)

This patient has Wilson's disease and is presenting with fulminant hepatic failure with severe coagulopathy and encephalopathy. Acute intravascular hemolysis is usually present in this situation. Unlike fulminant viral hepatitis, Wilson's disease is usually characterized by disproportionately low serum aminotransaminase levels, and the serum alkaline phosphatase level is in the normal or even low range. The serum bilirubin level is disproportionately elevated secondary to hemolysis. These patients do not respond well to chelation therapy and require urgent transplantation evaluation.

814   **E** (S&F, ch73)

The differential diagnosis of marked elevations of aminotransferase levels (>1000 U/L) includes viral hepatitis (A to E), toxin- or drug-induced liver injury, ischemic hepatitis, and, less commonly, AIH, acute Budd-Chiari syndrome, fulminant Wilson's disease, and acute obstruction of the biliary tract. The primary cause of ischemic hepatitis is tissue hypoxia, which may result from hypoperfusion secondary to cardiac failure, systemic hypoxemia from respiratory failure, or increased oxygen requirements from sepsis. Among all cases of extreme AST elevation (>3000 U/L), ischemic hepatitis accounts for approximately one half. Most cases of ischemic hepatitis are transient and self-limited. The overall prognosis depends primarily on the severity of the underlying predisposing condition, not the severity of the liver disease. Treatment for ischemic hepatitis is nonspecific and directed at improving cardiac output and systemic oxygenation.

815   **B** (S&F, ch73)

The first step in the evaluation of a patient with an isolated and asymptomatic elevation of the serum alkaline phosphatase level is to identify the tissue source (see figure for answer 801). The most precise way to do this is via fractionation through electrophoresis; each isoenzyme of alkaline phosphatase has different electrophoretic mobilities. An acceptable alternative method is to check either the serum GGTP or 5′-nucleotidase level; elevation of either verifies that the elevated alkaline phosphatase level is the result of hepatobiliary disease. Central to the evaluation of an elevated alkaline phosphatase level is imaging of the biliary tract. The absence of dilated intrahepatic bile ducts focuses the search on intrahepatic causes of cholestasis, whereas dilated ducts should lead to an evaluation of extrahepatic causes of cholestasis. Granulomatous liver disease can be caused by a number of disorders. Infectious etiologies must be excluded because treatment of many of the other causes of granulomatous liver disease is immunosuppressive therapy. Sarcoidosis is the most common etiology. The diagnosis is based on an elevated angiotensin-converting enzyme level and typical extrahepatic manifestations (see tables at end of chapter).

816   **A** (S&F, ch89)

Vitamin A deficiency, which can cause reduced night vision, and vitamin K deficiency, which can cause bruising and prolonged prothrombin time, can occur in patients with PBC. Many patients with advanced PBC have fat-soluble vitamin deficiency and should receive fat-soluble vitamin replacement therapy. Fat-soluble vitamin deficiency is almost always caused by malabsorption resulting from decreased amounts of bile salts in the intestinal lumen. When blood levels of vitamin A are low and the patient is symptomatic, replacement therapy with 100,000 IU/day of vitamin A orally for three days and then 50,000 IU/day for 14 days should be instituted. A trial of oral vitamin K (5 to 10 mg/day) should be given to determine whether the prothrombin time improves. If it does, the patient should be maintained on 5 mg/day of water-soluble vitamin K.

817 A (S&F, ch77)

The incidence of acute HAV has decreased by 90% since 1995. The greatest rate of decrease has been among children from states where routine vaccination of children was recommended in 1999. The highest rate of reported disease historically has been among children ages 5 to 14 years. Because of the rapid rate of decrease in children, however, rates are now similar among age groups, with adults ages 20 to 44 having the highest rate of disease in 2006.

818 D (S&F, ch91)

The diagnosis of SBP is made when there is a positive ascitic fluid culture and an increased ascitic fluid absolute PMN count (i.e., at least 250 cells/mm^3 [0.25 × 109/L]) without evidence of an intra-abdominal surgically treatable source of infection. Several antibiotics are now available for the treatment of ascitic fluid infection. Cefotaxime, a third-generation cephalosporin, has been shown in a controlled trial to be superior to ampicillin plus tobramycin for the treatment of SBP. Fully 98% of causative organisms were susceptible to cefotaxime, which did not result in superinfection or nephrotoxicity. Cefotaxime or a similar third-generation cephalosporin seems to be the treatment of choice for suspected SBP. Anaerobic coverage is not needed, nor is coverage for *Pseudomonas* or *Staphylococcus*. Elective surgical treatment of the hernia can be considered in patients with ascites, but it carries an increased risk compared with those patients without cirrhosis and ascites. Ascites should be minimized preoperatively to reduce the risk of hernia recurrence. There is no indication for TIPS placement or large-volume paracentesis in this patient.

819 A (S&F, ch88)

Preferred treatment regimens for AIH include combination therapy and single-drug therapy. Prednisone alone or at lower doses but in combination with azathioprine induces clinical, biochemical, and histologic remission in 65% of patients within three years. The average treatment duration is 22 months, and therapy improves survival. Single-drug therapy often consists of prednisone at a starting dose of 60 mg/day for one week, followed by slowly tapering doses. Combination therapy consists of prednisone at a starting dose of 30 mg/day for one week, followed by slowly tapering doses of prednisone with concomitant administration of azathioprine, starting at 50 mg/day. Cyclosporine and tacrolimus are not first-line therapy for AIH. UDCA has no role in the treatment of AIH.

820 A (S&F, ch90)

Patients with cirrhosis are at increased risk of specific abnormalities of pulmonary mechanics, hemodynamics, and ventilation-perfusion matching that can adversely affect both quality of life and longevity. Two of the most common pulmonary manifestations of cirrhosis are alterations in lung mechanics caused by the presence of ascites and intrapulmonary shunting and abnormal gas exchange, which together constitute HPS. HPS is defined as a widened age-corrected alveolar-arterial oxygen gradient (AaPo$_2$) of room air in the presence or absence of hypoxemia (AaPo$_2$ ≥15 mm Hg or ≥20 mm Hg in patients older than 64 years of age) as a result of intrapulmonary vasodilation. Classic clinical manifestations of HPS include platypnea (dyspnea worsened by an erect position and improved by a supine position), orthodeoxia (exacerbation of hypoxia and hypoxemia in the upright position), an insidious onset and slow progression of dyspnea, clubbing, and distal cyanosis. The diagnosis of HPS requires a high degree of clinical suspicion, measurement of arterial blood gases, detection of intrapulmonary shunting, and exclusion of intrinsic cardiopulmonary disease as the cause of hypoxemia. The most sensitive test for the diagnosis of intrapulmonary shunting is contrast echocardiography. Treatment options for HPS are limited. Currently, no established medical therapies exist, although case reports and small case series suggest that some treatments may improve oxygenation. Therefore, patients with well-preserved hepatic synthetic function who have hypoxemia are generally treated symptomatically until oxygenation worsens sufficiently to permit listing for liver transplantation.

821 B (S&F, ch91)

Spironolactone is the mainstay of treatment for patients with cirrhosis and ascites but increases natriuresis slowly. Single-agent diuretic therapy with spironolactone requires several days to induce weight loss. Although spironolactone alone has been shown to be superior to furosemide alone in the treatment of cirrhotic ascites, amiloride, 10 mg/day, can be substituted for spironolactone; amiloride is less widely available and more expensive than spironolactone but is more rapidly effective and does not cause gynecomastia. A 100:40 ratio of the daily doses of spironolactone and furosemide usually maintains normokalemia. The ratio of doses can be adjusted to correct abnormal serum potassium levels.

822 A (S&F, ch95)

Administration of a nucleoside/nucleotide analog in combination with HBV immunoglobulin has improved the outcome of liver transplantation in patients with liver disease due to HBV infection. When this regimen is not followed, recurrent HBV infection is the rule, and the graft is often lost as a result. Interferons are contraindicated in patients with decompensated HBV infection because in these patients interferons can lead to elevations in aminotransferase levels, loss of hepatocellular mass, and acute worsening of hepatic synthetic function. Immediate listing for liver transplantation may be appropriate for patients with fulminant HBV; not infrequently, there is an undetectable level of HBV DNA and there is a low risk of recurrent HBV. Prophylaxis with an oral nucleoside/nucleotide is indicated nonetheless.

823 D (S&F, ch85)

A lists typical findings in cases of AIH, B lists findings in cases of PBC, C lists findings in cases of α$_1$-AT deficiency, and E lists typical findings in cases of chronic HCV infection. Given her demographic profile, this patient is most likely to have NAFLD. D lists typical findings in cases of NAFLD.

824 A (S&F, ch95)
Renal toxicity is an unfortunate and very common adverse effect of using a calcineurin-inhibitor drug for immunosuppression. Although patients may be at risk of de novo malignancies after transplantation, other cancers are more common than renal cell cancer. Tacrolimus may incite diabetes, which can, in turn, lead to the other complications such as renal insufficiency; however, calcineurin inhibitor–associated hypertension is more common.

825 D (S&F, ch91)
This patient is gaining weight due to noncompliance with a low-sodium diet. The target sodium excretion should be 120 mEq/day on an 88 mEq/day sodium diet, so the diuretic dose is adequate. Fluid loss and weight change are related directly to sodium balance in patients with portal hypertension–related ascites. In the presence of avid renal retention of sodium, dietary sodium restriction is essential. The patient and the food preparer should be educated by a dietician about a sodium-restricted diet. Extremely sodium-restricted diets (e.g., 500 mg [or 22 mmol] of sodium per day) are feasible (but not palatable) in an inpatient setting but are unrealistic for outpatients. The standard dietary sodium restriction for both inpatients and outpatients is 2 g (88 mmol) per day.

826 D (S&F, ch74)
This patient does not have HH given his normal iron stores and normal ferritin on screening blood work. The fact that his cousin has been diagnosed does not mean that he too will have this disorder. At this point, only reassurance is necessary. Given normal iron levels, phlebotomy is incorrect because there is no need to deplete iron stores in patients who are not iron overloaded. Genetic testing for HH is also not necessary because he does not have elevated iron levels and is therefore very unlikely to be either C282Y/C282Y or C282Y/H63D, which are the most common genotypes for HH. A liver biopsy is only recommended in patients shown to have HH and especially in those who have a ferritin level greater than 1000 ng/mL, which has been shown to be predictive of advanced fibrosis. Patients with HH, especially those with cirrhosis, are at increased risk of developing hepatocellular cancer and should be screened. However, this patient does not have either and therefore does not need to be screened for hepatocellular cancer.

827 A (S&F, ch86)
An important aspect of the temporal relationship between ingestion of a drug and hepatotoxicity is the response to discontinuation of the drug or dechallenge. Dechallenge should be accompanied by discernible and progressive improvement within days or weeks of stopping the incriminated agent. Exceptions are ketoconazole, troglitazone, coumarol, etretinate, and amiodarone; with these agents, reactions may be severe and clinical recovery may be delayed for months. Although some types of drug-induced cholestasis also can be prolonged, failure of jaundice to resolve in a suspected drug reaction most often is indicative of

an alternative diagnosis. Rarely, deliberate rechallenge may be used to confirm the diagnosis of drug-induced liver disease or to prove the involvement of one particular agent when the patient has been exposed to several drugs; however, this approach is potentially hazardous and should be undertaken only with a fully informed and consenting (in writing) patient and preferably with the approval of an institutional ethics committee.

828 A (S&F, ch85)
Obesity is the condition most often reported in association with NAFLD. The health implications of the unremitting obesity epidemic are staggering, and NAFLD is a common by-product in both adults and children. NAFLD also is strongly associated with type 2 diabetes mellitus and glucose intolerance, with or without superimposed obesity. The presence of NAFLD in diabetic patients may also increase significantly the risk of cardiovascular disease. Most patients with NAFLD have multiple risk factors, including central obesity, type 2 diabetes mellitus, and hyperlipidemia, although some lack all recognized risk factors. The risk and severity of NAFLD increase with the number of components of the metabolic syndrome.

829 D (S&F, ch90)
The hyperdynamic circulation of cirrhosis is characterized by peripheral and splanchnic vasodilation, reduced mean arterial pressure, and increased cardiac output. Splanchnic vasodilation is caused in large part by relaxation of splanchnic arterioles and ensuing splanchnic hyperemia. Studies of experimental portal hypertension have demonstrated that splanchnic vascular endothelial cells are primarily responsible for mediating splanchnic vasodilation and enhanced portal venous inflow through excess generation of nitric oxide. This excess generation of nitric oxide and ensuing vasodilation, hyperdynamic circulation, and hyperemia in the splanchnic and systemic circulation contrasts with the hepatic circulation, in which nitric oxide deficiency contributes to increased intrahepatic resistance.

830 E (S&F, ch80)
HEV is an RNA virus endemic to developing countries such as those in the Indian subcontinent, Southeast Asia, and Central Asia. Overall attack rates range from 1% to 15% and are higher among adults. The outbreaks have been characterized by particularly high attack and mortality rates among pregnant women. In an epidemic in Kashmir, India, clinical HEV developed in 17.3% of pregnant women compared with 2.1% of nonpregnant women. Among the pregnant women, attack rates during the first, second, and third trimesters were 8.8%, 19.4%, and 18.6%, respectively. Fulminant hepatic failure developed in approximately 22% of the affected pregnant women, with an increased frequency of abortions, stillbirths, and neonatal deaths. The most recognizable form of HEV infection is acute enteric hepatitis. The clinical manifestations are similar to those of acute HAV infection. The onset of HEV infection is usually insidious, has a prodromal phase lasting one to four days, and is

characterized by a combination of flu-like symptoms, fever, chills, abdominal pain, anorexia, nausea, aversion to smoking, vomiting, clay-colored stools, dark urine, diarrhea, arthralgias, asthenia, and transient macular skin rash. Acute HAV infection is less likely in this patient given the presence of IgG antibody to HAV.

831 **E** (S&F, ch79)

Needlesticks are common in the health care setting and are underreported. Almost all surgical house-staff will sustain at least one needlestick, and in nearly one half, the needlestick will be from a high-risk patient. Fortunately, the risk of transmission of HCV is approximately 0.3% when exposure occurs from hollow-bore needles used to draw patients' blood, although deep injuries increase the risk of transmission. Postexposure treatment with interferon-α has been used after occupational exposure to HCV, but the experience to date is uncontrolled and no benefit has been shown (not surprisingly given the low risk of transmission in this setting). Although postexposure prophylaxis is not effective, early treatment of acute HCV infection is. Treatment should be strongly considered in patients with acute HCV infection. Therapy with peginterferon alone should be started between weeks 8 and 12 after presentation if HCV RNA has not cleared spontaneously from serum by that time.

832 **B** (S&F, ch95)

The development of ascites secondary to chronic liver disease is associated with a 50% two-year survival rate and should prompt evaluation for liver transplantation. Treatment of ascites and encephalopathy with diuretics and nonabsorbable antibiotics are necessary parts of care; however, listing for liver transplantation has the greatest impact on survival.

833 **D** (S&F, ch72)

The liver plays a central role in the synthesis of fatty acids for storage in distal sites and in the transport of lipids within the body. To transport lipids in the circulation, the liver synthesizes and extracts a large number of apolipoproteins. Apolipoproteins, in combination with triglycerides, phospholipids, cholesterol and its esters, and lecithins, constitute circulating lipoproteins. In addition to these protein- and lipid-synthesizing functions, the liver expresses cell surface receptors for circulating lipoproteins and modulates intravascular levels of these important macromolecules. Lipoprotein lipase is synthesized in fat and muscle cells; after synthesis, it traverses endothelial cells and binds to the luminal surface of the capillary bed. Found in adipose, lung, and muscle tissue, lipoprotein lipase promotes lipolysis of triglycerides present in very low density lipoproteins, chylomicrons, or high-density lipoproteins. Regulation of lipoprotein lipase involves multiple stimuli, including fasting and levels of various fatty acids, hormones, and catecholamines.

834 **E** (S&F, ch86)

Valproic acid–associated hepatic injury occurs almost exclusively in children, particularly those younger than three years of age. Also at risk are persons with a family history of a mitochondrial enzyme deficiency (particularly involving the urea cycle or long-chain fatty acid metabolism), Friedreich's ataxia, or Reye syndrome or with a sibling affected by valproic acid hepatotoxicity. Another risk factor is multiple drug therapy. Cases in adults have rarely been described. The overall risk of liver injury among persons taking valproic acid varies from 1 per 500 persons exposed among high-risk groups (children younger than three years of age, polypharmacy, genetic defects of mitochondrial enzymes) to fewer than 1 in 37,000 in low-risk groups.

835 **B** (S&F, ch87)

Pyrrolizidine alkaloids are found in approximately 3% of all flowering plant species throughout the world, and ingestion of such plants, often as medicinal teas or in other formulations, can produce acute and chronic liver disease, including sinusoidal obstruction syndrome, in humans and livestock. Sinusoidal obstruction syndrome was first reported in the 1950s as a disease of Jamaican children, manifesting with acute abdominal distention, marked hepatomegaly, and ascites, a triad that resembled Budd-Chiari syndrome. The disease was linked to consumption of "bush tea," made largely from plants of *Senecio*, *Heliotropium*, and *Crotalaria* species and taken as a folk remedy for acute childhood illnesses, and characterized histologically by centrilobular hepatic congestion with occlusion of the hepatic venules leading to congestive cirrhosis. Comfrey (*Symphytum officinale*) remains commercially available even though it is a dose-dependent hepatotoxin. In Afghanistan, ingestion of pyrrolizidine alkaloid–contaminated grains and bread led to a large epidemic of sinusoidal obstruction syndrome, affecting 8000 persons and innumerable sheep. The other choices are causes of acute hepatocellular injury.

836 **E** (S&F, ch90)

The approach to treating esophageal variceal hemorrhage also applies to acute gastric variceal hemorrhage and includes volume resuscitation, avoidance of overtransfusion, and antibiotic prophylaxis with 400 mg norfloxacin twice daily for seven days. Endoscopic variceal ligation is the preferred endoscopic modality for control of acute esophageal variceal bleeding and prevention of rebleeding; however, the utility of band ligation in the treatment of gastric varices is limited. The preferred endoscopic therapy for fundal gastric variceal bleeding is injection of polymers of cyanoacrylate, usually *N*-butyl-2-cyanoacrylate, but these tissue adhesives are not currently available in the United States. Band ligation of varices greater than 10 mm in diameter usually is unsafe. If endoscopic and pharmacologic therapies fail to control gastric variceal bleeding, then a Linton-Nachlas tube, which has a 600-mL balloon, may be passed as a temporizing measure. The commonly used Minnesota tube and Sengstaken-Blakemore tube, with only 250-mL gastric balloons, are not as effective as the Linton-Nachlas tube for controlling bleeding from gastric fundal varices. Nevertheless, most patients in whom endoscopic and pharmacologic treatment fails to control gastric variceal bleeding will require a TIPS, which can control bleeding in greater than 90% of patients, a rate of efficacy equivalent to that of TIPS in controlling esophageal variceal bleeding (see figure).

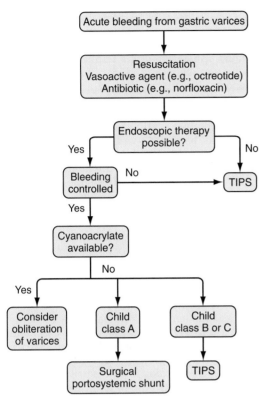

Figure for answer **836**

837 **B** (S&F, ch85)

There is no need for further testing to establish the diagnosis and no pharmacologic intervention is effective in cases of NAFLD. In these cases, biopsy is performed to stage the disease and help establish a prognosis. Large prospective studies are needed to define the natural history of NAFLD, but emerging evidence confirms that NAFLD can be progressive and associated with significant morbidity and mortality in some patients. The risks of liver-related morbidity and mortality are greatest in those with evidence of advanced NAFLD (steatohepatitis with necrosis and fibrosis) on the initial liver biopsy specimen. If clinical and biochemical risk factors for progressive disease can be established, a subset of patients can be identified in whom a liver biopsy will have the greatest prognostic and therapeutic value. For example, older age, obesity, diabetes mellitus, and an AST-to-ALT ratio greater than 1 were demonstrated in one study to be significant predictors of severe fibrosis (bridging/cirrhosis) in patients with NAFLD.

838 **E** (S&F, ch94)

The lesion in question is a hepatic adenoma, a benign tumor, but one that may rupture, especially if, as in this case, it is located peripherally. Because adenomas mimic normal liver tissue microscopically, needle biopsy and fine-needle aspiration may be of limited diagnostic value. Surgical resection is the recommended treatment for such tumors, whenever feasible. Arterial embolization should be reserved for lesions not amenable to surgical resection. Because of the risk of rupture and reports of malignant transformation, observation by repeat imaging is not an appropriate way to manage these tumors. Whether or not the tumor is removed, the patient must refrain from taking oral contraceptive steroids. If the adenoma is not resected, pregnancy should be avoided.

839 **C** (S&F, ch88)

Type 1 AIH can occur at any age and in either sex, although 78% of patients are women and the female-to-male ratio is 3.6:1. At initial presentation, fatigability is the most frequently reported symptom (86%). Hyperbilirubinemia is present in 83% of patients, and an elevated alkaline phosphatase level is found in 81%. Anti–smooth muscle antibodies, present in this patient, are characteristic of type 1 AIH. Increased IgG, but not IgM, fraction on serum protein electrophoresis would also support the diagnosis of type 1 AIH. IgM fraction elevation is more common in PBC. Liver/kidney microsome type 1 antibody is a classic finding in patients with type 2 AIH.

840 **A** (S&F, ch90)

The HVPG is the difference between the wedged hepatic venous pressure and the free hepatic vein pressure. The HVPG has been used to assess portal hypertension since its first description in 1951 and has been validated as the best predictor for the development of complications of portal hypertension. Measurement of the HVPG has been proposed for the following indications: (1) to monitor portal pressure in patients taking drugs used to prevent variceal bleeding; (2) as a prognostic marker; (3) as an endpoint in trials using pharmacologic agents for the treatment of portal hypertension; (4) to assess the risk of hepatic resection in patients with cirrhosis; and (5) to delineate the cause of portal hypertension (that is, presinusoidal, sinusoidal, or postsinusoidal) (see table for answer 759 at end of chapter), usually in combination with venography, right-sided heart pressure measurements, and transjugular liver biopsy. Although the indication for HVPG measurement with the most potential for widespread use is monitoring the efficacy of therapies to reduce portal pressure, HVPG monitoring is not done routinely in clinical practice because no controlled trials have yet demonstrated its usefulness.

841 **E** (S&F, ch79)

HCV infection is common in HIV-infected persons because the two infections share similar routes of transmission. Approximately 25% of HIV-infected persons are coinfected with HCV, and as many as 8% of HCV-infected patients are coinfected with HIV. HIV infection decreases the spontaneous rate of HCV clearance during acute HCV infection and leads to a correspondingly higher rate of chronic HCV infection. Progression of hepatic fibrosis is accelerated in HIV/HCV-coinfected patients when compared with HCV-monoinfected patients. SVR rates were lower in HIV/HCV-coinfected patients in clinical trials than in HCV-monoinfected historical controls. The safety and efficacy of peginterferon and ribavirin have not been established in patients with a CD4+ count less than 200/mm. Zidovudine, stavudine, and didanosine should not be used in combination with ribavirin because of the additive risk of mitochondrial toxicity.

842 C (S&F, ch78)

Several types of glomerulonephropathy have been described in patients with chronic HBV glomerular basement membrane. The immune complexes activate complement and production of cytokines with a subsequent inflammatory response. Nephrotic syndrome is the most common clinical presentation. Anti-HBV treatment has resulted in improved renal function and diminished proteinuria, sometimes completely.

843 E (S&F, ch91)

Renal impairment occurs in 33% of episodes of SBP. SBP leads to increased intraperitoneal nitric oxide production, which in turn further increases systemic vasodilation and promotes renal failure. Intravenous albumin (1.5 g/kg of body weight at the time the infection is detected and 1.0 g/kg on day 3) can increase intravascular volume and, in combination with cefotaxime, has been shown in a large randomized trial to reduce the risk of renal failure and improve survival compared with cefotaxime without albumin. Albumin seems to be effective by decreasing vasodilation. A confirmatory randomized trial is needed. Because of the survival advantage, however, the use of intravenous albumin as an adjunct to antibiotic treatment has been recommended.

844 A (S&F, ch76)

Hepatobiliary diseases noted in patients with CF can be grouped into three categories (see table at end of chapter). The pathognomonic lesion of CF, focal biliary cirrhosis, presumably results from defective function of the CF transmembrane regulator protein that is expressed in bile duct cells. Obstruction of small bile ducts leads to chronic inflammatory changes, bile duct proliferation, and portal fibrosis. At autopsy, FCC has been identified in 25% to 30% of patients older than one year of age. Progression to multilobular biliary cirrhosis occurs in approximately 5% to 10% of patients with CF and leads to symptoms associated with portal hypertension, such as splenomegaly and variceal bleeding. Hepatic steatosis also develops in approximately one half of patients but does not seem to correlate with outcome. Biliary abnormalities range from microgallbladder, which is largely asymptomatic and is found in as many as 20% of patients, to cholelithiasis and cholangiocarcinoma. Interestingly, the presence of liver disease does not correlate with the severity of pulmonary disease.

845 A (S&F, ch87)

Cocaine is a dose-dependent hepatotoxin. Acute cocaine intoxication affects the liver in 60% of patients, and many affected persons have markedly elevated serum ALT levels (>1000 U/L). Associated features include rhabdomyolysis, hypotension, hyperpyrexia, disseminated intravascular coagu-

lation, and renal failure. Hepatic injury is probably the result of toxic metabolites (e.g., norcocaine nitroxide) formed by the CYP system, specifically CYP2E1 and CYP2A, and enhanced hepatotoxicity is seen in persons who regularly consume alcohol. In animals, pretreatment with N-acetylcysteine decreases the risk of cocaine hepatotoxicity, although the usefulness of N-acetylcysteine for treating human cocaine-induced hepatic injury has not been determined. Ecstasy (3,4-methylenedioxymethamphetamine) is a euphorigenic and psychedelic amphetamine derivative that can lead to hepatic necrosis as part of a heatstroke-like syndrome that occurs as a result of exhaustive dancing in hot nightclubs ("raves"). Phencyclidine ("angel dust") is another stimulant that can lead to hepatic injury as part of a syndrome of malignant hyperthermia that produces zone 3 hepatic necrosis, congestion, and collapse, with high serum AST and ALT levels similar to those seen with ischemic hepatitis.

846 A (S&F, ch93)

Encephalopathy is a defining criterion for acute liver failure. The severity of encephalopathy can range from subtle changes in affect, insomnia, and difficulties with concentration (stage 1), to drowsiness, disorientation, and confusion (stage 2), to marked somnolence and incoherence (stage 3), to frank coma (stage 4). The pathophysiologic mechanisms underlying encephalopathy associated with acute liver failure are multifactorial. Many features of acute liver failure, including hypoglycemia, sepsis, hypoxemia, occult seizures, and cerebral edema, can contribute to neurologic abnormalities. Notably, neurologic conditions are the reason for excluding approximately 25% of patients with ALF from liver transplantation and for the deaths of more than 20% of patients who have undergone liver transplantation.

847 A (S&F, ch78)

The age at which a person becomes infected with HBV is a principal determinant of the clinical outcome. HBV infection in adults with intact immune systems is likely to cause clinically apparent acute HBV; only 1% to 5% of these persons become chronically infected. In contrast, as many as 95% of infected neonates become chronic HBV carriers because of immunologic tolerance to the virus. In adults, fulminant liver failure due to acute HBV occurs in less than 1% of cases, but this group still accounts for 5% of all cases of acute liver failure and approximately 400 deaths annually in the United States. Clinical symptoms and jaundice generally disappear after one to three months, but some patients have prolonged fatigue even after serum ALT levels return to normal. In general, elevated serum ALT levels and serum HBsAg titers decrease and disappear together, and in approximately 80% of cases, HBsAg disappears by 12 weeks after the onset of illness. In 5% to 10% of cases, HBsAg is cleared early and is no longer detectable by the time the patient first presents to a health care provider. Persistence of HBsAg after six months implies development of a carrier state, with only a small likelihood of recovery during the next 6 to 12 months.

848   **B** (S&F, ch94)

Intrahepatic cholangiocarcinoma represents approximately 10% to 20% of all primary liver cancers and 20% to 25% of cholangiocarcinomas. There is marked geographic variation in rates from 0.2 to 96 per 100,000 in men and from 0.1 to 38 per 100,000 in women due to the presence of known risk factors in the population. The highest rates are found in parts of Asia, most notably certain regions of Thailand, Hong Kong, China, Japan, and Korea. Chronic infestation of the biliary tree with one of the liver flukes is thought to be the cause of these high rates. The overall rate in the United States is 0.85 per 100,000, with the rate in men being 1.5-fold that of women. The rate in whites is approximately equal to that in African Americans and approximately half that in Asians. Although the underlying predisposing factor for most cases is unknown, there are a number of recognized risk factors. The strongest association is with *Opisthorchis viverrini*, a liver fluke endemic in parts of Southeast Asia and obtained by ingestion of raw or uncooked fish. The association with *Clonorchis sinensis*, a similar liver fluke, is less strong.

849   **A** (S&F, ch95)

Although histologic evidence of liver injury will develop in approximately one half of the patients within the first year after liver transplantation, severe graft dysfunction rarely occurs in the short term. With longer follow-up (five to seven years) after transplantation, HCV-related graft cirrhosis will develop in a substantial proportion of patients, ranging from 8% to 30%. Once the patient has reached the stage of clinically compensated cirrhosis, the risk of decompensation is approximately 40% per year. However, the development of histologic and biochemical cholestasis is a particularly ominous finding that may be a harbinger of rapid graft failure. In this setting, treatment may slow graft loss. Retransplantation for patients in whom graft failure develops due to recurrent HCV has not been widely advocated.

850   **B** (S&F, ch85)

Thiazolinedione treatment for NAFLD has been well tolerated and associated with improved insulin sensitivity and normalization of liver biochemistries. A drawback of both thiazolinediones, pioglitazone and rosiglitazone, is substantial weight gain and increased total body adiposity. Studies suggest that the beneficial effects of pioglitazone decrease when the drug is discontinued. A recent placebo-controlled European trial of rosiglitazone in 63 patients with NAFLD showed improvement in steatosis and transaminase levels, but not in necroinflammation or fibrosis.

851   **E** (S&F, ch79)

Patients with HCV infection may present with extrahepatic conditions, or these manifestations may occur in patients known to have chronic HCV. Classification of the extrahepatic manifestations of HCV is shown (see table at end of chapter) and is based on the strength of available data to prove a correlation. Types 2 and 3 cryoglobulinemia, characterized by polyclonal IgG plus monoclonal IgM and polyclonal IgG plus polyclonal IgM, respectively, can both be caused by HCV infection. Among HCV-infected patients, 19% to 50% have cryoglobulins in serum, but clinical manifestations of cryoglobulinemia are reported in only 5% to 10% of these patients and are more common in patients with cirrhosis. Symptoms and signs include fatigue, arthralgias, arthritis, purpura, Raynaud's phenomenon, vasculitis, peripheral neuropathy, and nephropathy.

852   **B** (S&F, ch82)

This patient has a pyogenic liver abscess resulting from inadequately treated diverticulitis. Most commonly, hepatic abscess is a result of cholecystitis or biliary obstruction but can be seen in poorly treated intra-abdominal infection as well. Most patients present with fevers, right upper quadrant pain, and leukocytosis. Imaging with ultrasonography, CT, or MRI is usually diagnostic. Although small abscesses can be sometimes managed with antimicrobial therapy alone, larger ones most always require percutaneous drainage along with antimicrobial therapy. Aspiration also allows identification of the microbe and helps tailor antibiotics according to sensitivities.

853   **D** (S&F, ch76)

The hepatic glycogen content is elevated in patients with glycogen storage disease type I, and the most accurate diagnostic measure is direct analysis of enzyme activity performed on fresh, rather than frozen, liver tissue. Analysis of fresh liver tissue is important to avoid disrupting microsomal glucose-6-phosphatase activity. Fasting serum glucose and lactate levels, a glucagon response test result, and the response to fructose or galactose administration (patients with glycogen storage disease type I do not show the expected increase in serum glucose concentration after administration of the substance) often provide supportive evidence but may not yield a definitive diagnosis. Intermittent severe neutropenia is noted in most patients with glycogen storage disease type Ib. DNA analysis-based approaches to diagnosis that integrate biochemical features and the presence or absence of persistent neutropenia have been proposed and may provide a diagnostic alternative to liver biopsy.

854   **D** (S&F, ch82)

This patient has risk factors for *Echinococcus* infection and a classic appearance of this infection on imaging. Infection occurs when humans eat vegetables contaminated by dog feces containing embryonated eggs. The eggs hatch in the small intestine and liberate oncospheres that penetrate the mucosa and migrate via vessels or lymphatics throughout the body. The liver is the most common destination (70%), followed by the lungs (20%), kidney, spleen, brain, and bone. In these organs, a hydatid cyst develops that produces numerous protoscolices, which reproduce asexually. Ultimately, the hydatid cyst ruptures and releases them to set up multiple additional daughter cysts. Characteristic cysts with ring-like calcifications along with septated cysts with multiple associated daughter cysts are seen on imaging.

855 E (S&F, ch83)

VOD is characterized by occlusion of the terminal hepatic venules and hepatic sinusoids. VOD most commonly occurs after bone marrow transplantation. A variety of antineoplastic drugs have been implicated as causes for VOD, including gemtuzumab ozogamicin, actinomycin D, dacarbazine, cytosine arabinoside, mithramycin, and 6-thioguanine. However, ingestion of alkaloids, as can be found in "bush tea," is reported as a common worldwide cause of VOD. Epidemics have been reported in India, Afghanistan, South Africa, the Middle East, and the United States. Classically, VOD presents with mild hyperbilirubinemia (concentration >2 mg/dL), painful hepatomegaly, weight gain, and ascites. On liver biopsy, sinusoidal dilation and severe hepatic congestion will be seen, the results of progressive occlusion of the sinusoids and venules. Inflammation is notably absent in VOD.

856 C (S&F, ch82)

In the United States, amebiasis is a disease of young, often Hispanic, adults. Amebic liver abscess is the most common extraintestinal manifestation of amebiasis. Typical symptoms include abdominal pain, fever, malaise, myalgias, and arthralgias. During its life cycle, *Entamoeba histolytica* exists in trophozoite or cyst form. After infection, amebic cysts pass through the gastrointestinal tract and become trophozoites in the colon, where they invade the mucosa and produce typical flask-shaped ulcers. The organism is carried by the portal circulation to the liver, where an abscess may develop. Aspiration of this abscess may yield a reddish brown, pasty ("anchovy paste") aspirate in which trophozoites are rarely identified. Treatment is with metronidazole. After treatment with metronidazole for seven to 10 days, eradication of residual amebae in the gut with agents such as iodoquinol, 650 mg three times daily for 20 days; diloxanide furoate, 500 mg three times daily for 10 days; and paromomycin, 25 to 35 mg/kg/day in three divided doses for seven to 10 days, is often recommended.

857 C (S&F, ch88)

A histologic hallmark of AIH is interface hepatitis, which is characterized by disruption of the portal tract by a lymphoplasmacytic infiltrate. Typically, lobular hepatitis (mononuclear inflammatory cells line the sinusoidal spaces) coexists with interface hepatitis and may be pronounced during an acute onset or during relapse after treatment withdrawal. Overall, histologic features are similar between symptomatic and asymptomatic patients, and both groups respond well to administration of glucocorticoid agents. Florid bile duct lesions are more characteristic of patients with early PBC. Fat and hyaline bodies are present in biopsy specimens of patients with steatohepatitis from alcohol.

858 B (S&F, ch89)

The initial lesion found on liver biopsy of a patient with PBC is damage to epithelial cells in the small bile ducts. The most important and only diagnostic clue in many cases is ductopenia (defined as the absence of interlobular bile ducts in >50% of the portal tract). The florid duct lesion, in which the epithelium of the interlobular and segmental bile ducts degenerates segmentally with formation of poorly defined, noncaseating, epithelioid granulomas, is nearly diagnostic of PBC, although this lesion is found in a relatively small proportion of patients, mainly those with early-stage disease.

859 C (S&F, ch88)

It has been reported that 38% of patients with AIH had concurrent extrahepatic immunologic diseases, the most common of which were autoimmune thyroiditis (in 12%), Graves disease (6%), and chronic ulcerative colitis (6%). Autoimmune thyroiditis is common in both type 1 and type 2 AIH. Additionally, type 1 AIH is most often associated with Graves disease and chronic ulcerative colitis, whereas type 2 AIH is more highly associated with vitiligo and type 1 diabetes mellitus. Rheumatoid arthritis, pernicious anemia, systemic sclerosis, Coombs-positive hemolytic anemia, autoimmune thrombocytic purpura, symptomatic cryoglobulinemia, leukocytoclastic vasculitis, nephritis, erythema nodosum, systemic lupus erythematosus, and fibrosis alveolitis also occurred but each in less than 1% of those with AIH. Cholangiography is warranted in all patients who have concurrent chronic ulcerative colitis to exclude primary sclerosing cholangitis.

860 D (S&F, ch92)

No specific laboratory findings indicate the presence of HE definitively. The most commonly used test to assess a patient with possible HE is the blood ammonia level. An elevation in the blood ammonia level in a patient with cirrhosis and altered mental status supports a diagnosis of HE. Blood ammonia levels may be elevated in the absence of HE, however, because of gastrointestinal bleeding or the ingestion of certain medications (e.g., diuretics, alcohol, narcotics, and valproic acid). In addition, blood ammonia levels may be elevated in the presence of HE, even in the absence of cirrhosis and portal hypertension, in patients with metabolic disorders that influence ammonia generation or metabolism, such as urea cycle disorders and disorders of proline metabolism (see table at end of chapter). Use of a tourniquet when blood is drawn and delayed processing and cooling of a blood sample may raise the blood ammonia level. Measurement of arterial ammonia offers no advantage to measurement of venous ammonia levels in patients with chronic liver disease.

861 D (S&F, ch93)

The diagnosis of acute liver failure is made clinically based on the physical examination (altered mental status) and supportive laboratory findings (hyperbilirubinemia, prolonged prothrombin time). Infrequently, acute liver failure may be confused with other clinical entities that are associated with jaundice, coagulopathy, and encephalopathy, such as sepsis, systemic disorders with liver and brain involvement (i.e., systemic lupus erythematosus, thrombotic thrombocytopenic purpura), and an acute decompensation of chronic liver disease. In particular, sepsis and acute liver failure have similar clinical profiles, and severe sepsis is frequently accompanied by a change in mental status; in this situation, jaundice and coagulopathy may result from intrahepatic cholestasis arising from high levels of proinflammatory cytokines and disseminated intravascular coagulation, respectively. Measurement of plasma factor VIII levels may help differentiate sepsis (low factor VIII level) from acute liver failure (factor VIII level generally not reduced). Alcoholic hepatitis and flares of chronic HBV infection may occasionally be mistaken for acute liver failure. In these instances, a careful review of the medical history, laboratory and imaging studies, and, in selected cases, liver biopsy findings is helpful.

862   **E** (S&F, ch73)
An increased ratio of AST to ALT may be seen in muscle disorders. The degree of elevation is typically less than 300 U/L, but in rare cases, such as rhabdomyolysis, levels observed in patients with acute hepatocellular disease can be reached. In cases of acute muscle injury, the AST-to-ALT ratio may initially be greater than 3:1, but the ratio quickly decreases toward 1:1 because of the shorter serum half-life of AST. The ratio typically is close to 1:1 in patients with chronic muscle diseases.

863   **B** (S&F, ch77)
HAV infection with prolonged cholestasis occurs rarely but can prompt the (inappropriate) performance of invasive diagnostic procedures because the diagnosis of acute hepatitis may not be readily considered in patients who have had jaundice for several months, even when they have detectable levels of IgM antibody to HAV. The cholestatic variant of HAV infection is not associated with increased mortality. The treatment is symptomatic. Complete clinical recovery is achieved in 60% of patients with acute HAV, regardless of the variant phenotype, within two months and in almost everyone by six months.

864   **A** (S&F, ch82)
Ascaris lumbricoides infection is present in at least one billion persons worldwide; it is most common among the poor. Humans are infected by ingesting embryonated eggs, usually in raw vegetables. The eggs hatch in the small intestine, and the larvae penetrate the mucosa, enter the portal circulation, and reach the liver, pulmonary artery, and lungs, where they grow in the alveolar spaces. From the alveolar spaces, they are regurgitated and swallowed and become mature adults in the intestine two to three months after ingestion, whereupon the cycle repeats itself. Symptoms generally occur in persons with a large worm burden; most infected persons are asymptomatic. Cough, fever, dyspnea, wheezing, substernal chest discomfort, and hepatomegaly may occur in the first two weeks. Chest radiography may show an infiltrate and eosinophilia may be present. ERCP is both diagnostic and therapeutic for ascariasis.

865   **C** (S&F, ch80)
Acute HEV infection is usually self-limiting. A few patients have a prolonged course with marked cholestasis, including persistent jaundice lasting two to six months, prominent itching, and a marked elevation in the alkaline phosphatase level, which resolves spontaneously. Mortality is very uncommon, with population surveys during outbreaks reporting mortality rates of 0.07% to 0.6%. There is no relationship between acute HEV and chronic hepatitis, cirrhosis, or hepatocellular carcinoma.

866   **C** (S&F, ch94)
Alpha fetoprotein is an α_1-globulin normally present in high concentrations in fetal serum but in only minute amounts thereafter. The reappearance of high serum levels of alpha fetoprotein strongly suggests the presence of hepatocellular carcinoma (or hepatoblastoma). This holds especially true in populations in which hepatocellular carcinoma is most prevalent: The great majority of Chinese and black African patients have an increased serum concentration of alpha fetoprotein (>10 ng/mL), and approximately 75% have a diagnostic level (>500 ng/mL). These percentages are lower in populations at low or intermediate risk of the tumor where the sensitivity ranges from 25% to 65%, with a specificity of 79% to 95% with cutoffs of 16 to 200 ng/mL.

867   **C** (S&F, ch95)
Angiotensin-converting enzyme inhibitors may exacerbate hyperkalemia to which the liver transplant recipient may be predisposed as a side effect of calcineurin-inhibitor therapy. Furosemide is an acceptable drug to treat hypertension after liver transplantation if it occurs in the setting of volume overload. A reduction in the doses of immunosuppressant drugs administered after transplantation usually does not significantly affect hypertension, so dose reduction should not be regarded as an appropriate initial approach to treating systemic hypertension after liver transplantation. Nifedipine is the initial treatment of choice for patients with hypertension after liver transplantation; unlike other calcium channel blockers, specifically verapamil and diltiazem, it will not interfere with the metabolism of calcineurin inhibitors.

868   **B** (S&F, ch71)
The caudate lobe of the liver is posterior to the transverse fissure. At the porta hepatis, the portal vein travels behind the hepatic artery and the bile duct. The falciform ligament contains the round ligament, which contains the obliterated umbilical vein. The fibrous capsule on the posterior aspect of the liver reflects on the diaphragm and posterior abdominal wall and leaves a bare area where the liver is in continuity with the retroperitoneum.

869   **D** (S&F, ch90)
Worsening renal function in a patient with cirrhosis and ascites can be the harbinger of HRS. However, this diagnosis can only be made based on signs and symptoms in patients with normal intravascular volume. Therefore, intravenous administration of fluids for volume expansion should always be attempted. Midodrine, an orally administered α_1-adrenergic agonist, and octreotide, a somatostatin analog that inhibits endogenous vasodilators, have been used in combination with

albumin for type 1 HRS in three small nonrandomized studies. In two studies, treatment with midodrine, titrated to cause an increase in mean arterial blood pressure, was associated with improved serum creatinine levels and improved survival compared with no treatment and was associated with few major side effects. This regimen has the advantage of ease of administration and seems to have a favorable safety profile; however, its efficacy has not been established in randomized, controlled trials.

870 D (S&F, ch81)

Like transfusion-transmitted virus, SEN virus is acquired predominantly by both the parenteral and fecal-oral routes. Neither virus is known to be sexually transmitted and neither virus causes chronic infection or end-stage liver disease. Most studies have shown no association between infection with either transfusion-transmitted virus or SEN virus and mortality or the response to treatment of chronic HCV infection.

871 C (S&F, ch83)

This patient has heart failure with resultant hepatic congestion. Heart failure causes an increase in the hepatic venous pressure that leads to congestion of the hepatic veins, central veins, and sinusoids. This results in progressive injury to the liver, which, in advanced stages, leads to central fibrosis, so-called cardiac cirrhosis. Sinusoidal hypertension and congestion can lead to the development of ascites. The ascites has a high SAAG, but unlike patients with advanced cirrhosis and portal hypertension, the protein concentration in congestive hepatopathy tends to be high.

872 E (S&F, ch91)

A urine sodium/potassium ratio less than 1 in a randomly obtained urine specimen suggests compliance with a low-salt diet and inadequate natriuresis despite diuretic therapy. The doses of both diuretics must be increased. Very low sodium diets are unrealistic for outpatients.

873 B (S&F, ch79)

Common risk factors for HCV infection and the associated frequency of infection in the United States are injection drug use (57.5%), blood transfusion before 1992 (5.8%), more than 50 lifetime sexual partners (12%), and family income below the poverty level (3.2%). The current prevalence of HCV infection in the United States may be underestimated because the National Health and Nutrition Examination Survey data did not evaluate persons who are homeless, incarcerated, or in the military. Among incarcerated persons, 12% to 35% are positive for HCV RNA serum, whereas those in military service have a seroprevalence rate for anti-HCV of 0.5%. An important mechanism of transmission worldwide has been the lack of sterilization of medical instruments such as syringes. Although the incidence of HCV transmission by medical instruments has also decreased markedly, the risk has not been eliminated, even in the United States. Currently, new HCV infections in the United States and other developed countries occur primarily as a result of injection drug use.

874 D (S&F, ch84)

The stellate cell is the major source of collagen production in the liver. It normally exists in a quiescent state and serves as a major storehouse for vitamin A. After activation, the stellate cell assumes a myofibroblast-like contractile phenotype and produces collagen. The cytokine transforming growth factor-β is a major stimulus for stellate cell activation and collagen production. Other cytokines implicated in the activation of stellate cells include platelet-derived growth factor and connective tissue growth factor. Oxidative stress plays a major role in stellate cell activation, and a variety of antioxidants can block both stellate cell activation and collagen production in vitro. Serum levels of 4-hydroxy-nonenal, a specific product of lipid peroxidation, are elevated in patients with alcoholic liver disease, serving to up-regulate both procollagen type I and tissue inhibitor of metalloproteinase-1 gene expression. Matrix metalloproteinase-1 plays a major role in degrading type I collagen. Tissue inhibitor levels of metalloproteinase-1 also are elevated in alcoholic liver disease. The result seems to be an increase in stellate cell activation and collagen production on the one hand and a decrease in matrix degradation on the other.

875 A (S&F, ch78)

Reactivation of HBV replication is a well-recognized complication in patients with chronic HBV infection who receive cytotoxic or immunosuppressive therapy. Suppression of the normal immunologic responses to HBV leads to enhanced viral replication. Most patients who experience immunosuppressive therapy–induced flares have been HBsAg positive, but some studies have reported the reappearance of HBsAg in patients who were initially positive for anti-HBs or anti-HBc, or both. Reactivated HBV in patients who are HBsAg negative and either anti-HBc or anti-HBs positive suggests the possible latency of HBV in liver and mononuclear cells and the large extrahepatic reservoir of HBV.

876 B (S&F, ch90)

Ligation initially should be at the bleeding site or immediately below the bleeding site. Other large varices should also be banded in the same session. If active bleeding is not noted, then ligation is performed beginning at the gastroesophageal junction and proceeding proximally at a distance of every 2 cm in a spiral fashion. If bleeding obscures the varices, then multiple bands are placed at the gastroesophageal junction circumferentially until bleeding can be controlled, but the long-term risks of esophageal stricture increase in such patients. Bleeding can be controlled in as many as 90% of patients by a combination of pharmacologic and endoscopic methods.

877 D (S&F, ch87)

Acute poisoning by copper leads to a syndrome resembling iron toxicity. Ingestion of toxic amounts (1 to 10 mg) usually is seen with suicidal intent, especially on the Indian subcontinent. Vomiting, diarrhea, and abdominal pain accompanied by a metallic taste are seen during the first few hours after ingestion. Gastrointestinal tract erosions, renal tubular necrosis, and rhabdomyolysis often accompany zone 3 hepatic necrosis by the second or third day. Jaundice results from both hepatic injury and acute hemolysis caused by high blood copper levels. The mortality rate is 15%, with early deaths resulting from shock and circulatory collapse and late deaths resulting from hepatic and renal failure.

878 **E** (S&F, ch89)
PBC is an autoimmune liver disease that generally affects middle-aged women from a variety of racial groups. It is the most frequently diagnosed cholestatic chronic liver disease in adults in the United States. It is characterized by ongoing inflammatory destruction of the intralobular bile ducts that leads to chronic cholestasis and biliary cirrhosis. The patient with PBC typically presents with symptoms of fatigue or pruritus. Other symptoms include right upper quadrant abdominal pain, anorexia, and jaundice. Widespread use of screening laboratory tests has led to the diagnosis of PBC at an asymptomatic stage in as many as 60% of patients with this condition. Such patients are identified by incidental findings of elevated serum alkaline phosphatase and antimitochondrial antibody levels in a serum specimen obtained during a routine health evaluation. In the case presented here, the patient is immune by previous vaccination to HBV and has no evidence of HCV. Symptomatic cholelithiasis is less likely than PBC; 50% of patients with PBC may have a positive ANA.

879 **B** (S&F, ch85)
MRI, ultrasonography, and computed tomography are all sensitive for the detection of hepatic fat, but none is able to distinguish simple steatosis from steatohepatitis. Liver biopsy remains the only reliable tool to make this distinction.

880 **A** (S&F, ch93)
The U.S. Acute Liver Failure Study Group identified the leading causes of acute liver failure to be acetaminophen (39%) and idiosyncratic drug reactions (13%), based on a study of 308 adults conducted between 1998 and 2001. Acetaminophen is a dose-dependent hepatotoxin that, when ingested in excessive doses, can lead to life-threatening liver injury characterized by hypoprothrombinemia, towering aminotransferase elevations, and a normal or minimally elevated serum bilirubin level (see table at end of chapter). Measurement of serum acetaminophen levels is helpful for assessing the risk of hepatotoxicity after an acute overdose, but falsely positive detection of acetaminophen in serum has been reported in some patients with

deep jaundice if a colorimetric assay for acetaminophen is used.

881 **C** (S&F, ch82)
Human infections with *Trichinella spiralis* are usually due to consumption of raw or undercooked pork containing *T. spiralis* larvae, which are released in the small intestine, penetrate the mucosa, and disseminate through the circulation. The larvae may then enter the myocardium, cerebrospinal fluid, brain, and, less often, liver and gallbladder. From these locations, the larvae re-enter the circulation and reach striated muscle, where they become encapsulated. Clinical manifestations of infection develop when the worm burden is high and include diarrhea, fever, myalgias, periportal edema, and leukocytosis with marked eosinophilia. The diagnosis is suggested by a characteristic history in a patient with fever and eosinophilia. A muscle biopsy may help to confirm the diagnosis. Treatment consists of glucocorticoids to relieve allergic symptoms, followed by albendazole 400 mg/day for three days or mebendazole 200 mg/day for five days.

882 **D** (S&F, ch86)
Aminopenicillins will often cause cholestasis with hepatocellular necrosis. Phenytoin causes a severe acute hepatitis. The range of liver diseases associated with nitrofurantoin includes acute hepatitis, occasionally with features of cholestasis, hepatic granulomas, chronic hepatitis with autoimmune phenomena, acute liver failure, and cirrhosis. The frequency of cholestasis with oral contraceptive steroids is 2.5 per 10,000 women exposed. The occurrence of cholestasis with oral contraceptive steroids is partly dose dependent and less likely with low-dose than high-dose estrogen preparations. Genetic factors influence the frequency of this complication, with a particularly high rate observed among women in Chile and Scandinavia. Persons with a history of cholestasis of pregnancy are also at risk (50%). The estrogenic component is most likely responsible. Symptoms develop two to three months, rarely as late as nine months, after oral contraceptive steroids are started. A mild transient prodrome of nausea and malaise may occur and is followed by pruritus and jaundice. The serum alkaline phosphatase level is moderately elevated, and serum aminotransferase levels are increased transiently, occasionally to levels exceeding 10 times the upper limit of normal. The serum GGTP level is often normal. Recovery is usually prompt, within days to weeks after cessation of the drug. Chronic cholestasis is rare.

Tables

ACUTE PORPHYRIAS	ENZYMATIC DEFECT	MODE OF INHERITANCE	CLINICAL FINDINGS	SITE OF EXPRESSION	MAJOR BIOCHEMICAL FINDINGS
Acute intermittent porphyria	PBG deaminase	Autosomal dominant	Neurologic	Liver	Urine: ALA < PBG
ALA dehydratase deficiency	ALA dehydratase	Autosomal recessive	Neurologic	Liver	Urine: ALA
Hereditary coproporphyria	Coproporphyrinogen oxidase	Autosomal dominant	Neurologic, cutaneous	Liver	Urine: ALA > PBG, coproporphyrin Stool: Coproporphyrin
Variegate porphyria	Protoporphyrinogen oxidase	Autosomal dominant	Neurologic, cutaneous	Liver	Urine: ALA > PBG, coproporphyrin Stool: Coproporphyrin, protoporphyrinogen
Cutaneous Porphyrias					
Congenital erythropoietic porphyria	Uroporphyrinogen III cosynthase	Autosomal recessive	Cutaneous	Bone marrow	Urine and stool: Coproporphyrin I
Erythropoietic protoporphyria	Ferrochelatase	Autosomal dominant	Cutaneous, rarely neurologic	Liver, bone marrow	Urine: None Stool: Protoporphyrin, coproporphyrin
Hepatoerythropoietic porphyria	Uroporphyrinogen III decarboxylase	Autosomal recessive	Cutaneous	Liver, bone marrow	Urine: Uroporphyrin, 7-carboxylate porphyrin Stool: Isocoproporphyrin
Porphyria cutanea tarda	Uroporphyrinogen III decarboxylase	Autosomal dominant or acquired	Cutaneous	Liver	Urine: Uroporphyrin, 7-carboxylate porphyrin Stool: Isocoproporphyrin

ALA, 5-aminolevulinic acid; PBG, porphobilinogen.

Table for answer 735 **Causes of Isolated Hyperbilirubinemia in Adults**

CAUSE	MECHANISM
Indirect Hyperbilirubinemia	
Hemolytic Disorders	Overproduction of bilirubin
Inherited	
Red cell enzyme defects (e.g., glucose-6-phosphate dehydrogenase deficiency)	
Sickle cell disease	
Spherocytosis and elliptocytosis	
Acquired	
Drugs and toxins	
Hypersplenism	
Immune mediated	
Paroxysmal nocturnal hemoglobinuria	
Traumatic: macro- or microvascular injury	
Ineffective Erythropoiesis	Overproduction of bilirubin
Cobalamin deficiency	
Folate deficiency	
Profound iron deficiency	
Thalassemia	
Drugs: Rifampin, Probenecid	Impaired hepatocellular uptake
Inherited Conditions	Impaired conjugation of bilirubin
Crigler-Najjar syndrome types I and II	
Gilbert's syndrome	
Other	
Hematoma	Overproduction of bilirubin
Direct Hyperbilirubinemia	
Inherited Conditions	
Dubin-Johnson syndrome	Impaired excretion of conjugated bilirubin
Rotor's syndrome	

Table for answers 759 and 840 **The Use of Hepatic Venous Pressure Gradient in the Differential Diagnosis of Portal Hypertension**

TYPE OF PORTAL HYPERTENSION	WHVP	FHVP	HVPG
Prehepatic	Normal	Normal	Normal
Presinusoidal	Normal	Normal	Normal
Sinusoidal	Increased	Normal	Increased
Postsinusoidal	Increased	Normal	Increased
Posthepatic			
Heart failure	Increased	Increased	Normal
Budd-Chiari syndrome	—	Hepatic vein cannot be cannulated	—

FHVP, free hepatic vein pressure; HVPG, hepatic venous pressure gradient; WHVP, wedged hepatic venous pressure.

Table for answer 780 **Laboratory Values in Urea Cycle Defects**

ENZYME DEFICIENCY	AMMONIA (PLASMA)	CITRULLINE (SERUM)	ARGININOSUCCINATE (URINE OR SERUM)	OROTIC ACID (URINE)	ARGININE/ ORNITHINE (SERUM)
Carbamyl phosphate synthetase	↑–↑↑↑	↓	↓	↓	↓
Ornithine transcarbamylase	↑–↑↑↑	↓	↓	↑↑	↓
Argininosuccinate synthetase	↑–↑↑↑	↑↑↑	↓	Normal–↑	↓
Argininosuccinase	↑–↑↑↑	↑↑↑	↑↑↑	Normal–↑	↓
Arginase	↑	↑↑	↑↑	Normal–↑	↑↑

Table for answer 790 **Classification of Ascites by Serum-Ascites Albumin Gradient**

HIGH GRADIENT ≥1.1 g/dL (11 g/L)	LOW GRADIENT <1.1 g/dL (11 g/L)
Alcoholic hepatitis	Biliary ascites
Budd-Chiari syndrome	Bowel obstruction or infarction
Cardiac ascites	Nephrotic syndrome
Cirrhosis	Pancreatic ascites
Fatty liver of pregnancy	Peritoneal carcinomatosis
Fulminant hepatic failure	Postoperative lymphatic leak
Massive liver metastases	Serositis in connective tissue diseases
"Mixed" ascites	Tuberculous peritonitis
Myxedema	
Portal vein thrombosis	
Sinusoidal obstruction syndrome	

Table for answer 798 **Reasons to Perform a Liver Biopsy in a Patient with Hepatitis C**

Assessment of the need for surveillance for hepatocellular carcinoma
Evaluation for concomitant liver diseases
Guidance for decisions regarding treatment of hepatitis C
Staging of fibrosis

Table 1 for answer 815 Intrahepatic Causes of Cholestatic Liver Enzyme Elevations in Adults

Drugs*
Bland cholestasis
  Anabolic steroids
  Estrogens
Cholestatic hepatitis
  Angiotensin-converting enzyme inhibitors: captopril, enalapril
  Antimicrobials: amoxicillin-clavulanic acid, ketoconazole
  Azathioprine
  Chlorpromazine
  Nonsteroidal anti-inflammatory drugs: sulindac, piroxicam
Granulomatous hepatitis
  Allopurinol
  Antibiotics: sulfonamides
  Antiepileptics: carbamazepine, phenytoin
  Cardiovascular agents: hydralazine, procainamide, quinidine
  Phenylbutazone
Vanishing bile duct syndrome
  Amoxicillin-clavulanic acid
  Chlorpromazine
  Dicloxacillin
  Erythromycins
  Flucloxacillin
Primary Biliary Cirrhosis
Primary Sclerosing Cholangitis
Granulomatous Liver Disease
Infections
  Brucellosis
  Fungal: histoplasmosis, coccidioidomycosis
  Leprosy
  Q fever
  Schistosomiasis
  Tuberculosis, *Mycobacterium avium* complex, bacillus Calmette-Guérin
Sarcoidosis
Idiopathic granulomatous hepatitis
Other
  Crohn's disease
  Heavy metal exposure: beryllium, copper
  Hodgkin's disease
Viral Hepatitis
Hepatitis A
Hepatitis B and C, including fibrosing cholestatic hepatitis
Epstein-Barr virus
Cytomegalovirus
Idiopathic Adult Ductopenia
Genetic Conditions
Progressive familial intrahepatic cholestasis
  Type 1 (Byler's disease)
  Type 2
  Type 3
Benign recurrent intrahepatic cholestasis
  Type 1
  Type 2
Cystic fibrosis
Malignancy
Hepatocellular carcinoma
Metastatic disease
Paraneoplastic syndrome
  Non-Hodgkin's lymphoma
  Prostate cancer
  Renal cell cancer
Infiltrative Liver Disease
Amyloidosis
Lymphoma
Intrahepatic Cholestasis of Pregnancy
Total Parenteral Nutrition
Graft-versus-Host Disease
Sepsis

*Categorized by histologic pattern. Drug lists are not meant to be comprehensive.

Table 2 for answer 815 Extrahepatic Causes of Cholestatic Liver Enzymes in Adults

Intrinsic
Choledocholithiasis
Immune-Mediated Duct Injury
   Autoimmune pancreatitis
   Primary sclerosing cholangitis
Malignancy
   Ampullary cancer
   Cholangiocarcinoma
Infections
   AIDS cholangiopathy
     Cytomegalovirus
     Cryptosporidiosis
     Microsporidiosis
   Parasitic infections
   Ascariasis
Extrinsic
Malignancy
   Gallbladder cancer
   Metastases, including portal adenopathy from metastases
   Pancreatic cancer
*Mirizzi's syndrome**
Pancreatitis
Pancreatic pseudocyst

*Compression of the common hepatic duct by a stone in the neck of the gallbladder.
AIDS, acquired immunodeficiency syndrome.

Table for answer 844 Spectrum of Hepatobiliary Disease in Patients with Cystic Fibrosis

Lesions specific to cystic fibrosis	Hepatic
	  Focal biliary cirrhosis with inspissation
	  Multilobular biliary cirrhosis with inspissation
	Biliary
	  Microgallbladder
	  Mucocele
	  Mucous hyperplasia of the gallbladder

Lesions secondary to extrahepatic disease	Hepatic lesions associated with cardiopulmonary disease
	  Centrilobular necrosis
	  Cirrhosis
	Pancreatic lesions
	  Fibrosis (leading to bile duct compression/stricture)

Lesions that occur with a higher frequency in patients with cystic fibrosis	Hepatic
	  Drug hepatotoxicity
	  Fatty liver
	  Neonatal cholestasis
	  Viral hepatitis
	Biliary
	  Biliary sludge
	  Cholangiocarcinoma
	  Cholelithiasis
	  Sclerosing cholangitis

Modified from Balistreri WF. Liver disease in infancy and childhood. In: Schiff ER, Sorrell MF, Maddrey WC, editors. Schiff's Diseases of the Liver, 9th ed. Philadelphia: Lippincott-Raven; 1999. p 1379.

Table for answer 851 **Extrahepatic Manifestations of Hepatitis C Virus Infection**

Proven Associations
Autoimmune thyroiditis
B-cell non-Hodgkin's lymphoma
Diabetes mellitus
Lichen planus
Mixed cryoglobulinemia
Monoclonal gammopathies
Porphyria cutanea tarda
Possible Associations
Chronic polyarthritis
Idiopathic pulmonary fibrosis
Non-cryoglobulinemic nephropathies
Sicca syndrome
Thyroid cancer
Renal cell carcinoma
Vitiligo

Table for answer 860 **Differential Diagnosis of Hyperammonemia**

Acute liver failure
Chronic kidney disease
Cigarette smoking
Cirrhosis
Gastrointestinal bleeding
Inborn errors of metabolism
    Proline metabolism disorders
    Urea cycle disorders (e.g., carbamyl phosphate synthetase
       I deficiency, ornithine transcarbamylase deficiency,
       argininosuccinate lyase deficiency, *N*-acetyl glutamate
       synthetase deficiency)
Medications
    Alcohol
    Diuretics (e.g., acetazolamide)
    Narcotics
    Valproic acid
Muscle exertion and ischemia
Portosystemic shunts
Technique and conditions of blood sampling
    High body temperature
    High-protein diet
    Tourniquet use

Table for answer 880 **Presenting Clinical Features of Acute Liver Failure***

PARAMETER	ACETAMINOPHEN ($N = 605$)	IDIOSYNCRATIC DRUG REACTION ($N = 156$)	INDETERMINATE ($N = 180$)	HEPATITIS B ($N = 102$)	HEPATITIS A ($N = 34$)	OTHER CAUSES ($N = 244$)
Age (yr)	36	46	38	42	49	42
Female (%)	75	68	57	43	44	73
Time to jaundice (days)	—[†]	9	9	6.5	3	7
Grade 3 or 4 encephalopathy (%)	51	37	49	53	53	41
Serum ALT level (U/mL)	4016	626	846	1702	2275	668
Serum bilirubin level (mg/dL)	4.5	20.4	22.4	18.5	12.3	15.7
Transplanted (%)	9	44	44	44	29	31
Spontaneous survival (%)	65	27	25	26	56	37
Overall survival (%)	73	68	66	64	82	64

*1321 consecutive adults enrolled in the U.S. Acute Liver Failure Study Group (1998 to July 2008). All data reported as median or percentage; survival determined at three weeks.

[†]Most patients do not develop jaundice.

ALT, alanine aminotransferase.

Data provided courtesy of Dr. William M. Lee and the U.S. Acute Liver Failure Study Group, September 2008.

CHAPTER
9

Small and Large Intestine

QUESTIONS

883 A 37-year-old woman with a history of Crohn's disease presents to the emergency department with one day of diffuse abdominal pain, vomiting, and absence of bowel movements and flatus. Until recently, she was asymptomatic and off all medications, but she reports having intermittent and progressively more frequent abdominal pain with occasional vomiting. She does not have fever or diarrhea and has had no previous surgeries. Findings of physical examination and abdominal series are consistent with small bowel obstruction (SBO); laboratory tests are significant for K^+ of 3.1, normal white blood cell (WBC) count, hemoglobin of 10.9 g/dL with a mean corpuscular volume of 101 fL; C-reactive protein and erythrocyte sedimentation rate are not elevated. She is admitted to the hospital and treated conservatively with only partial resolution. A small bowel series shows a severely narrowed fibrotic terminal ileum with minimal passage of barium into the cecum. Glucocorticosteroids are administered intravenously without effect after five days. What is the next best course of treatment?
A. Ileal resection
B. Methotrexate (MTX)
C. Infliximab
D. 6-Mercaptopurine (6-MP)

884 Patients with irritable bowel syndrome (IBS) are at a greater risk of which of the following?
A. Ischemic colitis
B. Colon cancer
C. Ulcerative colitis (UC)
D. Antibiotic-associated colitis
E. Pancreatic cancer

885 What is the approximate prevalence of celiac disease in the general population?
A. 1:3000
B. 1:1000
C. 1:100
D. 1:10

886 The smooth muscle cells within each muscle layer of the small intestine form a syncytium. Their activity is locally coordinated by which of the following?
A. Interstitial cells of Cajal (ICCs)
B. Enteric nervous system
C. Intrinsic neurons
D. Myenteric plexus
E. Extrinsic neurons

887 A patient with Crohn's disease who has had multiple resections is brought to the emergency department by his family with the chief symptoms of confusion and bizarre behavior. On physical examination, he has nystagmus and ataxia. Laboratory studies reveal a normal blood ethyl alcohol level and a normal toxin and drug screen results. There is a metabolic acidosis. Lactate levels are normal. The patient's diagnosis will be confirmed by which of the following blood tests?
A. Serum ammonia level
B. Blood copper level
C. Serum magnesium
D. Vitamin B_{12} level
E. D-Lactate level

888 With regard to the ICCs, which of the following is most accurate?
A. The distribution of these cells changes from infancy to adulthood.
B. These cells are present only in the small intestine.
C. They regulate intestinal motility by generating slow waves and determining the frequency of contractions.
D. Their number is regulated by dopamine.

889 Which following factor aids the host in defending against intestinal infections?
A. Adherence
B. Intestinal acidity
C. Intestinal microflora
D. Cytotoxin production

890 A 34-year-old woman who has had diabetes since the age of six years comes to your office with symptoms of diarrhea. After a thorough workup fails to reveal a cause of the diarrhea, it is believed that she has chronic diarrhea due to her diabetes. Although the exact mechanism of this type of diarrhea is unknown, which of the following is most accurate?
A. There is no correlation with glycemic control.
B. Often treatable diseases such as bacterial overgrowth, sprue, and pancreatic insufficiency can be associated.
C. Chronic diarrhea is more common in patients with type 2 diabetes.
D. Steatorrhea is an uncommon feature of chronic diabetic diarrhea.

891 What is the most common cause of large colon obstruction?
A. Colon carcinoma
B. Volvulus
C. Stricture form diverticulitis
D. Crohn's disease
E. Fecal impaction

892 All types of anesthesia have inhibitory effects on intestinal motility. One technique that may actually reduce postoperative ileus is
A. Lumbar epidural anesthesia
B. Midthoracic epidural anesthesia
C. Perioperative opioid therapy
D. Naloxone therapy postoperatively
E. General anesthesia

893 Which of the following statements regarding microsporidiosis is true?
A. *Enterocytozoon bieneusi* accounts for 90% of the cases and responds well to albendazole.
B. It occurs primarily in patients with impaired cell-mediated immunity.
C. Microsporidia are identified in less than 10% of acquired immunodeficiency syndrome (AIDS) patients with chronic diarrhea.
D. Unlike cryptosporidiosis, microsporidiosis is not associated with sclerosing cholangitis.

E. Highly active antiretroviral therapy (HAART) and immune reconstitution are not helpful in the control of microsporidiosis in AIDS patients.

894 Which of the following statements about small intestine bacterial overgrowth (SIBO) is most accurate?
A. Small intestinal bacterial overgrowth is a common cause of malabsorption in developed countries.
B. SIBO has been proven to cause IBS.
C. The gold standard for diagnosis is the ^{14}C-xylose breath test.
D. Treatment with antibiotics such as metronidazole, amoxicillin, clavulanate, and ciprofloxacin is usually ineffective.

895 A 75-year-old white man with a history of congestive heart failure comes to the emergency department because of abrupt onset of left lower quadrant pain and bloody diarrhea. His medications include digoxin and furosemide. Physical examination reveals a temperature of 100.5°F. His pulse rate is 110 beats per minute, and the rhythm is irregular. His blood pressure is 136/85 mm Hg. Moderate left lower quadrant tenderness is appreciated by palpation. No masses are noted. Rectal examination discloses bloody stool. His hemoglobin is 13.0 g/dL and leukocyte count is 14,000/mm^3. Gentle flexible sigmoidoscopy reveals a normal rectum and a localized area of mucosal erythema, friability, edema, and submucosal hemorrhage in the midsigmoid. Stool examination was positive for leukocytes, but no other infections or parasites were identified. Which of the following is the best plan of management at this time?
A. Laparotomy
B. Mesenteric angiography
C. Computed tomography (CT) of the abdomen and pelvis
D. Mesalamine and prednisone therapy
E. Supportive care and observation

896 What are mucosal folds of the small intestine called?
A. Columns of Morgagni
B. Appendices epiploicae
C. Plicae circulares
D. Rugae
E. Haustral folds

897 Carbohydrate digestion begins in the mouth where salivary amylase comes into contact with ingested starches. Which of the following statements regarding salivary amylase is true?
A. Salivary amylase cleaves ingested starches into its component monosaccharides.
B. Salivary amylase is activated by the low gastric pH.
C. Almost all dietary starch is digested by the time it reaches the duodenum.
D. The effect of salivary amylase is largely dependent on the proximity to ingested starches and the amount of time that the food bolus is in the mouth.

898 In reference to the dominant endoscopic finding (see figure) seen in a patient with UC who is undergoing his yearly surveillance colonoscopy, what is the next appropriate step in management?

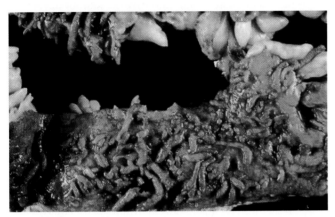

Figure for question **898**

A. Total proctocolectomy
B. Endoscopic removal of all polyps
C. Resection of affected portion of colon
D. Surveillance colonoscopy in one year

899 Which of the following statements regarding the transmural nature of the inflammation in Crohn's disease is most accurate?
A. It predisposes to the development of sinus tracts, fistulas, and fibrosis.
B. It is readily appreciated on endoscopic examination.
C. It occurs in continuous segments of bowel.
D. It is more commonly observed than Crohn's disease involving the mucosa and submucosa only.

900 With regard to azathioprine and 6-MP in the treatment of UC, which of the following is true?
A. There is ample evidence from randomized, controlled trials that 6-MP and azathioprine are effective in the induction and maintenance of remission for UC.
B. Metabolite testing is best used when patients are not responding or there is a question regarding compliance.
C. Bone marrow suppression is idiosyncratic, occurs in approximately 10% to 15% of patients, and primarily manifests with anemia.
D. The risk of non-Hodgkin's lymphoma is likely twofold that of the general population.

901 What is the most common cause of travelers' diarrhea?
A. *Salmonella*
B. *Aeromonas*
C. *Giardia*
D. Rotavirus
E. Enterotoxigenic *Escherichia coli*

902 Refractory celiac disease can be differentiated from celiac disease by which of the following?
A. Intraepithelial lymphocytes (IELs) lack expression of CD8 in celiac disease.

B. IELs lack expression of CD8 in refractory celiac disease.
C. IELs express CD8 in refractory celiac disease.
D. Many patients with refractory celiac disease have intestinal B-cell lymphoma.

903 A two-day-old infant is seen in the newborn nursery for failure to have passage of meconium. With regard to the pathogenesis of this disease, which of the following is true?
A. It results from the failure of splanchnic cells to migrate during organogenesis.
B. There is an absence of ganglion cells in the distal colon, resulting in a failure of the involved segment to relax.
C. A genetic basis for this disease has not been identified.
D. The abnormality is easily diagnosed by mucosal rectal biopsies.

904 Which of the following statements regarding the treatment of *Ascaris* infection is true?
A. Albendazole can be used safely in pregnancy.
B. Glucocorticoids should be used for pulmonary ascariasis.
C. Albendazole effectively kills worms within the bile duct.
D. Mebendazole is not an effective agent.

905 The hallmark serologic abnormality in paraneoplastic visceral neuropathy is which of the following?
A. Antinuclear antibody to ribonucleoprotein
B. Antineuronal nuclear antibody
C. Elevated creatine phosphokinase (CPK)
D. Abnormal creatine kinase levels
E. Anti-actin antibodies

906 The accuracy of fecal occult blood testing (FOBT) for colorectal cancer is affected by many factors. Which of the following statements is true?
A. Rehydration increases the specificity.
B. Ascorbic acid can affect the accuracy.
C. Tocopherol increases the sensitivity.
D. Ingestion of red meat need not be avoided.
E. Nonsteroidal anti-inflammatory drugs (NSAIDs) do not affect accuracy.

907 A 35-year-old woman with pan-UC for one year initially responded well to induction and maintenance therapy with mesalamine. However, two months ago, urgent bloody diarrhea several times daily and lower abdominal cramping developed; 40 mg/day prednisone allowed clinical remission to be achieved, but her symptoms have returned with prednisone tapering. The patient is otherwise healthy. Her medications are balsalazide, 2.25 g three times daily; prednisone, 15 mg/day; and calcium with vitamin D. Physical examination is normal. Laboratory studies reveal hemoglobin of 11.4 g/dL and plasma glucose of 140 mg/dL. Stool analysis for *Clostridium difficile* toxins A and B is negative. Which of the following is the most appropriate next step in the management of this patient?
A. Increase the prednisone dose to 60 mg/day.
B. Add olsalazine.
C. Add budesonide 9 mg/day.

  D. Increase the prednisone dose to 40 mg/day and add 6-MP.
  E. Start metronidazole.

908 Which of the following statements regarding the composition of human enteric bacterial flora is most accurate?
  A. Enteric flora are essentially identical in different individuals.
  B. The composition of an individual's enteric flora is usually unstable throughout adulthood.
  C. Environmental factors, including diet and sanitation, likely have a profound effect on early intestinal colonization with bacteria.
  D. In adulthood, dietary fluctuations induce changes in the relative populations of flora.
  E. Most human enteric bacteria can be cultured.

909 Severe diarrhea develops after a change in formula in a newborn. A diagnosis of a congenital galactose malabsorption is made after switching to a fructose-containing formula with resultant resolution of symptoms. With regard to this disease, which of the following is true?
  A. Blood and WBCs are commonly found in stool samples.
  B. Symptoms typically persist into adulthood.
  C. Supplemental enzymes typically need to be given.
  D. Stools are strongly positive for reducing substances.

910 Which of the following gastrointestinal signaling agents has been shown to increase appetite?
  A. Apolipoprotein A IV
  B. Cholecystokinin
  C. Ghrelin
  D. Leptin
  E. Peptide tyrosine-tyrosine

911 A 40-year-old woman with ileocolonic Crohn's disease previously maintained on mesalamime failed her second steroid taper. Her doctor wants to begin 6-MP in an effort to wean her completely off prednisone. What should he tell her with regard to this new medication?
  A. She is likely to be successfully tapered off the prednisone and taking only 6-MP within six weeks.
  B. She has a 70% chance of response.
  C. The risk of serious infection is less than 2%.
  D. If she gets pancreatitis, she can be rechallenged with azathioprine.

912 A five-year-old boy is brought to the emergency department by his concerned parents after they notice maroon-colored blood in the boy's stool. The child denies any pain, and he is hemodynamically stable. He has no other medical history, and the mother's pregnancy and his development have been otherwise unremarkable. Esophagogastroduodenoscopy and colonoscopy are performed, and the findings are unremarkable other than blood being seen throughout the colon. A presumptive diagnosis is made after a positive ^{99m}Tc-pertechnetate nuclear scan. Regarding the pathogenesis of this disorder, which of the following is most accurate?

  A. It results from the persistence of the ductal communication between the intestine and the yolk sac beyond the embryonic stage.
  B. It results from abnormal rotation of the primitive hindgut.
  C. Inadequate folate intake by the mother during her pregnancy most likely led to this condition.
  D. There is a genetic basis for this disease, and the patient's brothers and sisters should be subsequently screened.

913 Prolonged rectal storage of fecal material is made possible by an adaptive increase in rectal compliance allowing a previously empty rectal cavity to distend. Which of the following statements regarding this storage of fecal matter in the rectum is true?
  A. It provides a constant urge to defecate.
  B. It is mediated by excitatory nerves.
  C. Such rectal distention stimulates gastric emptying in a feedback mechanism.
  D. This type of rectal distention slows small bowel motility and reduces the frequency of proximal colonic propagating pressure waves.

914 An SBO develops in a patient during the postoperative period after laparoscopic cholecystectomy. What is the likely cause of obstruction?
  A. Richter's hernia
  B. Inguinal hernia
  C. Intra-abdominal adhesions
  D. Small bowel volvulus
  E. Metastatic gallbladder cancer

915 Which of the following statements regarding anal fissure is most accurate?
  A. Most anal fissures are located in the anterior position of the anus.
  B. The cause of anal fissures is likely related to trauma during defecation and reduced blood flow to the posterior anoderm.
  C. Patients with anal fissures commonly report the painless passage of bright red blood during defecation.
  D. Digital rectal examination must be performed during the initial evaluation of a patient with a suspected anal fissure.

916 What is the approximate prevalence of celiac disease in first-degree relatives?
  A. 1:200
  B. 1:100
  C. 1:50
  D. 1:20

917 Watery diarrhea without blood and only mild abdominal cramps develops in a 49-year-old person while on vacation in Mexico. Which organism is most likely to be responsible?
  A. Enteropathogenic *E. coli*
  B. Enterotoxigenic *E. coli*
  C. Enteroinvasive *E. coli*
  D. Enterohemorrhagic *E. coli*
  E. Enteroaggregative *E. coli*

918 What are the three cord-like smooth muscle layers that surround the colon?
  A. Plicae circulares
  B. Haustra

C. *Taeniae coli*
D. Rugae

919 Which of the following represent a correct pairing of genetics and/or serologic antibodies to disease behavior and/or location?
A. NOD2 and fistulizing subtype
B. Anti–*Saccharomyces cerevisiae* antibody and colonic inflammation
C. Anti-flagellin (Cbir1) and internal penetrating/ stricturing disease
D. Perinuclear anti-neutrophil cytoplasmic antibodies (pANCAs) and ileal disease

920 Which of the following is the most definitive environmental risk factor in the development of Crohn's disease?
A. Smoking
B. Breast-feeding
C. Working outside
D. Stress

921 This endoscopic picture (see figure) of the proximal small bowel is associated with all of the following diseases *except*:

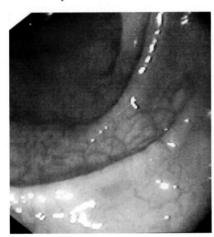

Figure for question **921**

A. Crohn's disease
B. Celiac disease
C. Tropical sprue
D. *Giardia* infection

922 The internal anal sphincter (IAS) and external anal sphincter (EAS) both have critical roles in regulating defecation. The EAS is a striated muscle and is located distal to the IAS. The IAS
A. Is composed of striated muscle under voluntary control and is innervated by the lumbar plexus, similar to the more proximal colon
B. Is composed of smooth muscle with a high resting tone that is modulated by both sympathetic and parasympathetic innervations
C. Is composed of striated muscle with a high resting tone that is modulated by the pudendal nerve (S3 and S4) similarly to other pelvic floor muscles
D. Is influenced by voluntary efforts to maintain continence

923 A 52-year-old man presents with five months of three to four loose, bloody stools with mild urgency and abdominal cramping and fatigue. He quit smoking 18 months ago and is otherwise healthy. Physical examination reveals normal vital signs and mild lower abdominal tenderness; examination of the rectum shows gross blood. Laboratory studies reveal a hemoglobin of 12.9 g/dL with a mean corpuscular volume of 78 fL. Stool culture is negative. Colonoscopic and histologic findings are consistent with mild UC of the rectum and sigmoid colon. Which of the following would be the most appropriate therapy for this patient?
A. Azathioprine
B. Ciprofloxacin
C. Metronidazole
D. Infliximab
E. Mesalamine

924 Paraneoplastic visceral neuropathy is associated with which of the following?
A. Gastric carcinoma
B. Breast cancer
C. Small cell carcinoma of the lung
D. Prostate carcinoma
E. Metastatic ovarian cancer

925 A 23-year-old man comes to see you for chronic diarrhea. Of note he has a history of Crohn's disease diagnosed at the age of 15 that has been under good medical control after an extensive ileal resection at the age of 18. After a thorough history and evaluation, you suspect that his diarrhea is due to bile salt malabsorption. Which medication should be your empiric drug of choice?
A. Loperamide
B. Diphenoxylate
C. Esomeprazole
D. Cholestyramine

926 Which is the true statement regarding genetic alterations in adenomas and colorectal cancers?
A. Somatic mutations of the *APC* gene occur in the majority of sporadic colorectal cancers.
B. Somatic mutations of the *APC* gene occur rarely in sporadic adenomas.
C. Mutations in the *K-ras* gene occur rarely in sporadic colorectal cancer.
D. Activation of the *p53* tumor suppressor gene leads to colorectal cancer.

927 What is the most common location of a nonspecific small bowel ulceration?
A. Duodenal bulb
B. Ligament of Treitz
C. Jejunum
D. Ileum

928 Which of the following pathogens causes a diarrheal illness that results from malabsorption?
A. Cholera
B. *Shigella*
C. *Campylobacter jejuni*
D. Enterotoxigenic *E. coli*

929 The peritoneum is derived primarily from the embryonic
A. Endoderm
B. Ectoderm
C. Vitelline duct
D. Mesoderm
E. Yolk sac

930 *Isospora belli* and *Cyclospora cayetanensis* share which of the following characteristics?
A. Do not stain with acid-fast stain
B. Readily treated with trimethoprim/sulfamethoxazole in immunocompetent patients
C. Protracted illness in immunocompetent and immunocompromised hosts
D. Peripheral eosinophilia with Charcot-Leyden crystals in the stool

931 Which of the following statements regarding vitamin B_{12} deficiency caused by SIBO is most accurate?
A. Vitamin B_{12} deficiency is caused by bacterial consumption of the vitamin within the intestinal lumen.
B. SIBO causes mucosal damage and greatly reduces the number of ileal binding sites for vitamin B_{12}.
C. Aerobic organisms are responsible for the vitamin B_{12} deficiency.
D. During the Schilling test, vitamin B_{12} deficiency is reversible by the addition of intrinsic factor.

932 Which of the following statements regarding anal cancer is false?
A. It accounts for 1.5% of gastrointestinal cancers.
B. Its incidence is decreasing in the United States.
C. Sixteen percent of cases are adenocarcinoma.
D. Tumors arising in the distal canal usually are keratinizing squamous cell carcinomas.
E. None of the above

933 NSAIDs are the most frequently administered drugs in the world. Features commonly associated with NSAID-induced small bowel ulceration include all of the following *except*:
A. Diaphragm-like strictures
B. Hypoalbuminemia
C. Anemia
D. Enteroenteral fistulas

934 The worm in Video 1 (see www.expertconsult.com) is harbored by as many as 25% of the world's population. Which of the following statements is true?
A. Most infected persons are symptomatic.
B. Worms are unable to enter the ampulla and cause biliary obstruction.
C. Intestinal obstruction is a rare intestinal presentation.
D. Pneumonia is usually self-limited.
E. Disease usually develops even in those with light worm burdens.

935 Which statement best describes the role of specific pathogens, gut flora, and immune response in the etiology of Crohn's disease?

A. The inflammation seen in Crohn's disease is more likely an inappropriate response to normal nonpathogenic gut flora rather than an appropriate response to a yet to be identified specific pathogen.
B. *Mycobacterium paratuberculosis* is believed to be the most likely culprit in the pathogenesis of Crohn's disease.
C. Healthy intestinal mucosa lacks any baseline inflammation.
D. Animal models of IBD demonstrate that specific pathogens introduced into the guts of genetically susceptible hosts will cause inflammation similar to that seen in IBD.

936 *Ascaris*, hookworm, pinworm, and whipworm are all sensitive to which of the following?
A. Praziquantel
B. Ivermectin
C. Metronidazole
D. Albendazole

937 A 20-year-old otherwise healthy man presents with three months of abdominal pain, diarrhea, a 10-lb weight loss, and diffuse arthropathy; he has not had any fevers. He has not traveled, takes no medicine, is a nonsmoker, and his family history is significant only for an uncle who had "some small intestine removed." His examination is remarkable for normal vital signs and right lower quadrant tenderness without a mass. What is the single next best test to confirm his diagnosis?
A. Stool studies
B. pANCA
C. Barium enema
D. Capsule enteroscopy
E. Colonoscopy with ileal intubation

938 Which group has the greatest risk of giardiasis in the United States?
A. Homosexual men who are not sexually active
B. Patients with AIDS
C. Children in day care
D. One whose drinking source is a treated deep well.

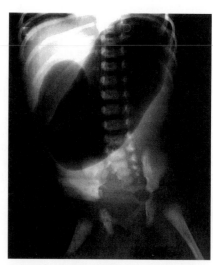

Figure for question **939**

939 A day-old infant girl is seen in the newborn nursery with severe bilious vomiting. The infant had normal meconium passage after delivery and is not jaundiced. The mother's pregnancy was uneventful. On examination, epigastric fullness is appreciated with tympany on percussion. An abdominal x-ray is obtained (see figure). What is the most likely diagnosis in this infant?
A. Hirschsprung's disease
B. Gastroschisis
C. Meconium ileus
D. Intestinal neuronal dysplasia
E. Duodenal atresia

940 High fever develops in the first few weeks of 6-MP therapy in a 38-year-old steroid-dependent female patient with Crohn's disease, and her doctor wants to start MTX. Which of the following statements regarding this treatment is most accurate?
A. It is equally effective in Crohn's disease whether given orally or parenterally.
B. This would be inappropriate therapy if this patient still wanted to conceive.
C. There is an approximately 60% chance that she will achieve a steroid-free remission.
D. She will respond to this medication within one month.

941 Dermatitis herpetiformis, a skin disease characterized by papulovesicular lesions on the extensor surfaces of the extremities, buttocks, trunk, neck, and scalp, is closely linked to which disease?
A. Tropical sprue
B. Crohn's disease
C. UC
D. Celiac disease

942 Which of the following statements regarding the epidemiology of UC is most accurate?
A. There is a distinct north-south gradient for the risk of developing UC.
B. The overall incidence of UC is increasing.
C. Incidence rates among various ethnicities are approximately equal.
D. Blacks have a much lower incidence of UC than whites.

943 Which of the following symptoms is not associated with IBS?
A. Continuous abdominal pain
B. Nausea
C. Bloating
D. Visible abdominal distention
E. Constipation

944 Acute onset of vomiting, diarrhea, fever, and abdominal pain develops in a 26-year-old pregnant woman. She is admitted to labor/delivery for dehydration and given fluids intravenously. You are consulted and asked to prescribe antimicrobial therapy. Stool cultures are pending. Which is the most appropriate antimicrobial agent?
A. Metronidazole
B. Tetracycline
C. Fluoroquinolones
D. Ampicillin
E. Trimethoprim/sulfamethoxazole

945 The enteric inhibitory motor neurons synthesize and secrete various neurotransmitters. In contrast, the enteric excitatory motor neurons synthesize and secrete only one neurotransmitter. This neurotransmitter is
A. Acetylcholine
B. Nitric oxide
C. Adenosine triphosphate
D. Vasoactive intestinal peptide
E. Epinephrine

946 The fat intake for all ages and sexes increased steadily from the 1940s to the 1980s before decreasing somewhat. With regard to the intraluminal digestion of fat, which of the following statements is true?
A. The majority of dietary lipid is absorbed in the distal ileum.
B. The majority of lipolysis occurs in the stomach with the help of gastric lipase.
C. Emulsification is critical for lipolysis to occur and is aided by gastric milling, dietary phospholipids, and bile salts.
D. Gastric lipase digests the majority of ingested phospholipids.
E. Pancreatic lipase is most active at an acidic pH.

947 An otherwise healthy 22-year-old woman presents with five months of low-grade fever, a 10-lb weight loss, and intermittent postprandial right lower quadrant pain associated with nonbloody diarrhea three to five times daily. She also notes mild bilateral knee pain that is worse on awakening or after prolonged sitting. The family history is noncontributory. Examination is notable for a temperature of 99.8°F and moderate right lower quadrant tenderness with no rebound, masses, or guarding. What is the most likely diagnosis?
A. Acute appendicitis
B. Crohn's disease
C. IBS
D. Meckel's diverticulum
E. UC

948 Which of the following statements regarding reperfusion injury is true?
A. It is the major cause of injury after a prolonged episode of ischemia.
B. It results in the production of superoxide, hydrogen peroxide, and hydroxyl radicals.
C. Thiopurine methyltransferase (TPMT) is the rate-limiting enzyme involved in the production of these oxygen radicals.
D. Leukotriene B_1 is a major cytokine involved in this type of injury.

949 The following test and interval have been widely advocated for colorectal cancer screening:
A. Biannual FOBT
B. Flexible sigmoidoscopy every three years
C. Optical colonoscopy every 10 years
D. Double-contrast barium enema every 10 years
E. Virtual colonoscopy every 10 years

950 Which statement regarding SBO secondary to hernias is true?
A. Internal hernias are a more common cause of obstruction than external hernias.

B. Hernias have a high risk of strangulation.

C. Inguinal hernias are more common in young adults.

D. Hernias are the most common cause of SBO.

E. Internal hernias are always congenital.

951 Which of the following statements regarding the pathogenesis of diarrhea caused by the following organisms is false?

A. *E. coli* heat-stable enterotoxin increases intracellular levels of cyclic guanosine monophosphate (cGMP).

B. *Vibrio cholerae* toxin increases levels of cGMP.

C. NSP4 enterotoxin released by rotavirus leads to an increase in intracellular calcium.

D. *Salmonella typhimurium* activates nuclear factor κB and interleukin (IL)-8 secretion.

E. *C. difficile* toxins A and B disrupt cytoskeletal architecture.

952 Which of the following is a metabolic property of enteric flora?

A. Biotransformation of bile acids

B. Breakdown of plant polysaccharides

C. Production of short-chain fatty acids (SCFAs) from carbohydrates

D. Conversion of prodrugs into active metabolites

E. All of the above

953 Which statement regarding a diverticular abscess is inaccurate?

A. *E. coli*, *Streptococcus* species, and *Bacteroides fragilis* grow most often.

B. Small pericolic abscesses can be treated with broad-spectrum antibiotics and bowel rest.

C. CT-guided percutaneous drainage may eliminate the need for a multiple-stage procedure with colostomy.

D. Urgent surgery is required in 5% to 10% of patients.

954 A 30-year-old man with ileal Crohn's disease status post-ileocecectomy seven years ago who is taking no medications reports chronic diarrhea and excessive gas and bloating; he has no abdominal pain, vomiting, fever, or extraintestinal manifestations (EIMs) of inflammatory bowel disease (IBD). Physical examination is unremarkable. Laboratory test results including C-reactive protein and erythrocyte sedimentation rate are within normal limits. A small bowel series shows a nonobstructive fibrotic stricture of the neoterminal ileum with some debris proximally and no active inflammation. What is the next best step in the management of this patient?

A. Start glucocorticosteroids and 6-MP.

B. Begin rifaximin therapy.

C. Surgical consultation for resection of the stricture

D. Begin infliximab therapy.

955 A patient with UC in whom mesalamine treatment is failing and who has required two rounds of steroids in six months is prescribed 6-MP. Her TPMT (thiopurine methyltransferase phenotype) shows that she has intermediate activity of this enzyme. Which of the following statements is true?

A. This phenotype corresponds to a heterozygous genotype (wild type/mutation).

B. Approximately 20% of the population has intermediate activity of TPMT.

C. 6-MP and azathioprine should not be used in patients with intermediate activity of TPMT.

D. She is at higher risk of hepatotoxicity.

956 Which of the following statements regarding colorectal cancer is true?

A. The incidence of colorectal cancer is high in undeveloped countries.

B. The rate of cancer death from colorectal cancer is second only to lung cancer in the United States.

C. Of the United States population, colorectal cancer will develop in 0.6%.

D. The incidence of colorectal cancer is higher in men.

957 A 27-year-old woman who is newly diagnosed with Crohn's disease asks you what the risk is that her future offspring will have the condition. What should you tell her?

A. Her children are no more likely to get Crohn's disease than if she did not have it.

B. Her children are more likely to be diagnosed with either Crohn's disease or UC.

C. If she has monozygotic (identical) twins and one is diagnosed with Crohn's disease, the other is virtually certain to have it as well.

D. Her children have a 14- to 15-fold greater risk of the development of Crohn's disease than the general population.

958 Current recommendations for treatment of Whipple's disease involve which of the following?

A. Penicillin G plus streptomycin followed by trimethoprim/sulfamethoxazole

B. Ciprofloxacin

C. Albendazole

D. Augmentin

959 Endogenous and exogenous opiates contribute significantly to the development of postoperative ileus. Through which of the following is the mechanism of action mediated?

A. Stimulation of sympathetic neural inhibitory activity

B. Direct inhibition of the pacemaker activity of the ICCs

C. Activation of intestinal mu-opioid receptors suppressing release of acetylcholine neurons

D. Stimulation of nitric oxide inhibitory activity

E. Stimulation of inflammatory cytokines release

960 Nausea, vomiting, and diarrhea after eating a well-done steak and canned vegetables develop in a 62-year-old man. Subsequently, he has constipation, dry mouth, double vision, dysphagia, and muscle weakness. Which treatment is crucial for his illness?

A. Antitoxin

B. Intravenous immunoglobulin

C. Intravenous fluids

D. Mechanical ventilation

E. Transcutaneous pacemaker

961 Which of the following is a factor that may reduce postoperative ileus?
A. Lumbar epidural anesthesia
B. Naloxone therapy postoperatively
C. Chewing gum
D. General anesthesia
E. Delayed oral feeding

962 The proposed mechanisms for acute intestinal pseudo-obstruction include which of the following?
A. Excess sympathetic motor input to the gut
B. Excess nitric oxide release from inhibitory motor neurons
C. Decreased stimulation of peripheral mu-opioid receptors by endogenous or exogenous opioids
D. Reflex motor excitation through splanchnic afferents in response to noxious stimuli
E. Reduced inflammatory response with reduced release of inflammatory mediators

963 Therapy for tropical sprue would include nutritional support as well as a trial of which of the following?
A. Tetracycline
B. Amoxicillin
C. Metronidazole
D. A gluten-free diet

964 A new class of compounds known as prostones (e.g., lupiprostone) has shown some promise in their ability to treat constipation. These medications work by which of the following methods?
A. Antagonizing 5-hydroxytryptamine (5-HT) 3 receptors
B. Stimulating 5-HT$_4$ receptors
C. Activating a type 2 chloride channel activator
D. Stimulating high-amplitude colonic propagating pressure wave sequences

965 A patient with steatorrhea, anorexia, abdominal cramps, and bloating, who was recently in Southeast Asia has a small bowel series as shown (see figure). This presentation is most consistent with which of the following?

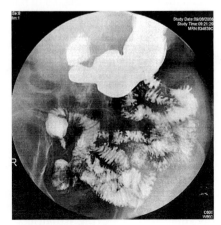

Figure for question **965**

A. Crohn's disease
B. UC
C. IBS
D. Tropical sprue

966 A patient is having recurrent gastric ulcers thought to be due to ischemia. Which of the following arteries will the interventional radiologist be most interested in examining?
A. Superior mesenteric artery
B. Inferior mesenteric artery
C. Arch of Riolan
D. The marginal artery of Drummond
E. Celiac axis

967 Which of the following statements regarding pANCA is most accurate?
A. pANCA titers directly correlate with disease activity.
B. pANCA is associated with the development of pouchitis after colectomy.
C. pANCA is never seen in patients with Crohn's disease.
D. pANCA is observed in more than 90% of UC patients.
E. pANCA likely has a direct pathogenic role in UC.

968 Which feature may distinguish rotavirus infection from norovirus infection?
A. The fecal-oral route is not the main mode of transmission for rotavirus.
B. Diarrhea lasts longer in rotavirus illness, as long as five to seven days.
C. Vomiting does not occur in norovirus illness.
D. Norovirus is a DNA virus.
E. Vaccination is available for norovirus.

969 Which of the following is postulated to be a major pathophysiologic consequence of an SBO obstruction?
A. Intestinal distention is primarily secondary to gases generated by bacteria and, to a lesser extent, swallowed air.
B. The translocation of enteric bacteria contributes to the septic consequences of an SBO.
C. Hypovolemia is primarily secondary to a lack of oral intake by the patient.
D. There is an inhibition of proinflammatory mediators including neutrophils, complement, and cytokines.
E. Normal intestinal motility is preserved in the setting of an SBO.

970 Colonic smooth muscle possesses intrinsic, oscillatory activity (even when external neural activity is blocked) that includes large-amplitude, slow membrane potential oscillations called slow waves. It also possesses small-amplitude, rapid membrane potential oscillations called which of the following?
A. Giant motor complexes
B. Accelerated fast waves
C. Migrating motor complexes (MMCs)
D. Myenteric potential oscillations

971 What is the most common anatomic position of the appendix relative to the cecum?
A. Anterior
B. Lateral
C. Medial
D. Retrocecal
E. Retrocolic

972 Which of the following regarding severe pseudo-membranous colitis is inaccurate?
A. It occurs in only 3% to 5%.
B. The mortality rate is as high as 65%.
C. Diarrhea may be minimal or absent.
D. Vancomycin is often used as first-line treatment.
E. Administer vancomycin intravenously in the presence of ileus.

973 Whipple's disease is an infection with *Tropheryma whippelii*. Which of the following statements concerning its epidemiology is true?
A. It is more common in women in their 50s.
B. It is more common in men in their 50s.
C. It is more common in women in their 20s.
D. It is more common in men in their 20s.

974 In addition to nutrient protein hydrolysis, which of the following is a function of pancreatic proteases?
A. Activating other pancreatic proteases from proenzymes
B. Splitting vitamin B_{12} from the R protein
C. Increasing the turnover of brush border membrane hydrolytic enzymes
D. Initiating the final steps in the processing of the sucrase-isomaltase complex
E. All of the above

975 What is the most predominant feature of tropical sprue in patients in Asia and the Caribbean?
A. Bloody diarrhea
B. Fat malabsorption
C. Hyperpigmentation
D. Alopecia

976 Which of the following medications has been approved to treat both UC and Crohn's disease?
A. MTX
B. Natalizumab
C. Infliximab
D. Adalimumab

977 What is the major anion transported in the colon?
A. Cl^-
B. HCO_3^-
C. Br^-
D. SCFAs

978 Abdominal pain in the right lower quadrant, fever, and diarrhea develop in a 25-year-old woman. Two weeks later, the diarrhea is resolved, but arthralgias develop. During the acute illness, stool examination shows white and red cells and a CT scan reveals mesenteric adenopathy and thickening of the ileum. What is the most likely etiology?
A. Enterotoxigenic *E. coli*
B. *V. cholerae*
C. *Yersinia enterocolitica*
D. *Salmonella typhi*
E. *C. difficile*

979 Causes of focal segmental ischemia (FSI) of the small intestine include which of the following?
A. Atheromatous emboli
B. Blunt abdominal trauma

C. Immune complex disorders
D. Oral contraceptives
E. All of the above

980 Which of the following is an accurate statement with regard to assessment of disease activity in UC?
A. Multiple indices to measure disease severity exist, most of which are specific and have been validated.
B. The Truelove and Witts activity index is a purely clinical classification of UC and characterizes disease activity as mild, moderate, or severe.
C. The UC disease activity index (or the Sutherland Index) gives a numerical score based on stool frequency, rectal bleeding, sigmoidoscopic appearance, and histologic severity.
D. Patients with fulminant colitis have fever, tachycardia, signs of peritonitis, and toxic megacolon on radiography.

981 The following is a characteristic of infection with *V. cholerae*:
A. The toxin increases cyclic adenosine monophosphate (cAMP) in intestinal cells leading to intestinal secretion.
B. The organisms invade the mucosa to activate cAMP.
C. The stool effluent is hypertonic.
D. The colon is primarily affected.
E. Hyperkalemic alkalosis occurs.

982 Which of the following statements regarding the EIMs of IBD seen in Crohn's disease is true?
A. Approximately 40% of patients with Crohn's disease will have at least one EIM.
B. EIMs seen in Crohn's disease may be categorized as those that are associated more with small bowel disease than with colonic disease.
C. Erythema nodosum and pyoderma gangrenosum are pathognomonic for Crohn's disease.
D. The risk of gallstones and kidney stones is not significantly different from that seen in UC.

983 A patient with UC taking 6-MP for five years experiences a flare and is started on prednisone. He responds initially, but then begins to flare on tapering of the steroids. Stool study results are negative. On sigmoidoscopy, deep ulcers are seen. Which of the following is the next best step in the management of this patient?
A. Begin a tumor necrosis factor α (TNF-α) antibody (e.g., infliximab).
B. Begin cyclosporine therapy.
C. Perform endoscopic biopsies of the ulcer bed and surrounding mucosa.
D. Increase the dose of 6-MP.
E. Colectomy

984 A 43-year-old morbidly obese woman comes to your office. She has tried various diets and weight loss programs but has been unable to lose weight. She is interested in having bariatric surgery, and after a long discussion, she is sent for Roux-en-Y gastric bypass (RYGB). Which of the following statements regarding this surgery is true?
A. Weight loss after RYGB results purely from the restrictive process.

B. Studies have shown a decrease in the circulating levels of ghrelin in patients undergoing RYGB.

C. Dumping syndrome is not known to occur after RYGB and is one of the advantages of this procedure.

D. The metabolic and nutritional deficiencies that occur after RYGB are often more severe than those seen in other bypass procedures.

985 Which of the following is the most common cause of SIBO?

A. Disorders affecting small intestine peristalsis, such as diabetes mellitus and scleroderma

B. Proton pump inhibitor use

C. Anatomic abnormalities resulting from abdominal surgery, such as blind loop

D. Atrophic gastritis

986 Regarding the prevalence of acquired primary lactase deficiency (adult-type hypolactasia), among which of the following subgroups does lactase persistence predominate?

A. Adults of Chinese heritage

B. Adults of Western European heritage

C. Adults of Native American heritage

D. Adults of Jewish heritage

E. Adults of Southern Italian heritage

987 Age at diagnosis of Crohn's disease can best be described by which of the following statements?

A. Crohn's disease is most commonly diagnosed between the ages of 10 and 20 years.

B. The median age at onset has been decreasing.

C. The median age at onset has been increasing, driven by more frequent diagnoses at an older age.

D. The median age at onset has remained stable.

E. Clinical and pathologic presentations are the same in older and younger populations.

988 Which of the following is the most accurate statement pertaining to the relationship between SIBO and IBS?

A. All patients with SIBO fulfill the Rome criteria.

B. The hypothesis that SIBO is the etiologic factor in IBS remains unproven.

C. The major benefit of antibiotic treatment is for the symptom of diarrhea.

D. A three-day course of treatment with rifaximin is usually adequate.

989 The "string of beads" appearance on an angiogram of the renal artery is typical of which of the following?

A. Fibromuscular dysplasia, medial type

B. Henoch-Schönlein purpura

C. Cogan's syndrome

D. Buerger's disease

E. Kawasaki's disease

990 Polyarthralgias of the knees, ankles, elbows, or fingers; uveitis; weight loss; diarrhea; abdominal pain; and skin hyperpigmentation are all associated with which disease?

A. Whipple's disease

B. Hemochromatosis

C. IBS

D. α_1-Antitrypsin deficiency

991 Which of the following regarding total proctocolectomy with ileal pouch anal anastomosis (IPAA) is true?

A. All patients facing colectomy for UC are candidates for IPAA.

B. The average number of stools is three to six per day.

C. Nocturnal seepage occurs in 20% of patients in the first year but is rare thereafter.

D. More than two decades after IPAA, approximately 20% of patients will experience some type of complication including pouchitis, obstruction, stricture, abscess, and fistula.

992 Which of the following patients with Crohn's disease is an appropriate candidate for treatment with natalizumab?

A. Newly diagnosed, as initial therapy for moderate ileal disease

B. Moderate to severe ileocolonic disease with elevated C-reactive protein and no response to infliximab and intolerance to azathioprine

C. A patient with fistulizing disease who has failed antibiotics, mesalamine, and immunomodulators

D. A patient with a narrowed fibrotic terminal ileum in whom adalimumab and MTX therapy has failed

993 A 60-year-old man with a medical history of congestive heart failure and intermittent atrial fibrillation presents to the emergency department reporting sudden onset of abdominal pain. For the previous three months he has had postprandial abdominal pain and a 20-lb weight loss. Physical examination is notable for a low-grade fever and mild to moderate diffuse abdominal pain without guarding or rebound. Stools are heme positive and brown. What is the most likely diagnosis?

A. Superior mesenteric artery thrombosis

B. Nonocclusive mesenteric ischemia

C. FSI

D. Mesenteric venous thrombus

994 A 25-year-old woman with UC for 13 years was recently diagnosed with low-grade dysplasia on surveillance colonoscopy, confirmed by an outside pathologist. Further, she has been symptomatic for more than a year despite various medical regimens. You recommend total proctocolectomy with IPAA given both the dysplasia and medically refractory disease. She has not had children yet and wants to know how this will affect her chances of getting pregnant. Which of the following do you tell her?

A. She is more likely to get pregnant after the surgery than before as she will feel better and be more receptive to sexual activity.

B. There is no difference in rates of fertility before and after IPAA.

C. Fertility rates do significantly decrease after IPAA and may be related to anatomic changes in the pelvis after surgery.

D. Rates of conception via in vitro fertilization are the same after IPAA compared with expected rates.

995 Yellow plaque-like lesions (lymphangiectasias) of the distal duodenum and jejunum with associated diarrhea are common in which disorder (see figure)?

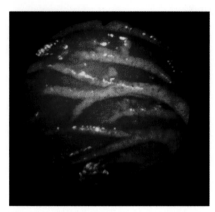

Figure for question **995**

A. Whipple's disease
B. Crohn's disease
C. UC
D. Celiac disease

996 Phosphatidylcholine is the predominant dietary phospholipid. What is the enzyme that is primarily responsible for its digestion?
A. Gastric lipase
B. PLA2
C. CEL
D. Pancreatic lipase–related protein 1
E. Pancreatic lipase–related protein 2

997 What is the most effective treatment for solitary rectal ulcer syndrome?
A. Cortisone enemas
B. Mesalamine suppositories
C. Mesalamine enemas
D. Biofeedback

998 A 15-year-old boy has recurrent respiratory, urogenital, and gastrointestinal infections. After a lengthy evaluation, he is diagnosed with a selective IgA deficiency. This immunodeficiency disorder has been strongly associated with which of the following?
A. Gluten-sensitive enteropathy
B. Chagas' disease
C. IBD
D. IBS

999 A 28-year-old man presents with a six-week history of frequent bloody urgent diarrhea. After appropriate evaluation including stool studies, flexible sigmoidoscopy, and biopsy, he is diagnosed with UC. He is started on glucocorticosteroids, but continues to be symptomatic. Further, his potassium levels frequently dip below 3. He is given supportive treatment with hyoscyamine for abdominal cramping. On hospital day 5, a low-grade fever of 99.8°F, tachycardia with a heart rate of 110 beats per minute, and hypotension with a blood pressure

95/60 mm Hg develop. Physical examination is significant for decreased bowel sounds. Laboratory tests reveal a WBC count of 13.1. A CT of the abdomen and pelvis shows diffusely thickened colon and dilation of the transverse colon to 9 cm. Which of the following statements about this patient's condition is true?
A. It is unusual to occur so quickly after a diagnosis with UC.
B. The patient should undergo colectomy without delay.
C. Pancolitis, anticholinergics, and hypokalemia are predisposing factors.
D. Antibiotics should be reserved for confirmed infection given the risk of *C. difficile*.

1000 A 33-year-old woman with UC for five years was previously well on mesalamine. She was recently admitted to the hospital after the development of urgent, frequent bloody bowel movements; stool study results and biopsy specimens from flexible sigmoidoscopy were negative for infection, including *C. difficile* and cytomegalovirus. She was started on intravenous steroids and has had a minimal response after one week. Cyclosporine therapy was initiated. With this treatment, which of the following is true?
A. Response is usually seen within two weeks.
B. Monitoring of drug levels is not required.
C. Patients can generally be transitioned back to mesalamine.
D. Cholesterol levels should be checked before initiation of therapy.
E. Adverse events are not dose dependent.

1001 A congenital hernia involving the umbilicus that is usually covered by an avascular sac (see figure) is referred to as which of the following?

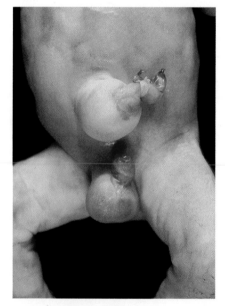

Figure for question **1001**

A. Gastroschisis
B. Omphalocele

C. Omphalomesenteric cyst
D. Failure of primary rotation

1002 A clinical picture of nutritional deficiencies that result in anemia, stomatitis, glossitis, pigmentation of the skin, and edema caused by hypoproteinemia is consistent with what infection?
A. Enterotoxigenic *E. coli*
B. *Campylobacter*
C. *Shigella*
D. Tropical sprue

1003 What is the most common cause of SBO?
A. Gallstone ileus
B. Inguinal hernia
C. Intra-abdominal adhesions
D. Neoplasms
E. Crohn's disease

1004 A 27-year-old obese woman sees you in the clinic. After various weight loss attempts, she is referred to a surgeon for RYGB. Postoperatively, she is most at risk of malabsorption of which of the following?
A. Vitamin D
B. Carbohydrate
C. Fat
D. Iron

1005 Which of the following does not aid in the diagnosis of *Ascaris* infection?
A. Endoscopy
B. Barium studies
C. Peripheral eosinophilia
D. Endoscopic retrograde cholangiopancreatography (ERCP)
E. Direct smears of the stool

1006 Which of the following EIMs of UC does not correlate with colonic symptoms?
A. Axial arthropathy
B. Peripheral arthropathy
C. Episcleritis
D. Erythema nodosum
E. Aphthous ulcerations

1007 In children intussusception is rarely caused by an anatomic abnormality; in adults, however, the most common cause is which of the following?
A. Small bowel neoplasm
B. Meckel's diverticulum
C. Crohn's disease
D. Idiopathic small bowel ulcers
E. Vascular ectasias

1008 A 35-year-old woman travels to Indonesia. Nausea, vomiting, and severe watery diarrhea develop. She is taken to the hospital six hours later and found to have poor skin turgor, dry mucous membranes, blood pressure of 84/50 mm Hg, pulse of 128, temperature of 99°F, and creatinine level of 2.2. Which statement is true about her treatment?
A. She is likely to respond to 1 L of intravenous dextrose 5% in water.
B. If she can tolerate hypotonic liquids and water, she can be discharged.
C. Antibiotics are unnecessary.

D. Due to massive fluid losses, intravenous and/or oral fluid replacement with isotonic solutions are needed.
E. Ciprofloxacin is not effective.

1009 An elderly patient presents with bloody diarrhea two days after elective surgery for an umbilical hernia. A sigmoidoscopy performed that day revealed the endoscopic image shown (see figure). The image is most consistent with which of the following?

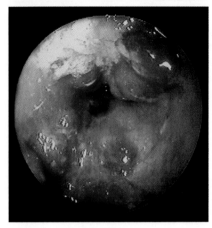

Figure for question **1009**

A. Ischemic colitis
B. IBD
C. NSAID colopathy
D. Pseudomembranous infectious colitis

1010 A deficiency of vitamin D in childhood can lead to the development of rickets. Which of the following statements regarding vitamin D absorption and metabolism is true?
A. Vitamin D_3 is the major dietary form of vitamin D.
B. Cow's milk contains adequate amounts of vitamin D to prevent rickets.
C. Both endogenous synthesis and dietary intake are required to avoid vitamin D deficiency.
D. Absorption of vitamin D is an active process.

1011 Surgical resection is the treatment of choice for colorectal cancer. Which statement regarding surgical treatment is correct?
A. A 92-year-old patient with large sigmoid cancer is too old for surgery.
B. A 64-year-old patient with liver metastases who is responding to chemotherapy should not have the primary tumor resected despite transfusion-requiring blood loss.
C. The number of lymph nodes evaluated after resection is associated with survival.
D. Carcinoembryonic antigen determination and CT scans every three months is the optimal surveillance strategy.

1012 Severe nausea, vomiting, and diarrhea develop secondary to viral gastroenteritis in a 70-year-old woman. She is seen in the emergency department.

Vital signs were notable for a blood pressure of 70/50 mm Hg before intravenous fluid replacement. One day later, she returns to the emergency department reporting sudden onset of crampy left lower quadrant pain and passage of bloody diarrhea. A limited sigmoidoscopy is performed, and the findings are as noted (see figure here and figure with question 1009). The cause of the new symptoms is likely which of the following?

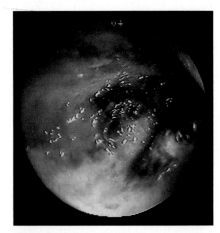

Figure for question **1012**

A. Recurrence of the viral gastroenteritis
B. Superimposed bacterial infection
C. Ulcerative proctitis
D. Colon ischemia

1013 Which stain will aid in the diagnosis of *Cryptosporidium* infection?
A. Trichrome stain
B. Periodic acid–Schiff (PAS) stain
C. Methylene blue stain
D. Modified acid-fast stain

1014 Diarrhea from cryptosporidiosis may be most severe in which group?
A. Human immunodeficiency virus (HIV)–positive men with a CD4 count above 700
B. Patients with immunoglobulin deficiency
C. Women of child-bearing age
D. Adolescents

1015 In the fasting state, interdigestive motor complexes are complex patterns of contractions that periodically sweep along the small intestine. Which of the following statements regarding the fed state is true?
A. "Fast" peristalsis replaces the "slow" peristalsis of the fed state.
B. Oral cecal transit time is greatly unchanged by the content of the food bolus.
C. Peristalsis, a coordinated contractile pattern, moves chyme along the small intestine to facilitate digestion and nutrient absorption.
D. Luminal contents have little impact on the development of peristalsis.

1016 In patients with presumed IBS without alarm features, the only proven cost-effective screening recommended is which of the following?

A. SeCAT test for bile salt malabsorption
B. p-ANCA and anti-*Saccharomyces cerevisiae* antibody for IBD
C. Anti-endomysial or tissue transglutaminase antibody for celiac disease
D. Serum trypsinogen for chronic pancreatitis
E. Lactose breath test

1017 Which of the following statements regarding diagnostic tests for *C. difficile* infection is false?
A. Tissue culture cytotoxicity assay is the gold standard.
B. Enzyme-linked immunosorbent assay (ELISA) is highly sensitive for toxins but less specific than the cytotoxicity test.
C. A stool culture for *C. difficile* has low sensitivity.
D. Sigmoidoscopic finding of pseudomembranous colitis in a patient with antibiotic-associated diarrhea is not pathognomonic for *C. difficile* colitis.
E. Colonic mucosal biopsies may be normal in mild disease.

1018 Diagnostic testing for amebiasis is complex. Which of the following statements is true?
A. Colonoscopy and biopsy are the gold standard.
B. Stool examination for ova and parasites is reliable.
C. Serum anti-amebic antibodies cannot differentiate *E. histolytica* from *Entamoeba dispar*.
D. Polymerase chain reaction testing is widely available.
E. Stool ELISA is the least specific test.

1019 What is the neurotransmitter thought to play a major role in the manifestations of IBS?
A. Norepinephrine
B. Nitric oxide
C. 5-HT
D. Acetylcholine
E. γ-Aminobutyric acid

1020 What is the most common symptom(s) early in the course of acute mesenteric ischemia (AMI)?
A. Abdominal distention
B. Fever
C. Abdominal pain
D. Nausea and vomiting
E. Bloody diarrhea

1021 Carcinoid tumors of the small intestine
A. Are the least common malignancy in the small intestine
B. Are usually located in the proximal small intestine
C. Are usually present at time of diagnosis of carcinoid syndrome
D. Are more likely to present with bleeding than gastrointestinal stromal tumors
E. Are most common in adults younger than 50 years old

1022 Which of the following drugs has been shown to be effective in the treatment of postoperative ileus?
A. Erythromycin
B. Metoclopramide

C. Naloxone
D. Alvimopan
E. Neostigmine

1023 A 45-year-old man with UC since age 22 has consulted you for surveillance colonoscopy. He has universal colitis with pseudopolyps. Multiple biopsy specimens are obtained randomly and of a 1-cm raised lesion in the sigmoid colon (see figure 1). The random biopsy specimens reveal chronic colitis and high-grade dysplasia of the sigmoid lesion (see figure 2). Which of the following should you recommend?
A. Aggressive medical treatment and another biopsy in three to six months
B. Endoscopic mucosal resection of the sigmoid lesion
C. Repeat colonoscopy and yearly biopsy
D. Left hemicolectomy
E. Proctocolectomy

1024 A 44-year-old man presents with diarrhea, fever, weight loss, and a cough. A colonoscopy is performed because a CT scan has shown a colonic mass. The colonoscopy shows an ileocecal stricture with hypertrophic folds. Which would be most useful in determining the diagnosis?
A. Anti-*Saccharomyces* antibody
B. Tuberculin skin test
C. Serology for ameba
D. Acid-fast stain of a biopsy specimen of the stricture
E. Carcinoembryonic antigen

1025 Which of the following statements regarding acute mesenteric venous thrombosis is true?

A. Thrombolytic agents are commonly used.
B. Intravenous heparin for seven to 10 days has been shown to improve survival.
C. One month of warfarin is usually adequate.
D. Even if peritonitis is present, laparotomy is unnecessary.

1026 Which of the following statements regarding glucocorticosteroid treatment in UC is true?
A. It is effective in the induction and maintenance of remission in patients with moderate to severe UC.
B. Doses above the equivalent of 40 to 60 mg/day are not associated with further clinical benefit.
C. Adrenocorticotropic hormone is a more effective and safer alternative to conventional glucocorticoid therapy.
D. Oral budesonide is an equally effective and safer alternative to conventional glucocorticoid therapy.
E. Topical (rectal) glucocorticosteroids are more effective than topical mesalamine in the treatment of distal disease.

1027 What is the most common cause of vitamin B_{12} malabsorption?
A. Pancreatic insufficiency
B. Bacterial overgrowth syndrome
C. Crohn's disease involving the terminal ileum
D. Pernicious anemia
E. Ileal resection

1028 A 25-year-old man who has mild-to-moderate ileal Crohn's disease is treated initially with mesalamine and budesonide with minimal response. A

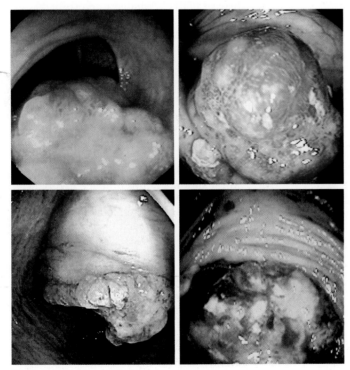

Figure 1 for question **1023**

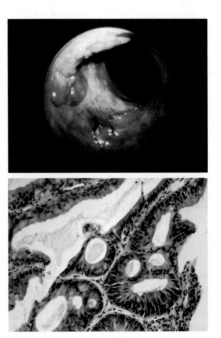

Figure 2 for question **1023**

decision is made to start prednisone. Which of the following statments regarding the use of glucocorticosteroids in Crohn's disease and UC is most accurate?
A. They should be started at an equivalent of prednisone more than 60 mg/day.
B. Low-dose prednisone is an effective maintenance treatment.
C. They should be given for only two to three weeks and tapered off quickly.
D. Approximately 80% of patients will have an initial response.

1029 A patient with diffuse small intestine ulcerations, celiac disease refractory to gluten withdrawal, and intestinal villous atrophy most likely has which of the following conditions?
A. Enteropathy-type intestinal T-cell lymphoma
B. Crohn's disease
C. NSAID-induced ulceration
D. Whipple's disease

1030 A 23-year-old man is being treated with infliximab for Crohn's disease. Approximately one hour into his fourth infusion, he experiences chest tightness, dyspnea, and hypotension. Which of the following is true with regard to this event?
A. Infusion reactions are more likely to occur with episodic therapy.
B. All patients receiving infliximab should be checked for antibodies to infliximab (ATI) and, if positive, should no longer be treated with this medication.
C. All patients receiving infliximab should be on concomitant immunomodulators.
D. Pretreatment medications do not decrease the risk of these symptoms.

1031 Which of the following statements regarding diverticulitis and fistulas is most accurate?
A. Fistulas occur in less than 5% of cases.
B. Colovesicular fistulas are the most common.
C. There is a 3:1 male predominance.
D. Colovaginal fistulas represent 25% of all cases.
E. All of the above

1032 Regarding imaging of acute appendicitis, which of the following facts are unreliable?
A. Ultrasound characteristic 7 mm or thicker noncompressible blind-ended loop of bowel identified
B. Abdominal CT is the imaging study of choice in nonclassic cases of appendicitis.
C. CT findings consistent with appendicitis include an inflamed, distended (>10 mm) appendix that fills with contrast medium.
D. Sensitivity and specificity of appendiceal CT is 92% to 100% and 87% to 98%, respectively.

1033 Tropical enteropathy has been detected in most tropical regions of Asia, the Middle East, the Caribbean, and Central and South America as well as which of the following?
A. Africa
B. Australia

C. New Zealand
D. Hawaii

1034 Malabsorption is most likely to occur from which of the following?
A. Amebiasis
B. Giardiasis
C. *Blastocystis hominis*
D. *Dientamoeba fragilis*

1035 Of the three subtypes of ICCs, which one is most likely the pacemaker for the small, rapid (12-20 per minute) oscillations in the membrane potential of the smooth muscle cells in the colon?
A. ICC_{MY}
B. ICC_{SM}
C. ICC_{IM}

1036 Which of the following statements regarding IBS is true?
A. It is the most frequent functional gastrointestinal disorder seen in gastrointestinal practices.
B. It is associated with abdominal pain that is continuous and not relieved with defecation.
C. It is not associated with noncolonic symptoms such as headache, backache, and impaired sleep.
D. It is not seen in patients with IBD.
E. Its occurrence is highest among middle-aged individuals.

1037 Which of the following is an accurate statement regarding the relationship between SIBO and chronic liver disease?
A. SIBO is more common in patients with advanced liver disease.
B. SIBO does not occur in cirrhotic patients in the absence of portal hypertension.
C. The etiology of SIBO in patients with chronic liver disease is likely related to motility disturbances.
D. Liver transplantation improves small bowel dysmotility in cirrhotic patients.
E. All of the above

1038 Peristalsis is the fundamental integrated motility pattern of the small intestine. Which of the following statements regarding this phenomenon is true?
A. Propagation always occurs in an aboral direction.
B. The exact mechanism and interactions of the various transmitters and hormones involved have been clearly elucidated.
C. It is initiated solely by the mechanical presence of food in the stomach or proximal small intestine.
D. Both sensory and motor aspects of the enteric nervous system play a key role in the initiation and propagation of peristalsis.

1039 Which of the following statements regarding the physical examination finding (see figure) is true?
A. This abnormality will resolve with sitz baths.
B. This abnormality is seen in approximately 50% of patients with Crohn's disease.

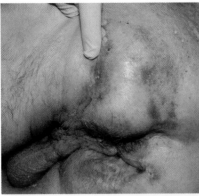

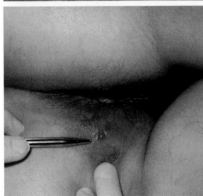

Figure for question **1039**

C. This abnormality is seen only in the setting of active rectal inflammation.

D. The release of proteases and matrix metalloproteinases is thought to contribute to its pathogenesis.

1040 Which group of susceptibility genes has been identified as conferring increased risk of the development of UC?

A. *NOD2/CARD15*, C3435T polymorphism for *MDR1*, *IL23R*

B. C3435T polymorphism for *MDR1*, *IL23R*, *ATG16L1*

C. *NOD2/CARD15*, *IL12β*, *IL23R*

D. C3435T polymorphism for *MDR1*, *IL12β*, *IL23R*

1041 One of the outcomes of bacterial metabolic activity includes increased gas production. Which of the following is not a gas produced by enteric bacteria?

A. CH_4

B. CO

C. CO_2

D. H_2

E. N_2

1042 Which of the following modalities is the most widely available study to assess small bowel wall motion?

A. Magnetic resonance imaging

B. Contrast fluoroscopy

C. Ultrasonography

D. Multichannel intraluminal impedance

1043 Which of the following is a finding on a gastrograffin upper gastrointestinal small bowel series that identifies patients in whom the SBO is likely to resolve with nonoperative management?

A. Documentation of a mid–small bowel intussusception

B. Complete distal SBO

C. Passage of contrast into the colon within six to 24 hours

D. Diagnosis of Crohn's disease

E. Meckel's diverticulum

1044 Which of the following would stimulate absorption from the gastrointestinal mucosa?

A. Increase in cAMP

B. Decrease in cAMP

C. Increase in cGMP

D. Increase in Ca^{2+} and/or activation of protein kinase C

1045 A 51-year-old man with three years of ileocolonic Crohn's disease presents with postprandial right lower quadrant and upper abdominal pain, diarrhea, and a 10-lb weight loss for six months. His disease was previously well controlled with azathioprine. He has never had any surgery. Laboratory tests are significant for hemoglobin level of 13.1 g/dL (14-17), albumin level of 3.9 g/dL (3.2-4.9), potassium level of 3.4 mmol/L (3.5-5), and normal ferritin, vitamin B_{12}, folate, magnesium, and zinc levels. C-reactive protein and erythrocyte sedimentation rate are elevated at 4.8 mg/dL (0.0-0.8) and 39 mm/hr (0-20), respectively. Results of stool studies including *C. difficile* toxins are negative. A colonoscopy shows moderate right-sided and splenic flexure inflammation; intubation of the terminal ileum shows minimal inflammatory changes. A CT enterography is normal. What is the most likely mechanism for his weight loss?

A. Malabsorption

B. Malignancy

C. Infection

D. Reduced oral intake

1046 A 75-year-old man with a 30-year history of left-sided UC is admitted to the hospital for the second time in six months for refractory disease. He has multiple comorbidities, including mild renal insufficiency, hypertension, and congestive heart failure. He was previously managed on only a 5-aminosalicylic acid (5-ASA) agent but recently has become steroid dependent, and bloody diarrhea has developed since his prednisone was tapered to 15 mg/day. Azathioprine was started three months ago and was not tolerated secondary to pancreatitis. Superimposed infection has been ruled out. His vital signs are within normal limits and he does not appear to be toxic. His abdomen is soft with only mild left lower quadrant tenderness. His laboratory study results are significant for hemoglobin of 10.5 g/dL (14-17), albumin of 3.4 g/dL (3.2-4.9), and glucose of 179 mg/dL (50-100). What is the next best step?

A. Total proctocolectomy with IPAA

B. Initiate cyclosporine therapy.

C. Initiate infliximab therapy.

D. Total proctocolectomy with Brooke (end) ileostomy

E. Subtotal colectomy with Koch pouch

1047 A "double bowel" sign on a CT scan is characterized by concentric rings of inner and outer bowel walls separated by hyperechoic fat. This sign represents which of the following?
A. Meckel's diverticulum
B. Intussusception
C. Carcinoid tumor
D. Acute appendicitis
E. SBO secondary to internal hernia

1048 A 30-year-old woman begins vomiting two hours after eating from a Chinese buffet. Her symptoms resolve in less than 10 hours. What is the most likely etiology?
A. *Aeromonas*
B. *Clostridium botulinum*
C. *Listeria*
D. *Bacillus cereus*
E. *Staphylococcus epidermidis*

1049 A seven-month-old infant boy is sent home from day care with diarrhea. You are told from several of the day care workers that the facility is experiencing an outbreak of rotavirus. What is the type of ion channels affected in this disease?
A. Calcium-activated chloride channels
B. Potassium transporters
C. Cystic fibrosis transmembrane conductance regulator (CFTR)
D. ClC_2 type chloride channels

1050 Which of the following statements regarding the location of Crohn's disease is the most accurate?
A. Approximately 50% of patients have disease confined to the terminal ileum.
B. Isolated jejunal involvement may be seen in approximately 15% of patients.
C. Approximately one third to one half of patients will have disease involving both the terminal ileum and the colon.
D. Upper gastrointestinal tract (esophageal, stomach, duodenal) occurs in approximately 20% of patients.

1051 What is the most important clinical feature differentiating early postoperative SBO from postoperative ileus?
A. Abdominal distention and pain
B. Nausea and vomiting
C. Occurrence of obstructive symptoms after initial return of bowel function and resumption of oral intake
D. Type of surgery performed
E. Cumulative dose of narcotics used postoperatively

1052 What is the treatment of choice for patients with *Strongyloides* infection?
A. Albendazole
B. Ivermectin
C. Praziquantel
D. Mebendazole

1053 Multichannel intraluminal impedance is a technique that
A. Measures differential resistances of luminal contents to monitor the bolus progression along the intestines
B. Measures the intraluminal pressures to determine the bolus progression along the intestines
C. Measures the differential conductivities of luminal contents to monitor bolus progression along the intestines
D. Measures the differential conductivities of luminal contents to monitor intraluminal pressures

1054 Celiac disease, also known as gluten-sensitive enteropathy, is an allergy to which of the following?
A. Barley, oats, and rye
B. Wheat, oats, and hops
C. Wheat, rye, and barley
D. Oats, wheat, and rye

1055 Which of the following statements regarding the Schilling test for vitamin B_{12} malabsorption is most accurate?
A. The Schilling test results are abnormal in patients with dietary vitamin B_{12} deficiency.
B. In patients with pernicious anemia, the results of the Schilling test normalize after oral administration of intrinsic factor.
C. In patients with ileal disease, the results of the Schilling test normalize after oral administration of intrinsic factor.
D. Pancreatic exocrine insufficiency does not cause Schilling test results to be abnormal.

1056 A 65-year-old woman is found to have sigmoid colon cancer. Findings on CT scan are normal, and after a left hemicolectomy, the cancer is determined to be Dukes stage B1. One year later, a CT scan shows liver metastases. Resection of liver metastases would be considered based on which of the following?
A. Only one lobe is involved
B. Only one metastatic lesion is present
C. More than four metastases are present
D. No extrahepatic disease is present

1057 The following pair of organisms can reside in the biliary tree:
A. *Clonorchis* and *Strongyloides*
B. *Opisthorchis* and *Necatur americanus*
C. *Ascaris* and *Fasciola*
D. *Fasciolopsis* and *Fasciola*

1058 Human leukocyte antigen (HLA)-DQ2 and HLA-DQ8 are associated with which disorder?
A. Tropical sprue
B. Celiac disease
C. UC
D. Crohn's disease

1059 There are two fundamental similarities of all gastrointestinal epithelial cells with regard to their ability to transport electrolytes and water. The first is a discrete polarity of the cell with apical and basolateral membranes with distinct biochemical properties. The second is the presence of a basolateral
A. Chloride pump
B. Sodium/potassium adenosine triphosphatase
C. Sodium/hydrogen pump
D. CFTR channel

1060 Tropical sprue is predominantly a disease of southern and southeast Asia, Central and South America, and which of the following?
A. England
B. Australia
C. Caribbean Islands
D. Hawaii

1061 A 56-year-old man goes to Mexico on business. He eats food from street vendors, drinks tap water, and eats a rare steak. Several days into his trip, he gets diarrhea and a low-grade fever. He calls you from Mexico and asks why he is ill and what he can take to allow him to get to an important meeting the next day. What regimen would be most effective?
A. Fluoroquinolone
B. Cefazolin
C. Metronidazole
D. Vancomycin

1062 Absorbed dietary lipids and cholesterol are resynthesized in the enterocytes before export into the bloodstream. During the fed state, chylomicrons are the predominant lipoprotein that emerges from the epithelium. What is the predominant form during the fasting state?
A. High-density lipoprotein
B. Low-density lipoprotein
C. Very low density lipoprotein
D. Chylomicrons

1063 A 60-year-old Guatemalan man moved to the United States a few months ago and now presents with dysphagia and shortness of breath. Chest x-ray shows congestive heart failure and an enlarged esophagus. Which of the following statements regarding the protozoon that caused this illness is true?
A. Cardiac symptoms are a rare presentation.
B. A bite from the reduviid bug is responsible for transmission.
C. Manometric findings are easily distinguished from achalasia.
D. Trimethoprim/sulfamethaxazole for four weeks readily treats this organism.
E. Diagnosis cannot be made by examining blood smears for the organism.

1064 Randomized, controlled trials of fiber supplementation therapy and diet manipulation for IBS have shown that
A. Wheat bran is better than placebo.
B. Fiber supplementation benefits constipation- and diarrhea-predominant IBS equally.
C. The key to fiber supplementation is to start at high doses and then taper to the lowest effective dose.
D. In most patients, a lactose-free diet improves typical IBS symptoms.
E. Exclusion of foods with a positive IgG antibody response may provide benefit in both diarrhea- and constipation-predominant IBS.

1065 Genetic testing is appropriate in which setting?
A. Family members of a patient with hereditary nonpolyposis colorectal cancer syndrome (HNPCC) whose tumor is negative for micro-satellite instability
B. A 67-year-old patient whose mother had colo-rectal cancer at age 70
C. A 67-year-old patient with a sporadic adenoma on consecutive examinations
D. Families with familial adenomatous polyposis (FAP)

1066 What statement most accurately reflects the natural history of UC after diagnosis?
A. Approximately 50% of patients will have intermittent flares between periods of wellness.
B. As many as 10% of patients will have such a severe first presentation of UC that ultimately a colectomy is needed.
C. Eighty percent of patients have a mild first presentation.
D. More than half of patients with the disease limited to the rectum and sigmoid will have disease extension at 10 years.
E. Fifteen percent of patients will require colectomy after 25 years of disease.

1067 Which of the following statments regarding genetic abnormalities in Crohn's disease is true?
A. At least two autophagy-related gene variants have been identified, both of which increase the risk of Crohn's disease.
B. Genetic variants of IL-23 and other related gene products represent an important pathway in the development of Crohn's disease.
C. A common variant of IL-23R is strongly protective in the development of Crohn's disease.
D. IL-12 shares a common p19 subunit with IL-23.

1068 A 55-year-old woman is newly diagnosed with Crohn's disease. Which of the following is true in considering treating her with a 5-ASA?
A. This is appropriate for moderate to severe disease.
B. It is more effective in patients with small bowel disease.
C. Mesalamine is a better choice than sulfasalazine.
D. Sulfasalazine may ameliorate arthropathy in addition to gastrointestinal symptoms.

1069 A 50-year-old woman with severe diarrhea-predominant IBS is placed on alosetron for management. Significant constipation developed within the first few days of its use. Which of the following regarding IBS and colon ischemia is true?
A. There does not seem to be an increased risk of colon ischemia with the use of a 5-HT$_3$ antagonist.
B. Dose reduction is all that is required.
C. There is a three to four times increased risk in these patients.
D. It generally occurs in men with IBS rather than women.

1070 What are the classic findings on x-ray for a sigmoid volvulus?

A. A distended ahaustral colonic loop with a bent inner tube appearance with the apex directed toward the patient's right shoulder
B. A distended colonic loop with a bent inner tube appearance with the apex directed toward the patient's left lower quadrant
C. A diffusely dilated colon with air throughout with a coffee bean appearance of a distended cecum
D. A colon cutoff sign at the splenic flexure
E. Nonspecific bowel gas pattern

1071 A 25-year-old man with no significant medical history is being evaluated for perianal pruritus. The patient reports that over the previous six months he has had worsening itching that occurs both after and unrelated to defecation. He has begun to vigorously clean his perianal area with a washcloth and soap several times daily, especially after bowel movements, without significant relief. The patient has no history of diarrhea, rectal bleeding, discharge, incontinence, or proctalgia. He denies participation in anal intercourse. The patient consumes approximately six alcohol-containing beverages weekly and three to five cups of coffee daily. An examination of the man's perianal area demonstrates no external hemorrhoids, anal fissures, skin tags, fistula tracts, or anal warts. No masses are appreciated on digital rectal examination. A stool sample is brown and tests negative for occult blood. A flexible sigmoidoscopy demonstrates normal rectosigmoid mucosa without evidence of internal hemorrhoids. What is the most likely cause of the patient's symptoms?
A. Human papillomavirus infection
B. Perianal Crohn's disease
C. Anal fissure
D. Idiopathic pruritus ani
E. Anal cancer

1072 What is the major etiology of short bowel syndrome (SBS) in adults?
A. Superior mesenteric artery ischemia
B. Crohn's disease
C. Tumor resection
D. Traumatic small bowel injury

1073 The risk of colorectal cancer is increased in patients with UC who have which of the following features?
A. Inflammation limited to the most distal 15 cm of colon
B. Primary sclerosing cholangitis
C. Disease of three years' duration
D. Mild inflammatory changes

1074 What is the most common finding on plain films of the abdomen early in the course of bowel ischemia?
A. Free air under the diaphragm
B. Normal results
C. Ileus
D. Thumbprinting of the right colon
E. Air in the portal vein

1075 Which region of the bowel is most commonly affected by celiac disease?
A. Duodenum
B. Stomach

C. Jejunum
D. Ileum

1076 Which of the following infections is least common in immunocompetent patients?
A. *Isospora*
B. Microsporidia
C. *Cyclospora*
D. *Cryptosporidium*

1077 Which of the following statements regarding *E. histolytica* is true?
A. Invasive disease develops in 90% of infected patients.
B. It occurs in a three-stage life cycle: infectious cyst, motile trophozoite, and larva.
C. The cecum and ascending colon are the most commonly affected sites.
D. Ten percent of infected individuals remain asymptomatic.
E. AIDS patients are at an increased risk of invasive amebiasis.

1078 Henoch-Schönlein purpura that presents with the rash shown (see figure):

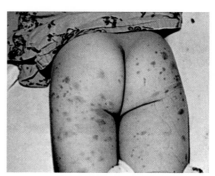

Figure for question **1078**

A. Typically affects adolescents 12 to 16 years of age.
B. Is characterized by IgG immune complexes.
C. Can be associated with intussusception.
D. Manifests as palpable purpura, typically involving the upper extremities.

1079 Which of the following patients is likely the best candidate for ileorectal anastomosis as opposed to total proctocolectomy with or without IPAA?
A. A young, otherwise healthy patient with medically refractory UC
B. An obese middle-aged patient with UC and multiple comorbidities and abdominopelvic surgeries who has quiescent disease
C. A patient with UC and high-grade dysplasia
D. A patient with rectal and perianal Crohn's disease

1080 Which of the following statements regarding pouch failure, which frequently requires pouch excision with creation of a Brooke ileostomy, is true?
A. It occurs in approximately 20% of patients.
B. Early and late complications of IPAA may result in pouch failure.

C. Pouchitis is the sole cause in most cases.

D. The majority of pouch failures occur approximately five years after the surgery.

1081 What is the gold standard for the diagnosis of Whipple's disease?

A. Sputum analysis

B. Stool analysis

C. Serologic antibodies

D. Small bowel biopsy of the duodenum with subsequent polymerase chain reaction

1082 A healthy 22-year-old woman reports three months of frequent and sometimes urgent bloody bowel movements with mucus; she has had one episode of fecal incontinence. She has had no recent travel or sick contacts and takes no medications. Physical examination findings are within normal limits except for gross blood on rectal examination. Laboratory test results are unremarkable except for a hemoglobin of 11.2 g/dL with a mean corpuscular volume of 79 fL. What is the most likely diagnosis?

A. Internal hemorrhoids

B. Infectious colitis

C. IBS

D. UC

1083 A young woman with medically refractory pan-UC recently consulted a surgeon with regard to a total proctocolectomy and IPAA. She has some concerns regarding the technical aspects and specifics of the operation and wants your advice. Which of the following would you tell her?

A. There is no clear difference in outcome or complication rate between hand-sewn IPAA and double-stapled IPAA, although the latter results in less nocturnal incontinence and better preservation of anal sphincter function.

B. She is likely to experience a decrease in sexual activity after surgery.

C. A two-stage operation is advised against because the risk of complications is increased by having a second surgery.

D. The risk of dysplasia or cancer is higher in patients undergoing double-stapled IPAA compared with the hand-sewn technique because a small rim of rectal cuff is left in place with the former.

1084 Observations on the serotonin receptor drug alosetron, a 5-HT$_3$ antagonist for IBS, have shown which of the following?

A. It has been associated with the development of ischemic colitis.

B. It can be used in patients with alternating diarrhea and constipation.

C. Alosetron (5-HT$_3$ receptor antagonist) is indicated in constipation-predominant IBS.

D. Alosetron is no longer available in the United States.

E. It can cause constipation in less than 10% of patients.

1085 The movement of ions and electrolytes across the epithelium occurs in a bidirectional manner and occurs via both paracellular and transcellular routes. With regard to these two modes of transport, which of the following is true?

A. Paracellular movement is a largely active process.

B. The characteristics of the tight junctions (tight vs. leaky) vary along the length of the intestine.

C. Net transport is termed absorptive if the serosal-to-mucosal flux is greater than the mucosal-to-serosal flux.

D. Net transport is termed secretory if the mucosal to serosal flux exceeds the serosal-to-mucosal flux.

1086 What is the best overall study to assess a patient suspected of having intestinal ischemia?

A. Duplex ultrasonography

B. Plain films

C. Tagged red blood cell scan

D. CT

E. Doppler flowmetry

1087 What is the most common cause of SBO secondary to neoplasms?

A. Carcinoid tumor

B. Advanced colorectal carcinoma

C. Metastatic breast cancer

D. Endometrial carcinoma

E. Melanoma

1088 What is the pathophysiologic defect in diabetes-induced chronic intestinal pseudo-obstruction (CIP)?

A. Degeneration of the myenteric and submucosal plexuses

B. Demyelination of the proximal vagus and sympathetic nerves supplying the bowel

C. Primarily a degeneration of the circular and longitudinal muscles

D. Proliferation of the ICCs

E. Bile salt malabsorption

1089 Which of the following statements regarding pro-inflammatory CD4$^+$ T cells is the most accurate?

A. T helper (Th) 17 cells produce highly expressed IL-23R, which, when activated by its ligand, has been shown to have a key role in the pathogenesis of mouse models of colitis.

B. Th1 cells mediate Crohn's disease.

C. Th2 cells mediate UC.

D. Regulatory T cells down-regulate Th1 but not Th2 cells.

1090 With respect to sex and age at onset of UC, which of the following statements is true?

A. Men more than women have UC, and the peak age at onset is bimodal, both in the second and third decades and then between the ages of 60 and 70 years.

B. Women more than men have UC, and peak age at onset is in the second and third decades.

C. No sex difference exists in UC, and the peak age at onset is in the second and third decades.

D. No sex difference exists in UC, and onset is equally distributed over all age groups.

1091 Which of the following statements is most accurate with regard to *NOD2/CARD15* as it relates to Crohn's disease?
A. Two allelic variants have been identified as most commonly associated with Crohn's disease in European and American populations.
B. Homozygotes for allelic variants of this gene have an odds ratio of 17 for the development of Crohn's disease, whereas heterozygotes have an odds ratio of 2.5.
C. As many as 50% of Crohn's patients have at least one allelic variant of this gene.
D. Abnormal variants of this gene predispose to colonic and perianal Crohn's disease.

1092 An 80-year-old woman with a medical history of coronary artery disease presents to her primary care doctor with four to six months of abdominal pain. Typically, it occurs 30 minutes postprandially and usually resolves in one to three hours. The severity of the pain has increased, and she is losing weight. Physical examination reveals a cachectic woman, but her abdominal examination is unremarkable. What is the most important symptom suggesting the diagnosis of chronic mesenteric ischemia?
A. Intermittent nausea and vomiting
B. Bloating
C. Fear of eating resulting in weight loss
D. Diarrhea

1093 Which of the following therapies has been shown to reduce the duration of postoperative ileus?
A. NSAIDs
B. Thoracic epidural injections with bupivacaine
C. Intravenous erythromycin
D. Intravenous metoclopramide
E. Nasogastric tube decompression

1094 The small intestine is innervated by both intrinsic and extrinsic neurons. Intrinsic neurons have their cell bodies within the wall of the small intestine and constitute the enteric nervous system. Extrinsic neurons
A. Outnumber the intrinsic supply
B. Have cell bodies that are outside the gut wall but have extensions that terminate in the intestinal wall
C. Belong to the autonomic nervous system when they are sensory
D. Are always afferent type neurons

1095 The gold-standard test for the diagnosis of celiac disease is which of the following?
A. Anti-endomesial antibodies
B. Anti–tissue transglutaminase antibodies
C. Resolution of symptoms on a gluten-free diet
D. Small bowel biopsy

1096 Cellular immune system abnormalities are characterized by which of the following?
A. An increased number of IELs (CD8$^+$)
B. Normal innate but abnormal adaptive cellular immunity

C. Normal adaptive but abnormal innate cellular immunity
D. Abnormal innate and adaptive cellular immunity
E. Normal nonspecific cellular immunity

1097 Factors thought to be related to small bowel adenocarcinomas include which of the following?
A. Adenocarcinomas of the duodenum develop only in patients with FAP.
B. A diet high in animal fat and protein is not associated with small bowel adenocarcinomas.
C. A different genetic mechanism underlies small bowel adenocarcinoma compared with large bowel adenocarcinoma.
D. Alcohol and tobacco use increase the risk of the development of small intestine cancer.
E. The relative resistance of the small bowel to adenocarcinomas is thought to be due in part to fewer bacteria and rapid transit.

1098 The glucose hydrogen breath test is commonly used to assess for SIBO. Which of the following statements regarding breath testing for SIBO is the most accurate?
A. An increase of 10 ppm above baseline is regarded as diagnostic of SIBO.
B. Sensitivity approaches that of a culture of intestinal aspirate.
C. Rapid transit has no effect on test results.
D. Patient preparation is important including avoiding smoking, eating bread or pasta, and avoiding exercise before the test.
E. An antibacterial mouthwash before testing is standard.

1099 Watery diarrhea, abdominal cramps, vomiting, and a temperature of 99.9°F develop in a 43-year-old man. The diarrhea becomes bloody, and he presents to the emergency department. Findings include abdominal tenderness, hemoglobin of 9.8 g/dL, WBC count of 15.3×10^3 /mL, platelet count of 90×10^3 /mL, and a creatinine level of 2.3 mg/dL. Five days earlier, he ate at a barbecue, and two of his friends are ill. Which organism is most likely to be responsible?
A. Enteropathogenic *E. coli*
B. Enterotoxigenic *E. coli*
C. Enteroinvasive *E. coli*
D. Enterohemorrhagic *E. coli*
E. Enteroaggregative *E. coli*

1100 Which of the following statements about diverticuli is false?
A. Right-sided diverticuli are more frequent than left-sided diverticuli in Asian countries.
B. Diverticuli are hernias of the mucosa and submucosa through a muscularis defect and are therefore pseudodiverticuli.
C. Diverticuli originate in four distinctive rows that correspond to penetration by major branches of the vasa recta.
D. Dietary factors suggest a major role in the pathogenesis.
E. None of the above

1101 At the time of initial presentation, what percentage of patients with UC have pancolitis?
A. 5%
B. 10%
C. 15%
D. 20%

1102 What is the minimal threshold cecal diameter to consider colonic depression in acute intestinal pseudo-obstruction after treatment of potential causes within the first 72 hours?
A. More than 6 cm
B. More than 9 cm
C. More than 12 cm
D. More than 15 cm
E. More than 18 cm

1103 In patients with short bowel syndrome, what is the length of remaining jejunum in patients with an intact colon that will likely lead a patient to require total parenteral nutrition?
A. 100 cm
B. 200 cm
C. 300 cm
D. 400 cm

1104 What is the initial test of choice to diagnosis giardiasis?
A. Stool ELISA for giardiasis
B. Stool for ova and parasites
C. Duodenal aspirate or biopsy
D. Stool acid-fast stain

1105 What are the immunologic abnormalities involved in the pathogenesis of UC?
A. They are related solely to the humoral immune system.
B. They are related only to cell-mediated responses.
C. They involve both humoral and cell-mediated responses.
D. They are related to increased IgG_2 synthesis.
E. They are not believed to be on the spectrum of autoimmune diseases.

1106 What is the test with the greatest diagnostic yield for detecting small bowel neoplasias?
A. CT scan of the abdomen
B. Enteroclysis
C. Push enteroscopy
D. Small bowel capsule endoscopy
E. Angiography

1107 A 75-year-old woman presents reporting abdominal pain. Recently she had a rash that she attributed to a bite from her dog. Her laboratory results indicate an eosinophilia. Which of the following statements is true?
A. The cellophane tape test will give the diagnosis.
B. Terminal ileum but not gastric biopsy specimens may show tissue eosinophilia.
C. Colonoscopy will reveal a normal ileum endoscopically and microscopically.
D. Eggs from the hookworm, *Ancylostoma caninum*, are easy to detect.

1108 Which of the following carbohydrates cannot be absorbed intact and requires hydrolysis by brush border enzymes in the duodenum and jejunum?
A. Galactose
B. Fructose
C. Lactose
D. Glucose

1109 The Rome III criteria for IBS is recurrent abdominal pain or discomfort for at least three days per month in the past three months associated with two or more of the following features:
A. Looser stool at pain onset, more frequent stools at pain onset, or abdominal distention
B. Passage of mucus, incomplete evacuation, abdominal distention
C. Pain relieved with defecation, onset associated with a change in stool frequency, or onset associated with a change in stool form
D. Bloating, anal fissures, or hemorrhoids from straining
E. Female sex, age younger than 30, pain relieved with defecation

1110 Which of the following is true about endometriosis, when defined as the presence of endometrial tissue outside the uterine cavity and musculature?
A. The rectosigmoid and appendix are the two most frequently involved intestinal organs.
B. Endometriosis is found almost exclusively in women of child-bearing age.
C. It is rare to see endometrial implants on the colonic mucosa except when there is hematochezia.
D. A barium enema aids in the diagnosis.
E. All of the above

1111 Diarrheal illnesses can be categorized into inflammatory and noninflammatory types. Which of the following statements regarding these types of illnesses is true?
A. Bleeding is common in both types.
B. The presence of fecal leukocytes helps differentiate the type.
C. The site of involvement is similar.
D. Patients with noninflammatory diarrhea appear more toxic.
E. Dehydration is more common with inflammatory diarrhea.

1112 Which of the following statements regarding *C. difficile* diarrhea recurrence after initial treatment is true?
A. Fifteen percent to 30% of cases that are successfully treated with metronidazole or vancomycin relapse.
B. Late recurrences occur as long as 5.5 months after stopping antibiotic treatment.
C. Diagnosis is confirmed by stool toxin assay.
D. Treat with a second course of the same antibiotic used to treat the initial attack.
E. Extend treatment for 14 days.

1113 Which of the following may be a deficient or inactive part of the adaptive immune system in Crohn's disease?
A. Tumor necrosis factor (TNF)
B. Nuclear factor κB
C. T-regulatory cells
D. IL-2

1114 Which of the following statements regarding asymptomatic diverticulosis incidentally found is a reliable conclusion?
A. No clear indication for any therapy or follow-up
B. A possible prophylactic benefit of a high-fiber diet in preventing new cases of symptomatic diverticulosis is widely accepted.
C. Diets high in fat and red meat are associated with an increased risk of diverticular disease.
D. A positive FOBT result should not be attributed to diverticulosis.
E. All of the above

1115 The autonomic nervous system plays a key role in the regulation of gastrointestinal motility. Postoperative ileus occurs partly as a consequence of altered autonomic nervous system function. What is the primary mechanism involved with impaired gut motility in the postoperative period?
A. An increase in inhibitory sympathetic efferent neural activity blocking the release of acetylcholine from the excitatory neurons in the myenteric plexus
B. Reduced parasympathetic nerve activity caused by irritation and inflammation of the peritoneum
C. Nonadrenergic, noncholinergic nerve activity
D. Release of inflammatory cytokines at the time of surgery
E. Endogenous and exogenous opiates

1116 What is the most common cause of ileus?
A. Abdominal surgery
B. Metabolic abnormalities
C. Drug induced
D. Gastroenteritis
E. Inactivity

1117 Which of the following facts regarding the anatomy of the anal canal are true?
A. Embryologically the dentate line represents the junction between endoderm and ectoderm.
B. Proximal to the dentate line, there is sympathetic and parasympathetic innervation; distally, the nerve supply is somatic.
C. A biopsy can be performed painlessly above the dentate line without the need for local anesthesia.
D. Venous drainage from the anal canal is by both systemic and portal systems.
D. All of the above

1118 A 50-year-old woman presents for colorectal cancer screening. Her father had colon cancer at age 45 and her sister at age 55. Her colonoscopy reveals a cecal adenocarcinoma. Which of the following statements regarding this syndrome is true?
A. It is inherited in an autosomal recessive fashion.
B. It causes less than 1% of all colorectal cancers.
C. There is increased frequency of cancer of the female genital tract.
D. Germline mutations in the *hMSH2* or *hMLH1* genes do not occur.
E. There is a predominance of distal tumors.

1119 The gross (endoscopic) pathology of UC (see figure) is best characterized by which of the following features?
A. Inflammation that is more severe proximally than distally
B. Continuous inflammatory changes that begin in the rectum and extend proximally
C. Periappendiceal inflammation in patients with left-sided UC is likely Crohn's disease, not UC
D. Rectum sparing is never seen in patients with UC

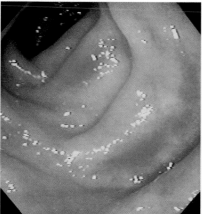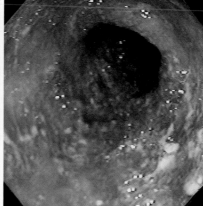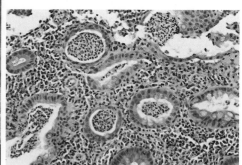

Figure for question **1119**

Continued

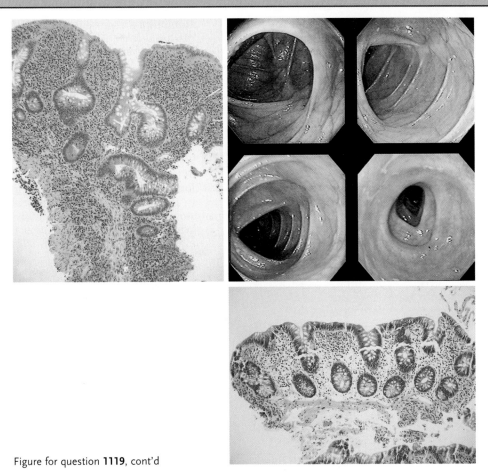

Figure for question **1119**, cont'd

1120 Which of these statements about small bowel neoplasms is true?
A. Small bowel neoplasms are more common in women.
B. Small bowel neoplasms are the second most common gastrointestinal malignancy.
C. Most small bowel neoplasms are malignant.
D. Small bowel neoplasms are more common in young adults.
E. The most common small bowel malignancies are sarcomas.

1121 A 60-year-old woman in India presents with mucoid bloody diarrhea, abdominal pain, fever, and rectal burning. Which statement about the treatment of this illness is most accurate?
A. Antidiarrheal agents will shorten the illness.
B. Antidiarrheal agents with a quinolone have been shown to shorten the illness.
C. Rehydration is rarely needed.
D. No need for attention to electrolytes.
E. Antibiotics are not needed.

1122 Which of the following regarding imaging studies and diverticulitis is false?
A. Barium enema: Use a water-soluble agent only.
B. CT is more sensitive and specific than a barium enema.

C. Endoscopy: Limited rigid or flexible sigmoidoscopy with minimal air insufflation may exclude alternative diagnoses.
D. Colonoscopy: Endoscopy is electively performed two to four weeks after the acute event.
E. Magnetic resonance imaging: Its usefulness in diverticulitis is not well established.

1123 A 27-year-old woman with Crohn's disease is seen in your office. She has a history of extensive bowel resections including an ileocecectomy. She is currently reporting diffuse watery diarrhea. She has been ruled out for infectious causes, and her most recent imaging studies have been unremarkable. Her diarrhea most likely is related to malabsorption of which of the following?
A. Bile acids
B. SCFAs
C. Fat
D. Complex carbohydrates
E. Disaccharides

1124 Well-established therapy for enteropathy-type intestinal T-cell lymphoma includes which of the following?
A. Glucocorticosteroids
B. Azathioprine
C. Cyclosporine
D. None of the above

1125 A 19-year-old patient with ileocolonic Crohn's disease presents with fever of 102°F, right lower quadrant pain, and a palpable mass on physical examination. He has been treated with glucocorticosteroids over the past few weeks for a flare; 6-MP was started concomitantly. His prednisone is being tapered by 5 mg/week and his current dose is 20 mg/day. What is the next best step in management?

A. Increase his dose of steroids and stop his 6-MP.

B. Small bowel series

C. Urgent CT scan of the abdomen/pelvis and empiric antibiotics

D. Start infliximab.

1126 The level of which vitamin tends to be high in patients with SIBO?

A. B_6

B. B_{12}

C. Folate

D. Vitamin D

E. Biotin

1127 Travelers to tropical countries in whom diarrhea develops are most likely infected with which of the following?

A. *Giardia*

B. Nontyphoid *Salmonella*

C. *Shigella*

D. *Yersinia*

1128 Visceral distention or discomfort of the small intestine is mediated by which of the following?

A. Sensory efferent neurons with cell bodies within the cerebellum

B. Spinal afferent fibers with cell bodies within the thoracic dorsal root ganglia and projections to the prevertebral ganglia and splanchnic nerves

C. The vagus nerve with cell bodies within the nodosa and jugular ganglia and projections to the intestinal wall

D. The vagus nerve with cell bodies within the dorsal root ganglia and projections to the intestinal wall

1129 Which patient may be at increased risk of nontyphoidal salmonellosis?

A. A 27-year-old person with sickle cell anemia

B. A 40-year-old person with iron and B_{12} deficiency anemia

C. A patient with gastroesophageal reflux who had a fundoplication

D. An HIV-positive patient with a CD4 count of 850

E. A 65-year-old person with a history of a knee replacement and a mitral valve replacement

1130 A 50-year-old Brazilian man with an upper gastrointestinal bleed is found to have esophageal varices. He has been living in the United States for 10 years, denies ethanol abuse, and is negative for hepatitis A, B, and C. Splenomegaly is present. On laboratory evaluation, the alkaline phosphatase and gamma glutamyl transferase are mildly elevated, but the other liver enzymes, albumin, and prothrombin time are normal. Thrombocytopenia and eosinophilia are present. Which statement about this disease is true?

A. The organism is transmitted by the reduviid bug.

B. Albendazole is the treatment.

C. Katayama fever is the classic presentation of acute infection.

D. Liver biopsy is diagnostic.

E. Cirrhosis develops in most patients.

1131 A 53-year-old woman presents with seven days of watery diarrhea, nausea, and abdominal discomfort after returning from a summer camping trip in the midwest. A modified acid-fast stain of her stool is positive for a small intracellular protozoan. What is the treatment that is most consistently effective?

A. Iodoquinol

B. Ciprofloxacin

C. Metronidazole

D. Nitazoxanide

1132 Pruritus ani develops in a seven-year-old girl. Which of the following will help her the most?

A. Checking for antibodies to this cestode

B. Treating only the symptomatic household members is necessary.

C. Treating her and all her family members with albendazole

D. Two doses of metronidazole 15 days apart is an alternative.

1133 Which of the following is a feature of chronic idiopathic intestinal pseudo-obstruction?

A. Sporadic, nonfamilial visceral myopathy

B. Rare form of intestinal pseudo-obstruction

C. Often associated with urinary tract impairment

D. Can result from various causes including drug toxicity, ischemia, radiation, and viral infection

E. Histologically, the myenteric plexus appears normal.

1134 A statistician consults you and wants to know precisely which test can prevent him from dying of colon cancer. Which of the following has been shown to decrease mortality from colorectal cancer?

A. Yearly FOBT

B. Double-contrast barium enema

C. Virtual colonoscopy

D. Yearly digital rectal examination

1135 The membrane of colonic smooth muscle cells is home to a variety of ion channels. The exact physiologic role of these channels is largely unknown. However, one of the following has been shown to play a crucial role in colonic motility:

A. Potassium channels

B. L-Type calcium channels

C. Chloride channels

D. Nonselective cation channels

1136 A 28-year-old man underwent total proctocolectomy with IPAA for medically refractory UC two years ago. He was doing well until one month ago when diarrhea, bleeding, urgency, and occasional incontinence developed. Stool studies are negative for infection. Pouchoscopy demonstrates friable

mucosa, erythema, and ulcerations of the pouch, with acute and chronic inflammation on histology. What is the best first-line treatment for this condition?
A. Imodium
B. SCFA enemas
C. Glucocorticosteroid suppositories
D. Metronidazole
E. Bismuth salicylate

1137 Observations on drug therapy for IBS have shown which of the following?
A. Anticholinergics are most useful for those with postprandial pain when taken before eating.
B. Sublingual anticholinergics are more effective than oral ones.
C. Loperamide is effective for abdominal pain and bloating as well as diarrhea.
D. Stimulant laxatives are not safe and should not be used in constipation-predominant IBS.
E. Codeine phosphate has a low side effect profile and low risk of dependency.

1138 Risk factors for the development of pseudomembranous enterocolitis in the absence of *C. difficile* infection are associated with which of the following?
A. Intestinal surgery
B. Intestinal ischemia
C. Neonatal necrotizing enterocolitis
D. Intestinal obstruction
E. All of the above

1139 Adjuvant therapy with 5-fluorouracil and leucovorin is considered standard treatment in advanced colorectal cancer. Which of the following statements regarding this regimen is true?
A. Prolongs disease-free survival, but not overall survival
B. 5-Fluorouracil and levamisole is superior in convenience and efficacy.
C. Prolongs disease-free and overall survival
D. Should not be used for stage 3 disease
E. Standard for all stage 2, node-negative disease

1140 Regarding laboratory findings in ischemic bowel, which of the following is true?
A. A normal WBC count excludes the diagnosis.
B. D-Lactate increases early in the course.
C. High intraperitoneal amylase is diagnostic of AMI.
D. Sensitivity and specificity of serum markers have not been established.

1141 There are several symptoms ("alarm features") that are thought not to be associated with IBS and should raise doubt in the diagnosis and prompt investigation to rule out organic disease. What is the one alarm feature that does not discriminate between IBS and organic disease?
A. Unexplained weight loss
B. History of rectal bleeding
C. Night-time or nocturnal symptoms
D. New-onset symptoms in older age
E. Dysphagia

1142 A 30-year-old HIV-positive man presents with watery diarrhea, weight loss, and abdominal pain of four weeks' duration. His CD4 count is 50. Which treatment has the greatest impact on his course with *Cryptosporidium* infection?
A. HAART
B. Nitazoxanide
C. Paromomycin
D. Azithromycin

1143 Vitamin B₁₂ malabsoption would not generally occur until more than how much of the ileum is resected?
A. 10 cm
B. 20 cm
C. 30 cm
D. 40 cm
E. 60 cm

1144 Which medication is approved by the U.S. Food and Drug Administration (FDA) for the reduction of polyps in familial polyposis?
A. Sulindac
B. Folic acid
C. Calcium
D. Celecoxib
E. Aspirin

1145 Which of the following is most accurate with regard to the epidemiology of Crohn's disease?
A. Incidence rates are increasing in all areas of the world.
B. The prevalence of Crohn's disease in adults in the United States is estimated to be approximately 50 per 100,000 adults.
C. There is a slight male predominance in adults.
D. Except for the white population of South Africa, Crohn's disease is exceedingly rare in Africa and South America.

1146 With regard to 5-ASAs in the treatment of UC, which of the following is true?
A. Doses higher than 2.4 g/day are more effective in patients with moderate compared with mild disease.
B. They are effective in the induction of, but not the maintenance of, remission.
C. They have established efficacy in severe disease.
D. Sulfasalazine is the oldest and most effective of the 5-ASAs.
E. There is no added benefit of combination oral and topical 5-ASAs in treating distal UC.

1147 A 25-year-old woman presents to you reporting intermittent left lower quadrant pain. On physical examination, you elicit a positive Carnett's test in that area. This finding is most consistent with the diagnosis of which of the following?
A. IBS
B. Inflammatory bowel disease
C. Pelvic inflammatory disease
D. Endometriosis
E. Abdominal wall pain

1148 Which of the following may mitigate colorectal cancer risk?

A. Obesity
B. Increasing physical activity
C. Diet high in fat and red meat
D. Cigarette use
E. Low-fiber diet

1149 One postulated mechanism for constipation-predominant IBS is which of the following?
A. Increased segmental nonpropulsive contractions
B. Increased rectal sensation
C. Hypertensive internal rectal sphincter
D. Enhanced gastrocolonic response to meals
E. Increased high-amplitude propagated contractions

1150 The beef and pork tapeworms *Taenia saginata* and *Taenia solium* occur when people eat raw and undercooked meat. Which statement is true?
A. Most colonized people are symptomatic.
B. Cysticercosis is a mild complication of *T. solium*.
C. Neurocysticercosis is a rare cause of epilepsy in endemic areas.
D. These tapeworms can be diagnosed by stool samples.

1151 Which of the following statements regarding hemorrhoids is a fact?
A. Hemorrhoids are not a normal part of human anatomy.
B. Hemorrhoids are dilated vascular channels located in four fairly constant locations: left lateral, right lateral, right posterior, left anterior.
C. Exact incidence of hemorrhoidal disease is unknown, but it is thought to be present in 10% to 25% of the adult population.
D. Second-degree hemorrhoids prolapse through the anal canal at any time but especially with defecation.

1152 This barium radiograph (see figure) from a patient with diarrhea and dermatitis herpetiformis shows findings consistent with which of the following?

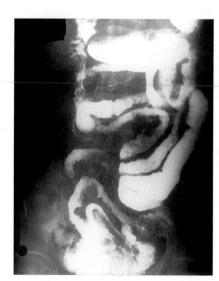

Figure for question **1152**

A. Crohn's disease
B. UC
C. Ulcerative enteritis
D. NSAID-induced ulcerations of the small bowel

1153 A 50-year-old healthy, asymptomatic man consults you for screening for colon cancer. He has no family history of colonic neoplasia and has a normal physical examination. You discuss the screening methods currently available. Which answer lists the tests recommended by current guidelines for average-risk individuals?
A. Colonoscopy, a single FOBT test during a yearly rectal examination, barium enema
B. FOBT, carcinoembryonic antigen determination, colonoscopy, sigmoidoscopy, virtual colonoscopy
C. FOBT, barium enema, sigmoidoscopy, colonoscopy, genetic testing
D. FOBT, barium enema, sigmoidoscopy, colonoscopy, virtual colonoscopy

1154 Which statement is true regarding other treatments for IBS?
A. Tricyclic antidepressants should not be used because the doses required exceed standard antidepressant dosing.
B. Selective serotonin reuptake inhibitors may be more beneficial in constipation-predominant IBS because they accelerate small bowel transit.
C. Colchicine has been used in diarrhea-predominant IBS.
D. Octreotide increases intestinal transit, secretion, and sensation in IBS.
E. Clonidine may be useful in constipation-predominant IBS.

1155 SIBO is associated with many different disease entities. Which of the following is not associated with SIBO?
A. Acne rosacea
B. Crohn's disease
C. Diabetes
D. Nonalcoholic steatohepatitis
E. UC

1156 Complications of celiac disease include which of the following?
A. T-cell lymphoma, colon cancer, and collagenous sprue
B. T-cell lymphoma, ulcerative jejunoileitis, and collagenous sprue
C. Collagenous sprue, B-cell lymphoma, and ulcerative jejunoileitis
D. Colon cancer, ulcerative jejunoileitis, and B-cell lymphoma

1157 The effect of smoking in UC can best be described by which of the following statements?
A. Smoking may be protective in the development of UC.
B. Smoking increases the risk of the development of UC and portends a worse outcome.
C. Ex-smokers do not have a greater risk of the development of UC than smokers.

D. There is no difference in the risk of the development of UC in light versus heavy smokers.

1158 Which of the following statements regarding familial visceral myopathy is true?
A. It is a disease characterized by degeneration of gastrointestinal neurons.
B. It is a primary disorder of the ICCs.
C. Hirschsprung's disease is a form of this disorder.
D. It may exhibit mitochondrial DNA abnormalities with associated lactic acidosis and peripheral neuropathy.
E. It is the most common cause of chronic intestinal pseudo-obstruction.

1159 What is the colonic gas produced by fecal flora associated with symptoms of constipation?
A. Hydrogen
B. Carbon dioxide
C. Nitrogen
D. Sulfur
E. Methane

1160 This PAS stain (see figure) is characteristic of what disease?

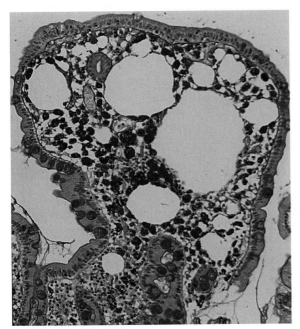

Figure for question **1160**

A. *Giardia* infection
B. *Cryptosporidium* infection
C. Whipple's disease
D. *Yersinia* infection

1161 Appendicitis is epidemiologically best linked to which of the following?
A. African countries
B. Highest incidence rate between ages of 15 and 19
C. Women

D. Third most common acute abdominal emergency in developed countries
E. None of the above

1162 Carcinoid tumors have been associated with a paraneoplastic form of CIP through which mechanism?
A. Acquired visceral myopathy
B. Familial visceral myopathy
C. Visceral neuropathy
D. Unknown mechanism
E. Mesenteric vasculitis

1163 Nonoperative management of patients with partial SBO is warranted based on which of the following reasons?
A. Surgery increases the risk of recurrent SBO.
B. Most patients will improve with nonsurgical management.
C. Gangrenous complications do not occur in patients presenting with partial SBO.
D. Partial SBO can always been distinguished from a complete SBO radiographically.
E. Oral gastrograffin is the treatment of choice to eliminate the need for surgery.

1164 What is the most common presenting symptom of a nonspecific small bowel ulceration?
A. Abdominal pain
B. Intermittent SBO
C. Perforation
D. Chronic gastrointestinal blood loss

1165 Psychological and psychiatric comorbidity is increased in those with IBS. Data have shown that
A. Patients with IBS are less likely to report greater lifetime and daily stressful events than are those patients with organic disease.
B. IBS patients report a history of sexual, physical, or emotional abuse more often than those without IBS.
C. When reported, adult stressful events are more important than childhood stressful events.
D. Animal studies show no effect of stress on colonic motility.
E. A history of abuse is associated with rectal hypersensitivity.

1166 After colectomy is performed for UC, which of the following are normal physiologic and functional sequelae?
A. Patients with ileostomies have obligatory sodium losses of 10 to 15 mEq/day.
B. A normal ileostomy discharge is 300 to 800 g of material daily, 50% of which is water.
C. A normal ileostomy water output is approximately 300 mL/day.
D. Patients with ileostomies have an increased risk of nephrolithiasis.
E. Malabsorption of vitamin B_{12} is common.

1167 A 30-year-old man presents to the emergency department with six weeks of urgent bloody diarrhea as many as eight times per day and sometimes awakens at night to have a bowel movement. In the past two days, he has had a fever as high as 101°F and abdominal pain. His examination is notable for a heart rate of 105 beats per minute, temperature of 99.9°F, blood pressure of 100/60 mm Hg, mild ten-

derness in the left lower quadrant, and gross blood on his rectal examination. Stool study findings are negative for *C. difficile*, culture, and ova and parasites. What is the next best step to try to make a diagnosis in this patient?
A. CT scan
B. Barium enema
C. Colonoscopy
D. Unprepped flexible sigmoidoscopy
E. IBD serologies

1168 *C. difficile* diarrhea and colitis are caused by toxins, not by bacterial invasion of the colonic mucosa. Which of the following is false?
A. *C. difficile* produces two structurally similar protein exotoxins, toxins A and B, which are the major known factors of these bacteria.
B. Toxin A is an inflammatory enterotoxin.
C. Toxin B is an extremely potent cytotoxin but has minimal enterotoxin activity in animals.
D. Toxin A is 10 times more potent than toxin B in causing injury and electrophysiologic changes in human colonic explants in vitro.
E. Toxin B is considered to be a major factor in the pathogenesis of *C. difficile* associated with diarrhea and colitis in humans.

1169 Which of the following is an example of an inflammatory neuropathy of the gut that can cause intestinal pseudo-obstruction?
A. Diabetes
B. Radiation injury
C. Amyloidosis
D. Myxedema
E. Paraneoplastic visceral neuropathy

1170 As feces enter the rectum, the rectoanal inhibitory reflex
A. Causes both the IAS and EAS to relax, leading to defecation
B. Causes both the IAS and EAS to contract, maintaining continence
C. Causes the IAS to relax, allowing feces into the proximal anal canal while continence is maintained by the EAS
D. Causes the EAS to relax, allowing feces into the proximal anal canal while continence is maintained by contraction of the IAS

1171 What is the best accepted risk factor for IBS?
A. Depression
B. Food intolerance
C. Bacterial gastroenteritis
D. Hypochondriasis
E. Oral glucocorticoid use

1172 Abdominal pain, fever, and malaise develop in a 53-year-old Chinese immigrant. He has been in the United States for 10 years. Liver enzymes are elevated, and an ultrasound scan shows a dilated bile duct. Which of the following is correct?
A. The organism will not be seen during ERCP.
B. Eosinophilia is not present.
C. Diagnosis cannot be made by stool examination.
D. *Opisthorchis viverrini* is a closely related parasite that also markedly increases the risk of cholangiocarcinoma.

1173 A 28-year-old woman recently returned from a visit to her family in Bangladesh. Abdominal pain, bloody diarrhea, and fever develop. Which of the following is the most effective regimen for her infection?
A. Single dose of iodoquinol
B. Nitazoxanide for seven days
C. Paromomycin for seven days
D. Ciprofloxacin and metronidazole for 10 days
E. Tinidazole for five days followed by paromomycin

1174 Which of the following statements is true with regard to complications that may be seen after a Brooke ileostomy?
A. Stomal output significantly decreases with obstruction.
B. Backwash ileitis predisposes to prestomal ileitis.
C. Obesity, steroid and/or immunosuppressant use, malnutrition, chronic respiratory disorder, malignancy, and older age are some of the predisposing factors in the development of a parastomal hernia.
D. Relocation of the stoma for the indication of a parastomal hernia is effective in most patients.

1175 A 47-year-old man comes to your office with symptoms of chronic diarrhea. He has a history of chronic pancreatitis secondary to alcohol abuse. His diarrhea is greasy and floats in the bowl. He also reports cramping and abdominal distention after a fatty meal. A diagnosis of fat malabsorption is suspected. Which of the following diagnostic tests would support that diagnosis?
A. A fecal fat excretion of 5 g/day with a fat intake of 100 g/day
B. A fecal acid steatocrit of 25%
C. A count of 150 fat globules per high-power field on microscopic examination of a random stool sample
D. A value of 15 mg/100 mL on measurement of serum photometric beta-carotene

1176 What is the primary manometric abnormality seen in myopathic forms of CIP?
A. Decreased amplitude of contractions in the affected small bowel segment
B. Increased gastric antral amplitudes
C. Disorganization and incoordination of motor activity with normal amplitudes
D. Absent or abnormal MMC activity
E. Cluster contraction pattern in diseased segment

1177 Which of the following statements regarding management of mild to moderately severe *C. difficile* diarrhea and colitis reflects sound clinical judgment?
A. Antimotility agents such as loperamide or narcotics are best avoided.
B. Vancomycin at doses of 125 mg four times daily may be as effective as 500 mg four times daily.
C. Avoid metronidazole and warfarin because of their prolongation of the prothrombin time.

D. Vancomycin should not be administered intravenously for *C. difficile* colitis.

E. All of the above

1178 A 35-year-old homosexual man presents reporting three weeks of diarrhea, bloating, and fatigue. He recently returned from a camping trip in the Rockies. Which of the following statements regarding his infection with *Giardia lamblia* is true?

A. Paromomycin may be used to treat this organism except in pregnancy.

B. Eighty percent to 95% of cases are eradicated with five days of metronidazole.

C. Nitazoxanide is effective but cannot be used in children.

D. Prolonged lactose intolerance does not occur.

1179 What is the most common clinical presentation of nontyphoidal *Salmonella*?

A. Chronic carrier state

B. Osteomyelitis

C. Typhoid fever

D. Bacteremia

E. Gastroenteritis

1180 A 29-year-old man experiences abdominal pain and bloody diarrhea for one week. Initial stool examination shows red and white cells. A sigmoidoscopy reveals erythema and erosions diffusely, and the biopsy sample shows an inflammatory infiltrate in the lamina propria with distortion and branching of the glands. What is the most likely diagnosis?

A. UC

B. *Campylobacter jejuni* infection

C. Salmonellosis

D. *Aeromonas* infection

E. Enterohemorrhagic *E. coli*

1181 Abdominal pain, nausea, vomiting, and diarrhea developed in a 60-year-old man two days after he attended a barbecue. Several others who attended the barbecue also became ill and all had eaten sausage. High fever, myalgia, and periorbital edema then developed. Which of the following is true regarding this infection?

A. Myositis only occurs in smooth muscle.

B. Eosinophilia and elevated CPK may occur.

C. Diagnosis can be made by examining stool samples.

D. The adult worms may be seen on a muscle biopsy specimen.

E. Treatment with praziquantel for 10 to 15 days is effective.

1182 A 70-year-old woman with UC for 27 years undergoes a surveillance colonoscopy; one of the biopsy specimens from the right colon is shown (see figure). What is your recommendation?

A. Immediate colectomy

B. Right hemicolectomy

C. Repeat colonoscopy in three months with extensive biopsies performed in the right colon.

D. Repeat colonoscopy in one year.

E. Confirm findings with a second pathologist and then recommend a total colectomy.

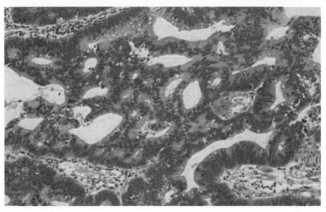

Figure for question **1182**

1183 Which occupations have been shown to have an increased risk of the development of Whipple's disease?

A. Dentists

B. Teachers

C. Farmers and carpenters

D. Sailors

1184 Treatment of small bowel ulcerations caused by NSAIDs includes which of the following?

A. Avoidance, metronidazole, sulfasalazine

B. Avoidance, metronidazole, imuran

C. Avoidance, sulfasalazine, imuran

D. No specific therapy has been shown to reduce inflammation and blood loss.

1185 Oculomasticatory myorhythmia and oculofacial skeletal myorhythmia are characteristic central nervous system signs of what disease?

A. Celiac disease

B. Crohn's disease

C. UC

D. Whipple's disease

1186 What feature is more consistent with mechanical obstruction as opposed to CIP?

A. Dysphagia

B. Constipation

C. Urinary retention

D. Symptom-free periods between attacks

E. Cachexia

1187 What is the initial treatment of choice for occlusive and nonocclusive forms of AMI without signs of peritonitis?

A. Immediate laparotomy

B. Intravenous heparin

C. Hyperbaric oxygen

D. Selected mesenteric angiography with possible infusion

1188 If a patient suspected of having colon ischemia undergoes a careful colonoscopy within 48 hours of symptom onset, typical findings that might be noted include which of the following?

A. A single line of erythema with ulceration oriented along its longitudinal axis of the colon (colon single-stripe sign)

B. Thumbprinting
C. Extensive rectal involvement with a single deep ulceration
D. Stricture formation in the sigmoid colon

1189 Which of the following statements about fluid load and the gastrointestinal tract is false?
A. The salivary glands produce 1500 mL of fluid daily.
B. The stomach produces 2500 mL of fluid daily.
C. Bile amounts to 1000 mL daily.
D. Pancreatic secretions total 1500 mL daily.

1190 What percentage of patients with UC have at least one family member with this disease?
A. 2% to 5%
B. 10% to 20%
C. 30% to 40%
D. More than 50%

1191 The majority of the digestive process is initiated in the duodenum, and, as such, delivery of chyme from the stomach into the duodenum is carefully controlled. Which of the following statements regarding the regulation of gastric emptying is true?
A. The process of trituration is one in which the gastric "mill" reduces the size of food particles to less than 2 mm so that they can be more easily digested.
B. High-viscosity meals empty more quickly than low-viscosity meals.
C. Gastric emptying is promoted when duodenal receptors detect an acidic gastric effluent.
D. The total calorie contents of meals have no bearing on the rate of gastric emptying.

1192 What is the principal factor restricting bacterial numbers in the small intestine?
A. Acid
B. Bile
C. Cytokines
D. Digestive enzymes
E. Peristalsis

1193 Which of the following statements regarding the development of pouchitis after IPAA is true?
A. Pouchitis is seen more commonly after IPAA performed for the indication of IBD compared with FAP.
B. Preoperative EIMs do not increase the risk of pouchitis.
C. Eighty percent of patients will have at least one episode of pouchitis.
D. Chronic inflammatory changes on histology are the hallmark of pouchitis.

1194 The risk of SBO from adhesions is more likely in patients who have undergone which of the following?
A. Appendectomy
B. Subtotal colectomy
C. Cholecystectomy
D. Tubal ligation
E. Laparoscopic Heller myotomy

1195 A patient with chronic hepatitis B presents with abdominal pain. An angiogram revealed an aneurysm in the mesenteric and renal vasculature. Which of the following medications have been shown to improve survival for patients with this disorder?
A. Infliximab
B. Ciprofloxacin
C. Cyclophosphamide
D. Mesalamine
E. MTX

1196 Intestinal pseudo-obstruction is a syndrome
A. Of impaired intestinal propulsion resembling intestinal obstruction without a mechanical cause
B. Involving the large colon only
C. That is chronic only
D. With a unique and specific pathophysiology
E. Primarily secondary to a myopathy

1197 Fast-track enhanced postoperative recovery protocols have been shown to do which of the following?
A. Reduce the duration of ileus
B. Increase the hospital readmission rate
C. Have no effect on length of stay
D. Have no effect on early oral intake
E. Have no effect on costs

1198 The only FDA-approved therapy for total parenteral nutrition–dependent short bowel syndrome is which of the following?
A. Thyroid-stimulating hormone
B. Octreotide
C. Glucagon-like peptide 2 (teduglutide)
D. Growth hormone (somatropin)
E. L-Glutamine

1199 A serpiginous urticarial foot rash develops in a 32-year-old man during a trip to Louisiana. He just finished a course of steroids for his asthma and reports abdominal pain, nausea, and worsening shortness of breath. *Strongyloides stercoralis* is suspected. Which statement regarding the diagnosis of this nematode is true?
A. ELISA for IgG antibodies is unavailable.
B. The larval form cannot be detected on an agar plate.
C. Intestinal biopsy is very insensitive.
D. Stool smear for rhabditiform larvae is more sensitive than ELISA.

1200 A 25-year-old woman comes to your office reporting that she has passed worms in her stool. She recently returned from a trip to Alaska where she frequently consumed salmon. *Diphyllobothrium latum* is diagnosed (see figure). Which statement is true?
A. This is one of the smallest parasites that infects humans.
B. It is acquired by eating undercooked or raw saltwater fish.
C. The treatment is ivermectin.
D. Patients are usually symptomatic.
E. Vitamin B_{12} deficiency may occur.

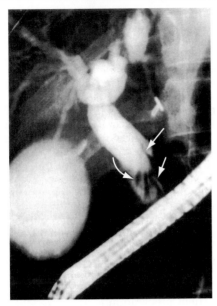

Figure for question **1200**

1201 Which statement regarding the treatment of nonty-phoidal *Salmonella* infections is true?
A. Antibiotics have no effect on the duration of illness in randomized trials.
B. Antibiotics decrease the duration and frequency of intestinal carriage.
C. Immunosuppressed patients should receive antibiotics.
D. Patients with joint replacements do not need antibiotics.
E. All patients with *Salmonella* infection should receive antibiotics.

1202 Observations of the Manning criteria for IBS have shown which of the following?
A. The criteria are only useful in women.
B. There are five major and five minor criteria.
C. Meeting three or more criteria correctly determined the diagnosis of IBS in more than 90% of patients.
D. All criteria have been shown to be statistically significant discriminators.
E. It is named for Peyton Manning, who has IBS and is a major supporter of IBS research.

1203 Which of the following statements regarding familial visceral neuropathies is true?
A. They are a group of genetic diseases characterized by degeneration of the ICCs.
B. They are a group of genetic diseases characterized by degeneration of the myenteric plexus.
C. They are disorders with effective therapy and a good prognosis.
D. They are inherited with incomplete penetrance, with most affected individuals being asymptomatic.
E. They only involve the small intestine.

1204 Screening families with HNPCC can include which of the following?
A. Colonoscopy every five years
B. Genetic testing for *APC* and *K-ras* mutations
C. Colonoscopy beginning at age 20 to 25
D. Yearly sigmoidoscopy starting at puberty and then colonoscopy every two years at age 40

1205 A 33-year-old man with ileocolonic Crohn's disease is seen urgently in your office with regard to several days of progressively worsening perianal and rectal pain. He also feels something "wet" sometimes in his underwear. He walks with an antalgic gait into the examination room and prefers to stand rather than sit. Perianal examination reveals a posterolateral abscess and an adjacent open draining fistula. In addition to surgical referral, which of the following medications is the next best step?
A. Ciprofloxacin and metronidazole
B. Rifaximin
C. Adalimumab
D. Mesalamine
E. Glucocorticosteroids

1206 The risk of colorectal cancer in UC is related to which of the following?
A. Age at disease onset
B. Disease activity
C. Severity of initial attack
D. Duration of disease
E. Number of pseudopolyps

1207 What is the most common human protozoal entero-pathogen recognized worldwide to cause chronic diarrhea and intestinal malabsorption and to be a contributing factor in the retardation of growth and development in infants and young children?
A. *I. belli*
B. *G. lamblia*
C. *C. cayetanensis*
D. *Cryptosporidium parvum*

1208 Which of the following statements regarding the incidence and mortality of colorectal cancer in the United States is true?
A. The mortality rate has increased since 1985.
B. The incidence has increased since 1985.
C. The incidence and mortality rate are higher in African Americans than whites.
D. Migration to the United States from areas of low incidence does not affect the risk.

1209 With regard to lactose malabsorption, which of the following is true?
A. Lactose malabsorption is seen with a similar prevalence across all ethnicities.
B. Primary lactase deficiency (adult-type hypolactasia) is caused by a mutation in the gene coding for intestinal lactase.
C. The diagnosis of lactose malabsorption is made by an increase in breath hydrogen concentration of greater than 20 ppm over baseline after ingestion of a lactose meal.
D. In young patients with lactose malabsorption, cystic fibrosis must be ruled out.

1210 Which of the following is true in a patient with AIDS and appendicitis?
A. Pain is common.
B. History of chronic abdominal pain is common.

C. Diarrhea is a more common presentation than HIV-negative patients.

D. Leukocytosis is relatively uncommon.

E. All of the above

1211 What are the intestinal pacemaker cells activating neuromuscular function?

A. Myenteric nerve cells

B. M cells

C. ICCs

D. IELs

E. Vagal crest cells

1212 Which of the following statements regarding scleroderma is correct?

A. The small bowel is the primary gastrointestinal organ involved.

B. Longitudinal muscles are more involved than circular muscles.

C. Pneumatosis cystoides intestinalis is a common association.

D. Bacterial overgrowth is an uncommon consequence.

E. There is absence of the interdigestive MMC.

1213 Abdominal pain, nausea, and bloody diarrhea developed in five people who attended a barbecue. *Salmonella* is diagnosed by stool culture. Which statement concerning the epidemiology of salmonellosis is most accurate?

A. Attack rates show no relationship to age.

B. A route of passage can include contaminated food and fomites.

C. Poultry is rarely involved.

D. Young children and the elderly do not have a high attack rate.

1214 Neoplasms of the small intestine can arise from any of the cells that compose it. Gastrointestinal stromal tumors are thought to arise from which cells?

A. Smooth muscle cells

B. Lymphocytes

C. ICCs

D. Argentaffin cells

E. Glandular mucosa

1215 Which of the following clinical and laboratory features are most consistent with a diagnosis of collagenous and lymphocytic colitis?

A. Fresh stools showed fecal leukocytes in 55% of cases of collagenous colitis.

B. Diarrhea is generally long-standing, with an average of eight stools each day.

C. Colonoscopic examination usually is normal.

D. More common in women

E. All of the above

1216 Celiac disease is associated with all of the following autoimmune disorders *except*:

A. Sclerosing cholangitis

B. Ulcerative proctitis

C. Insulin-dependent diabetes mellitus

D. Hypothyroidism

E. Wegener's granulomatosis

1217 A 64-year-old white woman with hypertension and non–insulin-dependent diabetes mellitus diagnosed 11 years previously is now referred for evaluation of abdominal discomfort and loose bowel movements. The patient reports postprandial bloating followed by loose bowel movements that she describes as "oily." She reports subjective weight loss over the past year. She denies a history of excessive alcohol consumption. Laboratory tests show macrocytic anemia with hemoglobin of 9.7 g/dL and a mean corpuscular volume of 106/mL. There is also evidence of mild hypocalcemia. Sudan stain of a stool specimen is positive for the presence of fecal fat. SIBO is suspected. A glucose breath test is ordered. Which of the following statements regarding the glucose breath test is most accurate?

A. In the presence of bacterial overgrowth, glucose absorption in the upper small intestine is greatly increased.

B. Within two hours of the ingestion of the glucose substrate, an increase of 20 ppm of hydrogen in exhaled breath is regarded as diagnostic of SIBO.

C. Patient preparation is not important for this test.

D. In general, breath testing in cases of suspected SIBO is prohibitively expensive, and therefore the glucose breath test is not widely used.

1218 Inhibitory neural reflexes play a role in postoperative ileus through which of the following?

A. Norepinephrine release by efferent sympathetic splanchnic nerves inhibiting acetylcholine release from excitatory neurons in the myenteric plexus

B. Serotonin release from neurons causing a direct inhibition of peristalsis

C. Somatostatin-induced inhibition of acetylcholine release

D. Nitric oxide production within the myenteric plexus

E. Reduction of endogenous opioids within myenteric plexus neurons

1219 Which of the following drugs stimulates small intestine motility when given after a meal?

A. Clonidine

B. Octreotide

C. Calcium channel antagonists

D. Antiparkinsonism drugs

E. Opiate analgesics

1220 One of the postulated mechanisms for diarrhea-predominant IBS is which of the following?

A. Inhibition of the gastrocolonic response after a meal

B. Increased high-amplitude propagated contractions

C. Reduced rectal sensitivity resulting in fecal urgency

D. Increased segmental nonpropulsive contractions

E. Hypertensive internal rectal sphincter

1221 What is the best predictor of a complete SBO versus a low-grade partial SBO?

A. Presence of feculent emesis

B. Borborygmi

C. Lack of stool evacuation

D. Crampy abdominal pain occurring every four to five minutes

E. Differential air–fluid levels in the same small bowel loop with a mean air–fluid level diameter of 2.5 cm or greater

1222 The intestine can tolerate what percentage of reduction of mesenteric blood flow and oxygen consumption for 12 hours without histologic change by light microscopy?
A. 10%
B. 25%
C. 50%
D. 75%
E. 90%

1223 What is the histologic feature that best discriminates between acute self-limited colitis (e.g., from infection) and chronic idiopathic IBD (see figure)?
A. Crypt architectural distortion (e.g., branching, bifid, shortened glands)
B. Edema of the lamina propria
C. Acute inflammatory cell infiltrate
D. Crypt abscesses

1224 What is the main treatment of celiac disease?
A. Avoidance of gluten
B. Glucocorticoids
C. Cyclosporine
D. Tetracycline

1225 With respect to environmental factors associated with UC, which of the following statements is true?
A. A single, yet to be identified organism is likely responsible for the development and continued inflammation in UC.
B. The risk of UC increases after appendectomy.
C. The normal intestinal environment may induce chronic inflammation via dysbiosis (an imbalance of protective and harmful bacteria) or by defects in the host immune system.

D. Bacteria do not seem to be an important contributor to chronic inflammation as there are no differences in rates of colitis in animals raised in germ-free environments and those colonized with bacteria.

1226 Which statement most accurately applies to complicated appendicitis?
A. The perforation rate is 10% to 30%.
B. Perforation rates vary widely with age but are most common with extremes of age.
C. The risk of perforation increases, particularly after 24 hours of illness.
D. Perforation is often the consequence of delay in diagnosis.
E. All of the above

1227 What is the most common presentation for benign small bowel neoplasms?
A. SBO
B. Overt gastrointestinal bleeding
C. Occult iron deficiency anemia
D. Perforation
E. Unexplained weight loss

1228 Malabsorption is not uncommon in SIBO. Vitamin deficiencies can occur. Which vitamin is least likely to be deficient in a patient with SIBO?
A. Vitamin A
B. Vitamin B_{12}
C. Vitamin D
D. Vitamin E
E. Vitamin K

1229 Which of the following statements regarding IPAA in the setting of indeterminate colitis is the most accurate?
A. The risk of developing subsequent Crohn's disease is approximately 30%.
B. IPAA should not be performed in patients with indeterminate colitis.

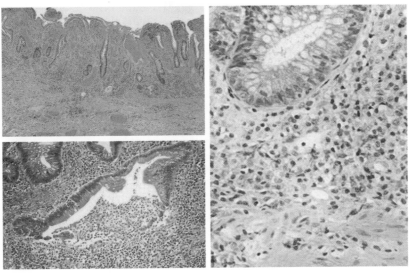

Figure for question **1223**

C. There is no difference in the rates of the development of Crohn's disease between those patients with indeterminate colitis and those with UC.

D. After IPAA, Crohn's disease will develop in approximately 15% of patients with indeterminate colitis compared with approximately 2% of patients with UC.

1230 EIMs of celiac disease include all of the following *except*:
A. Iron deficiency anemia
B. Ataxia
C. Osteopenia
D. Uveitis
E. Dermatitis herpetiformis

1231 When does vasoconstriction, the result of a major vessel occlusion, occur?
A. Immediately, elevating the pressure in the vascular bed, thus reducing collateral flow
B. After several hours, elevating the pressure in the vascular bed and reducing collateral flow
C. After 24 hours; it is readily reversible but has little to do with progressive bowel ischemia, even if cardiac function is fully restored
D. Days later, contributing to necrotic bowel

1232 A 75-year-old woman presents with chronic intermittent abdominal pain, distention associated with nausea, and vomiting. Imaging reveals a smooth stricture in the proximal ileum measuring 5 to 6 cm in length. What is the most likely diagnosis?
A. Crohn's disease
B. Idiopathic joint ileitis
C. Lymphoma
D. Small bowel adenocarcinoma
E. FSI

1233 Which of the following statements about the appendix is not well documented in the literature?
A. Appendectomy may protect against the development of UC.
B. The vast majority of appendiceal tumors are carcinoid tumors.
C. The lifetime risk of appendicitis at birth is approximately 1 in 12.
D. The greatest risk of appendicitis is in the first decade of life.
E. Persons between the age of 10 and 30 have the lowest perforation rates (10%-20%).

1234 Solitary rectal ulcers are most commonly located
A. On the posterior wall 2 to 3 cm from the anal verge
B. On the posterior wall 7 to 10 cm from the anal verge
C. On the anterior wall 2 to 3 cm from the anal verge
D. On the anterior wall 7 to 10 cm from the anal verge

1235 Which of the following is a primarily myopathic cause of CIP?
A. Diabetes
B. Parkinson's disease
C. Scleroderma
D. Multiple sclerosis
E. Amyloidosis

1236 A 34-year-old asymptomatic man states that his father died at age 52 of colorectal cancer and his paternal aunt had colon cancer at age 76. In addition to following your recommendations for colonoscopic screening, he wants your suggestions regarding chemoprevention. Which of the following has been shown in epidemiologic studies?
A. Calcium decreases the risk of metastases.
B. Folic acid decreases colorectal cancer mortality.
C. Vitamin C decreases colorectal cancer deaths.
D. Sulindac decreases the villous component of polyps.
E. Aspirin decreases the incidence of adenomas and colorectal cancer.

1237 Diversion colitis seems to be caused by which of the following?
A. Recurrence of IBD
B. Colonic epithelial changes due to luminal nutrient deficiency
C. Radiation
D. *C. difficile* infection

1238 Which of the following is not associated with *C. difficile* infection?
A. IBD
B. Elderly population
C. Antineoplastic therapy
D. HIV infection
E. None of the above

1239 Chemotherapy, radiation, and combined modality treatment are used to prevent postoperative recurrence of colorectal cancer. Which patient would benefit most from adjuvant therapy after curative intent surgery?
A. Patient with Dukes C1 sigmoid lesion
B. Patient with Dukes B1 transverse colon lesion
C. Patient with Dukes A rectal lesion
D. Patient with Dukes B2 ascending colon lesion
E. Patient with Dukes B1 rectal lesion

1240 What is the treatment of patients with complete SBO?
A. Urgent early laparotomy within 48 hours if no improvement or deterioration
B. Conservative management and laparotomy if signs of strangulation develop
C. Urgent surgery only in patients with inguinal hernias
D. Capsule endoscopy followed by surgery if capsule gets stuck
E. Therapeutic gastrograffin enteroclysis

1241 If you travel to the southeast Asian countries and experience diarrhea, the most likely cause would be which of the following?
A. Amebiasis
B. *Campylobacter*
C. *Salmonella*
D. Cholera

1242 Symptoms of rectal ulceration, erythema, or mass associated with straining at defecation, rectal prolapse, and a feeling of incomplete evacuation are most consistent with which of the following?
A. Solitary rectal ulcer syndrome
B. Ulcerative proctitis
C. Crohn's disease
D. Hemorrhoids

1243 A patient with Crohn's ileitis undergoes an ileocecectomy. Histologic examination of the specimen reveals the abnormality seen in the figure. Which of the following is true about this pathologic finding?

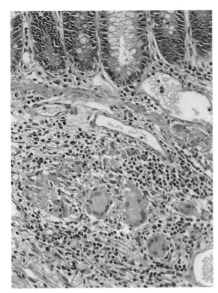

Figure for question **1243**

A. It generally occurs later in the course of the disease.
B. It is unique to Crohn's disease.
C. It is seen in approximately 15% of endoscopic specimens and as many as 70% of surgical specimens.
D. They are more commonly found outside the gastrointestinal tract.

1244 Epidemiologic studies in patients with IBS have found which of the following?
A. There is a male predominance with a 2:1 ratio.
B. Women have slower colonic transit and smaller stool output than men.
C. Prevalence is greater among African Americans than whites.
D. IBS is not seen in China or Japan.
E. Hispanics have the greatest prevalence compared with non-Hispanics.

1245 Which of the following methods has become the most common office treatment for second- and third-degree hemorrhoids?

A. Sclerosing agents
B. Rubber band ligation
C. Cryotherapy
D. Surgery
E. Infrared photocoagulation

1246 What is a factor that delays recovery from postoperative ileus?
A. Chewing gum
B. Early oral feeding
C. Laparoscopic surgery
D. Mobilization
E. Nasogastric tube placement

1247 Which of the following is a factor that may lower the risk of IBS?
A. Prolonged duration of diarrhea after bacterial gastroenteritis
B. Younger age
C. Oral glucocorticoid use
D. Affluent childhood environment
E. Postmenopausal estrogen use

1248 The prognosis in colorectal cancer is associated with some morphologic and some histologic factors. Which statement is correct?
A. Aneuploid tumors confer a better prognosis.
B. The size of the primary tumor correlates with the prognosis.
C. Perineural invasion is not important.
D. Venous invasion, but not lymphatic invasion, confers a worse prognosis.
E. Histologic grade, or degree of differentiation, correlates with the prognosis.

1249 You diagnose a hospitalized patient with acute colonic pseudo-obstruction. Abdominal x-ray reveals a cecal diameter of 9.5 cm. Your initial treatment modality is which of the following?
A. Colonoscopy with decompression
B. Treat reversible causes.
C. Administer intravenous neostigmine, assuming there are no contraindications.
D. Surgical decompression
E. Gentle water-soluble enema

1250 Seventy-two hours after your diagnosis and initial treatment of the patient in question 1249, the cecal diameter is now 10 cm. What should your next treatment option be?
A. Colonoscopy with decompression
B. Treat reversible causes.
C. Administer intravenous neostigmine, assuming there are no contraindications.
D. Surgical decompression
E. Gentle water-soluble enema

1251 What is the most specific early finding on a CT scan suggestive of intestinal ischemia in the setting of an SBO?
A. Small bowel feces sign
B. Whirl sign
C. Decreased small bowel wall enhancement
D. Pneumatosis intestinales
E. Pneumoperitoneum

ANSWERS

883 **A** (S&F, ch111)
This patient is presenting with SBO secondary to fibrostenotic Crohn's disease, which may occur suddenly after years of subclinical inflammation. The patient has no symptoms such as diarrhea and fever to suggest inflammation, and similarly her laboratory tests and small bowel series do not support an inflammatory component. Further, she does not respond to a trial of glucocorticosteroids. Because the stricture is fibrotic and not inflammatory, it will not respond to medications, and surgery is indicated. Although stricturoplasty can sometimes be performed, more commonly ileocecectomy is done, especially when there is only a single stricture without a history of resections. Of note, the patient has macrocytic anemia, which is likely secondary to vitamin B_{12} malabsorption.

884 **A** (S&F, ch118)
IBS is associated with a threefold increased risk of ischemic colitis. IBS is not known to be associated with an increased risk of the other illnesses listed.

885 **C** (S&F, ch104)
A Finnish study of 3654 schoolchildren aged seven to 16 years using two serologic screens with anti-endomysial and tissue transglutaminase antibodies in 1994 and 2001 demonstrated the heterogeneity of celiac disease. The prevalence of biopsy-proven celiac disease among schoolchildren was 1:99. The prevalence of schoolchildren who carried the HLA-DQ2 or HLA-DQ8 haplotype (which are strongly associated with celiac disease) and also were antibody positive was 1:67. A large multicenter study by Fasano and colleagues determined the prevalence of anti-endomysial antibodies in more than 13,000 at-risk and not-at-risk American subjects and found the prevalence of anti-endomysial antibodies to be 1:133 among 4126 not-at-risk individuals.

886 **A** (S&F, ch97)
The ICCs are cells that are interspersed within and between the muscular layers of the small intestine. These cells generate the electrical slow waves that determine the basic rhythm of the small intestine contractions. This intestinal pacemaking, by modulating the neurologic input to the smooth muscle cells, regulates contractile activity.

887 **E** (S&F, ch103)
D-Lactate acidosis is a rare complication of short bowel syndrome and only occurs in people with intact colons. Episodes occur by intake of refined carbohydrates. Malabsorbed carbohydrate is metabolized by colon bacteria to SCFAs and lactate, which lower the colon pH. Low pH promotes growth of acid-resistant, gram-positive anaerobes, which produce D-lactate. D-Lactate is absorbed from the colon and is metabolized to only a limited extent in humans because of lack of D-lactate dehydrogenase. The main excretory route for D-lactate is the kidney; absorbed D-lactate results in the development of a metabolic acidosis and characteristic neurologic signs and symptoms.

888 **C** (S&F, ch96)
The ICCs are the pacemaker cells of the intestine. They are mesenchymal cells located in the myenteric plexus, the muscularis propria, and the submucosa throughout the small intestine and colon (see figure). Their distribution is similar from infancy to adulthood, and they regulate intestinal motility through generation of slow waves and determine the frequency of contraction. They amplify neuronal signals, mediate neurotransmission from the enteric motor neurons to smooth muscle cells, and set the smooth muscle membrane potential gradient. Serotonin regulates the number of cells.

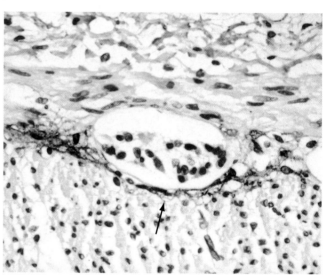

Figure for answer **888**

889 **C** (S&F, ch107)
Gastric acidity, intestinal motility, intestinal microflora, mucus, and other local and systemic immune factors comprise some of the host defenses against infection. Adherence, enterotoxin, cytotoxin, and mucosal invasion are the bacterial factors that help overcome the host defenses.

890 **B** (S&F, ch101)
Chronic diarrhea is quite common in patients with diabetes, particularly in those with long-standing type 1 diabetes. Mild steatorrhea is quite common even in patients who do not report diarrhea, and poor glycemic control is an important cofactor. The pathophysiology of this entity is not entirely understood, but most patients have autonomic dysfunction, which may play a role. Additionally, the presence of several very treatable diseases, such as sprue, bacterial overgrowth, and pancreatic insufficiency, is often seen in these patients and should not be overlooked.

891 A (S&F, ch119)

The most common causes of colonic obstruction are malignancy, volvulus, and strictures secondary to diverticulitis. Less frequent causes include Crohn's disease, endometriosis, intussusception, extrinsic tumors, and fecal impaction. Adenocarcinoma of the colon accounts for more than 50% of all cases of colonic obstruction.

892 B (S&F, ch120)

All general anesthesia agents can contribute to postoperative ileus. Reduction in postoperative ileus has been seen with midthoracic epidural anesthesia but not low thoracic or lumbar anesthesia. Opioids contribute to postoperative ileus. Naloxone is a nonselective opioid antagonist and has not been shown to be effective in reducing postoperative ileus.

893 B (S&F, ch109)

The two important species of Microsporidia are *Enterocytozoon bieneusi* and *Encephalitozoon intestinalis*. The former causes 90% of the cases but responds poorly to albendazole, whereas the latter accounts for 10% of the cases and responds well to albendazole. Disease from these organisms primarily occurs in patients with impaired cell-mediated immunity (i.e., AIDS patients and organ transplant patients). Some studies suggest that as many as 50% of HIV-positive patients with diarrhea are positive for microsporidiosis. Microsporidiosis, like cryptosporidiosis, can be associated with sclerosing cholangitis. Immune reconstitution is essential in the treatment of microsporidiosis.

894 A (S&F, ch102)

SIBO is probably second only to celiac disease as the most common cause of malabsorption in developed countries. Nowadays most patients do not present with the classic features of steatorrhea and megaloblastic anemia, and most patients do not have a blind loop or other predisposing anatomic abnormality. Many patients have nonspecific symptoms similar to those of IBS but have not yet been definitely proven to cause IBS. Although the glucose hydrogen and ^{14}C-xylose breath tests are simple and noninvasive, the gold standard for diagnosis is culture of an aspirate of small intestine contents. The aspirate may be collected easily at endoscopy, which usually is performed to obtain biopsy specimens of the small intestine wall during evaluation of malabsorption. Treatment with one of several broad-spectrum antibiotics is recommended and effective.

895 E (S&F, ch114)

The patient has typical findings of ischemic colitis. When colonic ischemia is diagnosed and there are no physical examination findings to suggest gangrene or perforation, expectant therapy is warranted. Fluids, bowel rest, and broad-spectrum antibiotics are also usually added to the treatment regimen. Urgent imagings of any type, including CT and angiography, are not warranted at this time. Because there are no peritoneal signs, laparotomy is not necessary. Mesalamine and steroids would have no role in ischemic colitis.

896 C (S&F, ch96)

Mucosal folds of the small intestine are called plicae circulares. These folds are more numerous in the proximal jejunum and gradually decrease in number in the distal small bowel. Haustra refer to colonic outpouchings between the taeniae coli. Appendices epiploicae are small peritoneal projections filled with adipose tissue; they are found on the surface of the colon. Columns of Morgagni are longitudinal folds within the anal canal that terminate in the anal papilla. Rugae refer to redundant gastric folds.

897 D (S&F, ch100)

Salivary amylase and pancreatic amylase are both endoenzymes and as such they cleave an internal bond of the polysaccharide chain producing shorter polysaccharides and maltose. The efficacy of salivary amylase is maximized by chewing food well and maximizing the amount of time that food is in the mouth. Salivary amylase is inactivated by the low gastric pH, and only a small portion of dietary starch is digested by the time food reaches the duodenum.

898 D (S&F, ch112)

The main pathologic finding of this endoscopic photo is pseudopolyps, also known as inflammatory polyps. These polyps are thought to result from epithelial regeneration after flares; although they are more characteristic of long-standing disease, pseudopolyps can certainly be seen acutely as well. In and of themselves, they are not believed to harbor any malignant potential and do not require a change in management, although if abundant, there may be concern about missing a true neoplasm.

899 A (S&F, ch111)

In contrast to UC, in which the inflammation is limited to the mucosa, the inflammation seen in Crohn's disease is characteristically transmural. The nature of this type of inflammation predisposes to the development of sinus tracts and fistulas, both of which are extensions of fissures: whereas sinus tracts end blindly, fistulas bear through the intestinal wall to connect to another epithelium-lined organ, such as the skin, bladder, or vagina. Fibrosis is observed macroscopically as irregular thickening of the bowel wall, which, when coupled with muscularis mucosae hypertrophy, often leads to the formation of strictures. Because endoscopic biopsies are superficial, one cannot appreciate the transmural nature of the inflammation via histologic samples. Transmural inflammation tends to be focal and is less commonly observed than disease that involves just the mucosa and submucosa.

900 B (S&F, ch112)

The randomized, controlled trials that have been conducted to examine the efficacy of azathioprine for the induction and maintenance of remission have been largely small and heterogeneous in design, had different outcome definitions, and, not surprisingly, reached different conclusions (see tables at end of chapter). The widespread use of azathioprine and 6-MP is mostly derived from its efficacy in Crohn's disease. Optimal levels of 6-thioguanine nucleotide, the active metabolite of 6-MP and azathioprine, have been shown to be greater than 230 pmol/8 × 10⁸. Checking metabolite levels (6-thioguanine nucleotide and 6-methyl mercaptopurine) as a means of monitoring whether a patient is receiving an optimal dose of medication is controversial to perform in all patients, and is probably best reserved for nonresponders and those with a question of nonadherence. Bone marrow suppression is dose dependent and not idiosyncratic, occurs in 2% to 5% of patients, and manifests primarily with leukopenia, although all lineages may be affected. A complete blood count should be checked at least every three months once the patient is on a stable dose. The risk of non-Hodgkin's lymphoma was reviewed in a meta-analysis of six studies, and a fourfold increased risk was found. Other adverse effects are reviewed (see table at end of chapter).

901 **E** (S&F, ch 107)
Enterotoxigenic *E. coli* accounts for approximately 40% to 60% of the cases of travelers' diarrhea. The table (at end of chapter) shows the relative frequencies of causes of travelers' diarrhea.

902 **B** (S&F, ch104)
Cellier and colleagues showed that the IELs in refractory sprue lacked the expression of CD8, which is commonly found on the lymphocytes of normal or celiac disease IELs. Many patients with refractory sprue have intestinal T-cell lymphoma.

903 **B** (S&F, ch96)
Hirschsprung's disease is caused by the failure of craniocaudal migration of neural crest cells, resulting in the absence of ganglion cells in both the myenteric plexus and submucosal plexus. This most commonly affects a short segment of the rectosigmoid colon, but the disease can extend more proximally and even rarely can affect the small intestine. The involved segment fails to relax, resulting in a functional colonic obstruction. Full-thickness or deep-suction biopsy specimens of the distal colon are required to demonstrate the absence of ganglion cells. Superficial mucosal biopsy specimens are not adequate. Several genetic mutations have been identified, including the *RET* proto-oncogene.

904 **B** (S&F, ch110)
Albendazole is teratogenic and should not be used during pregnancy. It does not penetrate the bile duct, and therefore worms are only susceptible when they migrate out of the ampulla into the intestine (see figure). Glucocorticoids, in conjunction with albendazole, are effective in reducing the pneumonitis.

905 **B** (S&F, ch120)
Patients with the paraneoplastic visceral neuropathy often have antineuronal nuclear antibodies that can be detected by immunofluorescence. This antibody is postulated to be directed toward an epitope that is shared by the neuronal elements within the enteric nervous system and the underlying malignancy.

906 **B** (S&F, ch123)
FOBT relies on the oxidation of a compound that will change from a colorless to a colored compound. Hemoglobin contains pseudoperoxidase activity. Rehydrating slides increases the sensitivity but decreases the specificity. Ascorbic acid may enhance or inhibit oxidation of the dye. The ingestion of red meat should be avoided during the collection of stool for testing as this may cause a false-positive result. Peroxidase-containing foods, such as turnips, cauliflower, broccoli, radishes, and cantaloupe, should be avoided. NSAIDs may cause frank or occult blood loss and will affect the accuracy of colorectal screening. Tocopherol is not known to interfere with occult blood testing (see three tables at end of chapter).

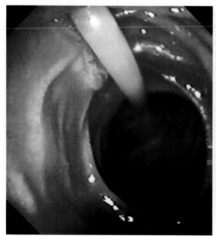
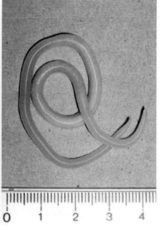

Figure for answer **904**

907 **D** (S&F, ch112)

Balsalazide is a type of mesalamine, 5-ASA, which is the first-line therapy for UC, and remission can often be induced and maintained with a 5-ASA only. When 5-ASA therapy is not effective initially or patients flare while in remission on 5-ASAs, often a short course of corticosteroids is required to induce or reinduce remission. However, corticosteroids are not effective as maintenance therapy and have many potential side effects, including hyperglycemia, osteoporosis, hypertension, mood instability, acne, infection, and osteonecrosis. Although some patients may maintain remission with continued 5-ASA therapy after corticosteroid taper, other patients become steroid dependent or resistant, as did this patient, and therapy with an immunomodulator such as 6-MP or azathioprine should be started. These agents are nucleotide analogs that interfere with DNA synthesis and induce apoptosis. Therapy with these agents may require as long as three months to provide clinical benefit, and, therefore, they are generally started with corticosteroids, which are then tapered. Because corticosteroids are not effective maintenance therapy, simply increasing the dose of prednisone without adding an immunomodulator would not be appropriate in this patient. The addition of another 5-ASA, such as olsalazine, will not provide any greater benefit. Antibiotic therapy has not been shown to be effective in the treatment of UC, and the patient's stool was negative for *C. difficile*. Further, budesonide, a nonsystemic corticosteroid that is useful in the induction of remission in patients with Crohn's disease involving the terminal ileum and right colon, would not be of added benefit in this patient.

908 **C** (S&F, ch102)

Most human enteric bacteria cannot be cultured because of a lack of truly selective growth media. Nonetheless, molecular profiling has shown that although different individuals have different flora, the population in each individual is relatively stable after weaning. Environmental factors such as diet and sanitation appear to have a profound effect on early intestinal colonization with bacteria. In adulthood, dietary fluctuations seem to induce changes in bacterial enzymes and metabolic activity rather than changes in the population of flora.

909 **D** (S&F, ch96)

Familial glucose/galactose malabsorption is characterized by an absence of the active transport carrier protein for glucose and galactose. Ingestion of formulas containing these sugars can lead to severe life-threatening diarrhea. Stool is strongly positive for reducing substances and free of WBCs and blood. A change in formula to a fructose-containing product is all that is typically needed to quell symptoms.

910 **C** (S&F, ch100)

Many enzymes and hormones have been implicated to influence food intake. CCK and apolipoprotein A IV have been implicated as transmitters of the satiety signal to the central nervous system. PPY is an anorectic peptide and has been shown to decrease appetite and promote satiety in both animals and human models. Leptin is a hormone released from fat cells and is an important peripheral signal from fat stores that modulates food intake. Leptin deficiency and leptin receptor defects produce massive obesity. Ghrelin, however, is the only signaling substance that has been shown to increase appetite.

911 **C** (S&F, ch111)

6-MP and its prodrug, azathioprine, are thiopurine antimetabolites used in the treatment of inflammatory bowel disease, with better data in Crohn's disease than UC. A Cochrane analysis found that 54% of patients treated with azathioprine or 6-MP will have a response to therapy, with an increased odds ratio after 17 weeks of therapy. Approximately two thirds of patients will maintain remission, with an increased odds ratio when appropriately higher doses are used (6-MP, 1.0 to 1.5 mg/kg, and azathioprine, 2.0 to 2.5 mg/kg). It is very unlikely that this patient will be off of steroids and on only 6-MP after six weeks of therapy; in clinical practice, it is generally accepted that these medications can take two to four months to have a full effect. The risk of serious infection is approximately 1.8% with long-term use, not necessarily related to leukopenia; this risk is greater with concomitant glucocorticosteroids and/or biologics. Pancreatitis is an idiosyncratic reaction that generally occurs within the first month of therapy and is seen in 3% to 7% of patients; patients should not be rechallenged with either medication if they experience pancreatitis.

912 **A** (S&F, ch96)

This child most likely has Meckel's diverticulum based on his positive nuclear scan. Meckel's diverticulum is one of several anomalies of the omphalomesenteric (vitelline) duct that develop when there is a persistence of the communication between the intestine and the yolk sac. Meckel's diverticulum is an antimesenteric outpouching of the distal ileum, usually occurring 2 feet from the ileocecal valve in 1% to 2% of the population. Ectopic gastrointestinal mucosa (typically gastric) is found in 50% of cases. Painless bleeding is the most common manifestation, although intestinal obstruction and diverticulitis can also occur. ^{99m}Tc-pertechnetate is taken up by mucus-secreting cells of the gastric mucosa and may aid in the diagnosis, although the diagnosis is often made at the time of surgery. Inadequate folate intake leads to neural tube defects and has no known association with Meckel's diverticulum. There is no known genetic predisposition to Meckel's diverticulum.

913 **D** (S&F, ch98)

The rectum has the ability to distend and store feces until a convenient evacuation can be achieved. Prolonged rectal storage is made possible by the ability of the rectum to accommodate an increasing volume without a corresponding increase in intrarectal pressure. This is mediated by inhibitory nerves and permits continence without a constant urge to defecate. This distention has a negative effect on the more proximal gastrointestinal tract and inhibits gastric emptying, slows small bowel transit, reduces the frequency of proximal colonic propagating pressure waves, and delays colonic transit.

914   A (S&F, ch119)
Richter's hernia is a herniation of the intestinal wall through a laparoscopic trocar site with resultant bowel obstruction. The incidence of this hernia after laparoscopic fundoplication or cholecystectomy is 1% to 3%. When an SBO develops in a patient shortly after a laparoscopic procedure, this needs to be looked for as the cause.

915   B (S&F, ch125)
An anal fissure is a longitudinal cut in the anoderm. More than 90% of anal fissures are located in the midposterior portion of the anus. It has been shown that the posterior area of the anoderm is less well perfused than other areas of anoderm. There is speculation that increased tone in the internal sphincter muscle further reduces the blood flow to this area. Based on these findings, fissures are thought to represent ischemic ulceration. Trauma during defecation, especially with passage of a hard stool, is believed to initiate the formation of a fissure. The history is classically one of severe pain during defecation. A digital examination causes inhumane pain, increases the spasm, and should be avoided. Once the fissure is healed or the pain has lessened, an examination can be performed to exclude associated problems.

916   D (S&F, ch104)
A large multicenter study by Fasano and colleagues determined the prevalence of anti-endomysial antibodies in more than 13,000 at-risk and not-at-risk American subjects. They found the prevalence of anti-endomysial antibodies to be 1:22 and 1:39 among first-degree and second-degree relatives of subjects with celiac disease, respectively. A prevalence of 1:56 was documented among patients with gastrointestinal symptoms of celiac disease or associated disorders. Of most significance, they found a prevalence of anti-endomysial antibodies of 1:133 among 4126 not-at-risk individuals.

917   B (S&F, ch107)
Enterotoxigenic *E. coli* is the most common cause of travelers' diarrhea in those traveling from North America or Northern Europe to the developing world. Although the diarrhea can be severe and cholera-like, it is often more mild and self-limited. Noninflammatory diarrhea occurs.

918   C (S&F, ch98)
The taeniae coli are the outer longitudinal smooth muscle layers that form three cord-like structures that run along the length of the colon. These are evenly spaced around the circumference of the colon. Between the taeniae the muscle layers are much thinner, and this allows the bulge. Irregularly spaced circumferential constrictions pinch the colon into pockets called haustra. The plicae circulares are the folds of the small intestine. The rugae are the redundant folds found in the stomach.

919   C (S&F, ch111)
NOD2 variants are associated with stricturing disease and ileal location. Anti–*Saccharomyces*

cerevisiae antibody positivity is also associated with ileal disease, whereas Cbir1 is seen more often in patients with internal penetrating and stricturing disease; anti–*E. coli* outer membrane porin (anti-OmpC) is likewise more common in patients with internal perforations. Observed more commonly in patients with UC, pANCA positivity in Crohn's disease patients predicts a UC-like inflammatory presentation.

920   A (S&F, ch111)
Smoking clearly increases the risk of the development of Crohn's disease, whereas it seems to be protective in UC. Further, continued smoking after a diagnosis of Crohn's disease portends a more difficult course, including a greater risk of surgery. The exact mechanism by which smoking plays a role in IBD is unclear, but effects on intestinal permeability, cytokine production, microvascular clotting, and carbon monoxide stimulation of immunosuppression are theorized. Breast-feeding seems to be protective against Crohn's disease, possibly by helping to develop the infant gut immune system and populate the gut flora. Crohn's disease seems to be less likely to develop in those who have outdoor occupations, but this association may be more tied to socioeconomic status and the hygiene theory, which proposes that less environmental antigenic exposure during childhood increases the risk of certain autoimmune diseases. Although patients often report increased symptoms during times of stress, and studies are starting to support this concept, Crohn's disease is not caused by stress or anxiety.

921   A (S&F, ch104)
Scalloping or absence of duodenal folds has been noted in some patients with celiac disease. Scalloping, however, is not specific for celiac disease, and other conditions that can cause duodenal scalloping include eosinophilic enteritis, giardiasis, amyloidosis, tropical sprue, and HIV enteropathy. In addition to scalloping or atrophy of the mucosal folds, the duodenal mucosa in untreated celiac disease may be marked by multiple fissures. A mosaic appearance also has been described in which the fissures circumscribe areas of mucosal nodularity in a manner similar to the grouting around mosaic tile. These mucosal features (atrophy and scalloping of the folds, fissures, nodularity, or a mosaic appearance) should alert the endoscopist to the need for a small intestine biopsy to evaluate for possible celiac disease. The mucosa of celiac disease, however, often appears normal at endoscopy, and the absence of the macroscopic features described previously does not eliminate the need for biopsy and histologic examination if celiac disease is suspected based on clinical grounds or positive serology.

922   B (S&F, ch98)
The IAS is a thickened band of smooth muscle with a relatively high resting tone that is in continuity with the circular smooth muscle of the rectum. The IAS is innervated extrinsically via the pelvic plexus and by lumbar sympathetic and sacral parasympathetic nerves, and it receives inhibitory innervation from enteric inhibitory

neurons with cell bodies in the enteric ganglia. Unlike the IAS, the EAS is influenced by voluntary efforts to maintain continence. The EAS and other pelvic floor muscles are innervated by the pudendal nerve (S3 and S4) and by motor neurons with cell bodies in the spinal cord.

923 **E** (S&F, ch112)
This patient has mild left-sided UC based on his clinical presentation and laboratory, endoscopic, and histologic findings. His ex-smoking status further supports this diagnosis. Mesalamine, a 5-ASA, is an effective agent for inducing and maintaining remission in this setting and, in mild cases, may be the only medication necessary. Its safety profile is excellent. Azathioprine, an immunomodulator, may require two to three months to have a therapeutic effect and is generally reserved for patients who require corticosteroids for a short period and then transition to this medication. Antibiotics, including both metronidazole and ciprofloxacin, have not been shown to be effective in UC. The role of infliximab, a chimeric antibody against TNF-α, in UC is evolving; in patients with severe disease or who do not respond to corticosteroid therapy for remission, infliximab may be effective, but it would

not be an appropriate first-line medication in mild UC.

924 **C** (S&F, ch120)
CIP is reported in association with small cell carcinoma of the lung, carcinoid tumors, and epidermoid carcinoma of the lip. This phenomenon represents a paraneoplastic syndrome caused by visceral neuropathy.

925 **D** (S&F, ch101)
A trial of cholestyramine or another bile acid–binding resin can be used to not only treat but to diagnose bile acid malabsorption as a cause of diarrhea. Failure of diarrhea to remit three days after the beginning of cholestyramine therapy makes bile acid malabsorption an unlikely cause of the diarrhea, but some patients will require very high doses.

926 **A** (S&F, ch123)
APC is a tumor suppressor gene found in 60% to 80% of sporadic adenomas and colorectal cancers. Mutations of the *Ras* gene are found in as many as 65% of sporadic colorectal cancers. However, deletions, and not activation, of the tumor suppressor gene *p53* mediate conversion of adenoma to carcinoma (see figure here and table at end of chapter).

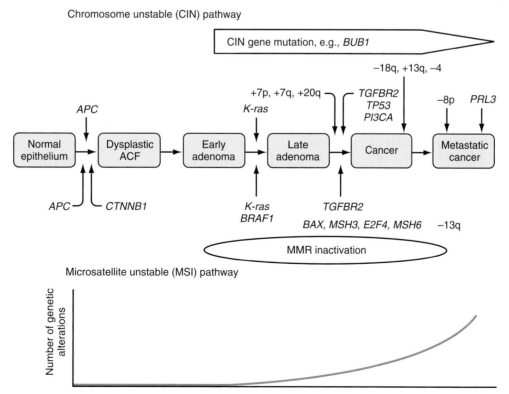

Figure for answer **926**

927 D (S&F, ch115)
In the Mayo Clinic series of 59 cases of small intestine ulcers, Boydstun and associates found that the ileum was the most common location of nonspecific ulceration (78%), whereas perforation (13 cases) occurred most commonly in the jejunum.

928 B (S&F, ch99)
Shigella causes dysentery through the release of Shiga cytotoxins. These toxins enter the epithelial cells, inhibit protein synthesis, impair absorption, and damage the mucosa. The other bacteria listed cause secretory diarrhea by elaborating enterotoxins that turn on the secretory machinery of the epithelial cell.

929 D (S&F, ch96)
The endoderm will eventually form the intestinal tube. During the fourth week of development, the mesoderm layers split during folding. The portion that adheres to the endoderm becomes the visceral peritoneum and the portion adherent to the ectoderm becomes the parietal peritoneum. The space between becomes the peritoneal cavity. The vitelline duct is the embryonic connection between the intestinal tube and the yolk sac.

930 B (S&F, ch109)
These two organisms share some characteristics. They both stain positive with acid-fast stains. Trimethoprim/sulfamethoxazole readily treats *Isospora* and *Cyclospora* infection in the immunocompetent patient. A self-limited illness usually occurs in the immunocompetent patient, but a protracted illness may ensue if the patient is immunocompromised. *Isospora* may cause a peripheral eosinophilia with Charcot-Leyden crystals in the stool, which does not occur with other protozoa such as *Cyclospora*.

931 A (S&F, ch102)
SIBO classically causes a megaloblastic anemia due to vitamin B_{12} deficiency that is not reversible by use of intrinsic factor. Vitamin B_{12} deficiency is caused by bacterial consumption of the vitamin within the intestinal lumen before it can be absorbed across the mucosa. Anaerobic organisms mainly are responsible for the vitamin B_{12} deficiency. Unlike aerobic bacteria, anaerobes can use vitamin B_{12} in both its free form and as a complex with intrinsic factor. Anaerobic bacteria deprive the host of ingested vitamin B_{12} and exacerbate its deficiency by using ingested vitamin B_{12} to produce inactive cobamides that then compete with dietary vitamin B_{12} for ileal binding sites, thereby decreasing absorption of the vitamin.

932 B (S&F, ch125)
Anal cancers account for 1.5% of gastrointestinal cancers in the United States, with 3500 new cases each year. Incidence has increased 2% to 3% every year in the United States since the early 1980s. Almost 80% are squamous cell cancers, 16% are adenocarcinomas, and 4% are other types. Tumors arising in the distal anal canal usually are keratinizing squamous cell carcinoma. Anal cancer has been associated with human papillomavirus and HIV infections, history of anal intercourse, cervical cancer, and the use of immunosuppressive medication after solid organ transplantation.

933 D (S&F, ch115)
Symptoms associated with NSAID-induced ulceration of the small bowel include hypoalbuminemia, anemia, and diaphragm-like strictures. In an autopsy study performed by Allison and associates, 8.4% of NSAID users had ulcerations of their small intestine compared with only 0.6% of NSAID nonusers. Three of these patients died of a small bowel perforation.

934 D (S&F, ch110)
A. lumbricoides has a worldwide distribution but is most prevalent in underdeveloped countries and areas of poor sanitation. Most patients infected are asymptomatic unless the worm burden is heavy. These worms can cause intestinal obstruction. Migration into the biliary or pancreatic ducts may cause jaundice, cholangitis, biliary colic, acalculous cholecystitis, or pancreatitis. A self-limited pneumonia can occur as the larvae migrate into the alveoli.

935 A (S&F, ch111)
Although there has been vigorous research to identify a specific pathogen responsible for causing an appropriate and sustained inflammatory response seen in Crohn's disease, to date no such pathogen has been identified. *M. paratuberculosis*, which is the bacteria responsible for causing Johne's disease, a similar granulomatous bowel disease found in ruminants, has received the most attention over the years. Attempts to isolate this organism from specimens from patients with Crohn's disease as well as empiric antibiotic treatment have yielded equivocal results. Mild physiologic inflammatory changes are seen in healthy intestinal mucosa exposed to normal gut flora, which may indicate a readiness to respond more aggressively to true pathogens. Many different animal models have demonstrated that in a genetically susceptible host, when normal commensal bacteria (and not necessarily a specific pathogen) are introduced into the gut, an inappropriate level of inflammation will be demonstrated, similar to that seen in IBD.

936 D (S&F, ch110)
All the nematodes listed can be treated with albendazole.

937 E (S&F, ch111)
This patient has signs and symptoms consistent with ileal and right-sided colonic Crohn's disease. Although stool studies should be done as part of his evaluation, given the duration of symptoms, he is unlikely to have an infection. IBD serologies may be supportive of a diagnosis of IBD, but are not diagnostic. Further, pANCA is more likely to be positive in patients with UC, although in patients with Crohn's disease, pANCA is associated with a UC-like phenotype. A barium enema will show inflammatory changes of the colon suggestive of Crohn's disease, but will not necessarily evaluate the terminal ileum, and biopsy specimens cannot be taken. Capsule enteroscopy is highly sensitive

in identifying the lesions of Crohn's disease, but is not specific and therefore should not generally be used as a first-line diagnostic study. Further, biopsy specimens cannot be taken, and the risk of capsule retention in the setting of a stricture can be as high as 25%. Colonoscopy with ileal intubation will not only allow macroscopic visualization of inflammatory changes in the colon and terminal ileum, but biopsies performed in both inflamed and noninflamed tissue will permit histologic mapping of Crohn's disease.

938   C (S&F, ch109)
Infants are infected more often than adults worldwide. In the United States, children in day care and sexually active homosexual men are at greatest risk. Other risk factors include drinking untreated surface water, a shallow well as a water source, swimming in natural fresh water, and contact with a person infected with *Giardia*. A severe protracted illness can develop in patients with common variable immunodeficiency. Giardiasis is not more frequent or severe in AIDS patients except perhaps when AIDS is in an advanced stage (see table at end of chapter).

939   E (S&F, ch96)
Duodenal obstruction in the newborn can result from atresia, stenosis, or an intestinal web. In the duodenum, 80% of atresias are contiguous or distal to the ampulla of Vater and develop due to a failure of recanalization of the solid stage of duodenal development. The diagnosis is usually made on imaging, which reveals the classic "double-bubble" sign with a paucity of small intestine air. Hirschsprung's disease is due to a lack of neural involvement in the colon and usually presents with no passage of meconium. Gastroschisis is a congenital abdominal wall defect.

940   B (S&F, ch111)
MTX is a folate antagonist that may be used as an alternate immunomodulator to 6-MP or azathioprine. In a randomized, controlled trial that compared weekly MTX 25 mg given intramuscularly with placebo in steroid-dependent Crohn's patients with active disease, almost 40% of MTX-treated patients compared with 19% of placebo patients achieved remission off steroids over 16 weeks. Most patients responded by the eighth week of treatment. Although studies in rheumatoid arthritis have shown equal efficacy in patients treated with subcutaneous as compared with intramuscular MTX, oral administration is not as reliable secondary to variable intestinal absorption, especially in patients with small bowel inflammation. MTX is an abortifacient and also teratogenic; further, it is toxic to sperm. Therefore, it is not appropriate for women or men who wish to conceive. Men should wait at least three months after therapy ends before attempting to conceive; highly effective birth control must be used while the patient is taking this medication. Side effects associated with MTX include stomatitis, nausea, diarrhea, hair loss, mild leukopenia, abnormal liver enzymes, and, rarely, liver fibrosis. Obesity, alcohol, and diabetes may increase the risk of hepatotoxicity.

941   D (S&F, ch104)
Dermatitis herpetiformis is closely associated with celiac disease. In fact, most, if not all, patients with dermatitis herpetiformis have at least latent celiac disease, whereas less than 10% of patients with celiac disease have dermatitis herpetiformis.

942   A (S&F, ch112)
There is a clear north–south gradient in UC rates, with the highest incidence and prevalence rates in North America, England, northern Europe, and Australia and significantly lower rates in Southern Hemisphere countries including Asia, Africa, and Central America. Although there is considerable geographic variation in incidence trends, the overall incidence of UC has remained stable over the past 30 years. Jewish populations across multiple geographic regions have higher incidences of UC than non-Jewish populations, and therefore incidence rates are not equal among various ethnicities. Although early studies found that UC was very rare in blacks, these data were likely flawed, and incidence rates between blacks and whites in the United States have been approximately equal since the late 1970s.

943   A (S&F, ch118)
Abdominal pain or discomfort that is continuous or unrelated to defecation or induced by menstruation, urination, or physical activity is unlikely to be caused by IBS. Nausea, bloating, abdominal distention, and constipation are all symptoms associated with IBS.

944   D (S&F, ch107)
Ampicillin or erythromycin is the appropriate drug in pregnancy. The others should be avoided. Diarrheal illnesses can cause dehydration and alter placental blood flow. Premature labor or spontaneous abortion can occur.

945   A (S&F, ch98)
Enteric excitatory motor neurons synthesize and secrete acetylcholine. Enteric inhibitory motor neurons synthesize and secrete various neurotransmitters including nitric oxide, adenosine triphosphate, and various peptides (e.g., vasoactive intestinal peptide). Epinephrine is not an enteric neurotransmitter.

946   C (S&F, ch100)
The intraluminal digestion of fat is a complex process and is driven by the insolubility of fat in water, with all the digestive mechanisms having evolved to overcome this fact. Emulsification is critical in overcoming the insolubility issue and is what allows lipolytic enzymes to gain access to the dietary lipids. Several factors, including gastric milling, ingested phospholipids, and bile salts, aid in the emulsification process. The majority of lipid absorption occurs in the upper two thirds of the jejunum. Gastric lipase accounts for only 20% to 30% of intraluminal lipolysis and has no activity in the digestion of phospholipids. Pancreatic lipase is activated at a neutral pH and thus is dependent on bicarbonate secreted from the pancreas and biliary tree.

947 **B** (S&F, ch111)

This young woman has a fairly classic presentation of ileal Crohn's disease, with pain in the right lower quadrant and diarrhea as well as systemic symptoms of fever and weight loss. Further, she has a pauciarticular arthropathy, an EIM of inflammatory bowel disease that tends to parallel the intestinal symptoms. IBS is incorrect because she has "alarm" symptoms including fever and weight loss. Acute appendicitis is also incorrect; although this can manifest with right lower quadrant pain and fever, the time course is too long and neither weight loss nor arthropathies would be expected. UC is also incorrect because this presents with bloody diarrhea, usually without systemic symptoms; if pain is present, it is generally not localized to the right lower quadrant, but tends to be more cramping lower abdominal pain. Meckel's diverticulum is incorrect because this generally presents with painless gastrointestinal bleeding, usually in infants or younger children.

948 **B** (S&F, ch114)

Reperfusion injury has been attributed to many factors, including formation of reactive oxygen radicals. Superoxide, hydrogen peroxide, and hydroxyl radicals are formed. The rate-limiting enzyme is xanthine oxidase, not TPMT. Leukotriene B_4 and platelet-aggregating factor are produced, not leukotriene B_1. Most injury from brief ischemia appears during reperfusion. After prolonged ischemia, hypoxia becomes more detrimental than reperfusion.

949 **C** (S&F, ch123)

The United States Preventive Services Task Force, the Agency for Health Care Policy Research, and the American Cancer Society are some of the groups that have advocated and published their screening guidelines. Virtual colonoscopy and barium enema are options but are suggested at five-year intervals. Although biannual FOBT has been shown to decrease mortality, an annual FOBT is more effective and is recommended. Sigmoidoscopy every five years is also an option (see table at end of chapter).

950 **B** (S&F, ch119)

Hernias are the second most common cause of SBO, accounting for 10% of cases. External hernias such as inguinal, umbilical, and femoral are more common than internal hernias. Inguinal hernias are more prevalent in the elderly. Internal hernias can be both congenital and acquired. SBO from hernias has a particularly high risk of strangulation, failure to resolve, and recurrence when not corrected surgically.

951 **B** (S&F, ch99)

E. coli heat-stable enterotoxin causes diarrhea by increasing intracellular levels of cGMP. *V. cholerae* releases cholera toxin that binds the GM_1-ganglioside receptor, leading to an increase in cytosolic cAMP, which ultimately results in the inhibition of Na/Cl coupled transport and increased chloride secretion. Rotavirus releases NSP4, which leads to an increase in intracellular calcium levels, thereby affecting calcium-sensitive ion channels.

S. typhimurium infection causes increased membrane permeability to calcium influx. The resulting increase in intracellular calcium might ultimately activate secretion of the cytokines nuclear factor κB and IL-8. *C. difficile* toxins A and B modify the Rho family of GTPases that are critical for maintaining cytoskeletal architecture.

952 **E** (S&F, ch102)

Although much remains to be learned about the metabolites of indigenous bacteria, these bacteria apparently benefit the host in several ways. In addition to producing regulatory signals for mucosal homeostasis, these flora have important metabolic functions not possessed by the host. These include biotransformation of bile acids, degradation of oxalate, breakdown of otherwise indigestible dietary components such as plant polysaccharides, and production of SCFAs, a major energy source for colonic epithelia, from fermentable carbohydrates. Other activities include synthesis of biotin, folate, and vitamin K. Clinicians also have exploited enteric bacterial enzymes such as azoreductase to convert prodrugs such as sulfasalazine to active drug metabolites (e.g., 5-ASA). Other examples of drug bioavailability due to the actions of bacterial flora include the metabolism of L-dopa to dopamine and degradation of digoxin.

953 **D** (S&F, ch117)

Most diverticular abscesses grow mixed aerobic and anaerobic infections. The most common single organism is *E. coli*, one of the *Streptococcus* spp., or *B. fragilis*. Small pericolic abscesses can often be treated conservatively with broad-spectrum antibiotics and bowel rest. Percutaneous drainage of abdominal abscesses has assumed a prominent complementary role with surgery; the immediate advantage is the rapid control of sepsis and patient stabilization without the need for general anesthesia and, often, elimination of the need for multiple-stage procedures with colostomy. Urgent surgical procedures are required in 20% to 25% of patients in whom the abscess is multiloculated, anatomically inaccessible, or unresolved with percutaneous drainage.

954 **B** (S&F, ch111)

This patient has diarrhea secondary to bacterial overgrowth from his nonobstructive stricture, and therefore a trial of a nonabsorbed antibiotic such as rifaximin is indicated. He has no signs or symptoms that indicate inflammatory changes, nor is there evidence of inflammation on his laboratory test results or imaging. Therefore, treating him with medications to reduce inflammatory changes such as glucocorticosteroids, 6-MP, and infliximab will not be helpful. Further, surgical consultation would not be indicated because he is not clinically or radiographically obstructed.

955 **A** (S&F, ch112)

TPMT is an enzyme that converts 6-MP to its inactive metabolites, 6-methyl mercaptopurine and 6-MP ribonucleotide. The FDA recommends checking either the genotype or activity level (phenotype) of this enzyme before initiating therapy with 6-MP or azathioprine. Eighty-nine percent of the population has homozygous wildtype TPMT, whereas 11% and 0.3% of the population have heterozygous (intermediate activity) and homozygous (no activity) mutations, respectively. Homozygous wildtype patients can be started on a full weight-based dose of 6-MP or azathioprine, although it is recommended that heterozygous or intermediate metabolizers should be started at half the weight-based dose. Only those who are homozygous for the mutation should avoid the medication entirely. In patients with TPMT mutations (and thus lower/intermediate enzyme activity), there is preferential shunting to the active metabolite 6-thioguanine nucleotide, which can be associated with leukopenia when levels are too high. 6-Methyl mercaptopurine is associated with hepatotoxicity, which thus should be seen less in these patients.

956 **B** (S&F, ch123)
Colorectal cancer will develop in 6% of the U.S. population. The death rate in the United States is second only to that of lung cancer. The incidence of colorectal cancer is equal in men and women in the United States. However, worldwide, there is a slight male predominance. The highest incidence is in North America, Australia, and New Zealand. The incidence is intermediate in Europe and low in Asia, South America, and sub-Saharan Africa (see two figures).

957 **D** (S&F, ch111)
Although Crohn's disease does not follow a mendelian genetic model, familial susceptibility lends clear support for a genetic predisposition. First-degree family members are 14 to 15 times more likely to be diagnosed with Crohn's disease than the general population. In families with multiple members who have inflammatory bowel disease, phenotypic concordance is generally observed; that is to say, all family members usually have either Crohn's disease or UC, although mixed kindreds can occur. In monozygotic twins, a concordance of up to 67% will be seen, which means that the environment plays a role in the development of Crohn's disease as well. Approximately one fifth of patients with Crohn's disease will report a family history of the disease.

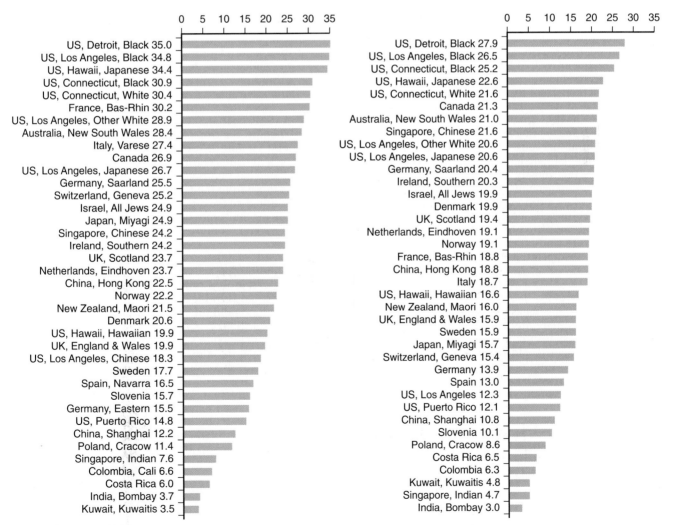

Figure 1 for answer **956**

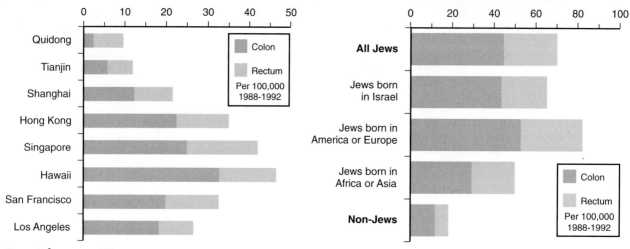

Figure 2 for answer **956**

---

958 **A** (S&F, ch106)
Based on these clinical observations, the current recommendation for treatment of Whipple's disease is to begin with an induction phase using either penicillin G plus streptomycin or a third-generation cephalosporin, such as ceftriaxone, followed by treatment with at least one drug that efficiently crosses the blood-brain barrier (e.g., trimethoprim/sulfamethoxazole) for at least one year.

959 **C** (S&F, ch120)
Of the three main classes of opiate receptors in the central nervous system and gastrointestinal tract (mu, kappa, lambda) the mu receptors are the ones that mostly modulate analgesia. Endogenous and exogenous opioids activate intestinal mu receptors suppressing release of acetylcholine from cholinergic neurons resulting in delayed intestinal motility. Sympathetic neural activity, nitric oxide, and inflammatory cytokines all play a role in postoperative ileus separate from opiate effects.

960 **A** (S&F, ch107)
This patient has ingested *Clostridium botulinum*. It can contaminate improperly canned foods. The initial illness results in gastrointestinal symptoms but then progresses to autonomic and cranial nerve symptoms. Administering botulinum antitoxin quickly is critical because once the toxin is bound to the presynaptic nerve endings, it cannot be displaced.

961 **C** (S&F, ch120)
Chewing gum as been shown to reduce the duration of postoperative ileus. All other choices either have no benefit or prolong postoperative ileus.

962 **A** (S&F, ch120)
The mechanisms proposed for acute pseudo-obstruction include (1) reflex motor inhibition through splanchnic afferents in response to noxious stimuli, (2) excess sympathetic (inhibitory) motor input to the gut, (3) excess parasympathetic (excitatory) motor input to the gut, (4) decreased parasympathetic (excitatory) motor input to the gut, (5) excess stimulation of peripheral mu-opioid receptors by endogenous or exogenous opioids, and (6) inhibition of nitric oxide release from inhibitory motoneurons.

963 **A** (S&F, ch105)
Therapy for tropical sprue would include parenteral vitamin B$_{12}$, oral folic acid, and iron as well as a broad-spectrum antibiotic, although this is somewhat controversial. Overland travelers, such as those from the United Kingdom, and patients in Puerto Rico are reported to improve on tetracycline, 250 mg four times daily, usually given over a period of several months.

964 **C** (S&F, ch98)
Lupiprostone activates a type 2 chloride channel. Activation of a type 2 chloride channel increases intestinal chloride secretion, resulting in increased intraluminal fluid accumulation, thereby accelerating intestinal transit, softening stool, and increasing spontaneous stool frequency in patients with constipation. Alosetron is an antagonist of 5-HT$_3$ and exerts a constipating effect by slowing colonic transit. Tegaserod is a drug that is a 5-HT$_4$ agonist and could treat chronic constipation, although this drug has been removed from the market secondary to cardiovascular side effects. Bisacodyl works by stimulating high-amplitude colonic propagating pressure wave sequences.

965 **D** (S&F, ch105)
This clinical presentation, along with recent travel to Southeast Asia, are consistent with tropical sprue. This similar presentation accompanied with recent travel to Africa would be consistent

with tropical enteropathy. The small bowel series shows an increase in the caliber of the small intestine and thickening of the folds. These changes are present throughout the small intestine, and the examination usually is notable for slow transit of the barium column through the gut.

966 **E** (S&F, ch114)
The celiac axis and its branches supply the stomach, duodenum, pancreas, and liver. None of the other arteries directly supply the stomach.

967 **B** (S&F, ch112)
pANCA is an IgG_1 autoantibody commonly seen in patients with UC. The height of the titer does not correlate to disease activity, but positivity for pANCA is associated with the development of pouchitis after colectomy. Crohn's disease patients with disease of the colon are more likely to have pANCA seroreactivity than those without colonic disease, which may characterize a UC-like Crohn's disease. In patients with confirmed UC, 60% to 85% will test positive for pANCA. The significance of pANCA in UC is unknown, but it is thought more likely to be a marker of susceptibility than having a direct pathogenic role.

968 **B** (S&F, ch107)
Both are RNA viruses, but rotavirus is double stranded and norovirus is single stranded. The illnesses are often indistinguishable because both cause vomiting, diarrhea, and abdominal cramps/pain. The diarrheal illness usually lasts no longer than 24 to 48 hours in norovirus but lasts five to seven days in rotavirus cases. Additionally, the illness and the dehydration can be more pronounced with rotavirus. The fecal-oral route is the main mode of transmission for both viruses. However, raw shellfish can be a major source of infection in norovirus. A rotavirus vaccine is available and recommended for infants (see figure here and table at end of chapter).

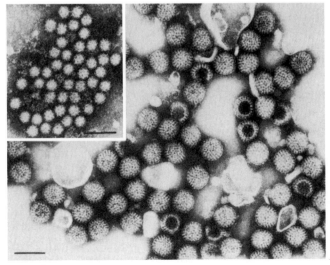

Figure for answer **968**

969 **B** (S&F, ch119)
Failure of normal intestinal motility causes bacterial overgrowth in the small intestine. Studies have shown that bacteria translocate to mesenteric lymph nodes and systemic organs, supporting the hypothesis that translocating bacteria contribute to the septic consequences of SBO. Hypovolemia primarily results from the loss of fluid into the intestinal lumen, bowel wall, and peritoneal cavity. The generation and activation of proinflammatory mediators have been linked to remote organ failure and mortality caused by intestinal ischemia during SBO.

970 **D** (S&F, ch98)
Myenteric potential oscillations are small-amplitude, rapid (12-20 per minute) oscillations that originate from the myenteric plexus and spread via gap junctions into both the longitudinal and circular muscular layers. In contrast, slow waves occur with a frequency of two to four per minute. When the colon is excited by neurotransmitters released from the excitatory enteric motor neurons, each myenteric potential oscillation or slow wave will reach the threshold potential for generating an action potential, resulting in powerful contractions lasting seconds. MMCs occur in the stomach and small intestine; in the fasting state, they occur every 60 to 90 minutes and sweep the luminal contents along the upper digestive tract. Giant motor complexes are powerful muscular contractile waves that propel luminal contents from the ileum into the colon.

971 **D** (S&F, ch96)
The vermiform appendix arises from the base of the cecum. It varies in length, averaging approximately 6 cm, and is anchored by the mesoappendix. It is most commonly retrocecal. It is rarely retrocolic, anterior, medial, or lateral to the cecum.

972 **E** (S&F, ch108)
Pseudomembranous colitis occurs in only 3% to 5% of patients with *C. difficile* infection but is associated with a mortality rate of as high as 65%. Diarrhea may be minimal or absent because of ileus and may be present with abdominal pain or peritoneal signs. Vancomycin is often used as the first-line agent in critically ill patients. In the presence of ileus, vancomycin may be administered via a nasogastric tube with intermittent clamping of the tube.

973 **B** (S&F, ch106)
Several studies indicate a statistically significant increase in recent decades in the age of patients at diagnosis. At present, patients are diagnosed at a mean age of 56 years, and approximately 80% are male.

974 **E** (S&F, ch100)
In addition to nutrient protein hydrolysis, pancreatic proteases have other functions. Trypsin activates the other proteases from zymogens. Pancreatic proteases split vitamin B_{12} from the R protein to which it is linked so that it can then bind to intrinsic factor. They increase the turnover of brush border membrane hydrolytic enzymes and initiate

the final steps in processing the sucrase–isomaltase complex.

975   **B** (S&F, ch105)
Approximately 90% of patients with tropical sprue in India and most patients in Asia and the Caribbean have impaired fat absorption. Absorption of micronutrients, particularly folic acid, is impaired, and as the enteropathy progresses to involve the ileum, vitamin B_{12} malabsorption often follows.

976   **C** (S&F, ch112)
MTX, a folic acid antagonist that has both antimetabolite and anti-inflammatory properties, has shown efficacy in the induction and maintenance of remission in Crohn's disease, but the same results have not been demonstrated in patients with UC. That being said, although the findings of the only randomized, controlled trial to date to evaluate MTX for the treatment of active UC were negative, only 12.5 mg per week given orally was used, in contrast to the 25 mg per week administered intramuscularly that showed efficacy in Crohn's disease. Although MTX is used to treat Crohn's disease, it is not approved by the FDA for this indication. Natalizumab is a new biological agent that is an IgG_4 monoclonal antibody to α_4-integrin, a lymphocyte adhesion molecule that blocks lymphocyte trafficking from the vascular space to the periphery. It is approved for the treatment of Crohn's disease and multiple sclerosis and is being studied in UC. Infliximab is a monoclonal chimeric (75% human and 25% mouse) anti–TNF-α monoclonal antibody that is approved for both the induction and maintenance of remission in Crohn's disease and UC. The ACT 1 and 2 studies established its efficacy in UC, with approximately one third of patients in remission at 30 weeks after treatment with infliximab 5 or 10 mg/kg. Adalimumab is a fully human anti–TNF-α antibody that has been approved for the treatment of Crohn's disease and is being studied at present for the treatment of UC.

977   **D** (S&F, ch99)
The major anion in the colon is SCFA. The magnitude of daily colonic load and absorption of SCFA is on par with that of colonic sodium. Bicarbonate and chloride are the predominant anions in the small intestine.

978   **C** (S&F, ch107)
Yersinia is a gram-negative rod that can lead to a mild gastroenteritis or an invasive ileitis or colitis. Enterocolitis is the most likely presentation. However, the illness can mimic appendicitis or Crohn's disease. A reactive arthritis associated with HLA-B27 and a rash can occur two to three weeks after the acute illness.

979   **E** (S&F, ch114)
Vascular insults of the short segments of the small bowel produce a broad spectrum of clinical features without the typical life-threatening complications of more extensive ischemia. With FSI, there is usually adequate collateral circulation to prevent transmural infarction. The most common lesion is partial bowel wall necrosis with translocation of

intestinal bacteria. FSI may present as acute enteritis, chronic enteritis, or a stricture. In the acute pattern, abdominal pain often seems like acute appendicitis and the physical examination findings are those of an acute abdomen. An inflammatory mass may be palpated. Chronic forms may resemble Crohn's disease or crampy abdominal pain, diarrhea, fever, and weight loss. FSI must be considered in patients with chronic SBO with intermittent abdominal pain, distention, and vomiting.

980   **B** (S&F, ch112)
The majority of the indices that have been developed to measure disease activity in UC are nonspecific and have not been prospectively validated. Indices may be purely clinical, endoscopic, or histologic, and some combine clinical and endoscopic assessment. Additionally, scores on these indices are often based on various symptoms and signs for which there is no unifed definition. The Truelove and Witts classification of UC is based on the frequency of bowel movements, the amount of blood, the presence of fever and tachycardia, anemia, and the erythrocyte sedimentation rate, all of which are clinical measurements; patients are classified as having mild, moderate, and severe disease. Although it is the oldest index, it is still one of the most commonly used because of its simplicity. The Ulcerative Colitis Disease Activity Index or Sutherland Index gives a numerical score that takes into account not only the clinical measures of stool frequency, rectal bleeding, and physician's global assessment, but also incorporates sigmoidoscopic appearance; it does not, however, include a histologic subscore. Patients are considered to have fulminant colitis when they have a toxic appearance, a fever higher than 101°F, tachycardia, abdominal distention, signs of peritonitis, and leukocytosis. Although these patients may also have toxic megacolon (radiologic measurement of the transverse colon >6 cm), this is not implicit in the definition of fulminant colitis.

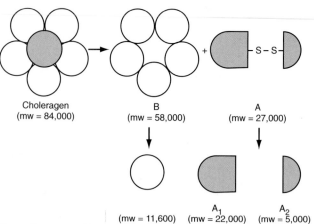

Figure for answer **981**

981 A (S&F, ch107)

V. cholerae is a gram-negative rod that produces enterotoxin. The toxin attaches to enterocytes, mostly in the upper small intestine, and activates cAMP. This in turn increases fluid secretion from the small intestine, which overwhelms the absorptive capacity of the colon. Isotonic fluid and significant potassium and bicarbonate are lost, leading to a hypokalemic acidosis. The organism does not invade the mucosa and does not affect the colon (see figure here and tables at end of chapter).

982 B (S&F, ch111)

One or more EIMs will develop in an estimated 6% to 25% of Crohn's disease patients, which may be categorized as those associated with small bowel disease versus colonic involvement as well as by those that occur independently of disease activity versus those that parallel disease activity. Neither erythema nodosum nor pyoderma gangrenosum is exclusive to inflammatory bowel disease. Patients with Crohn's disease have a higher risk of cholelithiasis, with the major risk factor being the number of ileal resections. They also have a higher risk of nephrolithiasis. Calcium oxalate kidney stones are seen in patients with Crohn's disease who have had ileal resections or who have extensive ileal inflammation and resultant fat malabsorption as free fatty acids bind to calcium, which then decreases the calcium available to bind and clear oxalate. Oxalate is then absorbed, and hyperoxaluria and calcium oxalate stones are formed. Uric acid stones may occur with significant volume depletion and hypermetabolic state.

983 C (S&F, ch112)

In patients with UC taking immunosuppressants and/or glucocorticosteroids, especially those with long-standing disease, the diagnosis of cytomegalovirus must be included in the differential diagnosis. On endoscopy, discrete deep ulcers may be seen, although inflammatory changes resembling UC can also be found. Biopsies of the ulcer bed and surrounding mucosa must be performed in the appropriate setting to look for giant cells with inclusion bodies. If there is no evidence of cytomegalovirus, then initiation of infliximab or cyclosporine might be appropriate. Increasing or optimizing the dose of 6-MP may be an option, but can take two to three months to have a clinical effect. Colectomy might be necessitated if the patient is either too sick to withstand further medical therapy or it is ineffective.

984 B (S&F, ch100)

Bariatric surgeries are typically classified as restrictive, malabsorptive, or both. RYGB results in weight loss by both restrictive and malabsorptive means. Levels of circulating ghrelin have been seen to be decreased in patients after RYGB and probably result from exclusion of the ghrelin-producing cells in the gastric fundus. Dumping syndrome can occur in any surgical procedure that bypasses normal pyloric function and results from the rapid passage of undigested food and nutrients to the ileum. The metabolic and nutritional deficiencies after RYGB are often less severe than in other previously common bypass procedures; this benefit is one of the appealing aspects of this weight loss surgery.

985 C (S&F, ch102)

The classic association of SIBO is with the blind loop resulting from abdominal surgery, such as Billroth II partial gastrectomy; other anatomic abnormalities that may cause SIBO include intestinal strictures and small bowel diverticulosis. Disorders affecting peristalsis in the small intestine, such as diabetes mellitus and scleroderma, are the next most common causes of SIBO after anatomic abnormalities. The ileocecal valve prevents reflux of colonic bacteria into the small intestine, and resection of the valve or development of fistulas between the colon and upper gastrointestinal tract may lead to reflux of colonic contents into the small intestine with ensuing bacterial overgrowth.

986 B (S&F, ch101)

The most common cause of carbohydrate malabsorption is late-onset lactose malabsorption due to decreased levels of the intestinal brush border enzyme lactase (adult-type hypolactasia, acquired primary lactase deficiency). Depending on ethnic background, lactase is present in less than 5% to more than 90% of the adult population. Lactase activity persists in most adults of Western European heritage. Some of the ethnic groups among which lactase deficiency predominates (60% to 100%) include Native Americans, African Americans, East Asians, and people of Near East and Mediterranean descent.

987 C (S&F, ch111)

Crohn's disease is most often diagnosed in patients between the ages of 15 and 30, but the median age at onset has been increasing overall, largely driven by a greater proportion of patients being diagnosed at an older age (older than 60). This trend has been seen in population studies in Minnesota, Sweden, and Denmark. For example, in Sweden, the median age of diagnosis increased from 25 to 32 from the early 1960s to the mid to late 1980s. In those studies that show such a second peak of incidence later in life, it has been theorized that more frequent contact of the older population with medical professionals may account for this finding. Although clinical presentation may vary between older and younger patients, pathologic findings overall are the same except for possibly more colonic and distal disease in older patients compared with more ileocolonic disease in younger patients.

988 B (S&F, ch102)

Although many articles have suggested so, the exact role of SIBO in patients with IBS has not been proven. Not all patients meeting with Rome criteria have SIBO. Abdominal bloating is the symptom for which patients achieved the most benefit after therapy. Rifaximin has been used in many recent SIBO trials because it is mostly nonabsorbable and therefore has a low side effect profile. The course is usually six to nine tablets for 14 days.

989 A (S&F, ch114)

The sign is only typical for fibromuscular dysplasia, especially in the renal arteries. Henoch-Schönlein purpura usually only affects children. Cogan's syndrome is a vasculitis of the conjunctiva cornea and cochlea and rarely involves the gastrointestinal tract. Buerger's disease, also called thromboangiitis obliterans, involves small to medium-sized peripheral veins and arteries, especially those of the lower extremities. Kawasaki's disease, also called infantile febrile mucocutaneous lymph node syndrome, manifests as fever and rash on the palms and soles along with a "strawberry tongue."

990 **A** (S&F, ch106)
These are all clinical manifestations of Whipple's disease. Arthralgias can precede intestinal symptoms by several years. Polyarthralgias are a common symptom. Skin hyperpigmentation can be found in 17% to 66% of patients. Dominant signs of Whipple's disease include diarrhea, weight loss, and abdominal pain.

991 **C** (S&F, ch112)
Many, but not all, patients who require colectomy for UC should be considered for IPAA. The elderly, those with multiple comorbidities or previous surgeries, and the morbidly obese may not be candidates for this type of surgery because it requires two to three surgeries and carries a higher risk of complications. Body habitus may preclude technical feasibility. The average number of stools per day is four to nine, with one to two at night. Nocturnal seepage occurs in 20% of patients in the first year but is rare thereafter. A large case series from the Mayo Clinic showed that although the pouch success rate is more than 90% over 20 years, the complication rate over time is high: pouchitis (48% at 10 years, 70% at 20 years), SBO (42% by 20 years), anastomotic stricture (39% by 20 years), abscess (16% by 20 years), and fistula (14% by 20 years).

992 **B** (S&F, ch111)
Natalizumab is the newest biological agent to be approved for the induction and maintenance of remission in patients with moderately to severely active Crohn's disease who have been intolerant of or failed other medications, including anti-TNF antibodies (i.e., infliximab, adalimumab, and certolizumab). Patients must have evidence of active inflammation as well. Therefore, none of the following patients would be appropriate for this therapy: a newly diagnosed patient who has not been on other medications, one with fibrotic (and not inflammatory) disease, and one who has never tried an anti-TNF agent. Natalizumab is an IgG_4 monoclonal antibody to α_4-integrin, a lymphocyte adhesion molecule that blocks lymphocyte trafficking from the vascular space to peripheral tissues including the gut. It is also approved for the treatment of multiple sclerosis. The most concerning adverse event associated with this medication is progressive multifocal leukoencephalopathy, a degenerative and usually fatal JC virus neurologic infection. Doctors and patients must participate in a mandatory patient registry and risk management program. As of the date of writing, there have been approximately 10 postmarketing cases of progressive multifocal leukoencephalopathy of approximately 52,000 patients treated.

993 **A** (S&F, ch114)
Patients older than 50 years old who have long-standing congestive heart failure, cardiac arrhythmias such as atrial fibrillation, recent myocardial infarction, or hypotension are at particular risk of AMI. The history of postprandial pain in the months before the acute episode is only associated with superior mesenteric artery thrombosis. Mesenteric venous thrombosis is far more indolent. Nonocclusive mesenteric ischemia is responsible for 20% to 30% of AMI cases and is usually due to splanchnic vasoconstriction consequent to a preceding cardiovascular event. The event may have occurred hours to days earlier than the presentation. Superior mesenteric arterial emboli are responsible for 40% to 50% of AMI episodes. Emboli usually originate from the left atrial or ventricular mural thrombus. FSI are vascular insults to short segments of the small intestine. The causes include arterial emboli, strangulated hernias, immune complex disorders, vasculitis, blunt abdominal trauma, segmental venous thrombosis, radiation therapy, and oral contraceptives. Patients typically present with signs and symptoms of an acute abdomen (see tables at end of chapter).

994 **C** (S&F, ch113)
Although women report higher rates of sexual activity after versus before IPAA, this does not translate into increased rates of fertility. Female fertility rates in a large Swedish population study decreased after total proctocolectomy and IPAA. Further, 29% of pregnancies that occurred in this population used in vitro fertilization compared with the expected 1%. This increase in infertility likely relates to adhesions that form in the pelvis after IPAA. If a woman has not yet completed her childbearing, some doctors may recommend subtotal colectomy with removal of the rectum and creation of the pouch only after she has completed her childbearing; this would minimize adhesions in the pelvis before conception and in theory may better preserve fertility, although this technique has not been studied.

995 **A** (S&F, ch106)
The histopathologic features of intestinal Whipple's disease are quite distinctive. On gross inspection, the mucosa of the distal duodenum and jejunum is abnormal in most patients. Whitish to yellow plaque-like patches are observed in approximately three fourths of patients; alternatively, the mucosa may appear pale yellow.

996 **B** (S&F, ch100)
Phosphatidylcholine is hydrolyzed by pancreatic phospholipase A_2, which is secreted in a zymogen form and is activated in the small intestine. It requires calcium for activation and bile salts for its activity. The rest of the answers have no role in phospholipid digestion.

997 **D** (S&F, ch115)
The most effective treatment for solitary rectal ulcer syndrome is biofeedback. It has been associated with an increase in local blood flow. Other treatments include local agents, improving bowel habits,

and surgery. Local agents such as topical steroids and sulfasalazine are not effective. Sucralfate enemas and human fibrin sealant have been effective in small studies. The addition of fiber as a bulking agent along with bowel habit training to reduce straining may result in symptomatic improvement in patients with mild disease. Behavioral therapy or biofeedback is the first line of therapy for patients with more severe disease and improves symptoms in more than 50% of patients, although ulcer healing is seen in a minority. This therapy aims at bowel habit training with normalization of pelvic floor coordination. Jarrett and associates demonstrated that biofeedback resulted in improved rectal blood flow, which was associated with a successful clinical outcome. Surgery is indicated in patients with severe disease who do not respond to medical or biofeedback therapy. Surgical procedures include operations for rectal prolapse, excision of the ulcer, and colostomy.

998 **A** (S&F, ch101)
Selective IgA deficiency is the most common primary immunodeficiency and results in nearly complete absence of secretory and serum IgA, which predisposes the individual to recurrent respiratory, urogenital, and gastrointestinal infections. It is common for autoimmune and allergic diseases to develop in this setting, and there is a 10- to 16-fold increased incidence of gluten-sensitive enteropathy. The rest of the answers listed have no association with IgA deficiency.

999 **C** (S&F, ch112)
Toxic megacolon has developed in this patient, defined as acute dilation of the transverse colon to 6 cm or more and loss of haustrations during a severe attack of colitis, which can be of varied etiologies. Approximately half of UC patients who develop toxic megacolon do so within the first three months of diagnosis, although overall this condition occurs in only 5% of patients with UC. It most often occurs in patients with extensive or pancolitis but can occur with disease limited to the left colon. Predisposing factors include electrolyte imbalance, use of drugs that slow motility such as anticholinergics and narcotics, and procedures such as colonoscopy and barium enema performed during an acute colitis attack. Clinically, patients may develop fever, tachycardia, hypotension, diffuse abdominal distention and tenderness, and hypoactive bowel sounds. Leukocytosis and metabolic alkalosis may be seen on laboratory tests. Although certainly a surgical consultation should be initiated when toxic megacolon develops, medical therapy remains the first-line therapy for this condition, unless perforation is suspected or imminent (increasing abdominal distention with peritoneal signs and/or hemodynamic instability). Medical therapy includes treatment of the underlying inflammation, bowel rest, volume/electrolyte repletion, cessation of any antimotility agents, and colonic decompression. Antibiotics are generally given empirically because the mortality risk greatly increases if sepsis develops. If patients do not improve in 48 to 72 hours, then colectomy should be performed. Approximately 50% of patients will generally require surgery.

1000 **D** (S&F, ch112)
Cyclosporin A inhibits cell-mediated immunity and is reserved for patients with severe steroid-refractory UC. The response time is rapid, with a mean of seven days in the only randomized, controlled trial of 20 patients, 82% of whom responded to initial therapy. Cyclosporine levels should be monitored daily during intravenous dosing, with a goal trough of 200 to 400 ng/mL. If response to intravenous therapy is achieved, patients should be transitioned to 6-MP or azathioprine, as this practice has been shown to reduce the rate of relapse and colectomy. Cholesterol levels must be checked before initiation of therapy as levels of 120 mg/dL or lower may increase the risk of seizures; nutritional therapy should be instituted to improve cholesterol levels when they are low. Adverse events are generally dose dependent, and thus a lower dose of 2 mg/kg/day may be considered if levels are still adequate. Adverse events include neurotoxicity (seizures, paresthesias, tremors, headache), hypertension, nephrotoxicity, and infection (see table at end of chapter).

1001 **B** (S&F, ch96)
An omphalocele is a congenital hernia that involves the umbilicus. Current theories suggest that an event during the first three weeks of gestation prevents return of the bowel to the abdomen and failure of lateral embryonic fold development. In larger omphaloceles, the liver and spleen are often found outside the abdominal cavity. Gastroschisis is an abdominal wall defect commonly located to the right of an intact umbilical cord, and there is no sac present. Omphalomesenteric cyst is an abnormality of the embryonic connection between the yolk sac and gut lumen.

1002 **D** (S&F, ch105)
Findings of nutritional deficiencies that result in anemia (vitamin B_{12}, folate), stomatitis (iron), glossitis (vitamin B_2), pigmentation of the skin (vitamin B_{12}), and edema caused by hypoproteinemia are all consistent with tropical sprue (see figure here and table at end of chapter).

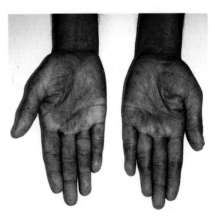

Figure for answer **1002**

1003 **C** (S&F, ch119)

All the choices are causes of SBO. The three most common causes are intra-abdominal adhesions, hernias, and neoplasms. Adhesions account for 50% to 75% of all cases.

1004 **D** (S&F, ch101)

Iron deficiency after gastric bypass is quite common, particularly in menstruating or pregnant women. Iron deficiency can develop for several reasons after gastric bypass (e.g., intolerance of red meat, diminished gastric acid secretion, and exclusion of the duodenum). Postoperatively, oral iron and vitamin C supplementation should be given because once iron deficiency develops, it may be refractory to oral iron supplementation.

1005 **C** (S&F, ch110)

A. lumbricoides can be seen on direct examination of the stool. Patients may see the worms on passage of a stool. If the worms are in the panceaticobiliary tree, they may be seen during ERCP (see figure). During an upper gastrointestinal series, *Ascaris* worms will retain barium after the gastrointestinal tract is cleared of the barium. Most patients do not have peripheral eosinophilia.

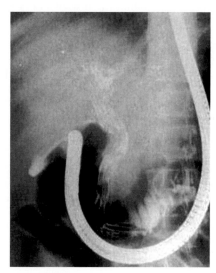

Figure for answer **1005**

1006 **C** (S&F, ch112)

EIMs of UC often parallel colonic disease activity. Various musculoskeletal abnormalities are seen with UC, including arthropathies. These are divided into both axial arthropathies, encompassing both sacroiliitis and ankylosing spondylitis, with the latter often being HLA-B27 positive. Sacroiliitis is more common, seen in 10% to 15% of UC patients, and patients either are asymptomatic or have mild low back pain; ankylosing spondylitis is seen in only 1% to 2% and may manifest with more severe symptoms and radiographic changes. Ocular EIMs include episcleritis and uveitis, with the former paralleling intestinal symptoms and the latter less predictably so. Episcleritis is seen in 5% to 8% of patients and presents with hyperemia of the conjunctiva and sclerae but is not painful and does not result in vision compromise. Uveitis, on the other hand, manifests with eye pain and blurry vision; immediate ophthalmologic examination and ocular glucocorticosteroid eyedrops are warranted. Erythema nodosum is one of the dermatologic manifestations that may be seen with UC; it usually parallels intestinal activity of UC. It occurs in 2% to 4% of patients and manifests with tender, raised erythematous nodules usually on the extensor surfaces of the lower extremities; biopsies should be avoided as scarring may be worse. Erythema nodosum usually remits with treatment of the underlying UC. Aphthous ulcerations of the mouth will be seen in approximately 10% of patients and generally occur simultaneously with colitis flares.

1007 **A** (S&F, ch119)

Although intussusception is most often recognized as a cause of SBO in children, approximately 5% of cases occur in adults. In children, there is rarely an anatomic abnormality, whereas in adults, an underlying pathologic process is present in more than 90% of cases. The most common cause is small bowel neoplasm. Inflammatory lesions and Meckel's diverticula account for most of the other cases.

1008 **D** (S&F, ch107)

V. cholerae is the prototypical toxigenic intestinal pathogen. It leads to massive fluid losses with as much as 15 to 20 L of diarrhea per day. Therefore, the presentation includes signs of dehydration and electrolyte imbalance, which can be severe. Death can occur within four hours of onset. Isotonic oral and intravenous fluid resuscitation is the mainstay of treatment. Additionally, tetracycline, ciprofloxacin, and trimethoprim/sulfamethoxazole are effective in decreasing stool output and shortening the duration of illness.

1009 **A** (S&F, ch114)

The findings described are typical of ischemic colitis. Presentation is usually 24 to 48 hours after another procedure that may have precipitated transient hypotension, which led to nonocclusive mesenteric ischemia.

1010 **A** (S&F, ch100)

Vitamins D_2 and D_3 are the only nutritionally important members of the vitamin D family, and vitamin D_3 is the major dietary form. Vitamin D_3 is found in a narrow list of foods but is sufficiently present in breast milk to prevent rickets. Normally enough vitamin D is produced endogenously in the skin during exposure to sunlight and the dietary intake of vitamin D is only critical when exposure to sunlight is low. The absorption of vitamin D is a passive process that occurs in the small intestine and is promoted by an acidic pH.

1011 **C** (S&F, ch123)

Age alone should not be the sole determinant for surgery. Surgical resection will prevent bleeding and obstruction and should be considered even when distant metastases are present. This is especially so if the patient is responding to chemotherapy. The optimal surveillance after curative-intent surgical resection has not been

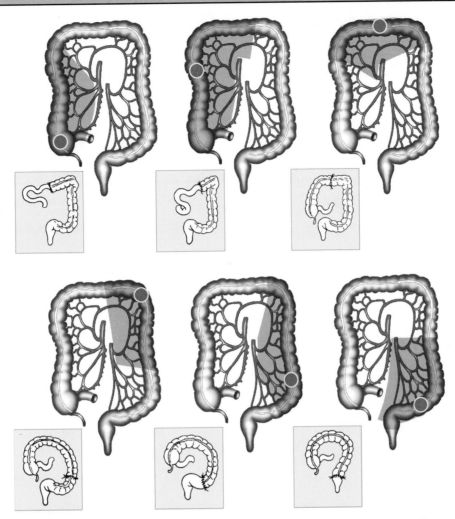

Figure for answer **1011**

determined. The postoperative carcinoembryonic antigen level is helpful. CT scanning, especially for those with resected rectosigmoid cancers, is useful to rule out pelvic recurrences. Additionally, colonoscopic surveillance is appropriate (see figure).

1012   **D** (S&F, ch114)
Colonic ischemia usually presents with sudden crampy mild left lower quadrant abdominal pain and an urge to defecate. This usually occurs within 24 hours of the precipitating event and is associated with bright red or maroon blood or bloody diarrhea. Bleeding is not significant enough to require transfusion. It is not likely that the patient's symptoms are secondary to recurrence of her virus or another superimposed viral infection. The findings seen endoscopically are not typical of ulcerative proctitis. These are hemorrhagic nodules typically seen during sigmoidoscopy that represent bleeding into the submucosa and are equivalent to thumbprints seen on barium enema studies.

1013   **D** (S&F, ch109)
Cryptosporidium, *Cyclospora*, and *Isospora* infection can all be diagnosed by examining stool specimens with a modified acid-fast stain.

1014   **B** (S&F, ch109)
The intracellular protozoon *Cryptosporidium* came to attention for the severe debilitating disease that it caused in AIDS patients before HAART. It is now recognized as a cause of self-limited diarrhea in the immunocompetent host. It is a more severe disease in those with immunoglobulin deficiency, lymphocytic malignancies, or low CD4 counts in HIV disease. Women of child-bearing age, adolescents, and HIV-positive patients with adequate CD4 counts generally have a milder self-limited course.

1015   **C** (S&F, ch97)
The predominant pattern seen in the fed state is that of peristalsis during which chyme is propagated aborally through the small intestine. Scintigraphic studies have shown wide variations in the time of small bowel transit depending on the type and quantity of food ingested. A segmenting pattern can also be observed in the postprandial states, which aids in the mixing of food and digestive enzymes but does not result in the net movement of the bolus through the gut lumen.

1016   **C** (S&F, ch118)
Decision analysis has shown that testing for celiac disease is cost-effective if the prevalence of celiac

disease in the population is greater than 1%. Bile salt malabsorption in the setting of IBS can occur, but a therapeutic trial of cholestyramine is more useful than the SeCAT test. Routine testing for IBD, chronic pancreatitis, or lactose tolerance is not recommended.

1017 D (S&F, ch108)
The gold standard diagnostic test to identify *C. difficile* toxin in the stool is a tissue culture cytotoxicity assay. The enzyme immunoassays are used widely for the detection of toxin A or toxins A and B of *C. difficile* in stool specimens. Although they have high specificity (75% to 100%) for toxins, the main drawback is that they are less sensitive than the cytotoxicity test (63% to 99%). Stool culture is sensitive (89% to 100%) but is not specific for toxin-producing strains to the bacterium. Sigmoidoscopic findings of colonic pseudomembranes are virtually pathognomonic for *C. difficile* colitis.

1018 A (S&F, ch109)
Colonoscopy and biopsy are the gold standard for diagnosis. Biopsy of the ulcer edge reveals the amebic trophozoites histologically. PAS stain aids detection. Noninvasive tests that are widely available include serum antibody titers and stool ELISA for amebic antigen, which are very specific. *E. dispar* is morphologically identical to *E. histolytica* but is not pathogenic. The stool examination for ova and parasite should not be relied on as it may only be 60% sensitive or less depending on delays in processing (see figure).

1019 C (S&F, ch118)
5-HT is released from enteroendocrine cells of the intestine after a meal. 5-HT then acts on primary intrinsic afferent neurons to initiate the peristaltic reflex mechanism. There is some evidence that an exaggerated release of 5-HT can occur after a meal in IBS. A leading hypothesis in IBS is that increased availability of mucosal 5-HT can induce diarrhea, but if there is desensitization of 5-HT receptors, this can lead to constipation or an alternating bowel pattern.

1020 C (S&F, ch114)
Almost all patients with AMI have acute abdominal pain. The pain may be out of proportion to the physical examination. The pain is often severe, but the abdomen is usually flat, soft, and nondistended. Nausea, vomiting, and bloody diarrhea would not be common early in an ischemic episode. This is also true of abdominal distention. When abdominal distention does occur, it is usually late and is the first sign of intestinal infarction.

1021 D (S&F, ch121)
Carcinoid tumors are usually located in the ileum, are more common in patients older than the age of 50, and are the second most commonly diagnosed small bowel malignancy. Carcinoid syndrome is generally absent, except with hepatic metastases. Gastrointestinal stromal tumors are more likely to present with gastrointestinal bleeding.

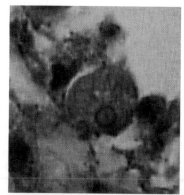

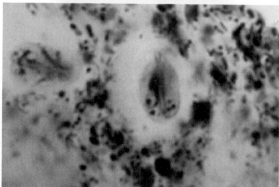

Figure for answer **1018**

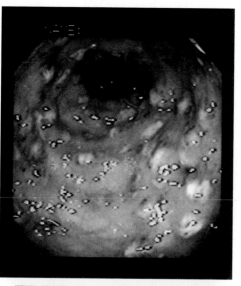

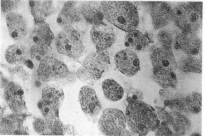

1022 D (S&F, ch120)

Alvimopan, a selective opioid antagonist, has been shown to shorten the time to gastrointestinal recovery and reduce length of hospital stay. Erythromycin, metoclopramide, naloxone, and neostigmine have not been shown to have a beneficial effect.

1023 E (S&F, ch123)

Dysplasia is the precursor to cancer in inflammatory bowel disease. Resected colons from IBD patients with colon cancer harbor dysplasia 90% of the time. Additionally, if high-grade dysplasia is present, there is a 30% chance of coexistent cancer. The highest risk of cancer is when high-grade dysplasia is found in a visible lesion, called a dysplasia-associated lesion or mass. Colectomy is advocated if severe dysplasia or a dysplasia-associated lesion or mass is present, as in this patient. The other choices are not appropriate due to the high risk of cancer in this lesion or elsewhere in the colon.

1024 D (S&F, ch107)

The patient has gastrointestinal tuberculosis. A positive tuberculin skin test result does not necessarily equate to active disease. The disease may resemble Crohn's disease, *Yersinia* infection, colon cancer, or amebiasis. Although some patients may require surgery for strictures or fistulas, standard antituberculosis medications achieve a high response rate.

1025 B (S&F, ch114)

Most patients with acute mesenteric venous thrombosis initially are believed to have some form of AMI and are treated as discussed and outlined in the algorithm (see figure on p. 256). Immediate heparinization for seven to 10 days has been shown to diminish recurrence and progression of thrombosis and improve survival. If peritonitis is present, laparotomy is necessary. Thrombolytic agents are not commonly used in this situation.

1026 B (S&F, ch112)

Although glucocorticosteroids are considered first-line agents for the induction of remission of moderate to severe UC, they have no benefit in the maintenance of remission. In those patients who have difficulty tapering off steroids or who become steroid dependent, a steroid-sparing agent such as an immunomodulator and infliximab are advised. There is no dose effect beyond the equivalent of prednisone, 40 to 60 mg/day, and doses higher than this result in increased side effects, which are numerous and can be serious (see table at end of chapter). Adrenocorticotropic hormone has been proposed as an alternative to traditional glucocorticosteroids for the treatment of UC, but the only randomized, controlled trial to date showed greater benefit of adrenocorticotropic hormone compared with hydrocortisone in steroid-naïve patients only. Further, this finding has not been replicated. Oral budesonide is a nonsystemic steroid with a pH-dependent release and high first-pass metabolism in the liver and erythrocytes; because of the low systemic availability, far less toxicity is seen. Although it is effective in the induction of remission for ileal and right-sided colonic Crohn's disease, oral budesonide has not shown efficacy in the treatment of UC. Budesonide enemas, on the other hand, have been shown to be effective for the treatment of distal UC, but are not available in the United States. Topical glucocorticosteroids are less effective than topical mesalamine for the induction of remission of distal UC, although the combination may be more effective than either alone.

1027 D (S&F, ch101)

Autoimmune gastritis (pernicious anemia) is the most common cause of vitamin B_{12} malabsorption. Cobalamin malabsorption in pernicious anemia is caused both by decreased intrinsic factor secretion due to parietal cell destruction in the stomach and blocking of autoantibodies, which inhibit intrinsic factor binding to vitamin B_{12}.

1028 D (S&F, ch111)

Glucocorticosteroids have multiple anti-inflammatory and immunosuppressive effects that make them effective in the induction of response/remission by one month for approximately 80% of patients with active Crohn's disease and UC. They are not effective in the maintenance of remission in inflammatory bowel disease and are wrought with a multitude of side effects, some of them potentially very serious, such as diabetes, osteonecrosis, and bone mineral density loss (see table at end of chapter). There are no data to suggest that doses beyond an equivalent of prednisone, 40 to 60 mg/day, are effective. Patients should not be underdosed either, which often leads to dose escalation and prolonged treatment. Further, glucocorticosteroids should not be given for either excessively short periods of time (3 weeks or fewer), as this is likely to lead to a rebound flare, or for long periods of time. If a taper fails, then a steroid-sparing immunomodulator or biological agent needs to be considered. When glucocorticosteroids are started, there should always be thought with regard to an "exit" strategy.

1029 A (S&F, ch115)

Enteropathy-type intestinal T-cell lymphoma has also been referred to as ulcerative jejunoileitis, idiopathic chronic ulcerative enteritis, and ETL. It occurs as a complication in established celiac disease or can present de novo with multiple intestinal ulcerations and malabsorption in patients without underlying celiac disease. These abnormal T cells express intracytoplasmic CD3, but lack cell surface expression of CD3-TCR complexes CD4 and CD8, thus setting them apart from uncomplicated celiac disease (CD3$^+$, CD4$^-$, CD8$^+$). These patients also have chromosomal imbalances in 87% of cases, with 58% showing gains on chromosome 9q and 16% on chromosome 1q. Most patients present in their 40s or later. Women are affected slightly more than men (1.6:1.0). Physical examination usually reveals profound weight loss, cachexia, and signs of severe malabsorption, steatorrhea, and protein-losing enteropathy.

1030 A (S&F, ch111)

This patient has demonstrated classic signs and symptoms of an acute infusion reaction to infliximab. Although patients who develop antibodies to

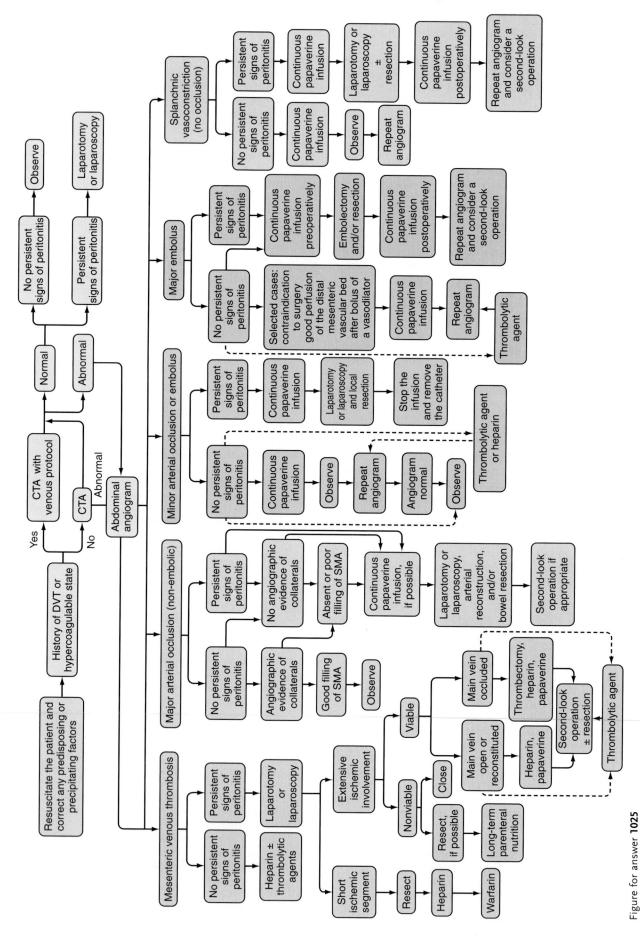

Figure for answer 1025

infliximab (ATI), formerly known as human anti–chimeric antibodies (HACA), are more likely to develop an infusion reaction, this likelihood does not mean they will necessarily develop it, and therefore ATI should not be checked as a matter of course in infliximab-treated patients. ATI will develop in approximately 13% of patients, and this is less likely to occur in those patients being treated with scheduled maintenance therapy rather than episodically. Glucocorticosteroids and immunomodulators decrease the formation of ATI. Combination infliximab and immunomodulator therapy also increases the risk of infection and has been linked to hepatosplenic T-cell lymphoma, a uniformly fatal disease that has been reported primarily in the pediatric male population. There have been some data to suggest that concomitant therapy could provide a therapeutic advantage over the use of infliximab alone in some patients. Therefore, the benefits and risks of treatment with combination anti-TNF therapy and an immunomodulator need to be weighed for each individual patient. Pretreatment with hydrocortisone has also been shown to decrease the risk of infusion reaction.

1031 E (S&F, ch117)
Fistulas are thought to develop in less than 5% of patients with diverticulitis and are present in approximately 20% requiring surgery for diverticulitis. Colovesicular fistulas are most common and account for 65% of fistulas in diverticular disease. A 3:1 male predominance is attributed to protection of the bladder in women by the uterus. Vaginal fistulas are the next most common internal fistula, representing approximately 25% of all cases.

1032 C (S&F, ch116)
Plain abdominal radiography is often the initial imaging study for patients with acute abdominal pain, although CT scans are considered the imaging study of choice in nonclassic cases of appendicitis. Findings consistent with appendicitis include an inflamed, distended (>6 mm) appendix that fails to fill with contrast or air, often accompanied by an appendiceal fecolith or wall thickening. Periappendiceal inflammation, cecal apical thickening, and a pericecal fluid collection are associated findings in appendicitis. A characteristic finding on ultrasound is a 7-mm or thicker noncompressible blind-ended loop of bowel.

1033 A (S&F, ch105)
Tropical enteropathy has been detected in most tropical regions of Asia, the Middle East, the Caribbean, Central and South America, and Africa.

1034 B (S&F, ch109)
Giardiasis causes a malabsorptive diarrhea, but the mechanism is unknown. The trophozoites adhere to the epithelium of the proximal small intestine, yet biopsies usually reveal normal histology. The pathogenicity of *B. hominis* and *D. fragilis* is unclear in humans. Although they may be associated with diarrhea, they are not clearly associated with malabsorption. Amebiasis usually affects the cecum and right colon and leads to colitis and not generally malabsorption.

1035 A (S&F, ch98)
In the human colon, there are three types of ICCs recognized and named based on their locations. ICC_{MY} is located in the plane of the myenteric plexus and is the pacemaker for the small, rapid (12-20 per minute) oscillations in membrane potential (myenteric potential oscillations). ICC_{SM} is located near the submucosal plexus and is the pacemaker for the large-amplitude slow waves. ICC_{IM} is located between the circular and longitudinal muscle layers. ICC_{IM} is a major target of neurotransmitters released from the axons of excitatory and inhibitory enteric motor neurons.

1036 A (S&F, ch118)
In the United States, 12% of patients seen by primary care physicians have IBS. In gastrointestinal practices, more than one third of patients have functional gastrointestinal disorders, with IBS being the most frequent diagnosis. IBS is associated with abdominal pain relieved with defecation, noncolonic symptoms, and a younger age group. Patients with inflammatory bowel disease can also have IBS.

1037 E (S&F, ch102)
SIBO seems to be common in patients with chronic liver disease. SIBO is more common in patients with advanced (Child-Pugh class C) liver disease and may be an independent risk factor for spontaneous bacterial peritonitis, although this latter association is controversial. There does not seem to be an association with any particular cause of chronic liver disease, but SIBO does not occur in cirrhotic patients if portal hypertension is absent. The etiology of SIBO in patients with chronic liver disease is likely related to disturbances in motility and possibly to the use of antacids, which might permit proliferation of bacteria. Small intestine dysmotility is more severe in cirrhotic patients with a history of spontaneous bacterial peritonitis, and treatment of SIBO improves motility. Liver transplantation also improves small bowel dysmotility in cirrhotic patients. Both antibiotic and prokinetic drugs are effective in SIBO-associated cirrhosis.

1038 D (S&F, ch97)
Peristalsis is a coordinated motility pattern that uses both sensory and motor aspects of the enteric nervous system. It can be initiated by both mechanical and chemical stimuli in the gut lumen and usually results in propagation in aboral direction; however, it can be reversed in the instance of luminal toxicity. The exact interplay of the various transmitters and hormones is not clearly understood.

1039 D (S&F, ch111)
A perianal fistula is pictured. It is typically treated with a combination of medical and surgical management. Perianal fistulas are estimated to occur in 15% to 35% of Crohn's disease patients and interestingly do not necessarily occur in the setting of active rectal inflammation. Proteases and metalloproteinases are released by the immune system and seem to be involved directly in tissue destruction, sinus tract formation, and penetration of adjacent tissue.

1040 **D** (S&F, ch112)

The *NOD2/CARD15* gene mutations on chromosome 16 that have been associated with Crohn's disease have not been linked to UC, except in some patients with "mixed" family histories (both UC and Crohn's disease). The C3435T polymorphism for human multidrug resistance 1 (MDR1) is linked to susceptibility for both UC and Crohn's disease: the *MDR1* gene codes for P-glycoprotein, expressed in intestinal epithelial cells, and defends against foreign antigens and bacteria. IL-12β on chromosome 5q33, which encodes the IL-12 receptor β$_1$ subunit (also known as p40) and is part of both the IL-12 and IL-23 receptors, as well as IL-23R on chromosome 1p31, which encodes the IL-23 receptor, are both identified as susceptibility genes for UC and Crohn's disease. The *ATG16L1* (autophagy-related 16-like 1) gene has an allelic variant that is protective against Crohn's disease.

1041 **B** (S&F, ch102)

CO is not a gas provided by enteric bacteria. N_2O_2, CO_2, H_2, and CH_4 make up 99% of flatus.

1042 **B** (S&F, ch97)

Contrast fluoroscopy is the most widely available wall motion study to assess small intestine wall motion. It provides in vivo information on time and space patterning of motor events and movements of luminal contents. Radiation exposure limits the use of this technique. The other choices are all suitable imaging methods for assessing wall motion and movement of intraluminal contents. They are not widely available, and all have limitations.

1043 **C** (S&F, ch119)

Multiple studies suggest that passage of orally administered gastrograffin into the colon within six to 24 hours may identify those patients most likely to respond to nonoperative management regardless of the cause of the obstruction.

1044 **B** (S&F, ch99)

Decrease in cAMP leads to net absorption. Other proabsorptive pathways include the inhibitor G-protein cascade and the phosphatidylinositol cycle. Secretagogues act through the signal transduction cascades such as those involving cAMP, cGMP, Ca^{2+}, and phosphatidylinositol.

1045 **D** (S&F, ch111)

Weight loss in Crohn's disease can be seen for multiple reasons. In patients with long-segment small bowel disease and/or multiple surgeries, malabsorption may result in not only weight loss but also nutritional deficiencies. This patient has minimal terminal ileal inflammatory changes and has not had any surgeries. Further, none of his laboratory test results support malabsorption, given normal levels of albumin, vitamin B$_{12}$, folate, ferritin, magnesium, and zinc. Although malignancy should always be considered in patients with Crohn's disease, his weight loss has not been out of proportion to his disease activity and he has no masses or strictures on endoscopic or radiographic examination that could harbor a cancer. Further, his disease is not long-standing. Although superimposed infection should always be considered with weight loss in inflammatory bowel disease, his stool studies have been negative and there is no evidence of intra-abdominal abscess. The most likely reason in this patient is decreased oral intake in an effort to avoid symptoms, which are largely postprandial. Inflammation in itself can also induce a catabolic state when it is severe enough.

1046 **D** (S&F, ch112)

This is an elderly patient with steroid-dependent UC. Cyclosporine would not be appropriate, given his renal insufficiency and inability to transition to an immunomodulator such as 6-MP and azathioprine, given his history of pancreatitis. Further, infliximab is relatively contraindicated because of his history of congestive heart failure. Remaining on high-dose steroids is also not an option because of multiple side effects including diabetes and hypertension. In addition, steroids are not effective maintenance medications. Therefore, surgery is the most appropriate option for this patient. A total proctocolectomy is the correct surgery, but the favored option would be an end-ileostomy, not IPAA (J pouch), given the patient's age and the potential complications such as pouchitis and incontinence that can occur with this surgery. Also, it generally requires two to three operations, which would increase the risk in this patient with multiple medical comorbidities. A Brooke or end-ileostomy is the correct choice because it permits the surgery to be done in one step and is associated with fewer complications. A subtotal colectomy (the rectum is left intact) is sometimes performed on an urgent basis when patients are sicker or have fulminant disease because removing the rectum is the more time-consuming part of the surgery. Generally, the rectum is then removed at a later date when the patient has recovered because it would still be at risk of disease and neoplastic changes. A Koch pouch or "continent" ileostomy has fallen out of favor and is rarely performed any more because of complications.

1047 **B** (S&F, ch119)

In adults, the imaging study of choice for intussusception is CT. A double-bowel sign characterized by concentric rings of inner and outer bowel walls separated by hyperechoic fat represents the intussusceptum, and the intussuscipiens along with mesentery fat is one of the diagnostic patterns seen.

1048 **D** (S&F, ch107)

B. cereus is a gram-positive organism that leads to two different illnesses depending on the toxin. A diarrhea or a vomiting syndrome can occur. The illness is likely due to the ingestion of preformed toxin because the incubation period is very short. The illness is usually mild and short-lived. Nearly all the cases of vomiting syndrome from *B. cereus* have been related to contaminated fried rice. *Staphylococcus aureus* can cause a similar illness; *Staphylococcus epidermidis* does not. *Listeria* is a much more dramatic illness. *Listeria* and *C. botulinum* can cause neurologic symptoms. *Aeromonas* causes a diarrheal illness (see three tables at end of chapter).

1049 **A** (S&F, ch99)
Multiple different classes of chloride channels exist in the mammalian intestine. The calcium-activated chloride channels are involved in the diarrhea caused by rotavirus. The rotavirus toxin NSP4 activates calcium-dependent chloride secretion in the colon leading to diarrhea.

1050 **C** (S&F, ch111)
Crohn's disease occurs most commonly in the terminal ileum and colon. Approximately one third to one half of patients will have inflammation involving both the terminal ileum and the colon. Approximately one third of patients will have disease isolated to the terminal ileum. Crohn's disease involving only the jejunum is rare; macroscopic disease of the esophagus, stomach, and duodenum is also unusual and usually occurs in association with ileal and colonic inflammation.

1051 **C** (S&F, ch119)
SBO in the early postoperative period may be very difficult to distinguish from normal postoperative ileus. The most important clinical feature differentiating early postoperative SBO from postoperative ileus is the occurrence of obstructive symptoms after an initial return of bowel function and resumption of oral intake. Symptoms of abdominal distention, pain, nausea, and vomiting can be seen in both cases. The type of surgery performed or cumulative dose of narcotics used will not help distinguish between an ileus and a mechanical SBO.

1052 **B** (S&F, ch110)
A single oral dose of ivermectin, 200 µg/kg, is the best treatment and better tolerated than thiabendazole. The others are not useful for treatment of *Strongyloides*. Successful treatment often leads to a decrease in antibody titers in six months.

1053 **C** (S&F, ch97)
Multichannel intraluminal impedance is a technique that depends on the differential conductivities of luminal contents to track the movement of the bolus along the intestines. When combined with manometry, this technique can provide real-time information about the pressure–flow relationship.

1054 **C** (S&F, ch104)
Celiac disease is characterized by small intestine malabsorption of nutrients after the ingestion of wheat gluten or related proteins from rye and barley. The reason that oats may be tolerated by patients with celiac disease is that oats contain a relatively smaller proportion of a toxic prolamin moiety compared with other gluten-containing cereals.

1055 **B** (S&F, ch101)
The Schilling test is used to clinically distinguish between gastric and ileal causes of vitamin B_{12} deficiency and to evaluate the function of the ileum in patients with diarrhea or malabsorption. It is performed by administering a small oral dose of radiolabeled vitamin B_{12} with a large intramuscular dose of vitamin B_{12}. If less than 7% to 10% of the administered oral dose is recovered in the urine at 24 hours, vitamin B_{12} malabsorption is diagnosed. To specify the site of malabsorption, a second phase of the test must be performed. This phase involves oral administration of intrinsic factor. In patients with pernicious anemia, the results of the Schilling test normalize after the oral administration of intrinsic factor, whereas in those with ileal disease, the abnormality persists. Results of the Schilling test are normal in patients with dietary vitamin B_{12} deficiency. Patients with pancreatic exocrine insufficiency may have an abnormal test result, but it will normalize if they are given pancreatic enzyme supplementation.

1056 **D** (S&F, ch123)
The liver is the most common site for colon cancer metastases. These patients have a poor prognosis, and therefore aggressive treatment is recommended. Resection of liver metastases is considered if the primary tumor has been removed with the intent to cure and no extrahepatic disease is present. Resection could be considered as long as there are no more than four metastatic tumors present, even if more than one lobe is involved.

1057 **C** (S&F, ch110)
Several worms may live in the biliary tree at some point during their life cycle. They include *Ascaris*, *Opisthorchis*, *Clonorchis*, *Fasciola*, and, rarely, *Taenia* species. The presentation can be that of biliary obstruction and cholangitis.

1058 **B** (S&F, ch104)
Understanding of the nature of the genetic predisposition of celiac disease began with the significant observation by Howell and coworkers that celiac disease was associated with specific HLA-2-DQ haplotypes. HLA class II molecules are glycosylated transmembrane heterodimers (α and β chains) that are organized into three related subregions (DQ, DR, and DP) and encoded within the HLA class II region of the major histocompatibility complex on chromosome 6p. The HLA-DQ (α1*501,β1*02) heterodimer, known as HLA-DQ2, is found in 95% of patients (compared with 30% of controls) and the related DQ (α1*0301,β1*0302) heterodimer, known as HLA-DQ8, is found in most of the remaining patients with celiac disease. Celiac disease actually develops in only a minority of individuals who express DQ2. In fact, HLA-DQ2 is common in Europeans and is expressed in 25% to 30% of the population.

1059 **B** (S&F, ch99)
A basolateral sodium pump is a fundamental property of all intestinal epithelial cells and helps to establish an intracellular electrochemical gradient with a low intracellular Na and a relatively negative intracellular charge. This pump is electrogenic, extruding three Na^+ ions in exchange for two K^+ ions (see figure on p. 260).

1060 **C** (S&F, ch105)
Endemic tropical sprue is not found universally in tropical and subtropical regions, a finding that strongly suggests that the etiologic factor or factors similarly are geographically restricted (see figure on p. 260).

1061 **A** (S&F, ch107)
Without knowing the organism and sensitivities, fluoroquinolones are generally the most effective.

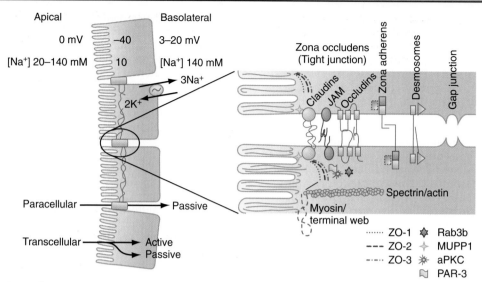

Figure for answer **1059**

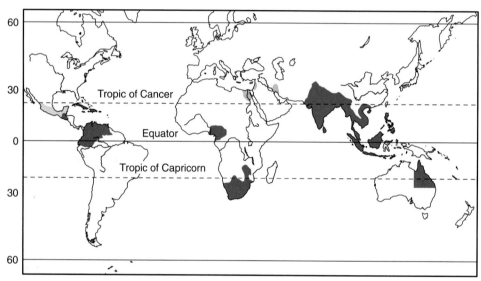

Figure for answer **1060**

Trimethoprim/sulfamethoxazole is also effective, but resistance in tropical areas has been reported. A combination of antimicrobial agents plus antimotility drugs was found to be the most effective regimen, halting diarrhea in one hour compared with 30 hours with either agent alone in a study of travelers to Mexico. Bismuth subsalicylate also helps to treat and prevent diarrhea with fewer side effects than antimicrobials (see table at end of chapter).

1062 C (S&F, ch100)
Triglycerides, cholesterol, and their esters and phospholipids are packaged in the enterocytes into either chylomicrons or very-low-density lipoprotein. During fasting, very-low-density lipoprotein is the predominant triglyceride-rich lipoprotein that emerges from the epithelial cells.

1063 D (S&F, ch109)
Chagas' disease is essentially confined to patients from Central and South America. However, with more people immigrating to the United States and the finding of large reservoirs in animals in the southern United States, it could become a significant health problem. The protozoon responsible, *Trypanosoma cruzi*, is transmitted by the bite of the reduviid bug. Acute Chagas' disease most often affects children with fever and edema, mostly in a periorbital distribution. Chronic Chagas' disease most often affects the heart, esophagus, and/or colon. The symptoms can be arrhythmias, heart failure, constipation, and typical achalasia-type symptoms. Manometrically, the disease is indistinguishable from achalasia. The diagnosis is made by finding the trypanosome on blood smears. Nitazoxanide or benznidazole can be used for treatment (see figure).

1064 E (S&F, ch118)
One randomized study measured IgG antibodies to foods and then excluded those IgG foods from the diet. The exclusion of foods with a positive IgG response benefited both diarrhea- and constipation-predominant IBS. Wheat bran is no better

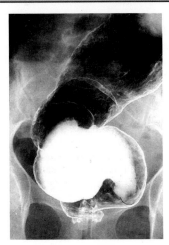

Figure for answer **1063**

than placebo. Soluble fiber benefits constipation-predominant but not diarrhea-predominant IBS and should be started at low doses to reduce side effects. In most patients with typical IBS symptoms, reducing lactose does not help.

1065 **D** (S&F, ch123)

Testing for alterations in the *APC* gene is available for FAP. Although alterations in the *APC* gene can be found in 60% to 80% of sporadic colonic adenomas and carcinomas, genetic testing is reserved for high-risk individuals. If HNPCC is suspected, testing the patient tumor for microsatellite instability can be explored. If present, then testing for the abnormality in family members should be performed. Genetic testing for those at risk of sporadic colorectal cancer is not recommended at the current time.

1066 **B** (S&F, ch112)

Approximately 80% of patients with UC will have a course of disease in which remission periods are interrupted by periodic flares. More than half will have mild symptoms with their first presentation, whereas approximately 10% will have such a severe course with their initial attack that colectomy is needed. Ten percent to 30% of patients with proctitis or proctosigmoiditis will have disease extension noted after 10 years. By 25 years, 30% with UC will have undergone a colectomy.

1067 **B** (S&F, ch111)

Autophagy is a cellular process that allows clearance of old or abnormal proteins and apoptotic bodies; further, autophagy also seems to be directly involved in innate immunity via multiple mechanisms. Two autophagy-related genes have been identified in relation to Crohn's disease: the autophagy-related 16-like 1 (*ATG16L1*) gene with an allelic variant that is protective against Crohn's disease and also the immunity-related GTPase family member M (*IRGM*), which seems to be important in the resistance to intracellular pathogens. IL-23 is a heterodimeric cytokine with two linked subunits, p19 and p40, the latter of which is also common to IL-12. The IL-23 receptor (IL23R) is up-regulated in response to IL-6 and transforming growth factor β (TGFβ), which activates Th17 cells to produce IL-17, an important inflammatory cytokine. An uncom-

mon variant of IL23R is protective against Crohn's disease. Allelic variants of the IL-12 receptor gene are associated with Crohn's disease as well; this gene encodes for the common p40 subunit of IL-12 and IL-23 (in addition to the *JAK2* and *STAT3* genes) and is important in IL-23 receptor signaling and Th17 cell differentiation.

1068 **D** (S&F, ch111)

5-ASAs are first-line induction and maintenance therapy in patients with mild to moderate UC. The data to support their use in Crohn's disease are equivocal and no 5-ASAs are approved by the FDA to treat Crohn's disease. That being said, sulfasalazine, in particular, may have a small margin of benefit in mild to moderate Crohn's disease of the colon. Sulfasalazine was originally used to treat rheumatoid arthritis, but was also found to decrease joint symptoms in patients with colitis. Therefore, it is a good choice for patients with IBD and associated arthropathy.

1069 **C** (S&F, ch114)

Alosetron (a 5-HT$_3$ antagonist) was taken off the market for general use (but is available through a special program) secondary to its increased risk of colon ischemia. This increased risk seems to be related to the serotoninergic antagonist rather than the serotonin agonist, although there have been a few case reports of the serotonin agonist. Dose reduction would not be adequate, and the medication must be stopped immediately. Because IBS is more common in women than in men, so would be the incidence of colonic ischemia.

1070 **A** (S&F, ch119)

The classic radiologic feature of a sigmoid volvulus is a distended ahaustral sigmoid loop (bent inner tube) appearance, the apex of which often is directed toward the patient's right shoulder. The classic features of cecal volvulus include a massively dilated cecum located in the epigastrium or left upper quadrant, a coffee bean appearance of the distended cecum, distended loops of small bowel suggesting SBO, and a single long air–fluid level present on upright or decubitus films. A colon cutoff sign is seen in pancreatitis.

1071 **D** (S&F, ch125)

Pruritus ani is an itch localized to the anus and perianal skin. Pruritus ani is categorized as either idiopathic or secondary. Idiopathic pruritus ani is diagnosed when no underlying etiology is found. Secondary pruritus ani results from an underlying disorder, and specific treatment leads to resolution of symptoms. Leakage of stool because of fecal incontinence and leakage of mucus because of prolapse of the rectum or hemorrhoids can cause irritation and itching. Other causes include contact dermatitis, infections (such as *Candida*), parasites, systemic diseases (diabetes mellitus), diet (coffee, cola, chocolate, milk, beer, and others), and some medications.

1072 **B** (S&F, ch103)

This is as a consequence of multiple small bowel resections. Vascular injuries secondary to venous or arterial thrombosis or embolism are other important causes.

1073 **B** (S&F, ch112)

The most important risk factors for colorectal cancer in UC are duration and extent of disease. In general, the risk is estimated to increase at a rate of 0.5% to 1% per year after eight to 10 years of disease in patients with extensive colitis. The risk of colorectal cancer is approximately 7% to 10% at 20 years and as high as 35% after 30 years. Primary sclerosing cholangitis, a chronic inflammatory disease of the biliary tree that progresses to fibrosis, cirrhosis, and end-stage liver disease, is seen in approximately 3% of patients with UC. These patients are at a significantly higher risk of colorectal cancer than those without it and need to begin surveillance immediately after diagnosis of primary sclerosing cholangitis. Other risk factors for colorectal cancer in UC include severity of inflammation, family history of colorectal cancer, age at diagnosis, smoking, and the presence of pseudopolyps (not explicitly stated in the chapter). Surveillance colonoscopy generally every one to two years should begin between eight and 10 years after symptom onset in those patients with disease beyond the rectum. Surveillance colonoscopy ideally should be done when patients are clinically in remission and four-quadrant biopsies should be performed every 10 cm with targeted biopsies obtained from any raised or suspicious-appearing lesions. At least 33 biopsies are required to achieve a 90% probability of identifying dysplasia, and 64 biopsies for a probability of 95%. Chromoendoscopy, high-magnification endoscopy, and narrow-band imaging may increase the yield of dysplasia detection but are not yet part of the standard of care.

1074 **B** (S&F, ch114)

Although poorly sensitive (30%) and nonspecific, plain films of the abdomen still are obtained in evaluating patients with suspected AMI. Most plain films are normal before infarction. Subsequently, formless loops of small intestine, ileus "thumbprinting" of the small bowel or right colon can be seen (see figure). Even later in the course, pneumatosis and portal or mesenteric vascular gas may be seen. Free air under the diaphragm would suggest perforation and would generally not be an early finding.

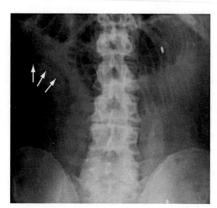

Figure for answer **1074**

1075 **A** (S&F, ch104)

Celiac disease affects the mucosa of the small intestine; the submucosa, muscularis propria, and serosa usually are not involved. The mucosal involvement of the small intestine in celiac disease may vary considerably in both severity and extent. This spectrum of pathologic involvement helps explain the striking variability of the clinical manifestations of the disease. Examination, by hand lens or dissecting microscope, of the mucosal surface of biopsy specimens from untreated celiac disease patients with severe involvement reveals a flat mucosal surface with complete absence of normal intestinal villi. Histologic examination of tissue sections confirms this loss of normal villous structure (see figure). Sparing of the proximal intestine with involvement of the distal small intestine does not occur.

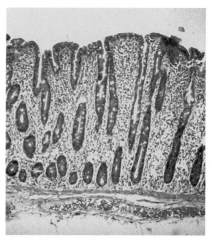

Figure for answer **1075**

1076 **B** (S&F, ch109)

Microsporidiosis is less common in immunocompetent patients. It is strongly associated with low CD4 counts, and 50% of AIDS patients with diarrhea harbor this protozoon. The other organisms can more commonly cause a self-limited diarrheal illness in the immunocompetent host.

1077 **C** (S&F, ch109)

Immigrants from endemic areas, institutionalized patients, and male homosexuals are at the greatest risk of amebiasis. Although infants, the elderly, pregnant women, and those receiving corticosteroids are at increased risk of fulminant disease, AIDS patients are not at increased risk of invasive disease. Invasive disease develops in only 10% of infected individuals, and 90% remain asymptomatic. The two-stage life cycle includes the infectious cyst, which is acquired by ingesting fecally contaminated food or water. The second stage is the trophozoite, which is responsible for tissue invasion. Amebic colitis may present like other colitides and most commonly affects the cecum and right colon (see figure).

1078 **C** (S&F, ch114)

Henoch-Schönlein purpura typically affects children four to seven years of age. It is characterized by an IgA, not an IgG, immune complex that is

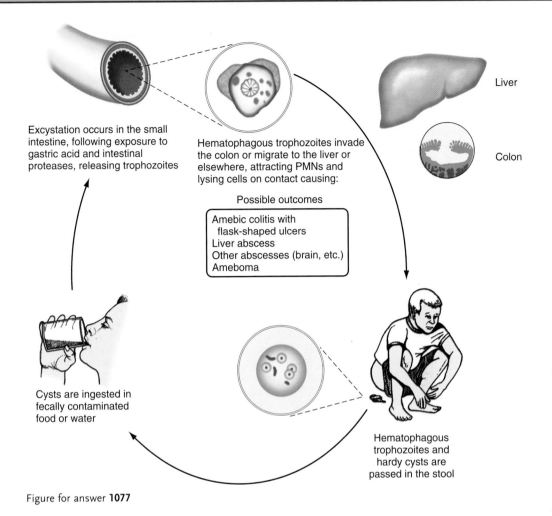

Excystation occurs in the small intestine, following exposure to gastric acid and intestinal proteases, releasing trophozoites

Hematophagous trophozoites invade the colon or migrate to the liver or elsewhere, attracting PMNs and lysing cells on contact causing:

Liver

Colon

Possible outcomes

Amebic colitis with
  flask-shaped ulcers
Liver abscess
Other abscesses (brain, etc.)
Ameboma

Cysts are ingested in fecally contaminated food or water

Hematophagous trophozoites and hardy cysts are passed in the stool

Figure for answer **1077**

deposited within the small vessels of the skin, gastrointestinal tract, joints, and kidneys. It is often preceded by an upper respiratory infection. The classic triad is palpable purpura (usually seen below the waist), arthritis (knees and ankles), and abdominal pain. The abdominal pain and bleeding are secondary to mucosal and submucosal hemorrhage. These submucosal hematomas may act as lead points for any intussusception.

1079 **B** (S&F, ch113)
An ileorectal anastomosis removes the vast majority of diseased colon, but preserves the rectum, to which the ileum is directly attached. This avoids a second surgery and a stoma and preserves continence. A noninflamed rectum will become distensible and capacious enough to handle the ileal contents so that patients have low stool frequency and minimal to no incontinence. Thus, a patient with inflammation of the rectum from either Crohn's disease or UC would not be a good candidate for this surgery. Because these patients need continued surveillance of the rectum for cancer, neither a young patient with no contraindication to IPAA nor one who is undergoing colectomy for a known history of high-grade dysplasia (and thus at higher risk of the development of subsequent dysplasia/cancer of the remaining rectum) would be an ideal candidate. The patient who is obese

(and thus may not be a good candidate for a stoma), who has had multiple abdominopelvic surgeries and other medical comorbidities (making the second surgery needed for a pouch more difficult and a higher risk), and who also has a noninflamed rectum is likely a good candidate for an ileorectal anastomosis.

1080 **B** (S&F, ch113)
Pouch failure is fortunately a rare event, occurring in an estimated 2% to 12% of patients who undergo IPAA. Approximately 6% of patients require pouch excision with end-ileostomy. Pouch failure is most often caused by one or a combination of the following early or late complications of surgery: pelvic sepsis, high output, Crohn's disease, intractable incontinence, and pouchitis. The latter was the only identifiable etiology in approximately 2% of patients. Seventy-five percent of pouch failure occurs in the first year, with the remainder occurring generally in the second or third year.

1081 **D** (S&F Chapter 106)
Almost all patients with Whipple's disease have involvement of the intestinal tract by this infection, regardless of whether gastrointestinal symptoms are present. Thus, the primary diagnostic approach to a patient with clinically suspected Whipple's disease is upper endoscopy (see figure for question

995) with mucosal biopsy. To avoid sampling errors in patients with patchy lesions, one should obtain approximately five biopsy specimens from regions as far distal as possible within the small intestine. Histologic examination with routine hematoxylin and eosin and PAS stains is usually sufficient to reach a diagnosis. In some cases, findings may be corroborated with silver stains; in contrast, the Gram stain is less useful in this infection. Traditionally, electron microscopy has been used as the gold standard for confirming the diagnosis of Whipple's disease. Currently, polymerase chain reaction analysis serves in this capacity.

1082   D (S&F, ch112)

Although internal hemorrhoids present with rectal bleeding, this is most typically limited to the toilet paper, on the surface of the stool, or dripping in the bowl and is not mixed with diarrhea and mucus. Although infectious colitis can have overlapping symptoms with UC, the time course would argue strongly against this diagnosis. Although IBS is commonly encountered in young women, classic symptoms include a change in bowel habits accompanied by abdominal pain/discomfort that is relieved by a bowel movement; bloody diarrhea with urgency and particularly incontinence are not characteristic of IBS and should raise suspicion of an inflammatory bowel disease such as UC. Generally, physical examination findings are normal, although rectal examination may be uncomfortable with a "velvety" mucosa and blood on the glove. Laboratory test results in mild to moderate UC are often normal, but a mild microcytic anemia may be seen.

1083   A (S&F, ch113)

There is some controversy about whether hand-sewn or double-stapled IPAA is the better surgery. In the former, a complete rectal mucosectomy is performed, whereas in the latter, 1 to 2 cm of the anal transition zone or columnar cuff is preserved. In a Mayo Clinic study comparing the two techniques, no differences in complication rates were found, although patients who had undergone the double-stapled IPAA had less nocturnal incontinence and better resting and squeezing anal tone. Sexual activity has been noted to increase significantly after IPAA in women, attributed to overall improved health. Two-stage IPAA is generally advocated: in the first part, the colon is removed, the pouch constructed, and a diverting ileostomy is created to allow the anal sphincter and ileal mucosa to recover before restoration of the fecal stream through the pouch. Further, although the presence of the diverting ileostomy does not protect against pelvic sepsis, it makes this most-feared complication easier to manage. Advocates of the one-stage procedure argue that this method precludes the temporary ileostomy and the second hospital stay and surgery. The only study to date comparing one- and two-stage surgeries did not find any differences in functional outcomes or complication rates. In experienced hands with a properly selected patient, a one-stage surgery may be a reasonable approach. The risk of dysplasia and cancer is no different in patients undergoing double-stapled or hand-sewn IPAA. The main risk

of the development of dysplasia after IPAA is whether a patient had cancer or dysplasia in the proctocolectomy specimen.

1084   A (S&F, ch118)

Cases of ischemic colitis have been reported in association with alosetron. Ischemic colitis occurs in 0.1% of patients and is drug related but dose independent. The ischemia is usually transient and without irreversible consequence, although as many as 50% of patients require hospitalization. Alosetron is indicated in patients with diarrhea-predominant IBS and is available in the United States under a restricted prescribing program. Constipation occurs in one third of patients treated with alosetron.

1085   B (S&F, ch99)

The fundamental characteristics of the tight junction (leaky vs. tight) vary along the length of the intestine and dictate how much of the paracellular transport will contribute to overall transport. Paracellular movement, as opposed to transcellular movement, is a largely passive process and is in response to a variety of gradients that are established. Absorptive transport is when the mucosal-to-serosal flux exceeds the serosal-to-mucosal flux. Secretory transport is the opposite.

1086   D (S&F, ch114)

CT scan has, for the most part, replaced plain film study of the abdomen for diagnosis and is used to identify both arterial and venous thrombosis as well as ischemic bowel. CT findings may include colonic dilation, bowel wall thickening, abnormal bowel wall enhancement, lack of enhancement of arterial vasculature with timed venous contrast injections, arterial occlusion, venous thrombosis, engorgement of mesenteric veins, intramural gas and mesenteric or portal gas (see figure), infarction of other organs, ascites, and signs related to the cause of the infarcted bowel (e.g., hernia). Tagged red blood cells would not be useful for making this diagnosis. Duplex ultrasonography and Doppler flowmetry may have some utility, but CT is still the best choice.

1087   B (S&F, ch119)

Neoplasms of the small intestine are a relatively unusual cause of SBO and account for approximately 5% to 10% of cases. In patients who present with an SBO without previous laparotomy or evidence of a hernia, approximately 50% will have malignant neoplasms as the cause. Most commonly, the small bowel becomes obstructed by extrinsic compression or local invasion or both from advanced gastrointestinal or gynecologic malignancies. The two most common malignancies are colorectal and ovarian adenocarcinomas.

1088   B (S&F, ch120)

Demyelination of the proximal vagus nerve and sympathetic nerves supplying the bowel occurs in diabetes. The intrinsic nervous system of the bowel seems unaffected because no morphologic abnormalities of the myenteric or submucosal plexus have been observed. In animal studies and in a single case report, there was degeneration of the ICCs. Most authorities believe that myopathy is not

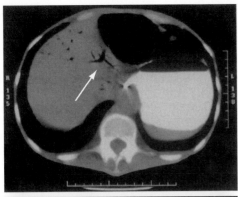

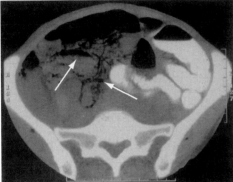

Figure for answer **1086**

a cause of the gastrointestinal dysmotility seen in diabetes.

1089 **A** (S&F, ch112)
Th17 cells are a relatively newly discovered important cell lineage involved in the pathogenesis of IBD. These cells produce IL-6 and IL-17, the latter of which is a key proinflammatory cytokine and not only activates T cells but also multiple other cell types, which then promote the production of a cascade of proinflammatory cytokines. It also expresses IL-23 receptor, activation of which by IL-23 is important in the development of colitis in mouse models. Traditionally, the Th1 cell pathway has been implicated in Crohn's disease and the Th2 cell pathway has been implicated in UC, but more recent data suggest that this represents an oversimplification of the Th cell role in the pathogenesis of IBD. T regulatory cells down-regulate both the Th1 and Th2 pathways via the production of IL-10 and transforming growth factor β.

1090 **C** (S&F, ch112)
The male-to-female ratio in UC is equal across all age groups. Although UC can present at almost any age, it is very uncommon before the age of 5 years and after the age of 75. The peak age at onset is in the second and third decades, and although there is a smaller peak between the ages of 60 and 70, this bimodal distribution is not as common as in Crohn's disease. The correct answer is therefore **C**.

1091 **B** (S&F, ch111)
With the ability of scientists to perform automated rapid DNA sequencing, genomewide association studies have uncovered more than 30 genetic loci that may be associated with Crohn's disease. The first such definitive genetic susceptibility locus was the *NOD2/CARD15* on chromosome 16 (nucleotide-binding oligomerization domain, also known as caspase-recruitment domain). Three allelic variants are most commonly associated with Crohn's disease in European and American populations and include two missense mutations and one frameshift insertion. These variants are contained within the leucine-rich repeat region of the gene and lead to interference of the binding of the gene product protein to muramyl dipeptide, contained within the cell walls of both gram-positive and -negative bacteria. Although the exact mechanisms are unclear, this leads to a defective innate immune response, which in turn might cause increased chronic activation of adaptive immunity. If an individual carries mutations on both chromosomes (homozygous), the odds ratio of development of Crohn's disease is 17 compared with 2.5 for a heterozygote. Twenty percent to 30% of Crohn's patients are believed to carry at least one allelic variant of this gene. Genetic polymorphisms of *NOD2/CARD15* are associated with a younger disease onset, the ileal location, and the stricturing subtype.

1092 **C** (S&F, ch114)
Abdominal pain with meals, leading to weight loss, characterizes this syndrome. The cardinal clinical feature of chronic mesenteric ischemia is abdominal cramping discomfort that occurs within 30 minutes after eating, gradually increases in severity, and then fully resolves over one to three hours. This usually progresses over weeks to months. Nausea, bloating, episodic diarrhea, malabsorption, or constipation may occur.

1093 **B** (S&F, ch119)
The epidural administration of local anesthetics blocks afferent and efferent inhibitory reflexes including inhibitory sympathetic efferent signals. Studies have shown that bupivacaine hydrochloride significantly reduced the duration of postoperative ileus. Studies have not shown any significant benefit from metoclopramide or erythromycin. NSAIDs have been shown to decrease the frequency of postoperative nausea and vomiting and improve gastrointestinal transit in several experimental and clinical studies. Its effect on reducing the duration of postoperative ileus has not been determined. Several randomized studies have shown that nasogastric tube decompression does not shorten the duration of postoperative ileus.

1094 **B** (S&F, ch97)
Intrinsic neurons greatly outnumber their extrinsic counterparts, which have cell bodies outside the gut wall with extensions that terminate in the intestinal wall. Both efferent (motor) and afferent (sensory) neurons compose the extrinsic neurons. Extrinsic sensory neurons do not belong in the autonomic nervous system and are classified as either vagal or spinal (see figure on p. 266). Extrinsic motor neurons are part of the ANS.

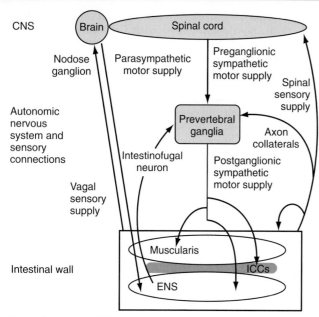

Figure for answer **1094**

1095 **D** (S&F, ch104)

The laboratory findings in celiac disease, like the symptoms and signs, vary with the extent and severity of the intestinal involvement. Serum IgA endomesial antibodies, tissue transglutaminase antibodies, and small bowel biopsy are the most accurate diagnostic tests for celiac disease. It is also important to document IgA deficiency, as this can lead to falsely negative serology results. Although the diagnosis of celiac disease may be suspected on clinical grounds or as a result of abnormal serologic test results, the current recommendation for confirmation of the diagnosis remains a biopsy of the small intestine. Several biopsy specimens should be obtained from the distal duodenum (second or third parts) to avoid the mucosal architectural distortion produced by Brunner's glands and changes caused by peptic duodenitis, both of which can cause difficulty in histopathologic diagnosis. Thus, shortening of the villi, crypt hyperplasia, cytologically abnormal surface cells, and increased lamina propria cellularity must be present to firmly make a diagnosis of celiac disease.

1096 **D** (S&F, ch112)

A normal or decreased absolute number of IELs, which are mostly CD8+ cells, is seen in UC. These cells are hypothesized to be cytotoxic and may be involved in suppressing local immune responses. Both innate and adaptive cellular immunity are likely abnormal in UC. The innate immune system is nonspecific and "untrained" and is mediated largely through pattern recognition receptors, which include Toll-like receptors and nucleotide-binding oligomerization domain–like receptors. These pattern recognition receptors are the "first responders" of the immune system and react immediately to foreign (and especially bacterial) antigens. The adaptive immune system is controlled by T- and B-cell responses, which also may be abnormal on various levels. Nonspecific cellular immu-

nity has also been implicated in the pathogenesis of UC, with an overproduction of circulating monocytes and mucosal macrophages and granulocytes.

1097 **E** (S&F, ch121)

It is thought that fewer bacteria in the small bowel limit bile acid conversion to carcinogens and the rapid transit limits contact between carcinogens and the mucosa. A diet high in animal fat and protein is associated with small bowel adenocarcinoma. Small and large bowel adenocarcinomas have similar genetic mechanisms of development. The most common cause of death in patients with FAP after colectomy is proximal small bowel cancer, but these cancers can occur in patients without FAP. Tobacco use and alcohol consumption did not affect the development of small intestine cancer.

1098 **D** (S&F, ch102)

Patient preparation is important. An increase to more than 20 ppm is what is used. Intestinal aspirate is still the gold standard. Rapid transit can lead to false-positive test results. Use of antibacterial mouthwash is not standard (although some recommend it).

1099 **D** (S&F, ch107)

Enterohemorrhagic *E. coli* is the most common pathogen isolated in patients with bloody diarrhea. The most common food to harbor this is hamburger meat. The O157:H7 serotype can be associated with hemolytic-uremic syndrome and thrombotic thrombocytopenic purpura. The organisms in choices **C** and **E** can cause bloody diarrhea but are much less common. The others usually cause a nonbloody, watery diarrhea. Only O157:H7 has been associated with hemolytic-uremic syndrome and thrombocytopenic purpura (see figure here and table at end of chapter).

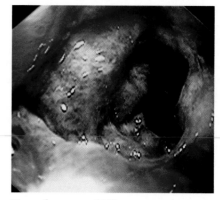

Figure for answer **1099**

1100 **E** (S&F, ch117)

Diverticulosis shows striking geographic variability. The disorder is extraordinarily rare in rural Africa and Asia; conversely, the highest prevalence rates are in the United States, Europe, and Australia. "Westernization" of diet increases the risk of diverticulosis, as in Asians who migrate. Diverticuli do not involve the muscle itself but are rather herniations of mucosa and submucosa through a defect in the muscularis. Common diverticula, strictly speaking, are pseudodiverticuli. In Western countries, diverticula occur mainly in the left colon, with as many as 90% of patients having involvement of the sigmoid and only 15% have right-sided involvement. In contrast, right-sided involvement is predominant in Asian countries.

1101 **D** (S&F, ch112)
Approximately 20% of patients have pancolitis at the time of diagnosis. Another 45% have inflammation limited to the rectosigmoid and 35% have disease beyond the sigmoid, but not involving the entire colon.

1102 **B** (S&F, ch120)
The mortality rate of patients with acute colonic pseudo-obstruction varies from 0% to 32%. The diameter of the colon may be a risk factor for mortality. When surgical decompression is used in mechanically obstructed patients with cecal diameters of 9 cm, there is a dramatic reduction in mortality. This is the basis for the use of the 9-cm cutoff as a sign of "impending perforation" in patients with acute colonic pseudo-obstruction.

1103 **A** (S&F, ch103)
Trying to keep as much of the colon intact as possible is highly beneficial for absorption; 100 cm or less of intact jejunum is insufficient for absorption leading to total parenteral nutrition for most of these patients.

1104 **A** (S&F, ch109)
The stool ELISA for giardiasis is the first test that should be done because it is more than 90% sensitive and nearly 100% specific. As cysts and trophozoites are only present in the stool intermittently, routine stool tests for ova and parasites are approximately 50% sensitive. Duodenal aspirate and/or biopsy are accurate but more invasive. The modified trichrome or iodine stains can be used to detect *Giardia*, but acid-fast stain cannot (see figure).

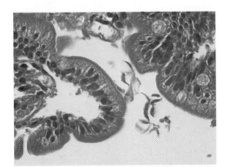

Figure for answer **1104**

1105 **C** (S&F, ch112)
The immune system of the intestine is in a constant state of mild inflammation in response to the ever-present bacteria and antigenic stimuli of the gut. Normally, this is a very well-regulated system, but in UC, abnormalities of both the humoral and cell-mediated immune systems contribute to the development of chronic uncontrolled inflammation. Increased production of plasma cells is seen in UC, and a disproportionate amount of IgG-producing plasma cells are seen: IgG_1 and IgG_3 are preferentially synthesized in UC, as compared with IgG_2 in Crohn's disease. UC is believed to be a type of autoimmune disease and is associated with other autoimmune disorders, including thyroid disease, diabetes mellitus, and pernicious anemia. Further, patients with UC are found to have various types of autoantibodies, with the best described being one that forms in response to a 40-kd epithelial antigen that is unique to the inflamed colonic mucosa in UC.

1106 **B** (S&F, ch121)
Over the past several years, studies have shown the superiority of capsule endoscopy over enteroclysis, push enteroscopy, and CT in detecting small intestine cancer. Angiography is of limited value.

1107 **B** (S&F, ch110)
A. caninum is a common hookworm in dogs and cats and has a worldwide distribution. See the figure for an example of the serpiginous rash. It may cause eosinophilic enteritis with eosinophils found on distal small bowel biopsy specimens and not gastric biopsy specimens, differentiating this from eosinophilic gastroenteritis. The ileum may reveal small aphthous ulcers. The worm does not lay eggs and is difficult to detect. The cellophane test is used to detect pinworm.

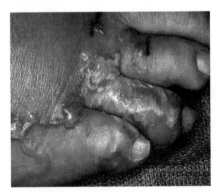

Figure for answer **1107**

1108 **C** (S&F, ch100)
The terminal products of luminal starch digestion, together with the major disaccharides in the diet (sucrose and lactose), cannot be absorbed intact and are hydrolyzed by specific brush border membrane hydrolases that are maximally expressed in the villi of the duodenum and jejunum. The three major diet-derived monosaccharides (glucose, galactose, and fructose) are absorbed by the saturable carrier-mediated transport systems located in the brush border membranes of enterocytes in the proximal and mid small intestine.

1109 **C** (S&F, ch118)
These are the Rome III criteria. Answers **A** and **B** are Manning criteria. Sex, age, anal fissures, or hemorrhoids are not part of any criteria.

1110 **E** (S&F, ch124)

The most frequent intestinal organs involved are the rectosigmoid (96%), appendix (10%), and ileum (5%). Clinical diagnosis may be difficult with onset usually between the ages of 20 and 45 years. Colonoscopy is often normal except for areas of extrinsic compression or strictures with intact mucosa. More helpful is a barium enema, which demonstrates submucosal polypoid masses or areas of circumstantial narrowing of the lumen (see figure).

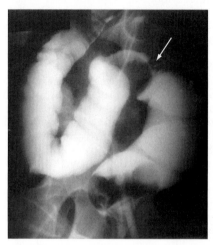

Figure for answer **1110**

1111 **B** (S&F, ch107)

Inflammatory diarrhea is usually characterized by small-volume, bloody, mucoid stools. The patient often has left lower quadrant pain and appears toxic. The site involved is usually the colon. Patients with noninflammatory diarrhea have large-volume, watery, nonbloody stool that more often leads to dehydration. This generally involves the small bowel. The distinction aids in determining the etiology and which patients require a further evaluation (see figure here and tables at end of chapter).

1112 **B** (S&F, ch108)

Approximately 15% to 30% of patients successfully treated with vancomycin or metronidazole relapse after completion of their initial antibiotic therapy. Recurrences may be seen for as long as two months after stopping the antibiotic therapy. Recurrence of *C. difficile* colitis and diarrhea is confirmed by stool toxin assay. Patients with recurrence typically are treated with a second course of the same antibiotic. Institute the initial plan, but treatment is usually for 14 days; the success rate is approximately 40%.

1113 **C** (S&F, ch111)

The adaptive immune response is a complex pathway (see figure) important in the pathogenesis

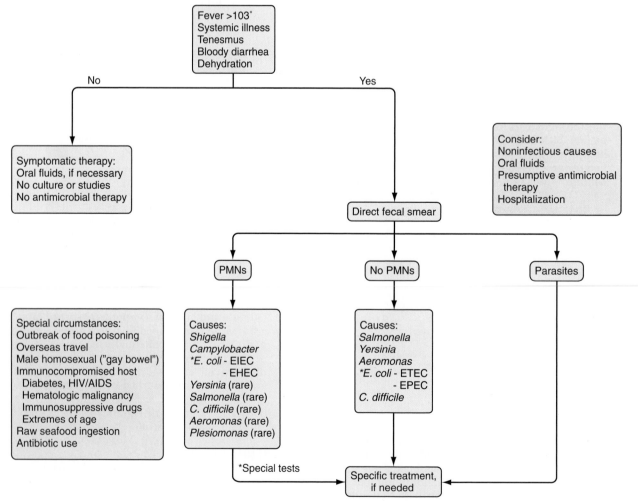

Figure for answer **1111**

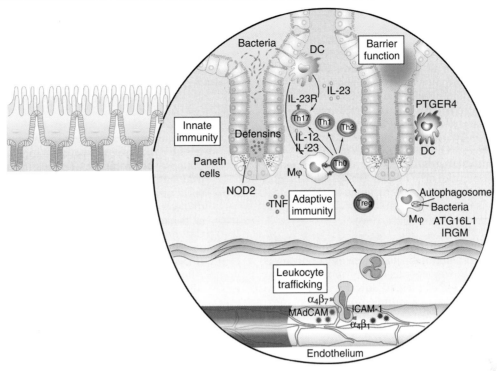

Figure for answer **1113**

of Crohn's disease. TNF is a key proinflammatory cytokine that has many different functions: granuloma formation, neutrophil activation, expression of both major histocompatibility complex class II on intestinal epithelial cells and adhesion molecules on intestinal endothelial cells, and binding of TNF to its receptor, which costimulates T-cell activation. Nuclear factor κB is a key nuclear transcription factor that regulates the transcription of IL-1, IL-6, IL-8, TNF, and other inflammatory peptides. IL-2 is an important growth factor for T cells. T-regulatory cells are the "policemen" of the adaptive immune response and help to keep the inflammatory response in check. If these cells are either deficient or ineffective, the proinflammatory response is not appropriately dampened and can lead to the inflammatory changes seen in Crohn's disease (see figure for overall scheme of pathogenesis of Crohn's disease).

1114   **E** (S&F, ch117)
There is no clear indication for any therapy or follow-up in patients incidentally diagnosed with diverticulosis. Diverticuli are common findings in increasing numbers of people undergoing endoscopic screening for colon cancer. A possible prophylactic benefit of a high-fiber diet has been suggested. Conversely, diets high in fat and red meat were associated with an increase of diverticular disease. Prospective, randomized trials are lacking, but some studies suggest that patients with asymptomatic diverticulosis may benefit from increasing fruit and vegetable fiber intake while decreasing their fat and red meat consumption.

1115   **A** (S&F, ch120)
The major mechanism for postoperative ileus is thought to be increased sympathetic neural activity

resulting in blockade of acetylcholine release from excitatory nerves. Surgical incisions and bowel manipulation can increase this activity. Nonadrenergic, noncholinergic activity, inflammatory cytokines, and opiates all play an additional role but are not thought to be primary.

1116   **A** (S&F, ch119)
The most common cause of ileus is abdominal or retroperitoneal surgery. Other causes of ileus are inflammatory, metabolic, neurogenic, and drug-related.

1117   **E** (S&F, ch122)
Embryologicially, the dentate line represents the junction between endoderm and ectoderm. Proximal to the dentate line, there is sympathetic and parasympathetic innervation; distally, the nerve supply is somatic. Therefore, above the dentate line, pain sensation is negligible and a biopsy can be performed painlessly. Venous drainage from the canal is by both the systemic and portal systems. The internal hemorrhoidal plexus drains into the superior rectal veins, which drain into the inferior mesenteric vein and then into the portal vein. The distal part of the anal canal drains via the external hemorrhoidal plexus through the middle rectal and pudendal veins into the iliac vein.

1118   **C** (S&F, ch123)
This family meets the Amsterdam criteria for HNPCC. This syndrome is inherited in an autosomal dominant fashion. There is a predominance of proximal tumors. Germline mutations in the *hMSH2* or *hMLH1* gene are present in 80% of colon cancers. There is an increased frequency of cancers of the female genital tract. This syndrome accounts for approximately 6% of all the colorectal cancers,

whereas FAP accounts for less than 1% (see three tables at end of chapter).

1119 **B** (S&F, ch112)

The inflammation of UC is generally more severe distally than proximally and is characterized by continuous inflammatory changes including hyperemia, edema, granularity, and ulcers. There is almost always a sharp demarcation between inflamed and normal colon, without the patchy, "skip" areas of Crohn's disease. That being said, as many as 75% of patients with left-sided UC will have periappendiceal inflammation or a "cecal red patch." Rectal sparing may be seen in patients treated with topical medications in the form of enemas or suppositories.

1120 **C** (S&F, ch121)

Two thirds of small bowel neoplasms are malignant. The most common neoplasm is adenocarcinoma. Small bowel neoplasms are more common in men and the elderly. Small bowel neoplasms are the least common gastrointestinal malignancy, occurring less commonly than those in the colon, esophagus, or stomach.

1121 **B** (S&F, ch107)

Shigellosis may cause 10% to 20% of all diarrheal illnesses worldwide. It causes classic dysentery, as described in this patient. Most transmission is person to person, although some foods can be vehicles. The treatment includes supportive care with rehydration, electrolyte repletion, and usually antibiotics. If a mild case occurs, it may be self-limited and antibiotics can be withheld. Antidiarrheals alone do not help and may aggravate the illness. However, it has been shown that ciprofloxacin with an antidiarrheal can shorten the duration and decrease the amount of diarrhea. The illness can be severe and may appear like UC (see figure).

1122 **D** (S&F, ch117)

Use of barium in intestinal perforation carries a risk of barium peritonitis. Only water-soluble contrast enemas (i.e., gastrograffin) should be used in the setting of acute diverticulitis. CT is more sensitive and specific than a barium enema. Endoscopy should be limited and generally avoided in the initial evaluation of patients with suspected acute diverticulitis. A limited rigid or flexible sigmoidoscopy with minimal insufflation may be helpful to exclude alternative diagnoses such as IBD, carcinoma, and ischemic colitis. When the acute setting has passed, however, colonoscopy should be electively performed to confirm the presence of diverticuli and to exclude competing diagnoses, particularly neoplasia, one to three months after the event.

1123 **A** (S&F, ch99)

When there is an increase of colonic bile acids, which can be seen in patients in whom there is ileal malabsorption (often due to surgical resection) or oral supplementation, diarrhea can result. Typically only 7α-dihydroxy bile acids, such as chenodeoxycholic acid, are associated with diarrhea. Bile salts cause colonic epithelial cells to secrete Cl^- via Ca^{2+} and PKC delta cascade.

1124 **D** (S&F, ch115)

After gluten withdrawal has failed, glucocorticosteroids are often tried, with varying success. Patients who do respond to glucocorticosteroids often remain steroid dependent. With the knowledge that refractory celiac disease and ulcerative enteritis are cryptic T-cell lymphomas, open-label studies using immunosuppressant therapy have been undertaken. In patients with refractory celiac disease, prednisone and azathioprine are more promising than cyclosporine, as demonstrated in separate trials (see figure).

1125 **C** (S&F, ch111)

This patient is presenting with classic signs and symptoms of a right lower quadrant abscess, including pain, fever, and a mass on physical examination. An estimated one fourth of Crohn's disease patients will present with an intra-abdominal abscess at some time in their disease course. He is at higher risk because he is being treated with glucocorticosteroids. The patient needs an immediate CT scan of the abdomen and pelvis to confirm this suspicion, and simultaneously empiric antibiotics should be started, generally a fluoroquinolone and metronidazole. Depending on the size and location, the abscess may be treated with antibiotics alone, percutaneous drainage, and/or surgery. A small bowel series is not the best study to assess for an intra-abdominal abscess because it assesses the luminal tract only. It is incorrect to increase his dose of glucocorticoste-

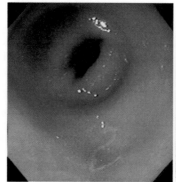
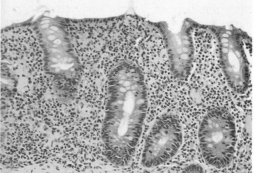

Figure for answer **1121**

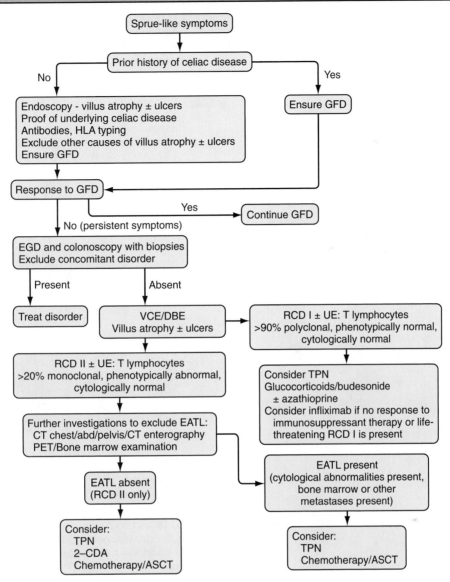

Figure for answer **1124**

roids or begin another immunosuppressant such as infliximab, both of which could worsen the abscess.

1126 **B** (S&F, ch102)
SIBO is associated with megaloblastic anemia, usually secondary to vitamin B_{12} deficiency. This occurs as a result of bacterial consumption of the vitamin within the intestinal lumen. Deficiencies of nicotinamide and thiamine have been reported. Folate tends to be high because bacteria synthesize folate.

1127 **A** (S&F, ch105)
Parasitic diarrheas (giardiasis and amebiasis) are the most common diarrheas in travelers to tropical countries. In a recent study of 17,353 travelers to tropical countries, acute diarrhea occurred in approximately 22% and chronic diarrhea occurred in 11.3%.

1128 **B** (S&F, ch97)
Splanchnic afferent nerve fibers are thought to mediate visceral distention via their connections with mural mechanoreceptors. Vagal afferent fibers are believed to be more important for physiologic homeostasis than for pain perception.

1129 **A** (S&F, ch107)
There are many predisposing conditions including hemolytic anemias, states of immunosuppression, and achlorhydria. Although patients with *Salmonella* and various implants, as in choice **E**, may need to receive antibiotics to prevent deep-seeded infections, they are not predisposed to acquiring *Salmonella* (see table at end of chapter).

1130 **C** S&F, ch110)
This man has schistosomiasis (see figure on p. 272). Different species are endemic to Africa, the Middle East, Central and South America, and parts of the Caribbean. The worms reside in the mesenteric vessels and can eventually reach the liver. Katayama fever is seen in acute infection from an early immune response to the eggs and leads to fever, malaise, arthralgias, myalgias, diarrhea, and cough. The eggs that lodge in the portal veins lead to presinusoidal portal hypertension. Synthetic function of the liver is intact, cirrhosis does not develop, and liver biopsy is not sensitive for the diagnosis. Praziquantel is the treatment. Chagas' disease is transmitted by the reduviid bug.

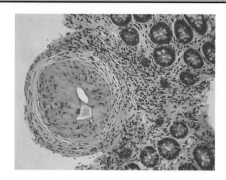

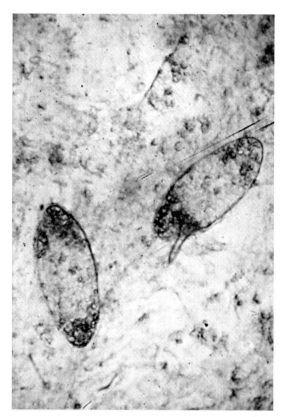

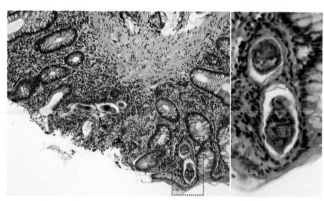

Figure for answer **1130**

1131 **D** (S&F, ch109)
Nitazoxanide has been shown to be consistently effective in the treatment of cryptosporidiosis in immunocompetent hosts. The other three medications listed are not effective.

1132 **C** (S&F, ch110)
Enterobius vermicularis is the most common worm encountered by physicians in developed countries (see figure and Video 3 [www.expertconsult.com]). The best treatment for this nematode should include treating the patient and all household members, whether or not symptoms are present, with mebendazole or albendazole. A second dose 15 days later helps prevent reinfection, which is common.

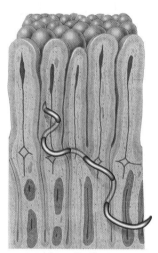

Figure for answer **1132**

1133 **D** (S&F, ch120)
Chronic idiopathic intestinal pseudo-obstruction is a sporadic nonfamilial visceral neuropathy which can result from injury to the myenteric plexus from drug toxicity, ischemia, radiation, or viral infection. Chronic idiopathic intestinal pseudo-obstruction is the most common diagnosis given to cases of intestinal pseudo-obstruction. Patients with chronic idiopathic intestinal pseudo-obstruction often have disturbed motility of the entire gastrointestinal tract without urinary tract impairment. Histologic examination of the myenteric plexus may reveal a reduction in the number or an abnormal morphology of neurons.

1134 **A** (S&F, ch123)
FOBT has been shown in large-scale, randomized, controlled studies to decrease mortality from colorectal cancer with yearly and biannual testing. A decrease in colorectal cancer mortality has been demonstrated with sigmoidoscopy. The National Polyp Study suggests that removal of adenomatous polyps reduces the mortality from colorectal cancer. Thus, it has been inferred that colonoscopy should have the same effect. The other choices have not been shown to reduce mortality (see table at end of chapter).

1135 **B** (S&F, ch98)
High-threshold, voltage-gated calcium channels (L-type) play a crucial role in colonic motility. These

channels open when the membrane potential of smooth muscle cells is depolarized beyond a voltage threshold and are responsible for the rapid up-stroke of smooth muscle action potentials. The exact physiology of the other channels as it pertains to colonic motility is not known.

1136 **D** (S&F, ch113)
This patient has signs and symptoms of pouchitis. Although antidiarrheals may be appropriate in this setting for patients who have only diarrhea without other clinical manifestations, they would not be the correct choice for this patient. Although it is believed that the normal colonic mucosa uses short-chain fatty acids (SCFAs) as a source of calories and diversion colitis results from deprivation of SCFAs and responds to SCFA enemas, ileal pouches contain high concentrations of SCFAs and therefore this is not an appropriate treatment for pouchitis. Glucocorticosteroid enemas, in addition to other treatments for IBD, may be used to treat pouchitis when patients do not respond to antibiotics, which are the first-line therapy. Metronidazole (500 mg orally twice daily for one month) is the mainstay of antibiotic treatment, but ciprofloxacin is also commonly used. Patients generally respond very well to such antibiotic treatment. Bismuth salicylate, 270 mg/day, may be effective in those patients with antibiotic-resistant pouchitis.

1137 **A** (S&F, ch118)
A meta-analysis of randomized, controlled trials concluded that antispasmodics were superior to placebo in the treatment of abdominal pain in IBS. They are more useful for postprandial abdominal pain when taken before meals. There is no proven advantage of sublingual anticholinergics. Loperamide is effective for diarrhea but not abdominal pain or bloating. Stimulant laxatives are safe in constipation-predominant IBS. Codeine phosphate should be avoided because of its side effects and high risk of inducing drug dependence.

1138 **E** (S&F, ch108)
Risk factors for development of pseudomembranous enterocolitis in the absence of *C. difficile* includes intestinal surgery, intestinal ischemia, and other enteric infections. Pseudomembranous enterocolitis is associated with a wide variety of other intestinal disorders, and reports have included associations with *Shigella* infection, Crohn's disease, neonatal necrotizing enterocolitis intestinal obstruction, Hirschsprung's disease, and chronic carcinoma. Before the identification of *C. difficile*, the most common cause of pseudomembranous colitis was *S. aureus* infection, identified in stool cultures of patients with postoperative pseudomembranous enterocolitis.

1139 **C** (S&F, ch123)
Advanced colorectal cancer has a high recurrence rate. Therefore, those with positive regional lymph nodes or whose primary tumor has extended into the serosa should consider adjuvant therapy. The standard regimen for stage 3 disease has been 5-fluorouracil and leucovorin. Controversy remains as to the appropriateness of adjuvant therapy in stage 2 disease. This regimen prolongs overall

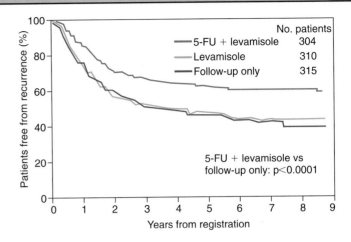

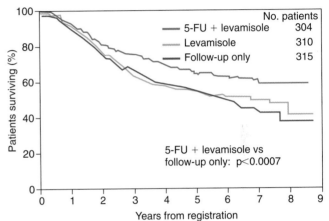

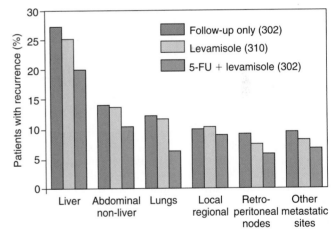

Figure for answer **1139**

disease-free survival. Additionally, this regimen is more convenient and efficacious than 5-fluorouracil and levamisole (see figure).

1140 **D** (S&F, ch114)
A normal WBC count cannot be used to exclude early AMI, just as a high WBC count does not make the diagnosis. However, it should be noted that 75% of patients have a leukocytosis greater than 15,000 cells/mm³. No serum markers, including phosphate, amylase, or D-lactate, have been shown to have adequate sensitivity and specificity. In

addition, serum markers, when elevated, usually indicate late-stage disease. Elevated intraperitoneal amylase as well as alkaline phosphatase is useful but not diagnostic of AMI. Amylase is not secondary to pancreatitis but rather rapid absorption of intraluminal amylase secondary to a defect in barrier function.

1141 **C** (S&F, ch118)
Contrary to what many clinicians believe, nighttime symptoms are common in IBS and do not discriminate IBS from organic disease, although weight loss, rectal bleeding, late age at onset, and dysphagia are alarm symptoms that warrant further investigation.

1142 **A** (S&F, ch109)
In the immunocompromised HIV-positive patient, immune reconstitution with HAART is the most important treatment. Nitazoxanide is effective in the immunocompetent host. Paromomycin, with or without azithromycin, is another option in the immunocompromised patient.

1143 **E** (S&F, ch103)
Resection of less than 100 cm of ileum causes moderate bile and malabsorption, whereas more than 100 cm causes severe malabsorption. More than 60 cm of resected ileum is usually required before vitamin B_{12} malabsorption occurs. Additionally, cholestyramine generally helps those with mild to moderate malabsorption but may worsen the diarrhea in patients with more intensive resection.

1144 **D** (S&F, ch123)
Celecoxib is the only FDA-approved medication for polyp reduction in familial polyposis. A double-blind, placebo-controlled trial showed a decrease in the number of polyps in patients with FAP treated with six months of celecoxib. The others do not have FDA approval, but many studies do show a benefit with these agents.

1145 **D** (S&F, ch111)
Incidence rates are increasing in some areas of the world such as South Korea and Denmark, but are stable in Olmstead County, Minnesota. Overall, similar to UC, there is a north–south risk gradient in Europe and the United States, with more northern countries and states having higher incidences of disease. The prevalence of Crohn's disease in the United States among adults is approximately 201 per 100,000, but only 43 per 100,000 in teens and children. There is a slight female predominance of Crohn's disease in adults, although this is reversed in the pediatric population. Crohn's disease is very uncommon in Africa and South America, except for the white population of South Africa.

1146 **A** (S&F, ch112)
5-ASAs are effective in the induction and maintenance of remission for mild to moderate UC. Recent data from the ASCEND I and II trials have shown a dose effect in patients with moderate disease, such that 4.8 g/day is more effective than 2.4 g/day; in patients with mild disease, this dose effect was not seen. 5-ASAs have not been evaluated in a randomized, controlled trial for the treatment of severe UC. Sulfasalazine was the first 5-ASA used to treat UC

and consists of a sulfapyridine moiety linked to the 5-ASA by an azo-bond that is cleaved by colonic bacteria azoreductase. The sulfapyridine has been linked to most of the side effects of this medication, and since then, multiple other non–sulfa-containing formulations and controlled-release systems have been developed. Overall, the efficacy of all the 5-ASAs is similar. Although topical (rectal) 5-ASAs including enemas for left-sided disease and suppositories for rectal and distal sigmoid disease are effective when used alone, greater benefit may be achieved when combined with oral 5-ASAs. The most recently developed 5-ASA is a multimatrix mesalamine formulated at a higher strength to allow for once-daily dosing.

1147 **E** (S&F, ch118)
Tensing the abdominal wall by flexing the chin on the chest or sitting up partially lessens tenderness that is caused by an intra-abdominal process. If tensing the abdominal wall increases abdominal tenderness, then a localized point of abdominal wall origin of pain should be sought (positive Carnett's test). Identification of such a point might enable treatment with an injection of lidocaine/triamcinolone.

1148 **B** (S&F, ch123)
Obesity, a high-fat and high–red meat diet, and cigarette smoking are associated with elevated risk, whereas a high-fiber diet and increasing physical activity are associated with lower risk (see table at end of chapter).

1149 **A** (S&F, ch118)
Constipation-predominant IBS may be secondary to increased segmental nonpropulsive contractions, decreased high-amplitude propagated contractions, or reduced rectal sensation. In IBS, diarrhea may occur from multiple colonic mechanisms including increased high-amplitude propagated contractions, an enhanced gastrocolonic response, and rectal hypersensitivity. A hypertensive internal rectal sphincter may be seen in Hirschsprung's disease.

1150 **D** (S&F, ch110)
Patients colonized with these tapeworms are usually asymptomatic. However, ingestion of the *T. solium* eggs leads to cysticercosis when the eggs disseminate. Local inflammation occurs in the nervous system and the heart and can be fatal. In endemic areas, neurocysticercosis is a common cause of epilepsy. The diagnosis can be made by finding eggs or proglottids in the stool, although multiple samples may be needed. A single oral dose of praziquantel, 10 mg/kg, is effective (see Videos 4 and 5 at www.expertconsult.com)

1151 **C** (S&F, ch122)
Hemorrhoids are a normal part of human anatomy, in contrast to hemorrhoidal disease, which presents as prolapse, bleeding, and itching. Hemorrhoids are dilated vascular channels located in three fairly constant locations: left lateral, right posterior, and right anterior.

Traditionally, internal hemorrhoids are classified into four grades: (1) first-degree hemorrhoids, which bleed with defecation; (2) second-degree hemorrhoids, which prolapse with defecation but return spontaneously to their normal position; (3) third-degree hemorrhoids, which prolapse through the anal canal at any time but especially with defecation and can be replaced manually; and (4) fourth-degree hemorrhoids, which are permanently prolapsed. Although the exact incidence of hemorrhoidal disease is unknown, it is thought to be present in 10% to 25% of the adult population.

1152 **C** (S&F, ch115)
This barium radiograph of the small bowel shows diffuse small intestine ulcerations in a patient with refractory celiac disease (ulcerative enteritis). There is diffuse involvement of the small intestine with multiple ulcerations and separation and thickening of the loops of jejunum and ileum.

1153 **D** (S&F, ch123)
Rectal examination may detect distal rectal cancers but is not recommended for screening by the current guidelines. Additionally, a single hemoccult test during a rectal examination has not been shown to be accurate for screening purposes. Carcinoembryonic antigen determination is not suitable for screening due to its low sensitivity and specificity but is useful in the preoperative staging and postoperative follow-up of patients with colon cancer. Genetic testing may be appropriate for certain high-risk groups but not for average-risk groups (see table for answer 949 at end of chapter).

1154 **B** (S&F, ch118)
Selective serotonin reuptake inhibitors accelerate small bowel transit and may be more beneficial in constipation-predominant IBS. Tricyclics are safe and effective, even at doses below full antidepressant dose levels. They are most beneficial for diarrhea-predominant IBS. Octreotide reduces intestinal transit, secretion, and sensation in IBS but is impractical to use for diarrhea in IBS. Clonidine may be useful in diarrhea-predominant IBS because it enhances rectal compliance and reduces fasting colonic motor activity. Colchicine increases spontaneous bowel movements and accelerates colonic transit and has been used in constipation-predominant IBS.

1155 **E** (S&F, ch102)
SIBO is associated with all diseases listed along with others such as scleroderma, pseudo-obstruction, and radiation injury (see table at end of chapter).

1156 **B** (S&F, ch104)
Malignancy, ulcerative jejunoileitis, and collagenous sprue are the major complications of celiac disease. In the past, patients with celiac disease or dermatitis herpetiformis had been reported to have a 10-fold increased risk of certain gastrointestinal tract malignancies and a 40- to 70-fold increased risk of non-Hodgkin's lymphoma. Recent studies, however, indicate that the risk of malignancy, and particularly lymphoma, is much less than initially thought. Small intestine lymphoma, often multifocal and diffuse, accounts for one half to two thirds of the malignancies complicating celiac disease and typically occurs after 20 to 40 years of disease (see Chapters 28 and 112). Whereas

in the general population, most small intestine lymphomas are of B-cell origin, intestinal lymphoma in celiac disease is typically of T-cell origin and the term enteropathy-associated T-cell lymphoma was coined to describe both the intestinal and extraintestinal lymphomas that complicate celiac disease. Carcinoma, particularly of the oropharynx, esophagus, and small intestine, complicates celiac disease.

1157 **A** (S&F, ch112)
Nonsmokers are more likely to get UC than smokers, with a relative risk of between two and six. UC patients who smoke may have a less severe course of disease, with fewer hospitalizations and decreased rates of pouchitis after colectomy. Those who quit smoking are especially at risk of the development of UC. A dose effect appears to exist as well, with light smokers at greater risk of UC than heavy smokers.

1158 **D** (S&F, ch120)
Familial causes of CIP such as familial visceral myopathy are rare. There are three types of FVM. In type II FVM, there are mitochondrial DNA disorders, and this condition is also called mitochondrial neurogastrointestinal encephalopathy. Histologically, all three types exhibit degeneration and fibrosis of gastrointestinal smooth muscle, not neurons. Hirschsprung's disease is an example of a familial visceral neuropathy characterized by aganglionosis within the IAS due to a disorder of colonization by migrating neural crest–derived neurons.

1159 **E** (S&F, ch118)
Methane gas production, which occurs in the minority of the population with methagenic fecal flora, is now well established to be associated with constipation.

1160 **C** (S&F, ch106)
PAS-positive cells reflect the presence of glycoprotein residue of degraded bacterial cell wall. They are associated with *Tropheryma whippelii*, *Mycobacterium avium* complex, histoplasmosis, macroglobulinemia, intestinal xanthelasmas, and pseudomelanosis duodeni.

1161 **B** (S&F, ch116)
Appendicitis is the most common acute abdominal emergency seen in developed countries, although the rate of appendicitis is as much as 10 times lower in many less developed African countries. Incidence of disease peaks between 15 and 19 years of age.

1162 **C** (S&F, ch120)
Carcinoid tumors, small cell lung cancer, and epidermoid carcinoma of the lip are associated with CIP through a paraneoplastic syndrome caused by a visceral neuropathy.

1163 **B** (S&F, ch119)
Partial SBO resolves with nonoperative treatment in 80% to 90% of patients; 85% to 95% of patients whose partial SBO ultimately resolves will show substantial improvement within the first 48 hours of treatment. Gangrenous bowel can occur, and

patients need to be monitored closely for any clinical signs. Partial SBO cannot always be distinguished from complete SBO radiographically. Oral gastrograffin administration may enhance resolution of a partial SBO but is not the treatment of choice.

1164   **B** (S&F, ch115)
Clinical presentations vary with location and degree of intestinal involvement and range from anemia and hypoproteinemia to abdominal pain, hemorrhage, obstruction, and perforation. Patients with nonspecific ulcers of the small intestine present most commonly with symptoms of intermittent SBO (63%). Symptoms may be present from a few days to many years before diagnosis. The average age at presentation is between the fifth and sixth decades of life, and no sex predominance was noted.

1165   **B** (S&F, ch118)
In patients with IBS, a history of sexual, physical, or emotional abuse is reported more often than in those without IBS. Abuse does not alter rectal sensation. Patients with IBS are more likely to report greater lifetime and daily stressful events. Childhood stress may be particularly more important. In rat studies, stress leads to accelerated colonic transit.

1166   **D** (S&F, ch113)
A normal colon absorbs 1 L or more of water and 100 mEq of sodium chloride each day. The colon can adjust its capacity for water absorption and sodium excretion depending on intake and losses. In patients who have ileostomies, however, this is not possible: they lose approximately 30 to 40 mEq of sodium per day. Further, ileostomies discharge approximately 300 to 800 g of material per day, 90% of which is water: this amounts to approximately 500 to 600 mL of water per day. Therefore, patients with ileostomies have chronic oliguria and also have altered urinary Na^+/K^+ ratios as the kidney tries to compensate for these higher water and sodium losses. As a result, these patients are more prone to develop kidney stones, usually calcium or urate. The ileum absorbs vitamin B_{12}, and thus those with colectomies performed for the indication of UC should not be at increased risk of vitamin B_{12} malabsorption because the ileum is not resected in this surgery as it might be in a patient with Crohn's disease who undergoes colectomy.

1167   **D** (S&F, ch112)
A CT scan may show thickening of the colon in patients with UC, but will not distinguish between different types of colitides (e.g., IBD vs. infection). If there is strong suspicion of a complication such as perforation, obstruction, and abscess, a CT scan may be warranted. Barium enema was previously one of the primary diagnostic tools for UC but has fallen out of favor with the advent of endoscopy. Findings seen with UC include mucosal granularity, thickened and irregular mucosa, and ulcerations; with long-standing disease, loss of haustral folds leads to a featureless "lead-pipe" appearance (see figure). Barium enema may still be superior to colonoscopy in delineation of strictures. A full colonoscopy is not necessary and may risk

perforation in patients with more severe disease. Colonoscopy should be undertaken after the patient has improved to establish the extent of gross and histologic disease and should include intubation of the terminal ileum to evaluate for Crohn's disease. An unprepped flexible sigmoidoscopy is the test of choice as UC always involves the rectum and extends proximally; further, biopsy specimens will lend histologic support to the diagnosis. It is best not to prep the bowel as this can lead to hyperemia, which may confound the gross changes. IBD serologies such as pANCA lack the sensitivity and specificity to be used as diagnostic tests.

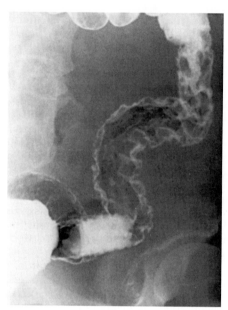

Figure for answer **1167**

1168   **D** (S&F, ch108)
Toxin A is an inflammatory enterotoxin and toxin B is an extremely potent cytotoxin but has minimal enterotoxin activity in animals. Initial studies suggest that toxin B did not contribute to diarrhea and colitis in humans. It is known, however, that toxins A and B cause injury and electrophysiologic changes in human colonic explants in vitro and that toxin B is 10 times more potent than toxin A in inducing both of these changes.

1169   **E** (S&F, ch120)
Paraneoplastic visceral neuropathy is an example of an inflammatory neuropathy. Inflammatory neuropathies are characterized by an intense inflammatory infiltrate of CD3+ lymphocytes that are composed of both CD4 and CD* lymphocytes and classically confined to the mesenteric plexus. The other choices are all examples of noninflammatory or degenerative neuropathies and are the result of dysfunctional mitochondria, altered calcium signaling, and accumulation of free radicals that leads to eventual degeneration and loss of neurons.

1170   **C** (S&F, ch98)
In response to distention of the rectum, there is simultaneous activation of the enteric descending inhibitory pathway. This causes relaxation of the

IAS and the extrinsic pathway, which leads to contraction of the EAS. This rectoanal inhibitory reflex allows entry of a small amount of feces into the proximal rectum while continence is maintained by the EAS. This allows the rectum to temporarily store material until defecation is desired.

1171 **C** (S&F, ch118)

The best accepted risk factor for IBS is bacterial gastroenteritis. Depression and hypochondriasis may increase the risk of postinfectious IBS. Food intolerance is another possible IBS risk factor. Glucocorticoid users may be at a lower risk of IBS.

1172 **D** (S&F, ch110)

The patient has the liver fluke *Clonorchis sinensis*, which is endemic to China, Hong Kong, Taiwan, and North Vietnam. *Opisthorchis* species are closely related and endemic to Thailand, Laos, Russia, and Ukraine. Both species cause a markedly increased risk of cholangiocarcinoma. Most infections are asymptomatic unless the worm burden is heavy. Peripheral eosinophilia does occur. Diagnosis is made by finding parasite eggs in the stool. Additionally, ultrasonography and ERCP (see Video 7 at www.expertconsult.com) may reveal evidence of the organism. The treatment of choice is praziquantel, although albendazole is an alternative.

1173 **E** (S&F, ch109)

Medications for amebiasis are either luminal or tissue amebicides. Luminal amebicides include iodoquinol, diloxanide furoate, and paromomycin. Paromomycin is preferred because it is safer and more effective and requires a shorter course. The tissue amebicides include metronidazole, tinidazole, nitazoxanide, erythromycin, and chloroquine. The first two are most efficacious. Luminal amebicides are used for noninvasive disease, and a tissue amebicide followed by a luminal agent is required for invasive disease (see table at end of chapter).

1174 **C** (S&F, ch113)

Stomal obstruction is not as commonly seen with newer surgical techniques, but results in cramping abdominal pain and increased ileal output (as much as 4 L/day) secondary to intestinal secretion from dilation of the proximal intestine. The etiology of prestomal ileitis is unclear, but in addition to possible obstructive symptoms, patients may also exhibit fever, anemia, and tachycardia. Punched-out ulcers are seen on mucosal inspection. Backwash ileitis is not a risk factor for prestomal ileitis and regresses with removal of the colon. Parastomal hernias are one of the more common complications seen with a Brooke ileostomy. Obesity, steroid and/or immunomodulator use, older age, malignancy, chronic respiratory disease associated with increased intra-abdominal pressure, wound infection, and malnutrition are risk factors for developing a parastomal hernia. Recurrence of the parastomal hernia is seen in as many as 76% of patients who undergo relocation of the stoma; prosthetic mesh for parastomal hernia repair has greatly reduced recurrence rates (as low as 10%).

1175 **C** (S&F, ch101)

Fat analysis by microscopic examination of a random stool sample is performed by placing the stool on a glass slide and adding drops of acetic acid as well as Sudan III stain. A count as high as 100 globules per high-power field is normal. Fecal fat excretion of less than 7 g per day with a fat intake of 100 g per day is usually considered normal. An acid steatocrit is calculated when a sample of stool is diluted 1:3 with distilled water in a test tube. The acid steatocrit is calculated by determining the ratio of fatty layer to the fatty layer plus the solid layer. A value of less than 31% is normal. A beta-carotene value less than 100 mg/100 mL suggests the presence of steatorrhea and a value less than 47 mg/100 mL is strongly indicative of steatorrhea.

1176 **A** (S&F, ch120)

In patients with smooth muscle dysfunction, manometry demonstrates a decrease in amplitude of contractions in the affected bowel segment. This pattern generally is found during both the fasting and fed periods. Antral and duodenal contraction amplitudes are usually reduced. The MMC is usually present but with diminished amplitudes.

1177 **E** (S&F, ch108)

The first step in the management of *C. difficile* diarrhea and colitis is to discontinue the precipitating antibiotics, if possible. Antimotility agents are best avoided because they may impair clearance of toxin from the colon and worsen toxin-induced colonic injury, precipitating ileus of the colon. Metronidazole is generally recommended as the drug of choice for acute *C. difficile* diarrhea and colitis and is generally inexpensive and highly effective. Metronidazole may potentiate the action of warfarin, resulting in prolongation of the prothrombin time and the combination should be avoided. Vancomycin, 125 mg four times daily, is as effective as vancomycin, 500 mg four times daily, and should be administered by mouth because effective colonic luminal concentrations are not achieved when given intravenously. Vancomycin is generally recommended for infections that fail to respond to metronidazole, for patients intolerant to metronidazole, or for patients with fulminant pseudomembranous colitis.

1178 **B** (S&F, ch109)

G. lamblia is ubiquitous and the most frequently found parasite in the United States. Metronidazole, 250 mg orally three times a day for five days, is 80% to 95% effective. Tinidazole, furazolidone, and quinacrine are alternatives. Paromomycin is the treatment of choice in pregnancy because it is not absorbed. Nitazoxanide is very effective and useful in children because it is available in a liquid preparation. Prolonged lactose intolerance may occur after infection.

1179 **D** (S&F, ch107)

All are possible presentations of *Salmonella* infections. Gastroenteritis accounts for 75% of the cases and is the correct answer (see table at end of chapter).

1180 **A** (S&F, ch107)

The key is the branching and distortion of the gland architecture. This only occurs in chronic colitis. In acute colitis due to an infection, the architecture of the glands is not distorted and branching does not occur. The first episode of UC can be mistaken for acute infectious colitis, but a biopsy can usually distinguish the two. A photomicrograph of an acute colitis is pictured (see figure).

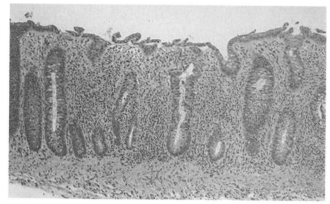

Figure for answer **1180**

1181 **B** (S&F, ch110)

Trichinosis is acquired by ingestion of undercooked contaminated meats, usually pork. The enteral phase occurs initially with nausea, vomiting, diarrhea, abdominal pain, and low-grade fever and is often misdiagnosed as food poisoning or viral gastroenteritis. The parenteral phase starts one week later as the larvae migrate into the muscle, heart, or nervous system. This leads to myalgias, headache, high fever, dysphagia, paresthesias, and periorbital edema. Eosinophilia and an elevated CPK level are present. The diagnosis can be made by finding larvae, not adult worms, on muscle biopsy specimens or by serology. *Trichinella* is not found on stool examination. Albendazole or mebendazole can be used for treatment.

1182 **E** (S&F, ch112)

The biopsy depicted in the figure (see question 1183) shows high-grade dysplasia. After confirmation by a second expert pathologist, a total proctocolectomy should be advised for this patient. Because significant interobserver variability exists among pathologists for the diagnosis of dysplasia and the recommendation for colectomy is not one to be taken lightly, a second opinion must always be obtained. Because there exists a significant risk of a synchronous cancer on colectomy in those patients with high-grade dysplasia (42% in a review study), it would be insufficient to recommend resection of only the part of the colon from which the high-grade dysplasia was found. Further, because of the significant risk of concomitant and future colorectal cancer, it would be incorrect to recommend following this patient with colonoscopy in three months or a year.

1183 **C** (S&F, ch106)

One remarkable epidemiologic feature in an analysis by Dobbin was the strong representation of patients with occupations in the farming and building trades involving work outdoors or frequent contact with animals or soil; of 191 patients for whom data were available, 43 (22%) were farmers and 10 (5%) were carpenters. Patients in all farming-related trades accounted for 34% of the total. By comparison, the proportion of farm workers among the total workforce in the analyzed countries was approximately 10%.

1184 **A** (S&F, ch115)

Avoidance is the most effective therapy for NSAID enteropathy. Experimental studies have also demonstrated that metronidazole reduces inflammation and occult blood loss without changing intestinal permeability. Sulfasalazine has also been shown to reduce inflammation. Healthy individuals taking cyclooxygenase-2 inhibitors compared with individuals taking naproxen had less small bowel injury noted on capsule endoscopy.

1185 **D** (S&F, ch106)

Central nervous system findings in Whipple's disease include progressive dementia and cognitive changes (28% to 71%), supranuclear ophthalmoplegia (32% to 51%), and altered level of consciousness (27% to 50%). Other less frequent signs are psychiatric symptoms, hypothalamic manifestations (e.g., polydipsia, hyperphagia, insomnia), cranial nerve abnormalities, nystagmus, seizures, and ataxia. Two signs are considered characteristic of central nervous system Whipple's disease: oculomasticatory myorhythmia and oculofacial skeletal myorhythmia. These have not yet been documented in other central nervous system diseases. Both consist of slow, rhythmic, and synchronized contractions (~1/sec) of ocular, facial, or other muscles; both occur in less than 20% of patients with central nervous system Whipple's disease.

1186 **D** (S&F, ch120)

Both diseases can have constipation. Urinary retention, dysphagia, and cachexia are features of CIP as opposed to mechanical obstruction. Mechanical obstruction is characterized by symptom-free periods between attacks, whereas CIP patients have more chronic persistent symptoms of abdominal pain, nausea, vomiting, and dysphagia.

1187 **D** (S&F, ch114)

If the patient does not have signs of peritonitis, laparotomy is not likely indicated early in the course. Papaverine infusion currently is the mainstay of diagnosis and initial treatment of both occlusive and nonocclusive forms of AMI and should be performed promptly if AMI is suspected or diagnosed on other imaging tests. Intravenous heparin and hyperbaric oxygen have no role in AMI. Prompt laparotomy is indicated in patients with suspected AMI if angiography cannot be performed expeditiously.

1188 **A** (S&F, ch114)

Thumbprinting is a finding seen on a barium enema or plain film. It corresponds to the hemorrhagic nodules seen at colonoscopy. The colon single-stripe sign has a 75% histopathologic yield in making the diagnosis of ischemic injury and signifies a milder course than that of a circumferential ulcer. Rectal sparing is typical of ischemic injury, and stricture formation is usually a late finding.

1189 **C** (S&F, ch99)
The total volume of endogenous secretions presented to the gastrointestinal tract daily is 7000 mL. Bile amounts to 500 mL. The small intestine produces 1000 mL of secretions. Of the total volume of fluid secreted daily, 98% of it is absorbed, mainly in the small intestine.

1190 **B** (S&F, ch112)
Genetics seems to play a key role in the multifactorial etiology of UC, as evidenced by the fact that family history is one of the most important risk factors for the development of UC. Although there is variation among epidemiologic studies, approximately 10% to 20% of patients with UC will have at least one family member affected, and most often these are first-degree relatives. The relative risk of the development of UC if one has a sibling with this condition is 7% to 17%. Clearly, the genetics of UC does not follow a mendelian model. In monozygotic twins, the concordance rate is approximately 6% to 16%, which is higher than that for dizygotic twins (~0% to 5%), but significantly less than concordance rates for Crohn's disease in monozygotic twins. Further, familial risk of UC is threefold higher in Jewish than non-Jewish populations. Additionally, there is a high degree of concordance of disease type (UC vs. Crohn's disease), extent of inflammation, and EIMs of IBD within families.

1191 **A** (S&F, ch100)
The control of gastric emptying is critical to ensure proper digestion, and, as such, there are several factors that play a role in regulating it, including consistency of the food, pH, osmolality, and lipid and calorie content (see figure). The pylorus prevents passage of food particles larger than 2 mm, and, as such, large particles are exposed to longer times in the stomach and are broken down to aid in proper digestion. Meals of low viscosity leave the stomach more quickly and when acidic stomach contents are neutralized in the duodenum by pancreaticobiliary juices, further gastric emptying is encouraged.

1192 **E** (S&F, ch102)
Although acid may have a role, peristalsis is the most important factor.

1193 **A** (S&F, ch113)
Although patients who undergo IPAA for FAP are not immune to pouchitis, this complication is much more common in patients with IBD. Preoperative extraintestinal manifestations portend a greater risk of pouchitis (39% vs. 26%). Forty percent of patients will never have an episode of pouchitis, 40% will have a single bout, 15% will have intermittently recurring pouchitis, and chronic pouchitis will develop in 5%. Chronic inflammation on histology is considered a normal finding

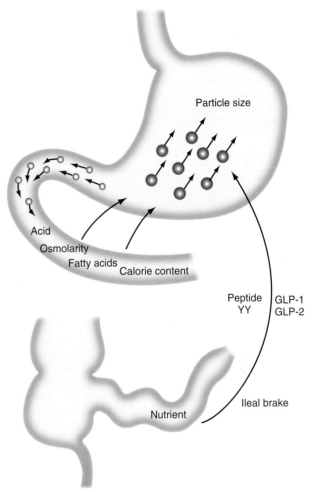

Figure for answer **1191**

after IPAA; patients with pouchitis generally also have acute inflammatory macroscopic and microscopic changes as well.

1194 **B** (S&F, ch119)
The risk of adhesive SBO is greatest after operations in which there is a resection and reanastomosis of the intestine. The risk of adhesive SBO after partial or subtotal colectomy is as high as 14%. Appendectomy and gynecologic surgery, such as tubal ligation, have a risk of only 1%. Upper abdominal surgery, such as cholecystectomy and Heller myotomy, have lower risks than lower abdominal or pelvic surgery.

1195 **C** (S&F, ch114)
Fifty percent of patients with classic polyarteritis are hepatitis B surface antigen–positive. Glucocorticoids and cyclophosphamide or azathioprine have improved survival greatly.

1196 **A** (S&F, ch120)
Intestinal pseudo-obstruction is defined as a syndrome characterized by impaired intestinal propulsion resembling intestinal obstruction without a mechanical cause. It may involve the small or large bowel and presents in acute, subacute, or chronic

forms. There are both myopathic and neuropathic forms. Its precise underlying pathophysiologic processes are unclear.

1197 **A** (S&F, ch120)
Fast-track postoperative protocols have been shown to reduce hospital stay, reduce costs, and reduce duration of ileus without increasing readmission rates.

1198 **D** (S&F, ch103)
Growth hormone was shown in double-blind, randomized, controlled trials to help reduce total parenteral nutrition requirements by 2 L per week. Although glucagon-like peptide 2 has shown promise in many recent studies, it is not yet FDA approved for short bowel syndrome. The other therapies listed are also not indicated or not approved.

1199 **C** (S&F, ch110)
Strongyloides stercoralis is endemic in tropical and semitropical areas but has been seen in the southeastern United States. It lives in the soil, and larvae can penetrate the skin. Larva currens is a serpiginous rash caused by the migrating larvae. Although most have no abdominal symptoms, pain, nausea, and occult gastrointestinal bleeding can occur. If the patient is immunosuppressed or receives glucocorticoids, a fulminant course can ensue, frequently leading to sepsis and death. Intestinal biopsy is very insensitive. ELISA is most sensitive for detection followed by inspection of agar plate and then direct stool smears.

1200 **E** (S&F, ch110)
Diphyllobothrium latum is the largest parasite that affects humans and may be as long as 40 feet. It is acquired by consumption of undercooked fresh-water, not saltwater, fish. Ivermectin may treat *Strongyloides*, whereas praziquantel or albendazole can be used for treatment of *D. latum*. The worms absorb nutrients from the intestinal contents of the host and have the ability to cleave vitamin B_{12} from intrinsic factor. Absorption of vitamin B_{12} by the worm can lead to vitamin B_{12} deficiency and thus megaloblastic anemia with neurologic symptoms.

1201 **C** (S&F, ch107)
Antibiotics have not been shown to alter the recovery in patients with *Salmonella* gastroenteritis. The intestinal carriage is more prolonged and more frequent, and relapse is more common in those treated with antibiotics. Therefore, antibiotics should not be used in most cases. However, certain situations do warrant treatment. See the table (at end of chapter) for a list of conditions for which antibiotics are suggested. Due to resistance to ampicillin and trimethoprim/sulfamethoxazole, fluoroquinolones are the drug of choice.

1202 **C** (S&F, ch118)
The Manning criteria are not sex specific and consist of six criteria: (1) abdominal pain that is relieved after a bowel movement, (2) looser stool at pain onset, (3) more frequent stools at pain onset, (4) abdominal distention, (5) sensation of incom-

plete rectal evacuation, (6) passage of mucus. Only four of these criteria were found to be statistically significant in the initial report. One study reported that three or more Manning criteria in the absence of alarm features correctly diagnosed 96% of cases of IBS.

1203 **B** (S&F, ch120)
Familial visceral neuropathies are a group of genetic diseases characterized by degeneration of the myenteric plexus. There are two distinct phenotypes: types I and II. Both forms are generally symptomatic, and there is no effective medical or surgical therapy available. Type I may involve both the large and small intestine, and type II is associated with hypertrophic pyloric stenosis.

1204 **D** (S&F, ch123)
Patients with a family history of HNPCC should be examined with colonoscopy as other screening methods are not as accurate in this high-risk group. Colonoscopic surveillance has been suggested to be performed every two years starting at age 20 to 25 or 10 years younger than the index case. Genetic testing for microsatellite instability testing can be performed. However, *APC* and *K-ras* mutations are found in the majority of colon cancers and not just in HNPCC. Sigmoidoscopy is an appropriate screening method in FAP and not HNPCC.

1205 **A** (S&F, ch111)
This patient has perianal Crohn's disease with both an abscess and a fistula. He should be referred to an experienced colorectal surgeon for incision and drainage and possible Seton placement and/or fistulotomy. Additionally, the patient should be started immediately on antibiotics; the two that are used most commonly and seem to have the most efficacy are ciprofloxacin and metronidazole, with the latter being more limited in terms of long-term treatment secondary to side effects. Rifaximin, a nonabsorbable oral rifamycin antibiotic approved for the treatment of travelers' diarrhea and also sometimes effective in treating IBS, may have efficacy in luminal Crohn's disease in patients with an elevated C-reactive protein level. Because it is not absorbed, however, it would not be appropriate treatment for perianal disease. Adalimumab, a fully human anti-TNF antibody, may be useful in closing the fistula after the abscess is drained, but would not be appropriate in the setting of active infection. Mesalamine and glucocorticosteroids do not have efficacy in treating perianal disease, and the latter might also exacerbate infection.

1206 **D** (S&F, ch123)
The risk of colon cancer in UC is related to the duration of disease. The risk increases after 7 years and may reach 30% after 25 years of disease. The risk is greatest in those who have universal disease. The other factors listed are not associated with increased cancer risk (see figure).

1207 **B** (S&F, ch105)
G. lamblia is the most common cause of human protozoon infection worldwide. It is also considered a contributory factor in the retardation of

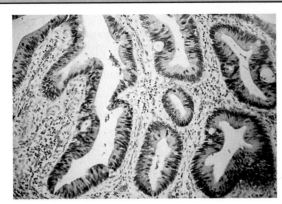

Figure for answer **1206**

growth and development in infants and young children. *I. belli* also produces chronic diarrhea and enteropathy, but is geographically restricted to the tropics and subtropics. *C. cayetanensis* is a recently recognized intracellular protozoon that has been identified in a number of tropical and subtropical locations as a cause of chronic diarrhea and enteropathy in immunocompetent and immunocompromised persons. *C. parvum* is a well-known cause of chronic diarrhea worldwide in immunocompetent persons, in whom the diarrhea usually is self-limited. It is also a major cause of chronic, intractable diarrhea in patients with HIV infection.

1208 **C** (S&F, ch123)
The incidence and mortality of colorectal cancer have decreased in the United States since 1985 by an annual rate of 1.6% and 1.8%, respectively. Colorectal cancer incidence and mortality rates are higher in blacks than whites. There is a rapid increase in the colorectal cancer risk when immigrants move from areas of low risk to areas of high risk.

1209 **C** (S&F, ch101)
Late-onset lactose malabsorption results from decreased levels of the intestinal brush border enzyme lactase and is the most common cause of carbohydrate malabsorption. Depending on the ethnic background, lactase can be present in less than 5% to more than 90% of the adult population. The hydrogen breath test is the noninvasive test of choice and exploits the fact that bacterial metabolism of carbohydrates results in the accumulation of hydrogen. A test result is considered positive when there is an increase in hydrogen concentration by more than 20 ppm over baseline after ingestion of a lactose meal. Lactase deficiency does not result from the mutation of the *LPH* gene but instead in a region upstream of the *LPH* gene. There is no association with cystic fibrosis.

1210 **E** (S&F, ch116)
Immunocompromised patients in general, and AIDS patients in particular, are a challenging group in which to diagnose appendicitis. Abdominal pain is common, with reported rates of 12% to 50%. Although patients with AIDS usually present with classic symptoms of appendicitis, there is also often a history of chronic abdominal pain. Leukocytosis is relatively uncommon.

1211 **C** (S&F, ch120)
The enteric nervous system consists of vast ganglionated plexuses located in the wall of the GI tract. The most important functionally are the myenteric and submucosal plexuses. In association with the muscle layers, the network of ICCs are recognized as the likely pacemakers activating neuromuscular function.

1212 **E** (S&F, ch120)
Intestinal pseudo-obstruction is a well-described complication of scleroderma. The small bowel is the second most frequently involved gastrointestinal organ after the esophagus. An uncommon but potentially serious finding is pneumatosis cystoides intestinalis, which usually signifies a poor prognosis. Degeneration of smooth muscle and its replacement by collagen is responsible for the small bowel dysmotility in scleroderma. The circular muscle is involved more often than is the longitudinal muscle layer. Small bowel dysmotility leads to bacterial overgrowth, resulting in steatorrhea, malabsorption, and weight loss. The hallmark dysmotility is the absence of the interdigestive MMC, low-amplitude clusters of propagated and nonpropagated contractions, abnormally prolonged MMC cycle, diminished activity of phase III, hypomotility of the fed pattern, and antral hypomotility.

1213 **B** (S&F, ch107)
The common routes of passage are indicated by the five Fs: flies, food, finger, feces, and fomites. The attack rates are strongly related to age with the highest rates in children younger than one year of age and the elderly. Foods that are commonly contaminated include poultry, meats, eggs, and dairy (see figure).

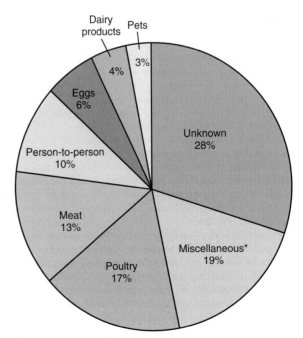

Figure for answer **1213**

1214 **D** (S&F, ch121)

Gastrointestinal stromal tumors were recently identified as arising from the ICC, which help control the motility of the intestine and have elements of both smooth muscle and neural differentiation. Carcinoid tumors arise from argentaffin cells. Adenomas/adenocarcinomas arise from glandular mucosa. Leiomyomas arise from smooth muscle cells and lymphomas from clonal proliferation of lymphocytes.

1215 **E** (S&F, ch124)

Patients with collagenous and lymphocytic colitis usually present with chronic watery diarrhea with an average of eight stools each day. Examination of fresh stools showed fecal leukocytes in 55% of 116 patients with collagenous colitis. Although nonspecific abnormalities including patchy edema, erythema, and friability are observed, findings of a colonoscopic examination are usually normal.

1216 **E** (S&F, ch104)

Autoimmune disease is associated strongly with celiac disease and has a prevalence of approximately 20% in adult patients. There is an established association between celiac disease and insulin-dependent diabetes mellitus. The frequency of celiac disease in patients with insulin-dependent diabetes mellitus ranges from 3% to 8%, and its frequency in celiac disease is approximately 5%. Celiac disease may also be associated with a variety of other autoimmune connective tissue diseases, including systemic lupus erythematosus, Sjögren syndrome, and polymyosis. Evidence also supports associations between celiac disease and inflammatory bowel disease (particularly ulcerative proctitis), chronic hepatitis, sclerosing cholangitis, primary biliary cirrhosis, IgA nephropathy, interstitial lung disease including chronic fibrosing alveolitis, idiopathic pulmonary hemosiderosis, and Down syndrome.

1217 **B** (S&F, ch102)

The glucose hydrogen breath test is the most widely used breath test in clinical practice: the substrate is inexpensive, and the hydrogen meter is economical, portable, and easy to use. Normally, glucose is absorbed entirely in the upper small intestine; if there is bacterial overgrowth, the glucose is cleaved by bacteria into carbon dioxide and hydrogen. The hydrogen is measured in the exhaled breath (at baseline, and every 30 minutes for two hours), and an increase of 20 ppm above the baseline is regarded as diagnostic of SIBO. Fasting breath hydrogen levels of more than 20 ppm are also considered positive, but high baseline hydrogen levels are common in patients with untreated celiac disease and normalize after gluten withdrawal. Patient preparation is important for this test. Patients must avoid smoking and eating nonfermentable carbohydrates such as pasta and bread the night before the test because they may increase the baseline breath hydrogen values; exercise may induce hyperventilation, thereby reducing baseline breath hydrogen values, and thus should be avoided for two hours before the test.

1218 **A** (S&F, ch119)

The pathophysiology of postoperative ileus involves a complex interaction of inhibitory neuroenteric reflexes including increased efferent inhibitory sympathetic activity, inflammation within the bowel wall, the local and systemic release of inhibitory gastrointestinal peptides and endogenous opioids, and the use of exogenous opioids for anesthesia and postoperative analgesia. Incision through the abdominal wall activates inhibitory sympathetic reflexes, releasing norepinephrine and inhibiting acetylcholine release from excitatory neurons in the myenteric plexus, causing relaxation of the intestinal wall. Serotonin stimulates peristalsis. There is increased endogenous opioid release in postoperative ileus. Evidence is lacking for a role for somatostatin and nitric oxide.

1219 **B** (S&F, ch120)

Many drugs affect gastrointestinal motility. Antiparkinsonism drugs decrease colonic and small bowel motility and can cause pseudo-obstruction. Opiate analgesics suppress motility throughout the gastrointestinal tract, particularly the colon. Calcium channel antagonists, especially verapamil, slow colonic transit and can cause constipation. They do not seem to have an effect on small bowel motility. Clonidine, an α_2-adrenergic agent, prolongs orocecal transit of liquids but recently has not shown any significant effect on gastric, small bowel, and colonic transit in healthy patients. Octreotide increases the frequency of MMCs by shortening the duration of phase II. It was shown to be useful in a small group of scleroderma patients with pseudo-obstruction by inducing phase III contractions and possibly reducing bacterial overgrowth. When given after a meal, intravenous somatostatin interrupts the fed pattern of motility and induces bursts of propagated activity similar to phase III in health and disease. Octreotide retards small bowel transit in health when given before a meal.

1220 **B** (S&F, ch118)

In IBS, diarrhea may occur from multiple colonic mechanisms including increased high-amplitude propagated contractions, an enhanced gastrocolonic response, and rectal hypersensitivity. Constipation may be secondary to increased segmental (nonpropulsive) contractions. A hypertensive internal rectal sphincter may be seen in Hirschsprung's disease.

1221 **E** (S&F, ch119)

In a study reviewing 12 abdominal radiologic findings associated with SBO, the combination of air–fluid levels of different heights in the same bowel loop and a mean air–fluid level diameter of 2.5 cm or more was most predictive of high-grade partial or complete SBO. The clinical and physical findings are not sufficiently reliable to predict the presence of a complete SBO.

1222 **D** (S&F, ch114)

The bowel can tolerate a 75% reduction in mesenteric blood flow and oxygen consumption for 12 hours with no change on light microscopy. This is because only one fifth of the mesenteric capillaries are open at any time and when oxygen delivery is decreased, the bowel adapts by increasing oxygen extraction. However, below a critical level of blood flow, these compensatory mechanisms will be overwhelmed.

1223 **A** (S&F, ch112)
Many of the histopathologic changes seen in UC are nonspecific and can occur in other colitides, including infection and ischemia. These more acute features include edema of the lamina propria and congestion of the capillaries and venules, followed by an acute inflammatory cell infiltrate. Neutrophilic infiltration of colonic crypts causes cryptitis and crypt abscesses. Histologic findings that characterize a chronic colitis such as UC include crypt architectural distortion, crypt atropy, increased intercryptal spacing, Paneth cell metaplasia, basal lymphoid aggregates, an irregular mucosal surface, and a chronic inflammatory infiltrate.

1224 **A** (S&F, ch104)
The mainstay of treatment of celiac disease is avoidance of gluten and gluten-containing foods; this includes wheat, rye, and barley. Although refractory celiac disease can be treated with glucocorticoids, the effect rarely persists once treatment is stopped. Therefore, glucocorticoids are not indicated in the routine management of celiac disease. Cyclosporine, azathioprine, and 6-MP can be used as a glucocorticoid-sparing agent in refractory sprue.

1225 **C** (S&F, ch112)
When referring to the "environment" as an etiology in the development of UC and Crohn's disease, it is the continuous antigenic stimulation by the normal intestinal flora that seems to be the most important factor. Although there have been numerous studies attempting to identify a single organism that causes IBD, to date, no definitive evidence exists to support this theory. Appendectomy likely confers protection against the development of UC, although the reason is not clear. Four mechanisms have been proposed to explain how the commensal microbiome induces inflammation in the intestine: (1) microbes adhere to or invade the intestinal epithelial cells and induce a proinflammatory cytokine cascade; (2) dysbiosis, a disturbance in the normal balance of "good" or protective and "bad" bacteria in the gut; (3) defects in host microbial killing and impairment of the normal barrier function; and (4) immunodysregulation causing abnormal responses to nonpathogenic microbes. One of the most important observations that lends credence to this theory is that mice and rats raised in germ-free environments do not develop inflammatory changes of the gut, but once colonized with bacteria, they do develop intestinal inflammation.

1226 **E** (S&F, ch116)
The perforation rate is between 10% and 30% in most series, most commonly at the extremes of age; patient rates as high as 90% have been reported in children younger than the age of two years. Adults older than the age of 70 have perforation rates between 50% and 70%. Perforation is often the result of delay in diagnosis; however, the delay is often a result in presentation to medical attention rather than delays in medical decision making.

1227 **A** (S&F, ch121)
SBO is the most common presentation for benign lesions secondary to either luminal constriction or intussusception. Gastrointestinal bleeding is the second most common symptom. Intestinal perforation is rare.

1228 **E** (S&F, ch102)
Vitamin B_{12} is often low, because of bacterial consumption of the vitamin. Vitamins A, D, and E (fat-soluble vitamins) can be low secondary to fat malabsorption. Vitamin K is rarely low because of production of this vitamin by luminal bacteria, offsetting any fecal fat losses.

1229 **D** (S&F, ch113)
In more than 1500 patients studied at the Mayo Clinic over a 14-year period, approximately 5% had features of indeterminate colitis. Of these patients, Crohn's disease developed in 15%, compared with 2% of patients with UC. At 10 years, this translated to 81% of patients with indeterminate colitis being Crohn's disease free compared with 98% of those with UC. That being said, patients with indeterminate colitis had long-term outcomes similar to those with UC, with 85% having a functioning pouch after a decade. Indeterminate colitis is thus not a contraindication to IPAA, but these patients do have a higher risk of the development of Crohn's disease, and thus physicians need to be even more vigilant about monitoring for signs and symptoms in this regard.

1230 **D** (S&F, ch104)
See table at end of chapter.

1231 **B** (S&F, ch114)
When major vessels are occluded, collaterals open immediately in response to the decrease in arterial pressure distal to the obstruction. After several hours, however, vasoconstriction develops in the obstructing bed, elevating its pressure and reducing collateral flow. This sustained vasoconstriction for a prolonged period can become irreversible and persist even after correction of the cause of the ischemic event.

1232 **E** (S&F, ch114)
The most common presentation of FSI is chronic SBO with intermittent abdominal pain, distention, and vomiting. Bacterial overgrowth in the more proximal dilated loops may produce a blind loop syndrome. Radiologic studies typically reveal a smooth, tapered stricture of variable length with an abrupt change to normal bowel distally and dilated bowel proximally. Treatment of FSI is resection of the involved bowel.

1233 **D** (S&F, ch116)
There are many epidemiologic studies suggesting that appendectomy may protect against the development of UC, a relationship not seen in Crohn's disease. Researchers have suggested that appendectomy may attenuate the course of active UC. Although appendiceal tumors are rare (<1% of

specimens), the vast majority of appendiceal tumors are carcinoid tumors. Common types of epithelial malignancies include mucinous and cystadenocarcinoma. Lifetime risk of appendicitis at birth is approximately 1 in 12 and decreases to 1 in 35 by age 35. The greatest risk of appendicitis in a given year occurs over the second decade of life when the risk is approximately 25% per year.

1234 **D** (S&F, ch115)
The anterior wall of the rectum, 7 to 10 cm from the anal verge, is the most common area of prolapse into the anal canal, and this area corresponds to the usual location of ulceration in solitary rectal ulcer syndrome (see figure).

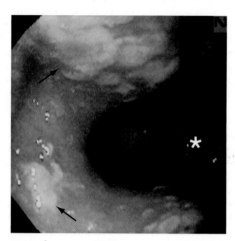

Figure for answer **1234**

1235 **C** (S&F, ch120)
Neuropathic causes include amyloidosis, diabetes mellitus, and Parkinson's disease. Scleroderma is an example of a myopathic form of CIP.

1236 **E** (S&F, ch123)
Chemoprevention is the use of agents that may reverse, suppress, or prevent progression or recurrence of cancer. Calcium has been shown to decrease the incidence and recurrence of adenomas at a dose of 1200 mg of elemental calcium. Additionally, there is the suggestion that calcium decreases the risk of colorectal cancer but not the risk of metastases. High doses of folate have been shown to decrease the incidence of colorectal cancer. In studies of FAP, sulindac decreased the number and size of polyps but not the villous component. Aspirin has been shown to decrease the incidence of both adenomas and colorectal cancer (see table at end of chapter).

1237 **B** (S&F, ch124)
Diversion colitis seems to be caused largely by the colonic epithelium having luminal nutrient deficiency. The principal nutrient substrates of colonic epithelium are luminal SCFAs, which are produced in negligible amounts in the excluded segments of colon. The numbers of obligate amounts are reduced in the excluded colon, consistent with reduced SCFA production.

1238 **E** (S&F, ch108)
Elderly patients and patients undergoing cytotoxic chemotherapy for malignancy are at increased risk of *C. difficile*–associated diarrhea and colitis. HIV-infected patients are also at risk due to multiple risk factors including frequent prophylactic and therapeutic antibiotic use, hospitalizations, and immunocompromised status. Patients with IBD are also predisposed. *C. difficile* is the most commonly identified specific pathogen in IBD in patients in North America and Europe and is present in as many as 5% to 19% of cases, with relapse in some case series. Many IBD patients without *C. difficile* infection do not have a history of recent antibiotic use, suggesting that IBD itself may cause sufficient alteration of the colonic microenvironment to negate the colonization resistance of the normal colonic microflora.

1239 **A** (S&F, ch123)
Dukes A and B1 lesions are not considered at highest risk of recurrence, and studies have not shown adjuvant therapy to be of benefit. Dukes B2 lesions may benefit from adjuvant therapy in certain situations, but the benefit is greater for Dukes C lesions. Only cancers of the rectum are considered for treatment with radiation, depending on their stage and the ability to obtain clear margins (see table at end of chapter).

1240 **A** (S&F, ch119)
Complete SBO necessitates early laparotomy. The rationale for early laparotomy in patients with complete obstruction is based on three observations: (1) the low likelihood of resolution with nonoperative management, (2) the risk of strangulation for complete SBO, and (3) the difficulty in detecting strangulation obstruction by clinical parameters until very late in the course of the disease.

1241 **B** (S&F, ch105)
Bacterial diarrhea is more common in travelers to Southeast Asian countries with *Campylobacter* > *Shigella* > nontyphoid *Salmonella*.

1242 **A** (S&L Chapter 115)
Solitary rectal ulcer syndrome is an uncommon disorder of evacuation affecting all ages characterized by the presence of rectal ulceration or erythema in association with straining at defecation, rectal prolapse, feeling of incomplete evacuation, and typical histologic features. It is also associated with occult or overt rectal prolapse with paradoxical contraction of the pelvic floor.

1243 **C** (S&F, ch111)
The pathologic finding in the figure (see question 1243) is a noncaseating granuloma. These lesions, like aphthous ulcers, are believed to be an early finding in Crohn's disease. Although they are highly characteristic of Crohn's disease, granulomas are not pathognomonic for this condition. Similar granulomas are seen in sarcoid and contain epithelioid histiocytes, various inflammatory cells, and occasional giant cells. They are sparse, scattered, and not well formed, without the central necrosis or acid-fast positivity seen in those of tuberculosis. Granulomas are reportedly found in

the range of 15% endoscopically to 70% in one surgical study. The more biopsies or the larger the sample, the more likely one will find granulomas. Although it is possible for granulomas to be seen outside the intestinal tract, such as in the skin, eye, and liver, it is rare.

1244 **B** (S&F, ch118)
Women are more likely to have IBS than men, with a 2:1 ratio. There is a similar prevalence of IBS in African Americans and whites. There is a lower prevalence in Hispanics, and IBS is commonly seen in China and Japan. Women have slower colonic transit and smaller stool output than men.

1245 **B** (S&F, ch122)
Rubber band ligation has become the most common office procedure for the treatment of second- and third-degree hemorrhoids. Sclerosing agents are injected as an irritant into the submucosa above the internal hemorrhoid at the anorectal ring. Approximately 75% of patients with second-degree hemorrhoids improve after injection therapy. Cryotherapy freezes tissues, thereby destroying the hemorrhoidal complex. The procedure can be painful, and healing prolonged. Infrared photocoagulation utilizes infrared radiation to coagulate, leading to fibrosis. Results are comparable to cryotherapy for first- and second-degree hemorrhoids. Surgical hemorrhoidectomy is the procedure of choice for fourth-degree, and some third-degree, hemorrhoids.

1246 **E** (S&F, ch120)
Nasogastric tube decompression is not recommended in routine abdominal operations, and it does not hasten recovery from ileus. All other choices have been shown to reduce postoperative ileus.

1247 **A** (S&F, ch118)
Oral glucocorticoid use may lower the risk of IBS. All other choices have been associated with an increased risk of the development of IBS.

1248 **E** (S&F, ch123)
Several morphologic and histologic characteristics of the primary tumor may correlate with the prognosis. The depth of invasion in the bowel wall and the presence of regional lymph node spread are most important. Lymphatic, perineural, and venous invasion have all been associated with local recurrence and decreased survival. The more poorly differentiated the tumor is, the worse the prognosis. Additionally, it seems that tumors with diploid DNA content fare better than those that are nondiploid or aneuploid. Unlike most cancers, the size of the primary tumor in colon cancer does not correlate with the prognosis (see figure here and table at end of chapter).

1249 **B** (S&F, ch120)
Initial therapy should always be the treatment of reversible causes unless there are signs of peritonitis, ischemia, or perforation. Infection should be excluded. Electrolytes and dehydration should be corrected. Medications that could aggravate the condition should be avoided. The other options are potential choices if initial therapy is not effective.

1250 **C** (S&F, ch120)
If there are no contraindications, then neostigmine is the next option if correction of reversible causes has not worked.

1251 **C** (S&F, ch119)
Decreased bowel wall enhancement is the most specific finding in intestinal ischemia; however, its sensitivity is relatively low. Portovenous gas, pneumoperitoneum, and pneumatosis intestinalis may be seen very late in the natural history of strangulated obstruction and suggest the presence of extensive necrosis. The small bowel feces sign refers to the presence of a mottled admixture of particulate matter and gas within the dilated bowel proximal to an SBO. The whirl sign suggests intestinal torsion or volvulus.

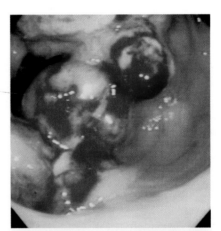

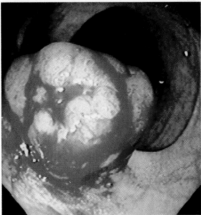

Figure for answer **1248**

Tables

Table 1 for answer 900 Randomized, Controlled Trials of Azathioprine for Ulcerative Colitis

REFERENCE	N	DOSE (MG/KG/D)	DURATION OF THERAPY (MONTHS)	RESPONSE (AZA)	RESPONSE (CONTROL)	P-VALUE	CO-THERAPY
Induction							
188	80	2.5	1	78%	68%	NS	Glucocorticoids in all
189	20	2.5	3	60%	80%	NS	None; control = 5-ASA
190	44*	2-2.5	6	NR	NR	NS	None
191	72*	2	6	53%	19%	.006	None; control = 5-ASA
Maintenance							
188	80	1.5-2.5	11	40%	23%	NS	Glucocorticoids for relapse
192	30*	1.5	6	NR	NR	NS	None
193	67	NR	12	64%	41%	.039	5-ASA in most AZA withdrawal
194	25	2.5	18	42%	62%	NS	Glucocorticoid induction Control = 5-ASA

*All patients in this study were glucocorticoid-dependent.
5-ASA, 5-aminosalicylates; AZA, azathioprine; mo, months; N, number of patients; NR, not reported; NS, not significant.

Table 2 for answer 900 Side Effects of Azathioprine and 6-Mercaptopurine

Abnormal liver biochemical test results
Bone marrow suppression
Hypersensitivity reactions (fever, rash, arthralgia)
Infections
Lymphoma
Nausea, abdominal pain, diarrhea
Pancreatitis

Table for answer 901 Relative Frequencies of Microbial Causes of Traveler's Diarrhea

PATHOGEN	FREQUENCY, %	
	AVERAGE	RANGE
Enterotoxigenic *E. coli*	40-60	0-72
Enteroadherent *E. coli*	15	NA
Campylobacter spp.	10	0-41
Shigella spp.	10	0-30
Rotavirus	5	0-36
Invasive *E. coli*	<5	0-5
Salmonella spp.	<5	0-15
Vibrio spp.	<5	0-30
Aeromonas spp.	<5	0-30
Giardia lamblia	<5	0-6
Entamoeba histolytica	<5	0-6
Cryptosporidium	<5	NA
Cyclospora cayetanensis	<5	NA
Hafnia alvei	<5	0-16
No pathogen identified	40	22-83

NA, not available.

Table 1 for answer 906 Costs of Screening Tests for Colorectal Cancer

PROCEDURE	COST (U.S.$)*
Fecal occult blood test	0
Flexible sigmoidoscopy	186.00
Colonoscopy	586.00
Colonoscopy with polypectomy	808.00
Air-contrast barium enema	194.00

*Costs are based on Medicare payments in 2008 at the University of Texas MD Anderson Cancer Center and may vary by institution. Charges to patients or other third-party payers are likely to be substantially higher.

Table 2 for answer 906 Proper Performance of the Slide Guaiac Test for Fecal Occult Blood

For three days before and during testing, patients should avoid the following:
  Rare red meat
  Peroxidase-containing vegetables and fruit (e.g., broccoli, turnip, cantaloupe, cauliflower, radish)
  Certain medications (e.g., iron supplements, vitamin C, aspirin and other NSAIDs)
Two samples of each of three consecutive stools should be tested. It is proper to sample areas of obvious blood.
Slides should be developed within 4 to 6 days.
  Slides should not be rehydrated before developing (for average-risk screening).
  If slides are rehydrated, the patient must have avoided eating red meat; otherwise, too many false-positive results will occur.

NSAID, nonsteroidal anti-inflammatory drug.

Table 3 for answer 906 Features of the Slide Guaiac Test for Fecal Occult Blood

Advantages
Readily available
Convenient
Inexpensive
Good compliance in motivated patients
Disadvantages
Depends on the degree of fecal hydration
Affected by storage (hemoglobin degradation can occur)
Affected by tumor location
Causes of False-Positive Results
Exogenous peroxidase activity
Red meat (nonhuman hemoglobin)
Uncooked fruits and vegetables (vegetable peroxidase: e.g., broccoli, turnip, cantaloupe, cauliflower, radish)
Any source of GI blood loss (e.g., epistaxis, gingival bleeding, upper GI tract pathology, hemorrhoids)
Certain medications (e.g., iron supplements, vitamin C, aspirin and other NSAIDs)
Causes of False-Negative Results
Storage of slides for a prolonged period
Degradation of hemoglobin by colonic bacteria
Ascorbic acid (vitamin C) ingestion
Improper sampling or developing
Non-bleeding lesion at the time of stool collection

GI, gastrointestinal; NSAID, nonsteroidal anti-inflammatory drug.

Table for answer 926 **Genes Altered in Sporadic Colorectal Cancer**

GENE	CHROMOSOME	FREQUENCY OF TUMORS WITH GENE ALTERATIONS (%)	GENE CLASS	FUNCTION OF GENE PRODUCT
K-ras	12	50	Proto-oncogene	Encodes guanine nucleotide-binding protein that regulates intracellular signaling
APC	5	70	Tumor suppressor	Regulation of β-catenin that is involved in activation of WnT/TcF signaling (activates c-myc, cyclin D1)*; regulation of proliferation and apoptosis; interaction with E-cadherin (cell adhesion?)
DCC	18	70	Tumor suppressor?	Netrin-1 receptor; caspase substrate in apoptosis; cell adhesion
SMAD4 (DPC4, MADH4)	18	?	Tumor suppressor	Nuclear transcriptase factor in transforming growth factor (TGF-β1) signaling; regulation of angiogenesis; regulator of WAF1 promoter; downstream mediator of SMAD2
TP53	17	75	Tumor suppressor	Transcription factor; regulates cell cycle progression after cellular stress; regulates apoptosis, gene expression, and DNA repair
hMSH2	2	†	DNA mismatch repair	Maintains fidelity of DNA replication
hMLH1	3	†	DNA mismatch repair	Maintains fidelity of DNA replication
hMSH6	2	†	DNA mismatch repair	Maintains fidelity of DNA replication
TGF-β1 RII	3	‡	Tumor suppressor	Receptor for signaling in the TGF-β1 pathway; inhibitor of colonic epithelial proliferation, often mutated in tumors with MSI

*β-Catenin mutations (downstream of APC) are found in 16%-25% of MSI colon cancers but not in MSS cancers.
†Approximately 15% of sporadic colorectal cancers demonstrate MSI associated with alterations in mismatch repair genes (principally hMSH2 and hMLH1 but also hMSH3, hMSH6, hPMS1, and hPMS2).
‡Mutated in 73%-90% of MSI colon cancers. Up to 55% of MSS colon cancer cell lines demonstrate a TGF-β signaling blockage distal to TGF-β1 RII.
MSI, microsatellite instability; MSS, microsatellite stable; RII, type II receptor; TGF-β, transforming growth factor-β.

Table for answer 938 **Frequency of Symptom(s) in Patients with Giardiasis[100,106,110]**

SYMPTOM(S)	FREQUENCY (%)
Diarrhea	32-100
Fatigue	22-97
Abdominal pain, cramps	75-83
Flatulence, bloating	58-79
Weight loss	60
Anorexia	45
Vomiting	17-26
Fever	12-21

Table for answers 949 and 1153 **Guidelines for Screening Average-Risk Persons for Colorectal Cancer**

SCREENING TOOL	U.S. PREVENTIVE SERVICES TASK FORCE*	AMERICAN CANCER SOCIETY, U.S. MULTI-SOCIETY TASK FORCE, AND AMERICAN COLLEGE OF RADIOLOGY JOINT GUIDELINES[†]
High sensitivity FOBT (guaiac-based or immunochemical)	Recommended annually as an option	Recommended annually as an option
Flexible sigmoidoscopy	Recommended every 5 yr + high-sensitivity FOBT every 3 yr as an option	Recommended every 5 yr as an option
Colonoscopy	Recommended every 10 yr as an option	Recommended every 10 yr as an option
Double-contrast barium enema	Not recommended	Recommended every 5 yr as an option
Computed tomographic colonography	Not recommended	Recommended every 5 yr as an option
Stool DNA testing	Not recommended	Recommended (interval uncertain)

*The U.S. Preventive Services Task Force recommends screening for adults of ages 50 to 75 years. Screening for adults of ages 76 to 85 years is not routinely recommended, and for adults older than 85 years, screening is not recommended.
[†]Testing options are divided into those that detect adenomatous polyps and cancer (flexible sigmoidoscopy, colonoscopy, double-contrast barium enema, computed tomography colonography), and those that primarily detect cancer (FOBT, stool DNA testing).
FOBT, fecal occult blood test.
U.S. Preventive Services Task Force. Screening for colorectal cancer: U.S. Preventive Services Task Force recommendation statement. Ann Int Med 2008; 149:627-637.
Levin B, Lieberman DA, McFarland B, et al. Screening and surveillance for the early detection of colorectal cancer and adenomatous polyps 2008: a joint guideline from the American Cancer Society, the U.S. Multi-Society Task Force on Colorectal Cancer, and the American College of Radiology. CA Cancer J Clin 2008; 58:130-60.

Table for answer 968 Medical Importance and Epidemiologic and Clinical Features of Human Gastroenteritis Viruses

VIRUS	MEDICAL IMPORTANCE DEMONSTRATED	EPIDEMIOLOGIC FEATURES	CLINICAL FEATURES	LABORATORY DIAGNOSTIC TESTS*
Rotavirus				
Group A	Yes	A major cause of endemic severe diarrhea in infants and young children worldwide (in winter in temperate zone)	Dehydrating diarrhea for 5-7 days; vomiting and fever are common	Immunoassay, electron microscopy, PAGE
Group B	Partially	Large outbreaks in adults and children in China	Severe watery diarrhea for 3-5 days	Electron microscopy, PAGE
Group C	Partially	Sporadic cases in young children worldwide	Similar to features of group A rotavirus	Electron microscopy, PAGE
Calicivirus	Yes	A cause of diarrhea in children; associated with ingestion of contaminated shellfish and other foods in adults	Rotavirus-like illness in children; Norovirus-like in adults	Immunoassay, electron microscopy
Norovirus	Yes	Epidemics of vomiting and diarrhea in older children and adults; occurs in families, communities, and nursing homes; often associated with ingestion of shellfish, other food, or water	Acute vomiting, diarrhea, fever, myalgias, and headache lasting 1-2 days	Immunoassay, immune electron microscopy
Norwalk-like viruses (small, round structured viruses)	Partially	Similar to characteristics of Norovirus-like illness	Acute vomiting, diarrhea, fever, myalgias, and headache lasting 1-2 days	Immunoassay, immune electron microscopy
Enteric adenovirus	Yes	Endemic diarrhea of infants and young children	Prolonged diarrhea lasting 5-12 days; vomiting and fever	Immunoassay, electron microscopy with PAGE
Astrovirus	Yes	A cause of diarrhea in children; reported in nursing homes	Watery diarrhea, often lasting 2-3 days, occasionally longer	Immunoassay, electron microscopy
Torovirus	Yes	A cause of acute and persistent diarrhea in children; increased risk in immunocompromised children; occurs in community and hospital settings	Dehydrating, watery, occasionally bloody diarrhea with vomiting and abdominal pain; usually lasts 5-7 days	Immunoassay, electron microscopy

*Laboratory diagnostic tests, other than those for rotavirus group A, are usually available only in specialized research or diagnostic referral laboratories. Immunoassays are usually enzyme-linked immunosorbent assays or radioimmunoassays.
PAGE, polyacrylamide-gel electrophoresis and silver staining of viral nucleic acid in stool.
Modified from Blacklow NR, Greenberg HB. Viral gastroenteritis. N Engl J Med 1991; 325:252.

Table 1 for answer 981 **Electrolyte Concentrations of Choleric and Nonspecific Fecal Fluid and of Intravenous Fluids Used to Treat Infectious Diarrheas**

TYPE OF FLUID	ELECTROLYTE CONCENTRATIONS (mmol/L)			
	SODIUM	POTASSIUM	CHLORIDE	BICARBONATE
Cholera Stool				
Adult	124	16	90	48
Child	101	27	92	32
Nonspecific Diarrhea (Child)	56	25	55	14
Intravenous Therapy				
Lactated Ringer's solution	130	4	109	28*
5:4:1 solution[†‡]	129	11	97	44
2:1 solution[§]	141	—	94	47

*Equivalent concentration after lactate conversion.
[†]Add glucose, 110 mmol/L (20 g/L).
[‡]Intravenous solution that is 5 g of sodium chloride, 4 g of sodium bicarbonate, and 1 g of potassium chloride per liter.
[§]Solution that has a carbohydrate-to-sodium ratio of 2:1.

Table 2 for answer 981 **Compositions of Some Oral Hydration Beverages**

BEVERAGE	SODIUM (mmol/L)	POTASSIUM (mmol/L)	CHLORIDE (mmol/L)	BASE (mmol/L)	CARBOHYDRATE (mmol/L)	OSMOLARITY (mOsm/L)
Rehydration						
WHO solution	90	20	80	10 (C)	111	310
Rehydralyte*	75	20	65	10 (C)	140	305
Maintenance						
Infalyte*	50	20	40	10 (B)	111	270
Lytren*	50	25	45	10 (C)	111	290
Pedialyte*	45	20	35	10 (C)	140	250
Resol*	50	20	50	11 (C)	111	270
Ricelyte*	50	25	45	11 (C)	30 (D)	200
Other Liquids						
Apple juice	3	28	30	0	690[†]	730
Chicken broth	250	8	250	0	0	450
Cola	2	0.1	2	13 (B)	730[†]	750
Ginger ale	3	1	2	4 (B)	500[†]	540
Tea	0	0	0	0	0	5

*Ready to use.
[†]Combination of glucose and fructose.
B, bicarbonate; C, citrate; D, rice-syrup solids (g/L); WHO, World Health Organization.
Modified from Avery ME, Snyder JD. Oral therapy for acute diarrhea: The underused simple solution. N Engl J Med 1990; 323:891.

Table for answer 1026 **Side Effects of Glucocorticoids**

Cutaneous
Acne
Impaired wound healing
Purpura, ecchymoses, petechiae
Striae
Endocrine
Adrenal insufficiency
Cushingoid appearance
Gastrointestinal
Dyspepsia
Dysphagia/odynophagia (candidiasis)
Infectious complications
Numerous pathogens
Metabolic
Electrolyte imbalance, hypokalemia
Fluid retention
Growth retardation
Hyperglycemia, secondary diabetes mellitus
Hyperlipidemia, altered fat distribution
Hypertension
Musculoskeletal
Myopathy
Osteonecrosis
Osteoporosis
Neuropsychiatric
Anxiety, mood swings
Depression
Insomnia
Psychosis
Ocular
Cataracts
Glaucoma

Table for answer 1028 **Safety Profiles of Agents Used to Treat Crohn's Disease**

AGENT	ADVERSE EFFECTS	PREGNANCY*	NURSING*
5-Aminosalicylates (5-ASA)			
Sulfasalazine	Anorexia, dyspepsia, nausea and vomiting; hemolysis, neutropenia, agranulocytosis; folate deficiency; reversible male infertility; neuropathy; see also sulfa-free 5-ASAs	No evidence of teratogenicity; normal fetal growth; give with folic acid	Negligible amounts; safe for term neonates
Sulfa-free 5-ASAs (mesalamine, olsalazine, balsalazide)	Headache; drug fever; rash; paradoxical disease exacerbation; pancreatitis; hepatitis; pericarditis; pneumonitis; nephritis; secretory diarrhea (olsalazine)	No evidence of teratogenicity, normal fetal growth	Found in breast milk in low concentrations; rare watery diarrhea in breast-fed infants
Antibiotics			
Metronidazole	Anorexia, nausea and vomiting, dysgeusia; disulfiram-like effect; peripheral neuropathy; reversible neutropenia	Questionable teratogenicity, normal fetal growth	Found in breast milk; with rare exception, should not be used
Ciprofloxacin	Nausea and vomiting; headache; restlessness; rash; pseudomembranous colitis; elevated serum aminotransferase levels; spontaneous tendon rupture	Theoretical teratogenic potential; insufficient data in humans	Found in breast milk, should not be used

Table continues on following page.

Table for answer 1028   **Safety Profiles of Agents Used to Treat Crohn's Disease—Cont'd**

AGENT	ADVERSE EFFECTS	PREGNANCY*	NURSING*
Glucocorticoids			
Classic	Sleep and mood disturbance; acne, striae, hirsutism; adrenal suppression; proximal myopathy; glucose intolerance; hypertension; narrow-angle glaucoma, cataracts, pseudotumor cerebri; infection; edema; impaired wound healing; growth retardation; bone loss, aseptic necrosis	No evidence of teratogenicity in humans, more frequent stillbirths and reduced fetal birth weight when used for other diseases; may be used as indicated by severity of disease	Safe for breast-feeding
Novel	Controlled ileal-release budesonide: Adrenal suppression at doses of 9 mg/day and higher in two divided doses, but occurrence of classic glucocorticoid adverse effects similar to placebo	No data available	No data available
Immune Modulators			
6-Mercaptopurine, azathioprine	Nausea; drug fever, rash, arthralgias; leukopenia, thrombocytopenia, bone marrow suppression; pancreatitis; hepatitis; infection; lymphoma?	Teratogenic in animals, but large series in renal transplantation and other diseases do not show increase in birth defects; evidence for fetal growth retardation and prematurity; isolated cases of neonatal immune and bone marrow suppression; outcomes appear favorable in limited series of patients with IBD; may be used when indicated because of disease severity	Small amounts excreted in breast milk; not recommended
Methotrexate	Anorexia, nausea and vomiting; leukopenia, megaloblastic anemia; alopecia; hepatic fibrosis; interstitial pneumonitis; neuropathy	Highly teratogenic, particularly in the first trimester; abortifacient	Small amounts excreted in breast milk; not recommended
Cyclosporine	Reversible or irreversible decrease in renal function; hypertension; tremor, headache, paresthesias, seizure; hypertrichosis; hepatotoxicity; infection; lymphoma; gingival hyperplasia	Significant levels in fetal circulation; does not appear to be teratogenic; intrauterine growth retardation and premature delivery increased, especially at higher doses; little reported experience in IBD	Excreted in breast milk; not recommended
Biological Response Modifiers			
Anti-TNF antibodies (infliximab, adalimumab, certolizumab pegol)	Upper respiratory tract and other infections; disseminated tuberculosis; increased risk of systemic fungal infection and other intracellular pathogens; acute or delayed hypersensitivity reactions; antinuclear antibodies, anti–double-stranded DNA antibodies, lupus-like reaction; demyelinating disease; contraindicated in heart failure because of increased mortality; lymphoma	Limited data in humans	Unknown safety in nursing. Early data suggest minimal infliximab levels in breast milk
Natalizumab	Headache, flushing, infections; progressive multifocal leukoencephalopathy; jaundice, liver failure	Teratogenic in animals	Unknown safety in nursing

IBD, inflammatory bowel disease; TNF, tumor necrosis factor.

*From Connell WR. Safety of drug therapy for inflammatory bowel disease in pregnant and nursing women. Inflam Bowel Dis 1996; 2:33, with permission.

Adapted from Sands BE. Therapy of inflammatory bowel disease. Gastroenterology 2000; 118(2 Suppl 1):S72, with permission.

Table 1 for answer 1048 **Estimates of Rates of Food-Borne Illnesses and Associated Mortality in the United States, 1999**

PATHOGEN	ESTIMATED TOTAL NO. OF CASES	FOOD-BORNE TRANSMISSION, %	NO. OF DEATHS	CASE-FATALITY RATE
Bacteria				
Brucella	1,554	50	11	0.0071
Campylobacter	2,453,926	80	124	0.0000
Escherichia coli				
O157:H7 (EHEC)	73,480	85	61	0.0008
Non-O157:H7 (non-EHEC)	36,740	85	30	0.0008
Listeria monocytogenes	2,518	99	504	0.2001
Salmonella typhi	824	80	3	0.0036
Nontyphoidal *Salmonella*	1,412,498	95	582	0.0004
Shigella	448,240	20	70	0.0002
Noncholera *Vibrio*	7,880	65	20	0.0025
Vibrio vulnificus	94	50	37	0.3936
Yersinia enterocolitica	96,368	90	3	0.0000
Toxins				
Bacillus cereus	27,360	100	0	0.0000
Clostridium botulinum (food botulism)	58	100	4	0.0690
Clostridium perfringens	248,520	100	7	0.0000
Food Poisoning				
Staphylococcal	185,060	100	2	0.0000
Streptococcal	50,920	100	0	0.0000
Parasites				
Cryptosporidium parvum	300,000	10	66	0.0002
Cyclospora cayetanensis	16,264	90	0	0.0000
Giardia lamblia	2,000,000	10	10	0.0000
Toxoplasma gondii	225,000	50	750	0.0033
Trichinella spiralis	52	100	0	0.0000
Viruses				
Astrovirus	3,900,000	1	10	0.0000
Norovirus and Norwalk-like viruses	23,000,000	40	310	0.0000
Rotavirus	3,900,000	1	30	0.0000
Hepatitis A virus	83,391	5	83	0.0010
Total	38,629,641	—	1,809	0.0000

EHEC, enterohemorrhagic *Escherichia coli*.
From Mead PS, Slutsker L, Dietz V, et al. Food-related illness and death in the United States. Emerg Infect Dis 1999; 5:607.

Table 2 for answer 1048 Features of Bacterial Food Poisoning

ORGANISM	COMMON VEHICLES	MEDIAN INCUBATION (HR) (RANGE)	PRIMARY TOXIN	CLINICAL FEATURES	MEDIAN DURATION, DAYS (RANGE)	SECONDARY ATTACK RATE, %	SOURCES OF DIAGNOSTIC MATERIAL
Bacillus cereus	Fried rice, vanilla sauce, cream, meatballs, boiled beef, barbecued chicken	2 (1-16) / 9 (6-14)	Heat stable / Heat labile	V, C, D / D, C, V	0.4 (0.2-0.5) / 1 (1-2)	0	Vomitus, stool, implicated food
Campylobacter jejuni	Milk, chicken, beef	48 (24-240)	Unknown	D, F, C, B, H, M, N, V	7 (2-30)	25	Stool, rectal swab
Clostridium perfringens	Beef, turkey, chicken	12 (8-22)	Heat labile	D, C (N, V, F rare)	1 (0.3-3)	0	Stool, rectal swab; food, food-contact surfaces
Escherichia coli spp.	Salads, beef	24 (8-44) / 96 (24-120)	Heat labile / Heat stable Verotoxin	D, C, N, H, F, M / F, M, D, C / B, C, F, hemolytic-uremic syndrome	3 (1-4)	0	Stool, rectal swab
Listeria monocytogenes	Milk, raw vegetables, cole slaw, dairy products, poultry, beef	?	Unknown	D, F, C, N, V, B	?	10	Stool, rectal swab
Salmonella spp.	Eggs, meat, poultry	24 (5-72)	Role of toxin unclear	D, C, N, V, F, H, B (rare), enteric fever	3 (0.5-14)	30-50	Stool, rectal swab from patients and food preparers; raw food
Shigella spp.	Milk, salads (potato, tuna, turkey)	24 (7-168)	Role of toxin unclear	C, F, D, B, H, N, V	3 (0.5-14)	40-60	Stool, rectal swab from patients, and food preparers; implicated food
Staphylococcus aureus	Ham, pork, canned beef, cream-filled pastry	3 (1-6)	Heat stable	V, N, C, D, F (rare)	1 (0.3-1.5)	0	Stool, vomitus; food or food-contact surfaces; nose, hands, purulent lesion on food preparer
Vibrio parahaemolyticus	Seafood (rarely saltwater) or salted vegetables	12 (2-48)	Role of toxin unclear	D, C, N, V, H, F, B (rare)	3 (2-10)	0	Stool, rectal swab; food, food-contact surfaces; seawater
Yersinia enterocolitica	Chocolate milk or raw milk, pork	72 (2-144)	Heat stable	F, C, D, V, pharyngitis, arthritis, mesenteric adenitis, rash	7 (2-30)	20	Stool from food preparer

B, bloody diarrhea; C, cramping abdominal pain; D, diarrhea; F, fever; H, headache; M, myalgia; N, nausea; NA, not available; V, vomiting.
From Snydman DR. Food poisoning. In Gorbach SL, Bartlett JG, Blacklow NR, editors. Infectious Diseases. Philadelphia: WB Saunders; 1992. p 771.

Table 3 for answer 1048 **Organisms and Food-Borne Diseases Associated with Specific Foods or Beverages**

Beef and Pork
Salmonella spp.
Staphylococcus aureus
Clostridium perfringens
EHEC
Bacillus cereus
Yersinia enterocolitica
Listeria monocytogenes
Brucella spp.
Trichinella spiralis
Chinese Food
Bacillus cereus (in fried rice)
Monosodium glutamate poisoning
Eggs
Salmonella spp.
Staphylococcus aureus
Fish
Clostridium botulinum
Ciguatera poisoning
Scombroid poisoning
Diphyllobothrium latum
Anisakiasis
Honey
Clostridium botulinum
Milk and Cheese
Salmonella spp.
Campylobacter spp.
EIEC and EHEC
Yersinia enterocolitica
Group A streptococci
Brucella spp.
Listeria monocytogenes
Poultry
Salmonella spp.
Staphylococcus aureus
Campylobacter
Clostridium perfringens
Listeria monocytogenes
Shellfish
Vibrio parahaemolyticus
Vibrio cholerae (O1 and non-O1)
Hepatitis A
Norovirus and Norwalk-like viruses
Paralytic shellfish poisoning
Neurotoxic shellfish poisoning
Vegetables
Clostridium botulinum
Salmonella spp.
Shigella spp.
Bacillus cereus
Norovirus

EHEC, enterohemorrhagic *Escherichia coli*; EIEC, enteroinvasive *E. coli*.
From Bishai WR, Sears CL. Food poisoning syndromes. Gastroenterol Clin North Am 1993; 22:579.

Table for answer 1061 **Drugs Used to Prevent Traveler's Diarrhea in Adults**

DRUG	DOSE*	COMMENTS
Bismuth subsalicylate	Two 262-mg tablets chewed well four times daily (with meals and at bedtime)	Not as effective as anti-microbial drugs but fewer side effects than other agents
Doxycycline	100 mg daily	Resistance is found in many areas of the world
Rifaximin	200 mg with meals	Because rifaximin is not absorbed in the intestine, serious side effects are rare
Trimethoprim-sulfamethoxazole	160/800 mg daily	Resistance is common in tropical areas
Fluoroquinolones		
Norfloxacin	400 mg daily	The most predictably effective antimicrobial drugs when susceptibilities are not known
Ciprofloxacin	500 mg daily	
Ofloxacin	300 mg daily	
Fleroxacin	400 mg daily	

*All drugs should be taken orally beginning on the day of arrival in the country one is visiting and continuing for 1-2 days after returning home, but none should be taken for more than 3 weeks. Modified from DuPont HL, Ericsson CD. Prevention and treatment of traveler's diarrhea. N Engl J Med 1993; 328:1821.

STRAINS	PATHOGENIC MECHANISMS	PERSONS AFFECTED	CLINICAL FEATURES
DAEC	Diffuse adherence to Hep-2 cells	Children in developing countries	Watery diarrhea (acute) and persistent diarrhea
EAEC	Aggregative adherence to Hep-2 cells	Children in developing countries	Watery diarrhea (acute) and persistent diarrhea
EHEC	Shiga-like toxin (large quantities) O serogroups (usually O157:H7)	Children and adults Persons who ingest contaminated food, especially hamburger (outbreaks)	Bloody diarrhea Hemolytic-uremic syndrome
EIEC	Shiga-like toxin Epithelial cell invasion	Children and adults Persons who ingest contaminated food and water (outbreaks)	Dysentery
EPEC	Attaching and effacing adherence O serogroups	Children Newborns in a nursery (outbreaks)	Watery diarrhea
ETEC	Heat-labile and/or heat-stable toxin Adherence	Children in developing countries; travelers	Watery diarrhea

DAEC, diffusely adhering *E. coli*; EAEC, enteroaggregative *E. coli*; EHEC, enterohemorrhagic *E. coli*; EIEC, enteroinvasive *E. coli*; EPEC, enteropathogenic *E. coli*; ETEC, enterotoxigenic *E. coli*; RBC, red blood cell; WBC, white blood cell.

Table 1 for answer 1111 **Characteristics That Help Distinguish Inflammatory from Noninflammatory Diarrhea**

CHARACTERISTIC	INFLAMMATORY DIARRHEA	NONINFLAMMATORY DIARRHEA
Clinical presentation	Bloody, small-volume diarrhea; lower quadrant cramps; patients may be febrile and toxic	Large-volume, watery diarrhea; patients may have nausea, vomiting, cramps
Site of involvement	Colon	Small intestine
Diagnostic evaluation	Indicated	Indicated only if the patient is severely volume depleted or appears toxic
Fecal leukocytes	Present	Absent
Causes	*Shigella* spp., *Salmonella* spp., *Entamoeba histolytica*, *Campylobacter* spp., *Yersinia* spp., invasive *Escherichia coli*, *Clostridium difficile*	Viruses, *Vibrio* spp., *Giardia lamblia*, enterotoxigenic *E. coli*, enterotoxin-producing bacteria, food-borne gastroenteritis

From Park SI, Giannella RA. Approach to the adult patient with acute diarrhea. Gastroenterol Clin North Am 1993; 22:483-97.

Table 2 for answer 1111 **Fecal Leukocytes in Intestinal Infections**

Usually Present
Campylobacter spp.
EHEC
EIEC
Shigella spp.
Present or Absent
Aeromonas spp.
Clostridium difficile (antibiotic-associated colitis)
EAEC
Salmonella spp.
Vibrio parahaemolyticus
Yersinia spp.
Usually Absent
Bacillus cereus
Clostridium perfringens
DAEC
Entamoeba histolytica
EPEC
ETEC
Food poisoning
Giardia lamblia
Staphylococcus aureus
Vibrio cholerae
Viruses
    Calicivirus, including norovirus
    Rotavirus
    Other viruses

DAEC, diffusely adhering *Escherichia coli*; EAEC, enteroaggregative *E. coli*; EHEC, enterohemorrhagic *E. coli*; EIEC, enteroinvasive *E. coli*; EPEC, enteropathogenic *E. coli*; ETEC, enterotoxigenic *E. coli*.

Table 1 for answer 1118 Amsterdam Criteria for Hereditary Nonpolyposis Colorectal Cancer

At least three relatives with colorectal cancer (one must be a first-degree relative of the other two)
Colorectal cancer involving at least two generations
One or more colorectal cancer cases before age 50 years

Criteria defined by the International Collaborative Group on Hereditary Nonpolyposis Colorectal Cancer.

Table 2 for answer 1118 Bethesda Guidelines for Testing of Colorectal Tumors for Microsatellite Instability[71]

Persons with cancer in families that meet the Amsterdam criteria (see Table 123-5)
Persons with two HNPCC-related cancers, including synchronous and metachronous colorectal cancers or associated extracolonic cancers*
Persons with colorectal cancer and a first-degree relative with colorectal cancer and/or HNPCC-related extracolonic cancer* and/or a colorectal adenoma; one of the cancers must be diagnosed before age 45 years and the adenoma diagnosed before age 40 years
Persons with colorectal cancer or endometrial cancer diagnosed before age 45 years
Persons with right-sided colorectal cancer with an undifferentiated pattern (solid/cribriform)[†] on histopathology diagnosed before age 45 years
Persons with signet ring cell-type colorectal cancer[‡] diagnosed before age 45 years
Persons with colorectal adenomas diagnosed before age 40 years

*Endometrial, ovarian, gastric, hepatobiliary, or small intestinal cancer or transitional cell carcinoma of the renal pelvis or ureter.
[†]Poorly differentiated or undifferentiated carcinoma composed of irregular solid sheets of large eosinophilic cells and containing small gland-like spaces.
[‡]Composed of >50% signet ring cells.
HNPCC, hereditary nonpolyposis colorectal cancer.

Table 3 for answer 1118 Comparison of HNPCC and Sporadic Colorectal Cancer

CLINICAL FEATURE	HNPCC	SPORADIC COLORECTAL CANCER
Mean age at diagnosis (years)	45	67
Multiple colon cancers	35%	4-11%
Synchronous colon cancers	18%	3-6%
Metachronous colon cancers	24%	1-5%
Proximal location*	72%	35%
Increased risk of malignant tumors at other sites	Yes	No
Mucinous and poorly differentiated colon cancers	Common	Infrequent
Prognosis	Favorable[†]	Variable

*Proximal to the splenic flexure; location of the initial cancer.
[†]Patients whose tumors demonstrate microsatellite instability have a more favorable prognosis than those with microsatellite-stable tumors.
HNPCC, hereditary nonpolyposis colorectal cancer.

Table for answer 1129 Conditions That Predispose to *Salmonella* Infection

Achlorhydria
   Autoimmune gastritis
   Gastroduodenal surgery
Hemolytic anemia
   Bartonellosis
   Louse-borne relapsing fever
   Malaria
   Sickle cell disease
Immunosuppression
   AIDS
   Chemotherapy
   Glucocorticoid therapy
   Radiation
Malignancy
   Disseminated carcinoma
   Leukemia
   Lymphoma
Schistosomiasis
Ulcerative colitis

AIDS, acquired immunodeficiency syndrome.

Table for answer 1134 Controlled Trials of Fecal Occult Blood Testing in Screening Asymptomatic People for Colorectal Cancer (CRC)

VARIABLE	TRIALS				
	MINNESOTA[99]	NOTTINGHAM[98]	GOTEBORG	FUNEN	NEW YORK
Size of study population	46,000	152,850	28,000	61,933	22,000
Age range	50-80 yr	50-74 yr	60-64 yr	45-74 yr	≥40 yr
Study design	Randomized: annual vs. biennial control	Randomized	Randomized	Randomized: biennial vs. control	Allocation by month assigned
Rehydration of test cards*	Yes, most	No	Yes, most	No	No
Compliance	Annual 75%; biennial 78%	50%	—	56%	—
Positivity rate	2.4% (nonhydrated) 9.8% (rehydrated)	1st screen: 2.1% 2nd screen: 1.2%	1st screen: 1.9%(nonhydrated) 5.8% (rehydrated) 2nd screen: 4.8% (prev. rehydrated) 8.0% (prev. nonhydrated)	1st screen: 1.0% 2nd screen: 0.8% 3rd screen: 0.9% 4th screen: 1.3% 5th screen: 1.8%	Regular attendees: 1.4% 1st screen: 2.6%
PPV for CRC	2.2% (rehydrated) 5.6% (nonhydrated)	1st screen: 9.9% 2nd screen: 11.9%	1st screen: 5.0% (nonhydrated) 2nd screen: 4.2% (rehydrated)	1st screen: 17.7% 2nd screen: 8.4%	10.7%
CRC mortality[†]	18-yr follow-up: 33% reduction for the annual group, 21% reduction for biennial group Mortality ratio: Annual: 0.67 Biennial: 0.79	7- to 8-yr follow-up: 15% reduction in cumulative CRC mortality Mortality ratio: 0.85	Not yet available	10-yr follow-up: 18% reduction in CRC mortality in the screened group Mortality ratio: 0.82	10-yr follow-up: 43% reduction in CRC mortality in the screened group

*Hemoccult test cards were used, rehydrated or nonhydrated.
[†]Reductions in mortality are relative risk reductions. A French trial[107] using biennial FOBTs yielded a 16% reduction in CRC-related mortality in the screened group. The mortality ratio was 0.84 (95% confidence interval, 0.71-0.99) with 11 years of follow-up.
PPV, positive predictive value; prev., previously.

Table for answer 1148 **Factors That May Influence Carcinogenesis in the Colon and Rectum**

Probably Causative
High-fat and low-fiber diet (adjusted for energy intake)*
Red meat consumption
Possibly Causative
Beer and ale consumption (especially for rectal cancer)
Cigarette smoking
Diabetes mellitus
Environmental carcinogens and mutagens
Heterocyclic amines (from charbroiled and fried meat and fish)
Low dietary selenium
Probably Protective
Aspirin, NSAIDs, and cyclooxygenase-2 inhibitors
Calcium
Hormone replacement therapy (estrogen)
Low body mass
Physical activity
Possibly Protective†
Carotene-rich foods
High-fiber diet
Vitamins C and E
Vitamin D
Yellow-green cruciferous vegetables

*Dietary fats and fiber are heterogeneous in composition, and not all fats or fiber components play a role in cause or protection.
†Based on limited data.
NSAIDs, nonsteroidal anti-inflammatory drugs.

Table for answer 1155 **Pathophysiology and Some Conditions Associated with Small Intestinal Bacterial Overgrowth**

PATHOPHYSIOLOGY	CONDITION
Anatomic abnormalities	Blind loop (Billroth II gastrectomy, end-to-side anastomosis)
	Small intestinal diverticulosis
	Small intestinal stricture (Crohn's disease, radiation enteritis, focal segmental ischemia)
Motility disorders	Diabetes mellitus
	Idiopathic intestinal pseudo-obstruction
	Scleroderma
Reduced gastric acid secretion	Acid-lowering medication
	Atrophic gastritis
	Previous vagotomy
Abnormal connection between colon and proximal bowel	Gastrocolic or enterocolic fistula
	Resection of ileocecal valve
Various mechanisms	Celiac disease
	Cirrhosis
	Chronic pancreatitis
	Chronic kidney disease
	Radiation enteritis
	Rheumatoid arthritis

Table for answer 1173 **Amebicidal Agents Currently Available in the United States**

AMEBICIDAL AGENT	ADVANTAGES	DISADVANTAGES
For Luminal Amebiasis		
Paromomycin (Humatin)	7-day treatment course; may be useful during pregnancy	Frequent gastrointestinal side effects; rare ototoxicity and nephrotoxicity
Iodoquinol (Yodoxin)	Inexpensive and effective	20-day treatment course; contains iodine; rare optic neuritis and atrophy with prolonged use
Diloxanide furoate (Furamide)		Available in the United States only from the CDC; frequent gastrointestinal side effects; rare diplopia
For Invasive Intestinal Disease Only		
Tetracyclines, erythromycin		Not effective for liver abscess; frequent gastrointestinal side effects; tetracyclines should not be administered to children or pregnant women
For Both Invasive Intestinal and Extraintestinal Amebiasis		
Metronidazole (Flagyl)	Drug of choice for amebic colitis and liver abscess	Anorexia, nausea, vomiting, and metallic taste in nearly one third of patients; disulfiram-like reaction with alcohol; rare seizures
Tinidazole (Tindamax)	Alternative to metronidazole; once daily dosing; now approved for distribution in the United States	Side effects are similar to those with metronidazole
Nitazoxanide (Alinia)	Useful alternative if the patient is intolerant of metronidazole or tinidazole	Limited clinical data for amebiasis; rare and reversible conjunctival icterus
For Extraintestinal Amebiasis Only		
Chloroquine (Aralen)	Useful only for amebic liver abscess	Occasional headache, pruritus, nausea, alopecia, and myalgias; rare heart block and irreversible retinal injury

CDC, Centers for Disease Control and Prevention.
Adapted from Huston CD, Petri WA. Amebiasis. In: Rakel RE, Bope ET, editors. Conn's Current Therapy, 2001. Philadelphia: WB Saunders; 2001. pp 50-4.

Table for answer 1179 **Relative Frequencies of the Clinical Syndromes of *Salmonella* Infection**

SYNDROME	FEATURES	FREQUENCY (%)
Gastroenteritis	Characterized by mild to severe and dehydrating (dysenteric) colitis	75
Bacteremia	With or without gastroenteritis, endocarditis, arteritis, or AIDS	5-10
Typhoid fever ("enteric fever")	With or without gastroenteritis	5-10
Localized infection	May involve meninges, bones and joints, wounds, gallbladder, and may form abscesses	
Carrier state (>1 yr)	—	<1

AIDS, acquired immunodeficiency syndrome.

Table for answer 1201 **Indications for Antibiotic Therapy in *Salmonella* Gastroenteritis**

Abnormal cardiovascular system
    Aneurysms
    Prosthetic heart valves
    Valvular heart disease
    Vascular grafts
Extreme ages of life
Hemolytic anemia
Immunosuppression
    AIDS
    Congenital and acquired immunosuppressive disorders
    Glucorticoid treatment
    Organ transplants
Lymphoproliferative disorders
    Leukemia
    Lymphoma
Malignancies
Pregnancy
Prosthetic orthopedic devices
Sepsis

AIDS, acquired immunodeficiency syndrome.

Table for answer 1230 Extraintestinal Manifestations of Celiac Disease

MANIFESTATION	PROBABLE CAUSE(S)
Cutaneous	
Ecchymoses and petechiae	Vitamin K deficiency; rarely, thrombocytopenia
Edema	Hypoproteinemia
Dermatitis herpetiformis	Unknown
Follicular hyperkeratosis and dermatitis	Vitamin A malabsorption, vitamin B complex malabsorption
Endocrinologic	
Amenorrhea, infertility, impotence	Malnutrition, hypothalamic-pituitary dysfunction
Secondary hyperparathyroidism	Calcium and/or vitamin D malabsorption causing hypocalcemia
Hematologic	
Anemia	Iron, folate, vitamin B_{12}, or pyridoxine deficiency
Hemorrhage	Vitamin K deficiency; rarely, thrombocytopenia due to folate deficiency
Thrombocytosis, Howell-Jolly bodies	Hyposplenism
Hepatic	
Elevated liver biochemical test levels	Unknown
Muscular	
Atrophy	Malnutrition due to malabsorption
Tetany	Calcium, vitamin D, and/or magnesium malabsorption
Weakness	Generalized muscle atrophy, hypokalemia
Neurologic	
Peripheral neuropathy	Deficiencies of vitamins such as vitamin B_{12} and thiamine
Ataxia	Cerebellar and posterior column damage
Demyelinating central nervous system lesions	Unknown
Seizures	Unknown
Skeletal	
Osteopenia	Malabsorption of calcium and vitamin D
Osteoarthropathy	Unknown
Pathologic fractures	Osteopenia

Table for answer 1236 Efficacy of Chemoprotective Agents for Colorectal Neoplasia

AGENT	OBSERVATIONAL STUDIES OF COLON CANCER INCIDENCE			RANDOMIZED HUMAN TRIALS		
	ANIMAL STUDIES	CASE CONTROL	COHORT STUDIES	REDUCTION IN MUCOSAL PROLIFERATION	REDUCED NUMBER OF POLYPS IN PATIENTS WITH FAP	REDUCED NUMBER OF SPORADIC ADENOMAS
Aspirin or other NSAID	+	+	+	NA	+	+
Cyclooxygenase-2 inhibitors	+	NA	NA	+	+	+
Vitamins A, C, E	+	+	+	+	~	~
Folate	~	+	+	+	NA	−
Calcium	+	+	+	~	NA	+
Fiber	+	+	+	+	~	−
Selenium	+	+	~	NA	−	NA
Fish oil	NA	+	NA	NA	+	NA
Organosulfur	+	NA	NA	NA	NA	NA
Difluoromethylornithine	+	NA	NA	+	+	+*

*In combination with sulindac.
+, Most studies are positive for efficacy; −, most studies are negative for efficacy; ~, studies are equivocal for efficacy; FAP, familial adenomatous polyposis; NA, not available; NSAID, nonsteroidal anti-inflammatory drug.

Table for answer 1239 **Dukes Staging of Carcinoma of the Rectum and Its Modifications for Colorectal Carcinoma**

STAGE	DUKES, 1932 (RECTUM)	GABRIEL, DUKES, BUSSEY, 1935 (RECTUM)	KIRKLIN ET AL, 1949 (RECTUM + SIGMOID)	ASTLER-COLLER, 1954 (RECTUM + COLON)	TURNBULL ET AL, 1967 (COLON)	MODIFIED ASTLER-COLLER (GUNDERSON, SOSIN), 1974 (RECTUM + COLON)	GITSG, 1975 (RECTUM + COLON)
A	Limited to bowel wall	Limited to bowel wall	Limited to mucosa	Limited to mucosa	Limited to mucosa	Limited to mucosa	Limited to mucosa
B	Through bowel wall	Through bowel wall	—	—	Tumor extension into pericolic fat	—	—
B1	—	—	Into muscularis propria	Into muscularis propria	—	Into muscularis propria	Into muscularis propria
B2	—	—	Through muscularis propria	Through muscularis propria (and serosa)	—	Through serosa (m = microscopic; m + g = gross)	Through serosa
B3	—	—	—	—	—	Adherent to or invading adjacent structures	—
C	Regional nodal metastases	—	Regional nodal metastases	—	Regional nodal metastases	—	—
C1	—	Regional nodal metastases near primary lesion	—	Same as B1 + regional nodal metastases	—	Same as B1 + regional nodal metastases	1-4 regional nodes positive
C2	—	Proximal node involved at point of ligation	—	Same as B2 + regional nodal metastases	—	Same as B2 + regional nodal metastases	>4 regional nodes positive
C3	—	—	—	—	—	Same as B3 + regional nodal metastases	—
D	—	—	—	—	Distant metastases (liver, lung, bone) or parietal peritoneum or adjacent organ invasion	—	—

GITSG, Gastrointestinal Tumor Study Group.

Table for answer 1248 **Pathologic, Molecular, and Clinical Features That May Affect Prognosis in Patients with Colorectal Cancer**

FEATURE OR MARKER	EFFECT ON PROGNOSIS
Pathologic	
Surgical-pathologic Stage	
Depth of colon wall penetration	Increased penetration diminishes prognosis
Number of regional nodes involved by tumor	1-4 nodes is better than >4 nodes
Tumor Morphology and Histology	
Degree of differentiation	Well-differentiated is better than poorly differentiated
Mucinous (colloid) or signet ring cell histology	Diminished prognosis
Scirrhous histology	Diminished prognosis
Invasion	
Venous	Diminished prognosis
Lymphatic	Diminished prognosis
Perineural	Diminished prognosis
Other Features	
Local inflammation and immunologic reaction	Improved prognosis
Tumor morphology	Polypoid or exophytic is better than ulcerating or infiltrating
Tumor DNA content	Increased DNA content (aneuploidy) diminishes prognosis
Tumor size	No effect in most studies
Molecular	
Loss of heterozygosity at chromosome 18q (*DCC, DPC4*)	Diminished prognosis
Loss of heterozygosity at chromosome 17p (*TP53*)	Diminished prognosis
Loss of heterozygosity at chromosome 8p	Diminished prognosis
Increased labeling index for p21WAF/CIP1 protein	Improved prognosis
Microsatellite instability	Improved prognosis
Mutation in *BAX* gene	Diminished prognosis
Clinical	
Diagnosis in asymptomatic patients	Possibly improved prognosis
Duration of symptoms	No demonstrated effect
Rectal bleeding as a presenting symptom	Improved prognosis
Colon obstruction	Diminished prognosis
Colon perforation	Diminished prognosis
Tumor location	May be better for colonic than for rectal tumors May be better for left colonic than right colonic tumors
Age <30 yr	Diminished prognosis
Preoperative CEA level	Diminished prognosis with a high CEA level
Distant metastases	Markedly diminished prognosis

CEA, carcinoembryonic antigen.

CHAPTER 10

Palliative, Complementary, and Alternative Medicine

QUESTIONS

1252 A 36-year-old man is evaluated for treatment of hepatitis C. He has not received interferon-based therapy, but is currently taking a complementary alternative medicine (CAM), the name of which he cannot recall. The patient's blood pressure is 156/92 mm Hg, and he has 1+ bilateral lower extremity edema. Laboratory studies are performed, and later that night, the laboratory calls because the serum potassium level is 2.6 mmol/L. The patient takes no other medication and has no history of hypokalemia. You suspect that the patient is taking which of the following?
A. Silymarin (milk thistle)
B. Chinese herbal medicine
C. Glycyrrhiza glabra (licorice)
D. Thymic extract

1253 A 41-year-old woman asks your opinion about colonic irrigation therapy. Which of the following statements regarding this treatment is the most accurate?
A. An administration device controls water flow, temperature, and pressure.
B. Serious adverse events have not been reported.
C. Randomized, controlled studies suggest a reduced incidence of adenomas.
D. The principle of autointoxication from colonic contents has been proven.

1254 A 66-year-old cachectic man with cirrhosis due to hepatitis C and alcohol is not a candidate for liver transplantation and is referred for hospice care. He is deemed a suitable candidate for hospice based on a history of hepatic encephalopathy refractory to therapy as well as laboratory studies demonstrating a prothrombin time international normalized ratio of 1.8 and serum albumin of 1.9 g/dL. Which of the following statements regarding this patient's care under the Medicare Hospice Benefit is most accurate?

A. Coverage for this benefit does not extend beyond six months of care.
B. The patient must relinquish heroic life-prolonging measures.
C. The patient agrees to avoid future hospitalization.
D. Care usually is provided in the patient's home.

1255 You are asked to be a medical director for a new company that will market an herbal product for the treatment of chronic liver disease. During the research conducted as part of performing due diligence, you learn many relevant facts about CAM therapies that influence your decision. Which of the following is the most accurate statement regarding CAM therapy?
A. Ten percent of outpatients with chronic liver disease have used some form of CAM therapy within the past month.
B. The U.S. yearly sales of herbal supplements are approximately $4 billion.
C. The 1994 Dietary Supplement Health and Education Act was developed to allow the U.S. Food and Drug Administration (FDA) to tightly regulate dietary supplements.
D. FDA approval is not required for a dietary supplement marketed before October 15, 1994.
E. Supplement manufacturers are required to report adverse events that occur with use of their products.

1256 A 60-year-old woman with advanced liver disease due to primary biliary cirrhosis is hospitalized and responding to treatment for subacute bacterial peritonitis. Using the Mayo Model for primary biliary cirrhosis, her survival rate is estimated to be 25% at one year. While deciding whether to undergo a transplantation evaluation or enter hospice, the patient has asked to be seen by the palliative care team. Which of the following is a contraindication for palliative care?

A. Entrance into hospice care
B. Acceptance as a transplantation candidate and placement on the transplantation list
C. Desire to undergo aggressive treatment for liver-related complications
D. This patient has no contraindication to palliative care.

1257 The National Center for Complementary and Alternative Medicine divides CAM into four domains. Which of these domains is most commonly used for gastrointestinal and liver diseases?
A. Mind–body medicine
B. Biologically based practices
C. Manipulative and body-based practices
D. Energy medicine

1258 The palliative care team is asked to evaluate a 40-year-old man with metastatic pancreatic cancer. The patient is having moderate pain throughout the day that is not responding to nonsteroidal medications, and a long-acting narcotic is recommended. What is the best initial approach to preventing constipation in this patient?
A. Begin Senokot before instituting narcotics.
B. Begin a fiber supplement before starting narcotics.
C. Begin methylnaltrexone before starting narcotics.

D. Begin polyethylene glycol before starting narcotics.

1259 Randomized, controlled trials suggest that probiotics may be effective for which of the following?
A. Reducing abdominal pain and flatulence in irritable bowel syndrome
B. Preventing radiation-induced diarrhea
C. Decreasing the number of flares of pouchitis in patients with chronic pouchitis
D. All of the above

1260 A 23-year-old woman with a very well controlled seizure disorder on phenytoin is referred for evaluation of nausea and vomiting. An extensive workup was performed and the findings are negative; the decision is made to treat the symptom. She refuses all prescription medications and wants a more "natural" approach. What is the most accurate information you can provide regarding CAM therapy for nausea and vomiting?
A. Relaxation therapy is effective in most patients.
B. The data supporting implementation of acupuncture/acupressure are impressive.
C. Ginger is a good option in the future if the patient becomes pregnant.
D. Pyridoxine often improves nausea and is very safe for this patient.

ANSWERS

1252 **C** (S&F, ch127)
All of these complementary alternative medications used to treat hepatitis C have been associated with adverse events. Licorice inhibits 11-β-hydroxysteroid dehydrogenase, and this may lead to a pseudoaldosterone effect resulting in hypokalemia, sodium retention, and hypertension. Although multiple adverse events have been reported with milk thistle, the most important relates to its ability to inhibit CYP3A4 and uridine diphosphoglucuronosyl transferase. This may lead to interactions with traditional prescription medications such as quinine, lidocaine, certain calcium channel–blocking agents, and cyclosporine, all of which are metabolized in part by CYP3A4. Chinese herbal medicine has been associated with possible hepatotoxicity, as well as pneumonitis, autoimmune hepatitis, and acute thrombocytopenic purpura. Finally, thymic extract has been reported to cause nausea, vomiting, and, rarely, thrombocytopenia.

1253 **A** (S&F, ch127)
Colonic irrigation therapy is not self-administered, but given by a practitioner via a device that controls water flow, temperature, and pressure. Serious adverse events, including perforation and amebiasis, have been reported. There are no randomized, controlled studies proving the efficacy of this therapy, and its theoretical basis that toxins originating in the intestine can enter the circulation and poison the body has not been proven.

1254 **D** (S&F, ch126)
Hospice care, under the Medicare Hospice Benefit, has defined regulations and admission criteria. Although admission is dependent on the physician certifying survival of less than six months, should the patient live longer, hospice service can be extended through recertification. Patients do not need to relinquish heroic life-prolonging measures, future hospitalization, or participation in research when they enter hospice care. Although many receive care in special residential facilities or long-term care facilities, most hospice care in the United States takes place in the patient's home.

1255 **D** (S&F, ch127)
Dietary supplements marketed before October 15, 1994, do not require FDA approval. However, no official list of supplements marketed before this date exists and the responsibility rests with the manufacturer. Supplement manufacturers are not required to report adverse events with their products. The Dietary Supplement Health and Education Act was developed to prevent "excessive" regulation of dietary supplements by the FDA. The market for CAM therapy is large and growing. One study reported 42% of outpatients with chronic liver disease used some form of CAM therapy within the preceding four weeks. The U.S. estimated annual expenditures for CAM therapies are in excess of $27 billion, and for herbal supplements, this figure is $13.9 billion.

1256 **D** (S&F, ch126)
Palliative care and hospice care share the same philosophy and are complementary but not identical.

The ultimate goal of palliative care is to prevent and relieve suffering and to optimize quality of life for patients and their families, regardless of the stage of disease or the need for curative or palliative therapies. Therefore, the patient may avail herself of the palliative care team regardless of the course of action she chooses with respect to her underlying liver disease.

1257 **B** (S&F, ch127)

Most of the therapies fall within the biologically based practices domain. They include substances within our natural environment, such as prebiotics, probiotics, and dietary supplements that are used to strengthen and heal the human body. The other domains are used for gastrointestinal and liver diseases, but to a much lesser extent overall.

1258 **A** (S&F, ch126)

Constipation will occur in more than 90% of patients started on opioid medications, which bind to mu receptors on smooth muscle and suppress peristalsis and increase anal sphincter tone. A bowel stimulant such as senna is usually necessary as a prophylactic agent for opioid constipation and may be used as a first-line treatment for established constipation. Low-dose osmotic agents such as polyethylene glycol are useful for constipation refractory to stimulant laxatives alone. Fiber should be avoided as it may lead to obstipation or obstruction in patients unable to ingest large amounts of fluids. Methylnaltrexone, which does not cross the blood–brain barrier and therefore does not reverse the analgesic effect of narcotics, is FDA approved for chronic opioid-induced constipation and should be used to manage constipation refractory to usual therapies.

1259 **D** (S&F, ch127)

All these have been demonstrated in published randomized, controlled trials. *Lactobacillus plantarum* reduced abdominal pain and flatulence in those diagnosed with irritable bowel syndrome. VSL #3 was effective in preventing radiation-induced diarrhea. This product was also effective in reducing both the frequency of pouchitis and the number of flares of pouchitis in those with chronic pouchitis after ileoanal anastomosis for Crohn's disease.

1260 **B** (S&F, ch127)

There are good data supporting the use of acupuncture and acupressure for treating nausea and vomiting. Relaxation therapy has primarily been used for chemotherapy-induced symptoms because they are somewhat conditioned and are developed as a form of associative learning. Ginger may be effective, but has been documented to be potentially mutagenic in laboratory assays, thereby raising questions about the safety of the herbal supplement in pregnancy. Finally, although pyridoxine is a popular CAM therapy for nausea and vomiting, it has been documented to decrease serum levels of levodopa, phenobarbital, and phenytoin when coadministered with these agents.

Illustration Credits

All figures and tables are original to the Sleisenger and Fordtran companion text except for those noted here.

Figure A for question 412 and Figure for answer 442
Courtesy of Pamela Jensen, MD, Dallas, TX.

Figure for question 437
Courtesy of Edward Lee, MD, Washington, DC.

Table 2 for answer 418
From Hundahl S, Philips J, Menck H. The National Cancer Data Base Report on poor survival of U.S. gastric carcinoma patients treated with gastrectomy: Fifth Edition American Joint Committee on Cancer staging, proximal disease, and the "different disease" hypothesis. Cancer 2000;88:921-932.

Table for answer 424
Adapted from Chey WD, Wong BC. American College of Gastroenterology guideline on the management of *Helicobacter pylori* infection. Am J Gastroenterol 2007;102:1808-1825; Peura, DA. Treatment of *Helicobacter pylori* infection. In Wolfe MM (ed): Therapy of Digestive Disorders. Elsevier, Philadelphia, 2006, p 277; and Jodlowski TZ, Lam S, Ashby CR. Emerging therapies for the treatment of *Helicobacter pylori* infections. Ann Pharmacother 2008;42: 1621-1639.

Table for answer 451
Adapted from Malfertheiner PF, Megraud C, O'Morain F, et al. Current concepts in the management of *Helicobacter pylori* infection: The Maastricht III Consensus Report. Gut 2007;56:772-781 and Chey WD, Wong BC. American College of Gastroenterology guideline on the management of *Helicobacter pylori* infection. Am J Gastroenterol 2007;102: 1808-1825.

Figure for answer 498
From Parkin DM. International variation. Oncogene 2004;23:6239-6240.

Figures for questions 519, 539, 570, 581, 611, 672, 686, and 700
Courtesy of David Loren, MD, Thomas Jefferson University, Philadelphia, PA.

Figures for questions 636, 651, and 714
Courtesy of Jason N. Rogart, MD, Thomas Jefferson University, Philadelphia, PA.

Figure 1 for question 708
Courtesy of Steve Burdick, MD, Dallas, TX.

Figure for question 722
Courtesy of Julie Champine, MD, Dallas, TX.

Figure for question 725
Courtesy of David Hurst, MD, Baylor Hospital, Dallas, TX.

Figure for question 746
Courtesy of Maha Guindi, MD, Toronto, Canada.

Figure for question 760
From Lucas SB. Other viral and infectious diseases and HIV-related liver disease. In MacSween RNM, Burt AD, Portmann BC, et al (eds): Pathology of the Liver, 4th ed. London, Churchill Livingstone, 2001, p 366.

Figure for question 799
Courtesy of Raphael Rubin, MD, Thomas Jefferson University, Philadelphia, PA.

Figure for answer 761
Modified from Poynard T, Naveau S, Doffoel M, et al. Evaluation of efficacy of liver transplantation in alcoholic cirrhosis using matched and simulated controls: 5 year survival. Multi-centre group. J Hepatol 1999;30:1130-1137.

Figure for answer 783
From Akriviadis EA, Runyon BA. The value of an algorithm in differentiating spontaneous from secondary bacterial peritonitis. Gastroenterology 1990;98:127. Copyright 1990 by the American Gastroenterological Association.

Table for answer 844
Modified from Balistreri WF. Liver disease in infancy and childhood. In Schiff ER, Sorrell MF, Maddrey WC (eds): Schiff's Diseases of the Liver, 9th ed. Philadelphia, Lippincott-Raven, 1999, p 1379.

Table for answer **880**
Data provided courtesy of William M. Lee, MD, and the U.S. Acute Liver Failure Study Group, September, 2008.

Figures for questions **898**, **1182**, **1223**, and answer **1180**
Courtesy of Feldman, online Gastro Atlas, Current Medicine.

Video 1 (question **934**)
From Jang MK, Lee KS. Images in clinical medicine. Ascariasis. N Engl J Med 2008;358:e16.

Figure for question **939**
Courtesy of J. Levenbrown, MD.

Figure for question **995**
Courtesy of Hans Jörg Meier-Willersen, MD, Heidelberg, Germany.

Figure for question **1039**
Courtesy of Lawrence J. Brandt, MD, Bronx, NY.

Figure for question **1152**
Courtesy of Christophe Cellier, MD, PhD, Paris, France.

Figure for question **1200**
From Veerappan A, Siegel JH, Podany J, et al. Fasciola hepatica pancreatitis: Endoscopic extraction of live parasites. Gastrointest Endosc 1991;37:473.

Figure for question **1243**
Courtesy of Gregory Lauwers, MD, Boston, MA.

Figure for answer **904**
From Esser-Kochling BG, Hirsch FW. Images in clinical medicine. Ascaris lumbricoides blocking the common bile duct. N Engl J Med 2005;352:e4.

Figure for answer **926**
From Grady WM. Genomic instability and colon cancer. Cancer Metast Rev 2004;23:11.

Figures 1 and 2 for answer **956**
Data from Parkin DM, Whelen SL, Ferlay J, et al. Cancer Incidence in Five Continents. [IARC Sci. Publ. No. 143]. Series. Lyon, International Agency for Research on Cancer, 1997.

Figure for answer **968**
Courtesy of A. Kapikian, MD. Previously published in Lennete EH, Schmidt NJ. Diagnostic Procedures for Viral, Rickettsial, and Chlamydial Infections, 5th ed. New York, American Public Health Association, 1979, p 933.

Table for answer **968**
Modified from Blacklow NR, Greenberg HB. Viral gastroenteritis. N Engl J Med 1991;325:252.

Figure for answer **981**
From Fishman PH. Action of cholera toxin: Events on the cell surface. In Field M, Fordtran JS, Schultz SG (eds): Secretory Diarrhea. Bethesda, MD, American Physiological Society, 1980, p 86.

Table 2 for answer **981**
Modified from Avery ME, Snyder JD. Oral therapy for acute diarrhea: The underused simple solution. N Engl J Med 1990;323:891.

Figure for answer **1005**
From van den Bogaerde JB, Jordaan M. Intraductal administration of albendazole for biliary ascariasis. Am J Gastroenterol 1997;92:1531.

Figure for answer **1011**
From Schrock T. Large intestine. In Way LW (ed): Current Surgical Diagnosis and Treatment, 10th ed. New York, Lange, 1994.

Figure for answer **1018** (*bottom right*)
From the photo collection of the late Harrison Juniper, MD.

Figure for answer **1025**
Modified from Brandt LJ, Boley SJ. AGA technical review on intestinal ischemia: American Gastrointestinal Association. Gastroenterology 2000;118:954; corrected version in Gastroenterology 2000;119:281.

Table for answer **1028**
From Connell WR. Safety of drug therapy for inflammatory bowel disease in pregnant and nursing women. Inflam Bowel Dis 1996;2:33. Adapted from Sands BE. Therapy of inflammatory bowel disease. Gastroenterology 2000;118(Suppl 1):S72.

Table 1 for answer **1048**
From Mead PS, Slutsker L, Dietz V, et al. Food-related illness and death in the United States. Emerg Infect Dis 1999;5:607.

Table 2 for answer **1048**
From Snydman DR. Food poisoning. In Gorbach SL, Bartlett JG, Blacklow NR (eds): Infectious Diseases. Philadelphia, WB Saunders, 1992, p 771.

Table 3 for answer **1048**
From Bishai WR, Sears CL. Food poisoning syndromes. Gastroenterol Clin North Am 1993;22:579.

Figure for answer **1060**
Modified from Klipstein FA. Tropical sprue in travelers and expatriates living abroad. Gastroenterology 1981;80: 590-600.

Table for answer **1061**
Modified from DuPont HL, Ericsson CD. Prevention and treatment of traveler's diarrhea. N Engl J Med 1993;328: 1821.

Figure for answer **1077**
From Petri WA, Sing U, Ravdin JI. Enteric amebiasis. In Guerrant RL, Walker DH, Weller PF (eds): Tropical Infectious Diseases: Principles, Pathogens, and Practice. Philadelphia, WB Saunders, 1999.

Figure for answer **1104**
Courtesy of the Carlo Denegri Foundation, Turin, Italy.

Figure for answer **1107**
Courtesy of the University of Iowa Department of Dermatology, Iowa City, IA.

Figure for answer **1110**
Courtesy of Mark Peterson, MD, Pittsburgh, PA.

Table 1 for answer **1111**
From Park SI, Giannella RA. Approach to the adult patient with acute diarrhea. Gastroenterol Clin North Am 1993;22:483.

Table 1 for answer **1118**
Criteria defined by the International Collaborative Group on Hereditary Nonpolyposis Colorectal Cancer.

Figure for answer **1121**
From Wilcox CM. Atlas of Clinical Gastrointestinal Endoscopy. Philadelphia, WB Saunders, 1995.

Figure for answer **1130** (*center*)
Courtesy of C. M. Knauer, MD, San Jose, CA.

Figure for answer **1130** (*bottom*)
Courtesy of P. Kirby and F. Mitros, University of Iowa, Iowa City, IA.

Video 3 (answer **1132**)
From Martines H, Fanciulli E, Menardo G. Incidental video-capsule diagnosis of small-bowel *Taenia saginata* in a patient with recurrent hemorrhage due to angiodysplasias. Endoscopy 2006;38(Suppl 2):e35.

Figure for answer **1139**
From Moertel CG, Fleming TR, MacDonald JS, et al. Fluorouracil plus levamisole as effective adjuvant therapy after resection of stage III colon carcinoma: A final report. Ann Intern Med 1995;122:321.

Video 4 (answer **1150**)
From Liao WS, Bair MJ. Images in clinical medicine. *Taenia* in the gastrointestinal tract. N Engl J Med 2007;357:1028.

Video 5 (answer **1150**)
From Park DH, Son HY. Images in clinical medicine. *Clonorchis sinensis*. N Engl J Med 2008;358:e18.

Table for answer **1173**
Adapted from Huston CD, Petri WA. Amebiasis. In Rakel R (ed): Conn's Current Therapy 2001. Philadelphia, WB Saunders, 2001.

Figure for answer **1213**
Redrawn from the Centers for Disease Control, Salmonella Surveillance, Annual Summary, 1976. Washington, DC, U.S. Department of Health, Education and Welfare, Public Health Service, 1977.

Table for answer **1230**
Modified from Trier JS. Celiac sprue and refractory sprue. In Feldman M, Scharschmidt BF, Sleisenger MH (eds): Gastrointestinal and Liver Disease, 6th ed. Philadelphia, WB Saunders, 1997, p 1557.